Comments on Type 1 Diabetes from reviewers

"This is far and away the best diabetes resource I have ever come across. It has information you will not find anywhere else and is well presented and indexed … If you are serious about managing your child's diabetes to the best of your ability, you cannot afford to do without this book."

Reviewer from London, featured on the Amazon website

"I have no hesitation in thoroughly recommending this book to adolescents and young people with Type 1 diabetes, their families, and also to all healthcare professionals involved in their care."

Professor Martin Silink in Diabetologia

"The information is clear, concise and extremely readable. All imaginable topics are covered from hypoglycaemia, through pregnancy and on to psychological issues! It is difficult to imagine anyone, including healthcare professionals, teachers and grandparents, not learning something helpful."

Practical Diabetes International

"It covers all aspects of living with diabetes and is one of the most useful and comprehensible books written for the person with diabetes."

Paediatric Nursing

"Congratulations to Dr Hanas on authoring a very comprehensive and informative book on type 1 diabetes. This is the most complete book on living with type 1 diabetes available and takes the reader from understanding basic information to the complex."

Pediatric Diabetes

**To my children
Mikael, Malin and Marie
and to my Karin**

You may well feel that there is an overwhelming amount of knowledge you must take in, but nobody expects you to memorize the entire contents of this book. If you use it as a reference, and read a little at a time, you will gradually get to grips with the information it contains.

TYPE 1 DIABETES

in Children, Adolescents and Young Adults

How to become an expert on your own diabetes

Dr. Ragnar Hanas, MD, PhD
Consultant Paediatrician

Sixth edition
fully revised and updated

CLASS PUBLISHING • BRIDGWATER

Printing history:
Authors: Ragnar Hanas, MD, PhD, Uddevalla, Sweden
First English edition, published by the author 1998
Second UK edition 2004, reprinted 2005
Third UK edition 2007
Fourth UK edition 2010
Fifth UK edition 2012
Sixth UK edition 2015

The author and publishers welcome feedback from users of this book. Please contact the publisher:

Class Health, The Exchange, Express Park, Bridgwater, Somerset TA6 4RR
Tel: 44(0)1278 427800; Fax: 44(0)1278 421077
Email: post@class.co.uk
Website: www. classhealth.co.uk

The information presented in this book is accurate and current to the best of the author's knowledge. The author and publisher, however, make no guarantee as to, and assume no responsibility for, the correctness, sufficiency or completeness of such information or recommendation. The reader is advised to consult a doctor regarding all aspects of individual health care.

Class Health is an imprint of Class Publishing Ltd.

A CIP catalogue record for this book is available from the British Library

ISBN 978-1-85959-566-4
Ebook ISBN 978-1-85959-567-1

10 9 8 7 6 5 4 3 2 1

Edited by Richenda Milton-Daws
Designed by David Penfold and Ragnar Hanas
Illustrations and figures are reproduced with the permission of the respective copyright owner (see page 411). Additional cartoons by David Woodroffe

Printed and bound in Finland by Bookwell, Juva

Contents

Preface to sixth edition

The number of children and adolescents with type 1 diabetes in the world is steadily increasing. There would appear to be something in the environment causing this, as genetic changes are not this rapid in humans. By contrast, the number of young adults developing type 1 diabetes seems to be constant, or even decreasing in some places. This would suggest that a particular group of individuals tend to get type 1 diabetes, but some environmental factor or factors are now causing it to appear earlier in the lifespan. Generally speaking, countries with a higher standard of living have a high percentage of children with type 1 diabetes. In the UK approximately 0.25% and in Canada close to 0.4% of all children can expect to develop diabetes before the age of 15 years. In Finland, the country where it is now most common, this figure is 0.6%.

Since I wrote the first edition of this book in 1998, a great deal has happened in the area of insulin treatment. New analogues, both rapid-acting and long-acting, have been developed and insulin pumps are used more often. These chapters have been extensively updated, allowing an individually tailored insulin regimen.

Today an intensive insulin regimen already from the start is standard regardless of age, and pre-school children may be given a pump already soon after the onset of diabetes. Teaching carbohydrate counting soon after the diagnosis is becoming increasingly more common. We have lowered the levels of what we consider as a normal blood glucose level to 4-8 mmol/l (70-145 mg/dl). If you check your mean glucose level on your meter at home, and contact your diabetes team if it goes above 8 mmol/l (145 mg/dl), it is quite possible to keep your HbA_{1c} below 52-58 mmol/mol (7.0-7.5%). Our advice on hypoglycaemia have changed in that we do not recommend more glucose than what is needed to raise blood glucose into the normal range (i.e around 4-5 mmol/l (70-90 mg/dl). If you eat more than this, you will need an additional dose of insulin. We stress always taking insulin before the meal (for breakfast preferably at least 15 minutes before) to get a sufficient effect.

I am always so impressed by the huge motivation that whole families put into the learning process. On being told their child has diabetes, they often go to an astonishing amount of effort to make life as good as possible for their child, learning to live with this new condition. Within a couple of weeks, they are able to manage everyday situations in relation to diabetes quite well on their own. In about a year's time, after having experienced the events of an ordinary family life including birthday parties, holidays and sports events but also infections, gastroenteritis and other things that can complicate life, they will have taken over the reins and become their own diabetes experts. It is from families like these that I have learned how to deal with diabetes in such a way that Professor Johnny Ludvigsson's saying becomes true: "It is not fun getting diabetes, but you must be able to have fun even while having diabetes".

I hope that this new, updated edition will make living with diabetes considerably easier for children, teenagers and young adults. Let me know your views and impressions of the contents of this book so that, together, we can improve the treatment of diabetes.

Ragnar Hanas, MD, PhD, Associate Professor, University of Gothenburg and Consultant Paediatrician, Department of Paediatrics, Uddevalla Hospital, S-451 80 Uddevalla, Sweden
E-mail: ragnar.hanas@vgregion.se

Foreword by Dr Fiona Campbell

Here at last is the eagerly awaited, fully revised and updated 6th edition of Type 1 Diabetes in Children, Adolescents and Young Adults by Dr Ragnar Hanas.

Since its first edition, published in 1998, this well loved book has been considered the 'go to' text book for use not only by every member of the multidisciplinary team caring for children and young people with type 1 diabetes, but most importantly, the patients themselves, their families and carers.

Type 1 diabetes remains an incurable lifelong condition and unfortunately the number of children living with this condition continues to increase world-wide. This disorder of blood glucose control impinges relentlessly and unpredictably on our patients' lives, every hour of every day. There is mounting evidence to suggest that achieving the best control of blood glucose, as soon as possible after confirmation of the diagnosis of diabetes, is of paramount importance to help minimise and even avoid the long- term complications of this condition. For this ambition to be achieved, it is clearly essential that the children and young people, along with their families, become the experts in managing their own diabetes and learn to understand that many factors influence their glucose profiles and insulin requirements on a day -to-day basis. They need to be given guidance on how best to frequently review and adjust their type 1 diabetes therapy by highly knowledgeable and caring healthcare professionals.

In this new 6th edition of his book, Dr Ragnar Hanas has once again demonstrated his complete understanding of the complexities of living with and successfully managing type 1 diabetes. He has succeeded brilliantly in writing a beautifully illustrated reference book that will, with no doubt, appeal to its many readers of all ages and with differing levels of diabetes knowledge, be it the patient and family on day 1 after diagnosis through to the healthcare professional with many years of clinical experience. I would commend this book to everyone with an interest in helping our children, young people and their families live the best life possible.

Dr Fiona M Campbell
MD, FRCPCH
Consultant Paediatric Diabetologist
Leeds Children's Hospital Diabetes Centre
Leeds
LS9 7TF
England
UK

Foreword by Dr Stuart Brink

The latest edition of Dr Hanas' book remains our favorite diabetes teaching manual at the New England Diabetes and Endocrinology Center (NEDEC). It is comprehensive, witty and informative while at the same time paying particular attention to the psychosocial issues of a chronic condition. With Type 1 diabetes (T1DM) increasing around the world, it is essential that families and health care personnel as well as teachers, coaches and school staff are well informed for T1DM to be recognized and treated correctly and for team work to optimize care. This is a disease where knowledge is a critical component of care. Not just knowledge, but up-to-date knowledge which brings research findings directly to providers and patients and facilitates the use of such knowledge. Such self-management skills are not so easy to elucidate, and even more difficult to put into practice but this manual continues to offer such advice.

The simple "rules" of diabetes suggest that too little insulin, too much food, too little activity or major illness or emotional upheaval cause high blood glucose, while too much insulin, too little food and/or too much activity cause hypoglycaemia. After all is said and done, the application of these few bits of information explains all of what we need to know about diabetes. However, the details and the intricacies as well as the variations of the themes of these "rules" are what diabetes self-management is all about. The application of such knowledge allows the possibility of excellent glucose control while the inability to afford such care or the misapplication of such knowledge is associated with both acute and chronic complications of type 1 diabetes mellitus.

The psychosocial aspects of self-care and the interplay with family issues are important concepts woven into the text. When appropriate self-care is not taking place, psychosocial problems are often key to understanding why problems persist. Acknowledging such a dilemma and applying research about empowerment and education coupled is a critical component of getting better results. How to discuss with friends and relatives, what to discuss and the interaction between home, school and other activities is presented in a friendly, sometimes humorous and frank manner throughout the text. What Dr Hanas does so well is to start with these basic premises and build the pieces of the self-care treatment puzzle step-by-step to elucidate what, why and how. The text moves from diagnosis and basics of treatment all the way to sophisticated insulin pumps and the newest information about continuous glucose monitoring with the hopes of an artificial pancreas and ongoing progress expected.

Dr. Hanas does not offer dogmatic suggestions but rather options to consider under different real life circumstances. In fact, this current edition, like the previous ones, accomplishes its goal of a diabetes teaching manual with attention to detail, and application of updated clinical as well as research findings from ISPAD and around the world. A tribute to the success of this manual is its translation into 13 other languages. School teachers, guidance counselors, therapists and all members of the diabetes medical community should have this book in their armamentarium as should those living with diabetes.

Stuart Brink, MD, Associate Clinical Professor of Paediatrics, Tufts University School of Medicine
New England Diabetes & Endocrinology Center
NEDEC, 40 Second Avenue Suite #170
Waltham MA, 02451-1136 USA

Acknowledgements

I am greatly indebted to the children and teenagers with diabetes and their parents who have contributed with experiences, tips, knowledge and drawings, to the diabetes nurses Catarina Andreasson, Pia Hanas, Elsie Johansson, Ann-Sofie Karttunen and Kristin Lundqvist for their many valuable contributions in discussions and clinical work, to my colleagues, collaborators and friends in Sweden and within ISPAD (International Society of Pediatric and Adolescent Diabetes) for joining me in increased efforts in intensive diabetes treatment and to Mats Bergryd for believing in the idea of writing a comprehensive diabetes manual for young people with diabetes and their parents. Without you there would have been no book.

My deep appreciation goes to Dr Kenneth Strauss for his enthusiastic and continued support of the book, to Dr Peter Swift, Dr Charles Fox, Dr Robyn Houlden, Dr Stuart Brink, Nancy Jones (mother of a child with diabetes), Gary Scheiner, MS, CDE, and Janette Apsley, RN, for reviewing and critically reading the English edition. Many thanks to the dietitians Ellen Aslander, Carmel Smart and Sheridan Waldron for their comments on the diet chapter. My sincere thanks to my editor Richenda Milton-Daws, my publisher Dick Warner, Judith Wise and Rebecca Hirst at Class Publishing for their endless patience in transforming my first English edition into a professional publication.

I am grateful to Louis Nitka for letting me use his drawings on pages 7 and 310 in the book. Illustrations and figures are all reproduced with the permission of the respective copyright owner. A full list is given on page 411.

For dosages and applications mentioned in this book, the reader can be assured that the author has gone to great lengths to ensure that the indications reflect the standard of knowledge at the time this work was completed. However, insulin needs and diabetes treatment must be individually tailored for each and every person with diabetes. Advice and recommendations in this book cannot be expected to be generally applicable in all situations and always need to be supplemented by individual assessment on the part of a diabetes team. The author cannot accept any legal responsibility or liability for any errors or omissions, or the use of the material contained herein and the decisions based on such use. Neither will the author be liable for direct, indirect, special, incidental or consequential damages arising out of the use, or inability to use, the contents of this book.

The use of general descriptive names, trade names, trademarks, etc. in this publication, even if not specifically identified, does not imply that these names are not protected by the relevant laws and regulations. NovoRapid, Levemir, Tresiba, Actrapid, Insulatard, Monotard, Mixtard, Ultratard, Penset, Novolin and Velosulin BR Human insulins are trademarks of Novo Nordisk A/S. Humulin, Humutard, Humaject and Humalog insulins are trademarks of Eli Lilly & Co. Lantus, Insuman Infusat, Insuman Rapid, Insuman Basal and Insuman Comb insulins are trademarks of Sanofi. The indwelling catheters Insuflon and i-Port are produced by Convatec A/S, Denmark. Please note that not all insulins and devices are available in all countries.

Introduction

"If you want something done properly, do it yourself." This is a wise old saying, but of course you need to know how to do it as well. If you have diabetes, you will need a thorough understanding of the disease and how to manage it. As anyone living with diabetes knows, it is an illness that is with you 24 hours of every day.

Traditionally, doctors have decided on the doses of insulin, and the times it could be given. Patients took the insulin as prescribed, neither less, nor more. But for 35 years now, we have been doing the opposite at our clinic. We begin

The diabetes clinic will often function as an information centre where the diabetes team can pass on good ideas from one family to another.

The underlying theme of this book is: "If you want something done properly, do it yourself". You are the only one who can be relied upon to be there 24 hours a day, and after a while you will be the greatest authority on your own diabetes. Learning to care for your diabetes from scratch, like learning anything else, is a matter of trial and error. And during the process, you are bound to make some mistakes. However, you can learn from each one of these; indeed you will learn more from your own mistakes than from the mistakes other people have made.

by teaching the fundamentals of diabetes management to our young patients. Then, gradually, we delegate more and more of the daily responsibility for diabetes care to the young people themselves, and where appropriate also to parents and other family members.

Usually, it takes about a year for someone to experience most of the day-to-day situations that can be affected by diabetes. These may include holidays, birthdays, parties, heavy exercise and periods of sickness. As you become more confident, you will begin to draw upon your own experiences and discover things about your condition that your diabetes team will find it helpful to know about. This sort of free exchange of information not only helps us to help you. It also enables the clinic to function as an information centre, passing on suggestions and knowledge from one family to another. Investigations into the father's role in diabetes show it is important for the diabetes team to take part in how he experiences the child's everyday life in the family, and to take this into consideration when setting up goals for the diabetes treatment.[131]

This is of course also true for the mother's experience, and it will not suit its purpose if we set a goal for diabetes treatment, for example long-term glucose control, and the family feels this is unrealistic to achieve. It is therefore our job to provide you with the tools you need to get a functioning life at home, and at the same time live up to the treatment goals that are set within your country and internationally for treating diabetes in young people.

Knowledge changes over time. What was advisable 10-15 years ago may not necessarily apply today. At one time I would hear from families whom I had just informed about some new development, "Well, we have been doing it that way for years, but we didn't dare tell anyone". Nowadays we share knowledge and learning with each other instead.

This book deals with type 1 diabetes in children, teenagers and young adults. It does not address the treatment of type 2 diabetes, except in the briefest of ways. If you have type 2 diabetes, you are referred to the companion book, *Type 2 Diabetes in Adults of all Ages* by Charles Fox and Anne Kilvert. The book in your hand describes methods of treating type 1 diabetes that are common in much of Europe as well as in North America and elsewhere in the world. However, the methods used may vary from one centre to another. The goal is to find a way of treating your diabetes effectively. There may be more than one way of reaching this goal.

Don't try to read the book from cover to cover, or memorize it. Use it as a reference book instead. A number of Latin medical terms are included, but their meaning should be obvious from the context, so you will not need to learn them unless you particularly want to. If you find some parts of the book difficult to understand, especially on the first reading, please don't let this discourage you. When you come back and read the text a second time, and when you have more experience of living with diabetes, it will all begin to fit together. More detailed information, aimed at those who want to learn a little bit more, can be found in the boxes in the text.

The small numbers raised above the lines of text (superscript) indicate the references which back up a particular piece of information. A full list of references, for those who are interested, is given at the end of the book.

Remember that you can learn things in many different ways. We usually arrange lessons around one aspect of diabetes at a time where we sit down with the whole family, and here we stress that both parents, if at all possible, should be present. If for some reason this is not possible, some other person in the close family can fulfil an important assignment by being

"*It is time to replace the old mistakes with more modern ones.*"

Grönköping's Weekly

"*The ability to think differently today than yesterday is what separates the wise from the stubborn.*"

John Steinbeck

We must be humble. What we look upon today as established knowledge, may appear as something quite different tomorrow.

involved and showing the child that this family has great resources when needed! However, you may also learn a great deal from a spontaneous conversation with a nurse, for example. The nurse's intonation, body language and expression may give you as much information as the spoken words. So, while you will be given official information during your more formal lessons, you will also hear unofficial views and additional information from other health professionals, fellow patients and others. Be aware of their body language, what they say and how they say it, and perhaps more importantly what they do not say. This type of information is also available from everyday contact with doctors. Body language can make more impact than words, and many people find that if it comes to a choice between remembering official information or informal information, they usually find it easier to remember informal information.[690]

If a member of your family has already been in contact with diabetes (perhaps through a relative or colleague) they may well have a clearly defined view of what diabetes is like. It is important to remember that this experience is not at all the same as having diabetes yourself or in your immediate family. Also, the treatment regimen is likely to be quite different for someone who has just been diagnosed compared with that for a person who has had diabetes for a number of years.

Many people are preoccupied by concerns about the future and the possible difficulties that may lie ahead. Your diabetes team will give you straightforward information about complications that might occur, and how to postpone them as long as possible or even avoid them. Our policy is to tell all there is to tell, not leaving any information out. Sometimes there is no straight answer to a question but we will tell you as much as we know.

During the first few weeks, you will need to get to know yourself all over again, and your parents will need to redefine their relationship with you too. You now know you have diabetes. To begin with, having to take this knowledge on board may make you scared about all sorts of aspects of your life. You may feel anxious and insecure, since you don't yet know how to tackle the different situations that daily life throws at you. But you will soon get to know yourself or your child in this new situation and you will gradually feel more confident about getting on with your life.

Getting to grips with diabetes

Managing diabetes involves lifelong treatment with insulin, but also permanent changes to your daily routine. Diabetes care includes both medical treatment and education. We want young people with diabetes, and their parents, to feel that they can assume responsibility for their own treatment and take charge of their own life. You can control your diabetes rather than let your diabetes control you. Once your diabetes has become manageable, so will other aspects of your life.

When you first find out you have diabetes

In Sweden and many other countries,[74] newly diagnosed diabetes is usually treated in hospital, where patients stay 1-2 weeks on the ward. In a few centres in the UK [1011] and many centres in the US [188] it is more usual to start your insulin treatment on an outpatient basis unless you are ill with ketoacidosis (see page 29). Now that healthcare costs are continually increasing, outpatient treatment at this stage is becoming more common.[187] This approach requires the diabetes team to be "on call" on a 24-hour basis for back up while you are getting used to coping with insulin treatment.[187] Long-term glucose control, which is measured by the level of a substance known as HbA_{1c}, appears to be just as good in patients who are treated as outpatients initially as in hospital.[1011] Whichever approach

"When a problem is too large and seems unsolvable, don't forget that you can eat an elephant, assuming it is cut it into small enough pieces".

Slavic saying

The first week is often chaotic, and it may be hard to understand how all the different facts fit together. Try to concentrate on one piece of information at a time. By the end of the second week, everything will become much clearer, and you will begin to understand how it all fits together.

you encounter, it is essential that you feel able to approach members of the diabetes team on a daily basis during the first week or two. It is their job to ensure you have the basic understanding and self-confidence necessary to give yourself the required doses of insulin.

The insulin requirement changes daily, and early on, the insulin dose will need to be revised continuously. During the first few days, patients need high doses of insulin, which will then be reduced by degrees. Many people feel much better immediately, and find they become ravenously hungry. This is natural if you consider that most young people who have been recently diagnosed with diabetes will have been insulin-deficient for several weeks before the diabetes was discovered, and are likely to have lost some weight. They can usually have as much food as they want at this stage, regulating the doses of insulin instead. The appetite usually settles down after a few weeks.

Keep a list of your questions to avoid problems recalling them when visiting us at the diabetes clinic.

During the first few days, many young people (and their parents too) may experience a feeling of resentment, disappointment and thoughts of "why me?/why my child?" If you are in this situation, you may have difficulty taking in the fact that you actually have diabetes. You will need time to examine your feelings and adjust gradually to this strange new situation that now faces you and the rest of your family. At this stage, you will probably find your doctors and nurses spend most of their time with you simply listening and answering questions. Then they will move on by degrees to teaching you more about diabetes. Most things will be new and you will often find them difficult to understand initially but, bit by bit, the different pieces of information will fall into place. By the end of the second week, you will be beginning to understand how insulin and blood glucose affect each other. You will discover that your blood glucose level fluctuates frequently, and that a perfect blood glucose level is a rare thing, even for those people whose diabetes is very closely supervised.

Parents can find they lose touch with each other if one is spending much more time than the

"Give a man a fish and he will not go hungry that day. Teach him how to fish and he will not be hungry for the rest of his life."

Chinese saying

It is important that you get used to handling your own (or your child's) diabetes early on. If you understand "why and how", you will be better prepared to meet different situations in life in harmony with your diabetes.

You will be feeling much better after a week or two with insulin. Now is the time to tell your friends at home and at school or work that you have diabetes. Then they will know and need not ask when you do something they don't understand, such as taking a blood glucose test. Even if you are worried about telling them, it often feels better once it is done.

other with the child. It is essential that both parents participate as much as possible in the daily care of the child with newly diagnosed diabetes. Taking time off work may help provide sufficient time to focus on diabetes care needs if this is possible.

Most people find that managing diabetes at home is easier than they had anticipated. To feel confident caring for yourself (or, in the case of parents, for your young child) at home, you should know what to do if the blood glucose level falls too low (see "Treating hypoglycaemia" on page 65). Having hypoglycaemia is not dangerous in itself, and it will help if you are aware from the earliest days that mild hypoglycaemia is a part of everyday life when you have diabetes. You can easily learn to manage it with glucose tablets.

You will have time during the early weeks to meet a dietitian several times, as well as a specialist diabetes nurse who can help you with many practical issues. Diabetes is an illness that can cause a lot of inconvenience, even in the most "normal" and well-adjusted families.

Knowledge and self-confidence are your best armour when you are confronted with other people's opinions about diabetes. They will help you to recognize and deal with the prejudice and out of date views that, unfortunately, you are likely to meet. It is important for patients and health professionals to help each other spread better knowledge and understanding about diabetes.

It can prove very valuable if you are able to see a child psychologist to discuss any difficulties that might arise. This way, if you do run into problems later on, you will already have an established contact should you wish to seek help.

Very young children

In the case of a baby or very young child having diabetes, the teaching will be directed at the parents, for obvious reasons. It is important, however, that children are given every opportunity to learn about diabetes themselves, and are given an increasing amount of responsibility for managing their illness as they grow. One way of helping to achieve this is by including young children in a diabetes holiday. Children who have reached or who are approaching the age of puberty should be encouraged to take an active part in managing their diabetes from the start. Parents' self-help groups can also be very helpful, so do ask if there are any in your area.

Our goal is for all children with diabetes, however young they were when diagnosed, to be able to take the greater proportion of responsibility for their diabetes before they enter puberty. If this applies to you, you can then begin to recognize diabetes as your own illness (not something your mum or dad uses to get you to do what they tell you). Then you can direct your energies towards other areas of life.

Routine check-ups

After the initial phase, you are likely to see your diabetes healthcare team for a check-up every second to third month. We prefer to see both parents joining in for the check-ups even after the initial teaching. It is important that parents are able to discuss the implications of their child's diabetes with each other. It is also important for the child to see both parents engaged in the practical care of the diabetes condition. This is of course equally, if not even more, important if the parents do not live together. Even if the child does not see much of one of the parents, for example the father, it is important that he also knows how to handle diabetes. An investigation of fathers' engagement in their child's diabetes showed that the single most important factor for the father taking an active part in his child's diabetes was that he had taken paternity leave together with his child, as it then was natural to become engaged also when the child fell ill.[132] If you are alone with the child, always think aloud. It helps you to shed light on the situation and what decisions you might need to take at that time. The child will also learn from taking part in your reasoning.

All children need love and care...

At the check-ups, your diabetes team can tell how your glucose control has been over the previous 2-3 months by measuring a substance in your blood called HbA_{1c} (see page 117). This has been reported in per cent (so called DCCT units), but from 2011 many countries will use the new IFCC units, which are reported in mmol/mol. See page 118 for conversion tables. It is important that you realize from the start that it is not possible to achieve perfect blood glucose levels every day. Everyone with diabetes has high blood glucose levels every now and then and, with the methods of treatment available today, this should not cause you too many problems. What is important is that your average blood glucose level is acceptable. More information about this will be found later in this book.

Older teenagers often prefer to come by themselves to their check-ups, or perhaps with a friend or partner for company. If you are in a steady relationship, it is very important that your partner comes with you when you visit your diabetes healthcare team. You may see the dietitian during team visits, but you can also contact him or her directly for further information. Once a year, you will usually have a more thorough check-up, including a full physical

If you don't have diabetes, your body will automatically work the way it should. Before you developed diabetes, your pancreas produced insulin without you having to give it a thought. Now you must listen to your body's signals and give yourself insulin in a way that is suitable for the different situations you are faced with.

examination. Several additional tests (mainly blood tests) may be included in your annual check-up (see page 350).

You need to be aware that the way your body changes during adolescence will affect your diabetes. During puberty your body will need a lot more insulin (see page 220). It is important to know when to increase the doses.

Hurrah, today is my birthday! This is a day for celebrating. For once you can be a bit more relaxed about routines and rules. Young people should be allowed to remember their birthdays and other special occasions as joyful and happy days, without undue restrictions.

We check your weight and height at every visit to make sure that you continue to grow as well as you did before having diabetes. If you don't get enough insulin you will lose weight and may even experience growth retardation. If, on the other hand, you get too much insulin (and food) you will gain too much weight.

Living the life you choose

Diabetes is a chronic illness that will affect you every day for the rest of your life. Try to become friends with your diabetes (or at least not to see it as an enemy) since you can't escape it and there is no currently known cure. It will probably be easier to manage diabetes well if you have a life with some sort of regular routine. If you are accustomed to a lifestyle that is neither regular nor predictable, you may find it more difficult (though by no means impossible) to combine this with diabetes.

It is essential, however, that from the very beginning you plan how to carry on with your life in a manner that suits you. Don't let your diabetes dictate the type of life you should live. A lot of people find themselves thinking: "I can't do such and such any more, now that I have diabetes. But I used to enjoy it so much before my diagnosis". However, most activities are not only "allowed", but you can do them perfectly well. Nothing is absolutely forbidden, but you would be wise to think things through more carefully than you used to, in all sorts of situations. It is important to experiment and learn by trial and error. If you choose the life you want to live, it is our job as diabetes profes-

"It is much easier to have a strong opinion if you don't know all the facts involved".

You and your family will find that many people you come in contact with think they know a great deal about diabetes. Often their knowledge about diabetes treatment is far from up to date. Be a bit sceptical when you hear generalized statements about diabetes, especially early on before you have your own knowledge and experience to rely upon.

sionals to tailor an insulin regimen that will enable you to do this. However, there are a few limitations on what sort of work you can do; for example it may not be possible to join the army or police force, or be a pilot (see "Choice of job or employment" on page 332).

Caring for your own diabetes

Goals for managing diabetes

A number of international authorities have put together recommended guidelines for the treatment of diabetes in young people. One of these is the International Society of Pediatric and Adolescent Diabetes (ISPAD, see page 339).[4] Other national and international programmes for the treatment of diabetes in childhood and adolescence are to be found in the Handbook on Childhood and Adolescent Diabetes from APEG (Australasian Paediatric Endocrine Group),[968] the St Vincent Declaration,[206] and the American Diabetes Association's Clinical Practice Recommendations,[26] among others.

An important goal of diabetes management is to reduce the number and severity of the symptoms and side effects you may experience. It is particularly important that young children grow and develop normally, and we ensure this by referring to standard weight and height development charts at every stage of treatment. In the past, insulin treatment plans were inadequate and prevented many children from growing properly, but this is no longer acceptable.

"My home is my castle", as the saying goes. Build yourself a castle of knowledge and motivation so you can feel safe and comfortable while dealing with your diabetes.

During puberty, insulin treatment plans need to be looked at and modified regularly.

Diabetes should not disrupt schooling or working patterns. It is difficult to study if your blood glucose is too high or too low, as this disturbs concentration. During puberty, your peer group becomes ever more important. Teaching teenagers how to balance an enjoyable social life with good diabetes management becomes a key goal at this time. As the young person matures into adulthood, having a family and children becomes increasingly important. In the long run, it is essential to prevent side effects and complications from diabetes.

How can you achieve these goals?

Traditionally there are three cornerstones of diabetes management: insulin, meal planning and exercise. The use of insulin is essential as this hormone is more or less missing from your body and it is essential for life. However, the

Goals of treatment

♠ No symptoms or discomfort in everyday life.

♠ Good general health and well-being.

♠ Normal growth and development.

♠ Normal puberty and peer-group relations.

♠ Normal schooling and professional life.

♠ Normal family life including the possibility of pregnancy.

♠ Prevention of long-term complications.

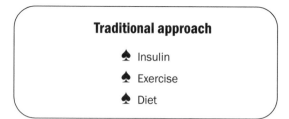

Traditional approach

♠ Insulin

♠ Exercise

♠ Diet

Diabetes today

Professor Johnny Ludvigsson, Sweden:

♥ Insulin
♥ Love
♥ Care

"It is no fun getting diabetes, but you must be able to have fun even if you have diabetes."

I would like to add a fourth cornerstone:

♥ Knowledge

Motivation of your own ➠ Self-care

If you want to manage well with diabetes you must:

① Become your own expert on diabetes.

② Have more knowledge about diabetes than the average doctor.

③ Accept your diabetes and learn to live with it.

other two cornerstones are being questioned by modern diabetes specialists, especially where children and teenagers are concerned. Eating sensibly is essential but meals that are appropriate for people with diabetes need not be very different from the sort of ordinary healthy meals that everyone can benefit from. Similarly, exercise is recommended for everyone and will help you achieve a good general level of fitness. In the past, exercise was an important part of diabetes treatment; however newer studies of diabetes and exercise do not indicate that it improves glucose control.[1093] If your blood glucose levels are high with not enough insulin, it may not be a good idea to exercise. So exercise is no longer considered as a part of actual diabetes treatment, although it is recommended for more general reasons.[480] See also the chapters on healthy eating and physical exercise.

Dr Johnny Ludvigsson, Professor of Paediatric Diabetology in Sweden, has re-defined the cornerstones of diabetes treatment as: insulin, love and care.[690] These goals coincide well with our clinic's view of diabetes treatment. Diabetes is a deficiency disease and it is natural to replace what is missing, i.e. insulin. Love and care are essential parts of every child's upbringing, and will be even more important for a child with a chronic illness.

I would like to introduce a fourth cornerstone in the treatment of diabetes, namely knowledge. A Chinese saying goes "Give a man a fish and he eats for a day. Teach him how to fish and he will eat for a lifetime".

Becoming your own expert

The more motivated you are, the better you will be able to manage your own diabetes. It is important you realize the treatment is for your own sake, not for your parents' or your family's, and certainly not to benefit your doctor or nurse. Your motivation for the best possible self-treatment might be to be as good (or better...) at football as you were before, to achieve good grades in school without getting hypoglycaemic, or to get the job you want and make it run smoothly despite irregular working hours. If you have diabetes you must become your own expert, learning to handle whatever life may throw at you in a satisfactory way.

The treatment of diabetes has changed a great deal in recent years, but public awareness has not necessarily caught up. So you are likely to come across a lot of people with out of date or fixed ideas, who think they know a great deal more than they actually do. But you need to be able to rely on your own knowledge. Indeed, to live your life in the way you want without too many unpleasant symptoms, you will actually need to know even more about diabetes than the average doctor does! To gain this knowledge you will have to ask questions and find out information if any aspect is less than crystal clear. Be sure to contact your consultant or diabetes nurse if you have questions on insulin dosages or other issues. If you save the question until your next visit, which might be 3 months away, you may simply forget all about it.

Becoming fully engaged with your diabetes and your own care is vitally important. Because you have to live with diabetes 24 hours a day, it is crucial that you decide as early as possible whether you are going to adjust your life around your diabetes, or whether you prefer to decide on a particular lifestyle and then adjust your diabetes treatment to enable you to achieve it. We encourage young people to be as active as possible in the management of their own diabetes from the start and aim to ensure that children have a good grasp of their diabetes by the time they reach puberty. This is important as there is so much else to occupy the mind of a young person during the teenage years. Children who have already come to grips with the basis of their own diabetes care before this stage will find they have more confidence to enjoy the increased freedom that adolescence should bring.

Can you take "time off" from diabetes?

Well, this really isn't possible since your diabetes is with you 24 hours a day. But you can make a distinction between everyday life and having a good time on special occasions. Most people (with or without diabetes) will allow themselves something extra once in a while, even if they know that this little extra is not necessarily terribly healthy. If your usual lifestyle is appropriate for diabetes, you too can allow yourself to be a bit "more relaxed" with

"To dare is to lose foothold for a short while — not to dare is to lose yourself."

Sören Kierkegaard, Danish philosopher 1813-1855

It is not easy to take individual responsibility for your own diabetes. On the other hand you are the only one who can do it. Only you can be there 24 hours a day, and this is what it takes to make your diabetes function well both today and in the future.

food if you are celebrating for example (see also "Party-time" on page 255).

If you go on holiday or a school trip, your routine is bound to differ from the one you have at home. The goal on these occasions should not be to have perfect control over your blood glucose. The important thing is that you feel well enough to participate in all activities. This may mean you have to accept having a slightly higher blood glucose level than usual, but of course you shouldn't let it get so high that it affects your well-being.

It is better to have 15 "bad" and 350 "good" days and feel happy about life, than 75 "half-bad" and 290 "good" days but feel miserable all the time. Many people with diabetes choose to have a slightly higher blood glucose level when they are about to do something important, such as an examination in school or an interview for a new job. And there are good reasons for this. In certain situations it is much more important to avoid hypoglycaemia than to have a perfect blood glucose level.

Alternative and complementary therapies

Sometimes we encounter questions about complementary or alternative treatment methods. In Sweden it is forbidden to treat children below the age of 8 with so called "alternative medicines" according to the law of quackery. Many parents have told us that despite this they have been informed about different types of treatment for children when they have consulted an alternative practitioner. In Finland, a 5-year-old boy died in 1991 after his parents stopped giving him insulin and instead gave him different types of herbal and steam baths. Both the parents and the person responsible for the treatment were prosecuted for causing the death of the child.

Four cases have been reported in the UK of insulin doses being decreased or stopped completely and different types of alternative treatment being given instead (prayers, healing, special diet and treatment with vitamins and trace elements). Three of the people involved developed ketoacidosis, while the fourth suffered from high blood glucose levels and weight loss.[400] Parents of an 11-year-old girl in the US were found guilty of reckless homicide after they treated her symptoms (of undiagnosed diabetes and ketoacidosis) with prayer alone.[663]

Unlike an alternative therapy, which is used instead of a conventional one, complementary therapy means exactly what its name implies. It should be used in addition to medical treatment, to complement, rather than replace it. So, while a complementary therapy cannot be a substitute for insulin you may benefit from it in

Sometimes you may feel like this when everything you have planned goes wrong and your blood glucose level ends up much too high or low. At a time like this, it might be a good idea to put your monitoring and adjustments "on hold" for a week and just take time off. Then, you can start afresh with renewed enthusiasm. Check your blood glucose only to avoid hypoglycaemia. Most things in life are learned this way, in "waves". As you become more familiar with your diabetes, these moments of exasperation will occur less and less often.

other ways, for example to help you to cope with the anger you feel at having to organize your life rather differently from your peers.

I have discussed this topic with parents on several occasions. In my opinion, three issues are especially important:

① We must talk frankly with each other about this subject. If you want to try an alternative or complementary treatment for your diabetes despite recommendations not to, it is better that you do this openly so that your doctor and diabetes nurse know about it.

② Children and adults with diabetes must continue taking their insulin and other medical treatment as prescribed by the doctor, otherwise their health will be in serious danger.

③ The alternative or complementary treatment must not be in any way dangerous or harmful to the person with diabetes.

Diabetes: some background

Diabetes mellitus, usually referred to simply as "diabetes", has been known to mankind since ancient times. Diabetes means "flowing through" and mellitus means "sweet as honey". Diabetes used to be described as either "insulin-dependent" (IDDM) or "non-insulin-dependent" (NIDDM). Nowadays, you are more likely to hear the terms "*type 1 diabetes*" and "*type 2 diabetes*".

Egyptian hieroglyphic findings from 1550 BC illustrate the symptoms of diabetes. Some people believe that the type of diabetes depicted was type 2 and that type 1 diabetes is a relatively new disease, appearing within the last two centuries.[139]

In the past, diabetes was diagnosed by tasting the urine. No effective treatment was available. Before insulin was discovered, type 1 diabetes always resulted in death, usually quite quickly.

Type 1 diabetes

If you are going to get type 1 diabetes, you are likely to know before your 35th birthday. Most people whose diabetes is diagnosed in childhood or the teenage years used to be type 1 diabetes, but now there is an alarming increase in type 2 diabetes in young people.

Type 1 diabetes is insulin-dependent, meaning that treatment with insulin is necessary from the time the disease is first diagnosed. In type 1 diabetes, the insulin-producing cells of the pancreas are destroyed by a process in the body known as "autoimmunity" (i.e. in which the body's cells attack each other, see page 376). This leads eventually to a total loss of insulin production. Without insulin, glucose remains in the bloodstream, so the blood glucose level increases, especially after eating meals. Glucose is then passed out of the body in the urine.

Type 2 diabetes

Type 2 diabetes is also called adult-onset diabetes as the onset usually takes place after the age of 35. Although type 2 diabetes is also called non-insulin-dependent diabetes, many people need treatment with insulin at a later stage in much the same way as people with type 1 diabetes. Diet and reduction of overweight are very important when treating type 2 diabetes. In type 2 diabetes, the ability to produce insulin does not disappear completely, but the body becomes increasingly resistant to insulin, so tablets are needed to balance this. It is rare for insulin injections to be necessary in the early stages of type 2 diabetes. The pills used for treating type 2 diabetes do not contain insulin, but act by increasing the body's sensitivity to insulin, or by increasing the release of insulin from the pancreas. Primary treatments are metformin and sulphonylurea tablets.

Insulin history

♠ The first human to be treated with insulin was a 14-year-old boy, Leonard Thomson, in Canada in the year 1922. James Havens was the first American treated with insulin in 1922. In the UK, insulin was first given as part of a research trial later the same year. In Sweden, the first insulin injections were given in 1923 to, among others, a 5-year-old boy who subsequently lived almost 70 years with his diabetes.

♠ In the early days, insulin was distributed as a powder or tablets which were mixed with water before being injected.

♠ Insulins with a longer action time (intermediate-acting insulins) were invented in 1936. Before this, regular insulin was given with each main meal and a late night injection was given at 1 AM to cover the night.

♠ It was considered quite a demanding insulin regime at that time. In 1941 Dr Robin Lawrence (who had diabetes himself) wrote: "The most continuously normal blood sugar can best be obtained by four to six small injections of soluble (short-acting) insulin in the 24 hours...but the insistence on such physiological perfection would produce a distorted existence and mental invalidism".

♠ In 1960 a study was presented, comparing individuals with a diagnosis between 1922 and 1935 with a strict diet and multiple daily injections (including regular insulin at night), with those diagnosed between 1935 and 1945 having a free diet and 1 or 2 injections per day. After 15 years of diabetes, 9% of those with diagnosis before 1935 had retinopathy compared with 61% of those diagnosed after 1935.

♠ Not much attention was given to these results as just about everyone preferred the "modern" insulin regime with only 1 or 2 injections per day. One exception was the American paediatrician Robert Jackson, who continued to give his patients regular insulin for each meal and a bedtime dose of NPH insulin.[553] It was not until the 1980s that taking insulin before each meal was reintroduced as the physiological way of treating diabetes.[568] Research has now proven beyond doubt that this decreases the long-term risk of diabetes complications significantly (see page 366). Even young children start with this type of regimen and find no problems complying with it (see page 124).

A new generation of medication for type 2 diabetes (glitazones) is now being used in adults. These pills make the body more sensitive to insulin, and may also be helpful in other ways, for example by lowering the level of fats in the blood and reducing blood pressure. However, they are not yet approved for use in children.

An increasing number of reports from North America, Japan, the UK and other parts of the industrialized world indicate that overweight teenagers are now beginning to develop type 2 diabetes. This appears to be more common in girls than in boys.[322,1109] In North America, type 2 diabetes and heart disease among young and middle-aged people from the members of the native American population is reaching epidemic proportions.[904]

In certain groups, the number of cases of type 2 diabetes as a proportion of the total number of newly diagnosed diabetes among children is extremely high. This proportion varies between 10% and 100% in different native American tribes, is approximately 30% in Mexican Americans, and 70-75% in African Americans.[1109] Type 2 diabetes is often diagnosed in African Americans after they become ill with the symptoms of ketoacidosis (see page 29).[1109]

Being overweight will make you more vulnerable to type 2 diabetes as, in the long run, your body will not be able to produce the large amounts of insulin necessary to keep your blood sugar normal. Japanese sumo wrestlers with a body weight of 200-260 kg have an increased risk of type 2 diabetes when they stop their intensive training.

Other risk factors for type 2 diabetes in children and young people are low birth weight, type 2 diabetes in the family, ethnic origin (Canadian and American First Nation's people, Hispanic, African American, Japanese, Pacific Islander, Asian and Middle Eastern), a diet that is high in fat and low in fibre, lack of exercise, high blood pressure and dark velvety discolouration of the skin (known as acanthosis nigricans).[322,904]

A possible reason for the increase in type 2 diabetes in young people may be that some people were "programmed" thousands of years ago to survive famine by conserving energy compared with periods when there was better access to food.[904] Today, when we have easy access to food, these "survival capacities" may cause problems instead. For example, the number of young people with type 2 diabetes is much higher in African Americans than among Africans still living in their home continent, although the genetic make-up of these two groups is very similar. This suggests that lifestyle and diet may be particularly important.[1109]

Principles of treatment for type 2 diabetes in young people [1109]

⟼ Change what you eat to include smaller portions with less fat and carbohydrate.

⟼ Take up a form of regular exercise that involves your friends too. Walking, jogging and team sports can all be fun in groups.

⟼ Get your school on board. Changing the type of food offered in the school canteen and regular physical exercise on the school timetable will help.

⟼ You are likely to need insulin in the first week or so, especially if you had ketones or ketoacidosis when your diabetes was diagnosed.

⟼ The use of oral anti-diabetic agents such as metformin can be effective for treating type 2 diabetes in young people.[572]

Other types of diabetes

LADA (Latent Autoimmune Diabetes in the Adult) is a form of type 1 diabetes that appears in adults and is caused by the body's own immune mechanisms. These individuals are relatively thin and are very insulin sensitive. They usually produce insulin of their own for many years, much longer than the typical remission or "honeymoon" period seen in children and adolescents. Perhaps as many as 15% of people who are believed to have type 2 diabetes (and up to 50% of those who are not overweight) may have LADA.[1131] One way of finding out whether someone actually does have LADA is to measure the level of certain antibodies that attack the insulin-producing beta cells in the pancreas (ICA and GAD, see page 376).[1131]

Some children and adolescents have a rare form of genetic diabetes (MODY, maturity-onset diabetes of the young [1065]). This is associated with a definite family history of diabetes. One type of MODY (MODY2) has a modest increase in blood glucose levels, which often does not need any treatment at all besides a diet. People with MODY 2 seldom get complications from their diabetes. Some forms of MODY can be treated successfully with drugs (sulphonylureas), while people with other forms of MODY are likely to need insulin. Ask your doctor about taking a genetic test if diabetes is present in several generations of your family.

A special form of diabetes has been discovered in approximately half of the children with an onset of permanent diabetes below the age of 6 months.[355] The difficulty in secreting insulin is caused by a problem on a part of the beta cell (called Kir 6.2), responsible for regulating the release of insulin from the pancreas. This type of diabetes can be treated with a high dose of sulphonylurea tablets.[468] Genetic testing is done for free (shipping costs only) if the diabetes onset was before age 6 months, even if the person is an adult today. See www.diabetes-genes.org for more information.

How common is diabetes?

The number of individuals with diabetes varies enormously from country to country. According to 2012 data, 55 million in Europe and 25.8 million people in USA have type 1 or type 2 diabetes. The risk of a child developing type 1 diabetes before adulthood is approximately 0.3-0.5% in the Scandinavian countries.[623] This incidence varies between countries, and an estimated 497,000 children and adolescents aged under 15 years are thought to have diabetes worldwide.[549] Each year, another 79,000 children in this age group are estimated to develop diabetes,[549] as are a further 119,000 aged 15 years or more.[548]

In the US, approximately 13,000 new cases of diabetes are diagnosed in children every year.[29] Some 154,000 American individuals below the age of 19 years have diabetes (1 out of every 523 young persons), making this the second most common chronic disease in school-age children (the first being asthma).[668] Type 2 diabetes is rare below the age of 9 years, but in older youth the proportion of type 2 diabetes varies greatly among racial and ethnic groups (American Indian 76%, Asian/Pacific Islanders 40%, African American 33%, Hispanic 22% and Non-Hispanic white 6%).[668] In the UK there are at least 20,000 children under 15 years with diabetes (type 1 and type 2).[557] In Sweden there were approximately 7,500 children and adolescents with type 1 diabetes in 2007 and there are around 700 new cases of diabetes every year below the age of 18 years.[673]

There is a slow but steady increase in the number of cases of type 1 diabetes diagnosed per year in most countries, especially in the younger age group.[232,389] The overall annual increase in Europe in the age group 0-14 years from 1989-1999 has been 3.2%.[417] The same trend of a continuing rise (around 6% per year)

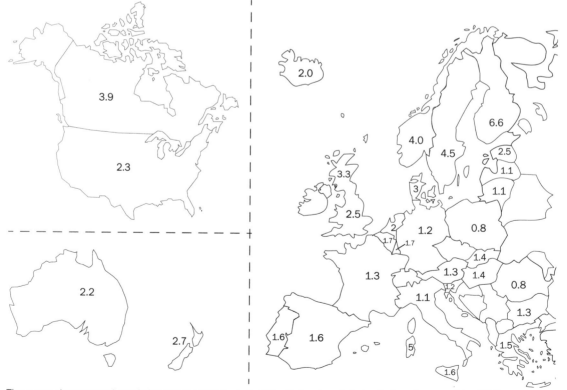

The maps show approximately how many children in 1,000 will develop diabetes before the age of 15.[416,592]

in the number of new cases in the ages 0-14 years over the last 20 years – (but not for young adults aged 15-29) – has been found in the UK.[351]

Finland has the highest incidence of childhood and adolescent diabetes in the world, and Sweden comes in third after Sardinia. In Japan childhood and adolescent type 1 diabetes is very uncommon. Although 120 million people live in Japan (compared with Sweden's 8 million) the actual number of Japanese children and teenagers with diabetes does not exceed the number in Sweden.[606]

We don't know why there is such a difference from one country to another, but it depends at least partly on cultural and environmental differences. For example, diabetes is more common among Asian immigrants living in the UK than in their relatives remaining in their countries of origin.[108] See also "What causes diabetes?" on page 375.

Juvenile diabetes is most common in the Nordic countries. In spite of having 15 times the population of Sweden, Japan has approximately the same number of children and teenagers with type 1 diabetes as Sweden.[602]

Can you catch diabetes?

Diabetes is not infectious. This may be obvious to adults but young children may be less confident. It is very important to get the message across to all friends, both at home and at school, that they cannot "catch" diabetes off you or anyone else. The best way may be to explain this to the whole class when going back to school. Ask the diabetes nurse to come to school and talk to friends and teachers about diabetes, and show them how injections and blood glucose tests are performed. Also tell them about the symptoms of hypoglycaemia and what they can do to help. It is especially important for teenagers with newly diagnosed diabetes to tell their friends. If, for whatever reason, you don't do this shortly after you are diagnosed, it becomes increasingly likely you will not tell them at all. Telling other people is a very important part of accepting your own diabetes.

Does eating too many sweets cause diabetes?

No! Eating sweets will not influence your risk of getting type 1 diabetes in adolescence or childhood. If you are the parent of a young child, remember to tell this to your child's friends as younger children in particular often wonder whether sweet-eating will give them diabetes too. Parents can fall into the trap of thinking: "If we only had done this or that differently, perhaps our child wouldn't have diabetes". But they shouldn't blame themselves like this. Generally speaking, there is nothing a parent could have done differently to prevent his or her child from developing type 1 diabetes.

Type 2 diabetes is rather different however. While sweets do not in themselves cause type 2 diabetes, excess calories of any kind (sweets, cake, potatoes, sugary drinks), or just insufficient physical exercise coupled with eating too much, is clearly related to obesity. And if you have a genetic susceptibility to type 2 diabetes, obesity will greatly increase your likelihood of developing it.

How your body works

It is important to understand how the body works in order to understand the difference in the way it works when you have diabetes. If you are not familiar with medical terms, or not interested in learning them, you can skip the terms in brackets. You do not need to know them to understand what is being said.

The three most important things making up the food we eat are sugar or starch (carbohydrates), fat and protein. When we eat, the digestion of starch (long chains of sugar, see page 232) begins immediately in the mouth with the help of a special enzyme (saliva amylase). An enzyme is a protein compound that breaks the bonds holding chemicals together. The food collects in the stomach, where it is mixed and broken down by the acidic gastric juice. The stomach then empties this mixture, a little at a time, into the small intestine through the lower opening of the stomach (pylorus, see illustration on pages 22 and 70).

As soon as you see food your mouth will water and your body will begin to prepare to digest it.

Phases in glucose metabolism

① **Storing at meals:**
During a meal and for the following 2-3 hours glucose from the meal will be used as fuel by the cells. At the same time the stores of glycogen (glucose in long chains, see picture on page 232), fat and protein are rebuilt.

② **Fasting between meals**
After 3-5 hours the carbohydrate content of the meal is consumed and the blood glucose level starts to decrease. The glycogen stores in the liver will then be broken down to maintain a constant blood glucose level. The glucose produced in this way provides fuel for the brain during fasting as, unlike the rest of the body, the brain cannot make use of the free fatty acids produced by fat tissue for its fuel.

Once the food is in the small intestine, it will be broken down even more by digestive enzymes from the pancreas and suspended in bile produced by the liver. If you eat sugar (for example, if you have hypoglycaemia, see page 65) it cannot be absorbed into the blood until it has entered the small intestine. A study on adults indicates that glucose cannot be absorbed from the mouth (oral cavity) [430] or from the stomach.[368] In this sense the emptying rate of the stomach will have a considerable impact on how quickly the sugar you eat enters the bloodstream and increases your blood glucose level (see page 231).

The carbohydrates we eat are broken down into the simple sugars (mono-saccharides), glucose (dextrose, grape-sugar), fructose (fruit sugar) and galactose. Fructose must first be transformed into glucose in the liver before it can affect your blood glucose level. Food proteins are broken down into amino acids, and fat into very tiny droplets (known as chylomicrons, and composed mainly of triglycerides). Simple sugars and proteins are absorbed directly into the blood while the fat droplets are absorbed into the lymph system and enter the bloodstream through the lymph vessels.

How insulin works

① Insulin opens the door for glucose to enter the cells.

② It stimulates the storage of glucose in the liver (as glycogen).

③ It stimulates the development of fat from excess carbohydrates.

④ And it stimulates the development of protein compounds in the body.

The smallest building blocks in your body are called cells. All the cells in your body need glucose to function well. With the help of oxygen, glucose is broken down into carbon dioxide, water and the vital energy to make cells work throughout the body (see "A healthy cell" on page 25).

Insulin

Many of the different things your body does are controlled by hormones. Hormones act through the blood and work like keys, "opening doors" to different functions in the body. Insulin is a hormone that is produced in the pancreas in special types of cells called beta cells. The beta cells are found in a part of the pancreas known as "the Islets of Langerhans", which also contain alpha cells producing the hormone glucagon (see picture on page 24). Other hormones are also produced by the islets, and help the islet cells to communicate with each other. The pancreas has another very important function. It produces enzymes to help you digest your food. This part works quite well, even in a person with diabetes.

The venous blood draining the stomach and intestines passes through the liver before reaching the rest of the body. A large amount of glucose will be absorbed by the liver with the help of insulin, and then stored as a reservoir as glycogen (see page 34). These stores can be used between meals, during the night, and when a person is starving. Only glucose that is not absorbed by the liver can reach the peripheral bloodstream (reaching all over the body), and it is through this that glucose is delivered to the rest of the body. This glucose can be measured by a finger prick or a blood test from the vein.

The muscles can also store a certain amount of glucose as glycogen. Whereas the glycogen store in the liver can be used to raise the blood glucose level, the store in the muscles can only be used by the muscles themselves during exercise. The body's ability to store glucose is very limited. The glycogen stores are only sufficient for 24 hours without food for an adult and 12 hours for a child.[974]

The glucose content of the blood is surprisingly constant during both day and night in a person without diabetes (approximately 4-7 mmol/l, 70-125 mg/dl). In adults, this blood glucose level corresponds to only about two lumps of sugar. If you think about it this way, you won't find it surprising that even a small amount of sugar, a few sweets for example, can disturb the balance of glucose in the body of a person with diabetes.

The reason that insulin is so important is that it acts as the key that "opens the door" for glucose to enter the cells. As soon as you see or smell food, signals are delivered to the beta cells to increase insulin production.[336] Once the food has gone into your stomach and intestine, other special hormones send more signals to the beta cells to continue increasing their insulin production.

The beta cells contain an inbuilt "blood glucose meter" that registers when the level of glucose in your blood goes up and responds by sending the correct amount of insulin into your bloodstream. When a person without diabetes eats food, the insulin concentration in their blood increases rapidly (see figure on page 23) to take

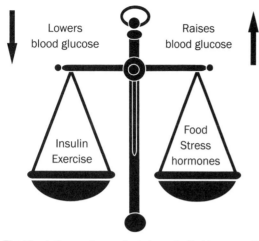

The blood glucose in your body is controlled by many different actions that balance each other to achieve an as even a level as possible throughout the day.

care of the glucose coming from the food, transporting it into the cells. This person's blood glucose level will normally not rise more than 1-2 mmol/l (20-35 mg/dl) after a meal.[336]

Insulin follows the bloodstream to the different cells of the body, sticking to the cell surface in special insulin receptors. This makes it possible for glucose to travel through the cell wall made penetrable to glucose. Insulin causes certain proteins inside the cell to come to the cell surface, collect glucose and then release it inside the cell. In this way, the blood glucose level is kept at a constant level.

Not all cells require insulin to transport glucose into their interior. There are "insulin-independent" cells that absorb glucose in direct proportion to the blood glucose level. Cells like this can be found in the brain cells, nerve fibres, retina, kidneys and adrenal glands, as well as in the blood vessels and the red blood cells.

It may seem illogical that certain cells can absorb glucose without insulin. However, in a situation where there is not enough glucose in the body, the insulin production will be stopped, reserving the glucose for the most important organs. If you have diabetes and

your blood glucose level is high, the cells that don't need insulin will absorb large amounts of glucose. In the long run this will poison the cells, making those organs susceptible to long-term damage from having diabetes.

The body needs a small amount of insulin, even between meals and during the night, to accommodate the glucose coming from the liver (see page 34). This is often referred to as the "basal insulin level" to distinguish between the need for insulin in the background between mealtimes, and the "boluses" of insulin needed to accommodate the eating of meals or snacks. Around 40-50% of the total amount of insulin produced by a person without diabetes, over any 24-hour period, will be released as basal insulin between meals.[110]

A large amount of carbohydrate from a meal will be stored in the liver (as glycogen, see page 34). If you eat more than you need, the excess carbohydrate is transformed into fat and stored in the fat tissue. The human body has an almost unlimited ability to store fat, so fat left over from a meal is stored in the same way. Proteins (amino acids) from the meal can be used by different body tissues. There is no specific way of storing amino acids. The liver can produce glucose from amino acids, for example if you haven't eaten for some time. But this means that the body tissues themselves are broken down since the body has no way of storing amino acids.

All the organs in the body are built of cells, which are like the bricks in a house. Each organ contains specialized cells to enable it to perform its function, so there are identifiable kidney cells, liver cells and muscle cells.

Your body doesn't realize it has diabetes

When you read about how your body functions if you have diabetes, remember that it always "thinks" and reacts as if it did not actually have diabetes, that is to say, as if the insulin production was still working as well as it should. Your body doesn't understand why things go wrong when you become insulin-deficient, because it doesn't realize what has happened (see page 26). On the other hand your brain can help you by thinking through what will happen when your insulin production stops working. It is very important therefore that you remember to stop and think about how your body reacts in particular situations, why it reacts like this, and how you can influence these reactions.

Your insulin doses will vary from day to day since you rarely conduct your life in the same way from one day to another. If you did not have diabetes, your beta cells would make automatic adjustments for this. But now it is up to you to notice how your body reacts on different days, and how much insulin you need in different situations.

What happens to the carbohydrates in the food?

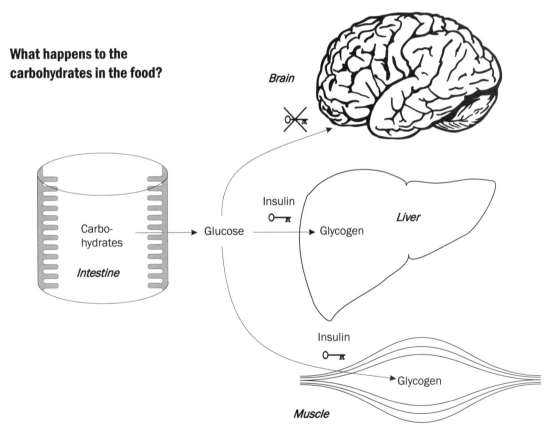

The complex carbohydrates in food are broken down to simple sugars in the intestine. Glucose is absorbed into the bloodstream and stored as glycogen in the liver and muscles. The key hormone insulin is needed to transport glucose into the cells of these organs. The brain cannot store glucose, so it has to depend upon a regular supply if it is to function well. The nervous system and some other cells (for example, those in the eyes and kidneys) can take up glucose without the help of insulin. There are advantages to this in the short term as the nervous system will not experience a lack of glucose, even if no insulin is present. However, in the long term, there are disadvantages for a person with diabetes, as the nervous system will be exposed to high levels of glucose inside the cells when the blood glucose level is high.

The anatomy of your body

When you eat, the food passes from your mouth through your gullet on its way down to your stomach. Sugar cannot be absorbed into your blood until the food has passed the lower opening of your stomach (pylorus) and entered the intestine. In the intestine, it will be digested by enzymes from your pancreas and intestinal lining.

The small intestine is very long (3-5 metres or 9-15 feet in an adult) and is folded or coiled in order to fit comfortably inside your abdominal cavity (belly). The first part of the small intestine, the duodenum, is 25-30 cm (10-12 inches) long.

After leaving the small intestine, the food passes into the large intestine (or colon) which is approximately 1.5 metres (4-5 feet) long. The large intestine passes around the abdominal cavity before entering the rectum.

Pancreas

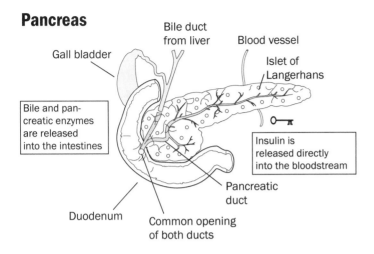

Gall bladder

Bile duct from liver

Blood vessel

Islet of Langerhans

Bile and pancreatic enzymes are released into the intestines

Insulin is released directly into the bloodstream

Pancreatic duct

Duodenum

Common opening of both ducts

"I am now your pancreas but one day, when you are older and learn to take care of yourself, your brain will become your pancreas."

The mother of Maria de Alva, former president of IDF (International Diabetes Federation).

Your pancreas is about the size of the palm of your hand. It is positioned under the left rib cage in the back of the abdominal cavity, close to the stomach. The pancreas has two main functions: it produces enzymes which help you digest food, and it produces insulin which helps control blood sugar. The digestive enzymes from the pancreas reach the intestine through the pancreatic duct. This drains into the duodenum together with the duct from the liver and gall bladder. There are approximately 1 million islets of Langerhans in the pancreas. Insulin produced in the beta cells of the islets is released directly into the small blood vessels passing through the pancreas.

Insulin and blood glucose

A person without diabetes

If an individual doesn't have diabetes, the insulin concentration in the blood will increase rapidly after a meal.[808] When the glucose in the food is absorbed from the intestine, and the blood glucose has returned to normal levels, the insulin level will drop back to baseline once again. However, the insulin level will never go right down to zero, as a low level of basal insulin is needed to take account of the glucose coming from the reserve stores in the liver between meals and during the night.

The resulting blood glucose level will be very stable in a person without diabetes as this graph illustrates.[714] The normal blood glucose level is between about 4 and 7 mmol/l (70-125 mg/dl).

Islets of Langerhans

If you look at an islet of Langerhans through a microscope, you will find it contains beta cells, which produce insulin, and alpha cells, which produce glucagon. Both of these hormones are released directly into the blood. The beta cells contain a sort of "built-in" blood glucose meter. If the blood glucose level is raised, insulin will be released. If it is lowered, the secretion of insulin stops. If it falls below the normal level, glucagon is released. Other hormones are also produced by the islets, and help the islet cells to communicate with each other.

The islets of Langerhans are very small, only 0.1 mm (four thousands of an inch) in diameter.

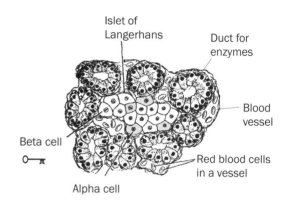

All the islets together contain approximately 200 units of insulin in an adult. The volume of them all combined is no larger than a fingertip.

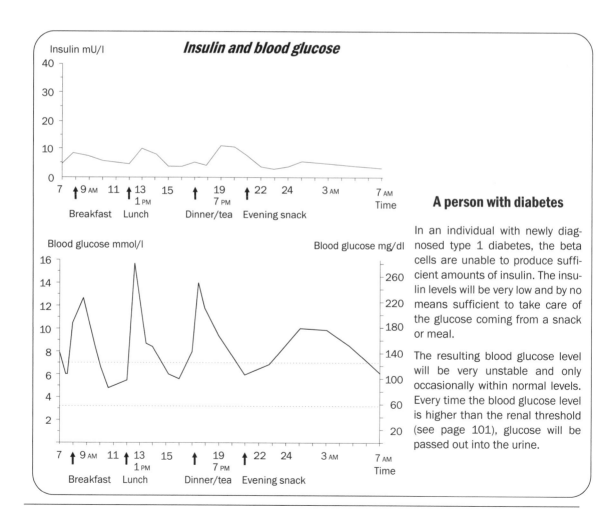

A person with diabetes

In an individual with newly diagnosed type 1 diabetes, the beta cells are unable to produce sufficient amounts of insulin. The insulin levels will be very low and by no means sufficient to take care of the glucose coming from a snack or meal.

The resulting blood glucose level will be very unstable and only occasionally within normal levels. Every time the blood glucose level is higher than the renal threshold (see page 101), glucose will be passed out into the urine.

Cellular metabolism

A healthy cell

Sugar in the food is absorbed from the intestine into the blood in the form of glucose (dextrose) and fructose. Glucose must enter the cells before it can be used for producing energy or other metabolic processes. The hormone insulin is needed to "open the door", i.e. make it possible for glucose to penetrate the wall of the cell. Once it is inside the cell, glucose is converted with the help of oxygen into carbon dioxide, water and energy. The carbon dioxide travels to the lungs, where it is exchanged for oxygen.

Energy is vitally important to the cell if it is to function properly. In addition, glucose is stored (in the form of glycogen) in liver and muscle cells for future use. The brain, however, is not capable of storing glucose as glycogen. It is therefore dependent on an even and continuous supply of glucose from the blood.

Starvation

When no food is available, there is a shortage of glucose in the blood. In this case, opening the "cell door" with the help of insulin will not do any good. In a person who does not have diabetes, the production of insulin will be stopped almost completely when the blood glucose level goes down. The alpha cells in the pancreas recognize the lowered blood glucose level and secrete the hormone glucagon into the blood-

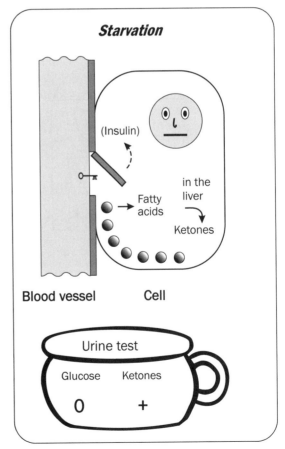

stream. Glucagon acts as a signal for the liver cells to release glucose from the reserve supply of glycogen. Adrenaline, cortisol and growth hormone are other hormones that are produced when the body is starving (see page 33).

If starvation continues, the body will use the next reserve system for glucose supply. Fat is broken down into fatty acids and glycerol with the help of the stress hormone adrenaline. The fatty acids are transformed into ketones in the liver (these are known as "starvation ketones") and glycerol is changed into glucose. These reactions will take place if you are fasting or if you are too ill to eat, for example if you have gastroenteritis.

All the cells of the body (except the brain) can use fatty acids as fuel. Only the muscles, the heart, the kidneys and the brain, however, can use ketones as fuel. As fasting continues, ketones may supply up to two-thirds of the brain's energy needs.[644] In children, starvation ketones develop more quickly and reach higher levels than in adults.[471] The cells will retrieve some energy from this but less than when glucose is available. If the body is without food for too long, proteins from muscle tissue will start to break down too, so that they can be converted into glucose.

Diabetes and insulin deficiency

Type 1 diabetes is a "deficiency disease" in which the hormone insulin is missing. The result of this is that glucose is unable to enter the cells. The cells then act exactly as they would in the starvation situation described above. Your body will try to raise your blood glucose to even higher levels since it believes that the reason for the lack of glucose inside the cells is a low glucose level in the blood (see "Your body doesn't realize it has diabetes" on page 21). The hormones adrenaline and glucagon (see page 35) will give signals to the liver to release glucose from the glycogen stores.

In this situation, however, the starvation takes place in the midst of plenty. The bloodstream already contains an excess of glucose, which is being passed out into the urine. Inside the cells, fatty acids are being produced. These are then transformed into ketones in the liver ("diabetes ketones"), and the ketones are also passed out into the urine. If this continues without treatment for a longer period of time, there is a risk that the person will end up with ketoacidosis (see page 29). When insulin is supplied, the cells can function properly again and this "vicious cycle" will be broken.

"Starvation ketones" and "diabetes ketones" are chemically identical but they are often referred to differently depending on how they originate (see page 109).

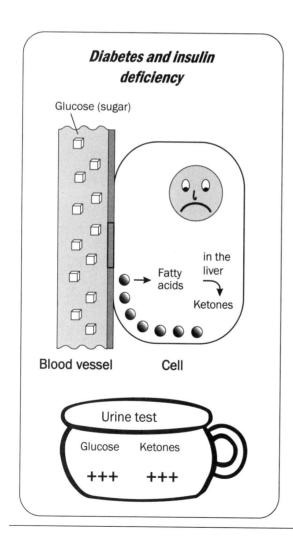

Diabetes and insulin deficiency

Glucose (sugar)

in the liver

Fatty acids

Ketones

Blood vessel   Cell

Urine test

Glucose   Ketones

+++   +++

High blood glucose levels

Vomiting with diabetes is a warning sign, as it is often the first sign of insulin deficiency. A child who is unable to drink may go downhill very quickly and soon become seriously ill. Contact your diabetes healthcare team or the hospital if you are at all unsure as to how to handle the situation (see sick day rules on page 301).

If your blood glucose level rises temporarily (e.g. following a large meal), you may not even notice. Many people feel fine, even with a blood glucose level of 16-18 mmol/l (290-325 mg/dl). You may be a bit more tired and thirsty than usual, but the symptoms are not nearly as obvious as when your blood glucose level is low. One study of adults found no difference in neuro-psychological function (simple motor abilities, attention, reaction time, learning and memory) when comparing blood glucose levels of 8.9 and 21.1 mmol/l (160 and 380 mg/dl).[304] However, if the rise in your blood glucose level is caused by a lack of insulin, you are likely to feel unwell even if your blood glucose is not higher than 12-15 mmol/l (215-270 mg/dl) if your level of ketones is raised. It is the lack of insulin that makes you feel unwell, not the high blood glucose level as such.

What happens in the body when there is not enough insulin?

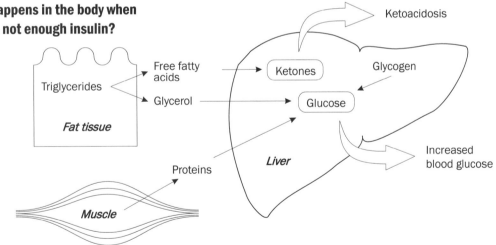

The reaction of a person's body without diabetes to shortage of insulin is quite logical if you remember that the levels of insulin are normally low only when the blood glucose is low too. So low insulin levels make the body "think" it must send more energy to the blood. This process in turn triggers the hormones adrenaline, cortisol, glucagon and growth hormone to stimulate the production of both glucose and ketones. Ketones can be used as fuel by your brain if you are starving. However, if you have diabetes which is untreated or undertreated, insulin levels will be low at the same time as your blood glucose level is high. Your body will be confused by this, and will respond by trying to increase the blood's supply of energy in the same way as it would have done before you developed diabetes. The amount of ketones in the blood will increase, which can lead to ketoacidosis. The blood glucose level will go right up, even if you don't eat anything.

What happens in the body when there is not enough insulin?

Insulin deficiency results in a lack of glucose inside the cells (see figure on page 26). This causes ketones to be produced, which can be used as fuel. If a lot of ketones are produced, however, they will have some very unpleasant effects. In smaller children, nausea and vomiting are often the first symptoms when the level of ketones in the blood increases. For example, if a child's bedtime insulin is forgotten, he or she may feel sick or vomit in the morning. If a child with diabetes vomits, you should **always** consider whether a lack of insulin may be to blame (for example forgotten injections). Alternatively, the sickness may indicate the start of an illness which will cause the child to need more insulin than usual. Either situation could rapidly become critical if the correct measures are not taken! See the chapter on Fever and sick days on page 303 for further information.

Remember that your blood glucose level will rise when your insulin level is low, even if you don't eat anything. This is because the lack of insulin in itself stimulates the liver to release more glucose through an increased level of hormones (see "Regulation of blood glucose" on page 33) to make up for the lack of glucose inside these cells. This is logical if you remember that, before you had diabetes, there was a lack of glucose inside the cells only when your blood glucose level was low.

Symptoms of insulin deficiency

These symptoms will develop more quickly if you take a smaller proportion of your daily insulin dose as intermediate- or long-acting insulin. If you use an insulin pump you will be even more sensitive to insulin deficiency as the pump uses only rapid- or short-acting insulin.

① **Production of ketones**

➡ Vomiting, feeling sick.

➡ Tiredness.

➡ Abdominal pain.

➡ Heavy breathing, the smell of acetone on the breath.

➡ Pain in the chest or stomach, difficulty breathing.

➡ Drowsiness.

➡ Diabetes coma (unconsciousness caused by ketoacidosis).

② **Depletion of energy stores, breakdown of muscle tissue**

➡ Weakness.

➡ Weight loss.

➡ Decreased growth (long-standing insulin deficiency).

How to treat a high blood glucose level

We usually recommend to correct a blood glucose level that is high (>8 mmol/l, 145 mg/dl) by a correction dose (see page 146). However, if it is high on repeated monitoring, you should always check for ketones in your blood or urine. If there are no ketones, it is unlikely that

the cells are "starving" (see page 109). If you feel well, measure your blood glucose level once again before the next meal and add insulin according to the correction factor to your pre-meal dose if the level is still high (see page 147 for further advice).

If your blood glucose level continues high for several hours and you have ketones in your blood or urine, it is likely that your insulin level is low (see page 111), and you should take an

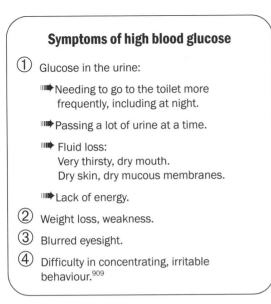

Symptoms of high blood glucose

① Glucose in the urine:

⮕ Needing to go to the toilet more frequently, including at night.

⮕ Passing a lot of urine at a time.

⮕ Fluid loss:
Very thirsty, dry mouth.
Dry skin, dry mucous membranes.

⮕ Lack of energy.

② Weight loss, weakness.

③ Blurred eyesight.

④ Difficulty in concentrating, irritable behaviour.[909]

extra dose of 0.1 U/kg. See page 115 for more information on interpreting blood ketone tests. If the ketone level increases in spite of your taking extra insulin, you should always contact the hospital or your diabetes specialist. Blood levels of ketones above 3 mmol/l, or urine ketones increasing to large amounts, indicate that you are at risk of developing ketoacidosis.[1082] Don't

hesitate to seek advice from your diabetes healthcare team if you feel unwell or are worried about your glucose or ketone levels. See also "What to do if your blood glucose level is high" on page 147.

When insulin levels are low, the blood glucose level will be high and blood and urine tests will show ketones. Once you have taken extra insulin, however, it will be more difficult to interpret your urine tests. Blood tests for ketones will give you more correct information in this situation. There are two types of ketones (beta-hydroxybutyric acid and acetoacetate) but only one type (acetoacetate) will show on the urine ketone strips. Often both types of ketones are increased when insulin levels are low. When extra insulin is given, further production of ketones is blocked. Early on in treatment, it may appear that there is a rise in ketones in the urine. This is because beta-hydroxybutyric acid is transformed into acetoacetate, giving the impression of an increase in ketones on the urine test strip.[644] Actually, however, the total amount of ketones in the blood has gone down (see also page 112).

Ketoacidosis

Ketones are produced when fat is broken down in the body for any reason. In normal circumstances, ketones are used as fuel by your muscles, heart, kidney and brain. If you have diabetes, ketones are produced in excess when there is a lack of insulin in your body, for example when insulin is omitted or not increased sufficiently during an illness or growth spurt. Too many ketones make your blood acidic, causing ketoacidosis.[280] Your body tries to get rid of these ketones by excreting them, either in the urine or in the form of acetone, which is breathed out through the lungs, giving a fruity smell to the breath. Your breathing becomes faster (called Kussmaul breathing) as your body tries to get rid of as much acetone as possible.

Ida
12

Ketoacidosis is treated with intravenous insulin and fluids. It is always caused by a deficiency in insulin and it is not uncommon to be in ketoacidosis if you have had symptoms of thirst and increased urine output for a longer period of time before the diagnosis is made.

Ketoacidosis can rapidly develop into a life-threatening condition. This must be treated adequately in a hospital with intravenous fluid and insulin.

General abdominal pain and tenderness may be caused by ketoacidosis, but these could have other causes (not related to diabetes), so it is important that other possible medical problems are not dismissed until they have been ruled out.[1116] If you cannot increase the intake of fluid to compensate for the increased amount of urine you are passing, you will become dehydrated. If this continues without treatment, you will become unconscious and fall into a coma (diabetic coma).

Ketoacidosis is a life-threatening condition that must be treated with intravenous fluid and insulin in hospital.[661,1116] Although effective treatment is now available, there are still people who die from ketoacidosis, ranging from less than 1% in developed countries [308] to 6-24% in developing countries.[661]

Ketoacidosis can occur at the onset of diabetes, though the likelihood of this happening varies considerably (between 15% and 67%) from one country to another.[308] It can also occur if you are unable to take your insulin for 12-24 hours, for some reason. Another situation which can cause ketoacidosis is if your body suddenly needs more insulin than usual, for example if you have an infection accompanied by a high temperature. Alcohol intake may cause ketoacidosis to develop much more quickly.[952] In Sweden, about 18% of new onset diabetes in children and adolescents have ketoacidosis,[929] while in other parts of the world as many as 70% have ketoacidosis at onset.[308]

Insulin deficiency and ketoacidosis will develop more quickly if a smaller part of your daily insulin dosage consists of intermediate- or long-acting insulin. This is because the insulin depot will be much smaller if you are using rapid- or short-acting insulin, compared with when you use intermediate- or long-acting insulin. See "Depot effect" on page 86. With an insulin pump the depot is very small since the pump delivers only rapid- or short-acting insulin. Some people, therefore, can feel sick or vomit after only one night without insulin if the pump fails (see page 197). With the use of rapid-acting insulin (Humalog, NovoRapid) in pumps, the depot will be even smaller, resulting

Causes of diabetic ketoacidosis (DKA)

Ketoacidosis is always caused by a relative or absolute deficiency of insulin. Relative insulin deficiency occurs if, for example, you don't increase your insulin doses when you are ill with fever, or during the growth spurt of puberty. The increased blood glucose level, along with other contributing factors, results in increased insulin resistance (i.e. a decreased sensitivity to insulin, see page 223). Much larger doses of insulin are needed to achieve the same blood glucose-lowering effect as before the change.

Do high glucose levels affect the brain?

♠ The brain volume increases up to about 6 years of age, but the maturation is not complete until adolescence or early adulthood. This development is vulnerable to long-term high glucose levels, which are not an uncommon problem among teenagers. Certain regions of the brain are more susceptible to damage from high glucose levels.[48] These are the same regions that are affected in early Alzheimer's disease, for which diabetes is thought to be a risk factor.

♠ In an Australian study, the IQ in a group of children dropped approximately 10% when blood glucose levels were raised to 20-30 mmol/l (360-540 mg/dl).[256]

♠ When the blood glucose was normalized, the IQ also returned to the normal level. However, ketoacidosis seems to be able to damage intellectual function in a way that is not reversible.

♠ An American study found the IQ to be permanently lowered by approximately one point for every time a person needed hospital treatment for ketoacidosis.[369]

♠ In a Swiss study, ketoacidosis at onset and long-term high HbA_{1c} were the main contributing factors to lower results on cognitive testing, but only in boys, not girls. Severe hypoglycaemia was not found to be related to impaired test results in this study.[951]

♠ Adults with type 1 diabetes and damage to blood vessels (caused by long-term high HbA_{1c}) have decreased functional connectivity between brain regions involved in working memory, language, attention, motor control and visual processing.[1063]

Blurred eyesight and diabetes

Blurred eyesight can be a symptom of a high blood glucose level. This is caused by difference between the glucose content of the lens, compared with that of the blood. The lens contains no blood vessels (if it did they would block the passage of light into the eye). Glucose from the blood must therefore be transported into the lens through the surrounding fluid (aqueous humour, see figure on page 358). So, when the glucose content of the blood is changing rapidly, the glucose content of the lens is bound to be different. If the glucose content of the lens is higher than that of the blood, the lens will try to absorb water, and this will make it swell. The lens will then refract the light differently, causing temporary shortsightedness. It affects your vision in very much the same way as if you borrow someone else's glasses.

The eye itself won't be damaged by this phenomenon, and vision often returns to normal within a few hours. If you borrow a friend's glasses, you will probably be able to focus but your eyes will find the effort of focusing makes them very tired. This type of visual disturbance is common at the onset of diabetes and usually happens when the glucose level is changing rapidly. It has nothing to do with the eye complications that can occur after many years of diabetes. See also page 360.

in even faster symptoms of insulin deficiency if the delivery is interrupted (see page 214).

Symptoms of a low blood glucose level are usually fairly easy to recognize. However, when the blood glucose level is high many people won't have any symptoms at all. Try to train yourself to recognize the sensation of going into "autopilot", warning you when the blood glucose level is rising. If you can do this, you are less likely to need to rely on blood glucose tests. Thirst and the need to pass a lot of urine both occur when your blood glucose level goes above the renal threshold, but remember that this level can vary from one person to another (see page 101). Other common symptoms are apathy and a sense that everything is "slowing down". One study of children and adolescents aged 9-18 years found that higher blood glucose levels were reflected in impulsive behaviour.[909] What signs can you see to indicate your own blood glucose level is high?

Regulation of blood glucose

If you are not eating, the chances are your entire bloodstream will contain only about 5 g (1/5 ounce) of glucose (barely two lumps of sugar). If you are not fully grown, it will be even less. At the same time, your blood needs to deliver about 10 g (1/3 ounce) of glucose every hour to the tissues of the body.[6] Obviously, if something happens to the supply of glucose you will very quickly run out, resulting in a severe shortage of glucose in your blood within an hour.

Counter-regulation

In someone who does not have diabetes, the body is able to regulate its own blood glucose levels within narrow boundaries, normally between approximately 4 and 7 mmol/l (70-125 mg/dl). When your blood glucose falls below 3.5-4.0 mmol/l (65-70 mg/dl) you will feel unwell. A drop in your blood glucose level affects all your bodily reactions, as your body struggles to give your brain access to what little glucose is left. The body tries to get the remaining glucose moving, while the cells outside the brain attempt to economize by decreasing the amount of glucose they use. The brain is unable to store glucose, so it has to depend on an even and continuous supply from the blood. However, if no food has been eaten for a while, the

CHRIStoPHer

brain adapts and uses other types of fuel, mainly ketones.

While the hormone insulin lowers your blood glucose level, there are other hormones in your body which can raise it. The body reacts to low

---

Where does the glucose in your blood come from?

① From your food.

② From the breakdown of glucose stored as glycogen in the liver (called glycogenolysis).

③ From protein and fat used for the production of glucose (called gluconeogenesis).

Counter-regulating hormones that increase blood glucose levels

① Adrenaline	Increases the blood glucose for 2-4 hours after hypoglycaemia.[129]
② Glucagon	
③ Cortisol	The effect starts after 3-4 hours, and lasts for 5-12 hours after hypoglycaemia.[129]
④ Growth hormone	

Effects of insulin

⇒ Insulin is produced in the beta cells in the pancreas.

① Insulin decreases blood glucose by:
  ⇒ increasing the uptake of glucose into the cells.
  ⇒ Increasing the body's ability to store glucose as glycogen in liver and muscle.
  ⇒ Decreasing the production of glucose from the liver.

② Insulin counteracts the production of ketones from the liver. It stimulates the utilization of ketones in the cells.

③ Insulin also increases the production of muscle protein.

④ It increases the production and decreases the breakdown of body fat.

Body reserves during fasting and hypoglycaemia

⇒ The store of glycogen in the liver is broken down to glucose.

⇒ Fat is broken down to free fatty acids that can be used as fuel. Fatty acids can be transformed into ketones in the liver. Ketones can also be used as fuel, mainly by the brain.

⇒ Proteins from the muscles are broken down to be used in the liver in order to produce glucose.

blood glucose with a defensive reaction known as counter-regulation. In counter-regulation, the autonomic nervous system cooperates with a number of different hormones to raise the blood glucose level. This defence against hypoglycaemia is extremely important to your body. The symptoms associated with hypoglycaemia are caused by the brain's response to a lack of glucose as well as by the direct effects of the counter-regulatory hormones.

Children are generally more sensitive to hypoglycaemia than adults. In one study on healthy children and adolescents, hypoglycaemic symptoms and adrenaline responses were evident when the blood glucose level was 3.8 mmol/l, compared with 3.1 mmol/l (68 vs. 56 mg/dl) observed for adults.[574]

It may be difficult to understand the biochemistry of the hormones and which hormone is doing what. The figures on page 25 give you a short summary of what you need to know to begin with when you are new to diabetes.

The liver

The liver functions as a bank for glucose. In times of plenty, you deposit glucose in the liver, and in times of fasting you will be able to withdraw it. The excess of glucose from a meal will be stored as a "reservoir" in the liver and muscle cells in the form of glycogen (see illustration on page 232). Insulin is needed to transport the glucose into both liver and muscle cells.

The liver can also produce glucose from fat and proteins to raise the blood glucose level (by a process called gluconeogenesis). The adult liver produces about 6 g (1/5 ounce) of glucose per hour in between meals.[974] The majority of this glucose will be consumed by the brain, which can make use of glucose without the help of insulin. A smaller child's liver will produce up to six times as much glucose per kg body weight. The liver of a 5-year-old will produce as much glucose in an hour as an adult. After a longer period without food, the kidneys can produce glucose in the same way as the liver does.[349] Recent research suggests that the kidneys can contribute as much as 20% of the body's total glucose production after a night without food.[183]

People with diabetes can also use the stores of glycogen when their blood glucose is low. If you

Liver and muscle stores

♠ Liver cells can release glucose into the blood from the store of glycogen.

♠ Muscle cells can only use the glucose released from the glycogen stores as fuel inside the cell.

♠ An adult has about 100-120 g (3.5-4.2 ounces) of glucose stored in the liver.[570]

♠ The glycogen store can be broken down to glucose when the blood glucose is low (glycogenolysis) and can compensate for about 24 hours without food in an adult.[974]

♠ In children, glycogen stores are smaller and can compensate for a shorter time without food.

♠ A preschool child has enough glycogen for about 12 hours without food, a smaller child even less.

♠ A child will use up glucose faster than an adult will, even when not very active. This is because a child's brain is larger in relation to body mass than an adult's brain.

have emptied your stores of glycogen, for example during a game of football when the body needs a lot of extra glucose, you will have smaller reserves for dealing with any hypoglycaemic episode that might occur later, including during the night. This leads to an increased risk of hypoglycaemia several hours after physical exercise (see page 284).

A healthy pancreas produces insulin. Since the blood flow from the pancreas goes to the liver first, this organ will have the quickest and highest concentration of insulin. When insulin is injected into the subcutaneous tissue, it will enter a superficial blood vessel and reach the liver only after the blood has passed through the heart. Because of this, people with diabetes have a much lower insulin concentration in the liver than people without diabetes.

Glucagon

During the day you tend to feel hungry at intervals of about 4 hours, whereas during the night you can do without food for up to 8 or even 10 hours. This is because glycogen from the liver is broken down into glucose during the night, with the help of the hormones glucagon and adrenaline. Small children have small stores of glycogen, so they need to eat more often.

The glucagon production in the pancreas won't necessarily be affected in your early days with diabetes. However, within 5 years of diagnosis, your body's ability to produce sufficient amounts of glucagon in response to hypoglycaemia will usually disappear.[127] This happens in children as well as in adults.[22,37] It is probably

The liver acts like a bank for glucose in your body. When times are good, i.e. during the hours after a meal, glucose is deposited in the "liver bank" to be stored as glycogen.

When times are bad, i.e. a couple of hours after the meal and during the night, glucose is withdrawn from the "liver bank" to keep the blood glucose level adequate.

not a long-term complication as such, but rather a reflection of the way your body adapts to repeated episodes of hypoglycaemia.[218] Those individuals who still produce some of their own insulin appear to be better able to carry on secreting glucagon in response to hypoglycaemia ("the glucagon defence").[22,218,817] Some research results suggest that the glucagon defence can be at least partly restored if you manage to avoid hypoglycaemia[342,587] (see also "Hypoglycaemia unawareness" on page 52).

In a person who doesn't have diabetes, the production of glucagon goes down when the blood glucose and insulin concentration rise after a meal. But this doesn't happen when a person has diabetes, even though their blood glucose level goes up. This is because insulin from injections into the subcutaneous tissue is less concentrated by the time it reaches the glucagon-producing alpha cells in the pancreas. In addition to the glucose derived from a meal, blood from the liver will contain glucose derived from glycogen, also contributing to an increase in blood glucose after a meal.[292]

The effects of glucagon

⇒ Glucagon is produced in the alpha cells in the pancreas.

① Glucagon raises blood glucose by:
  ⇒ Releasing glucose from the glycogen stores in the liver.
  ⇒ Activating the production of glucose from proteins.

② Glucagon stimulates the production of ketones in the liver.

Glucagon injections

If a person with diabetes is unconscious or unable to eat or drink, you can give an injection of glucagon to stimulate the breakdown of glycogen in the liver. This will raise the blood glucose level. Glucagon injections are not difficult to administer. It would be a good idea, for example, to encourage a teacher or youth leader to learn how to do this before school outings or activity holidays.

Glucagon is given as a subcutaneous injection in the same way as insulin. If you are using an indwelling catheter (Insuflon) you should not

Glucagon directly affects your quality of life. Whenever you have a glucagon kit with you, you are armed with your own emergency treatment. You can go camping, hiking in the mountains or sailing with minimum danger. It is a good idea to take glucagon with you if you go on holiday abroad, so you will not need to depend on local healthcare if you develop severe hypoglycaemia. Make sure that your travelling companion knows where you store your glucagon, and how it should be used.

Give a glucagon injection if a person with diabetes develops severe hypoglycaemia and becomes unconscious or has a seizure. If the person has not woken up within 10-15 minutes, call an ambulance. However, if the person has woken up and has a normal blood glucose level by the time the ambulance arrives, it won't be necessary for them to go to hospital.

It may be difficult to mix glucagon for the first time in a situation where you really need it. In order to avoid panic at such a time, check the contents of the kit and read through the instructions as soon as you bring them home. Indicate the dose you would need on the syringe with a felt tip pen, so you will not have to worry about this when you are stressed. When the expiry date has passed and you have a new glucagon kit, you can use the old one for practising the mixing and drawing up of glucagon. Write in your own words the directions for administering glucagon on a small piece of paper and put this with the kit.

use this for glucagon as the effect will be reduced if the catheter is not working properly. The dose of glucagon is 0.1-0.2 mg per 10 kg (20 lb) body weight.[23,218] The blood glucose-raising effect starts within 10 minutes and lasts for at least 30-60 minutes.[23] The effect will be just as good after a subcutaneous injection as after an intramuscular one, so it does not matter how deep you insert the needle.[23] The higher dose (0.2 mg/10 kg or 20 lb) will give a slightly higher rise in blood glucose, but it may also increase your risk of side effects.[23]

Everyone who has diabetes and is using insulin should have glucagon available.[4,513,694] Check the expiry date! When the expiry date has passed and you have picked up a new injection kit from the pharmacy you can use the old one for practising and demonstrating mixing procedures. Don't eat anything for at least 30 minutes after taking a glucagon injection, or you may feel sick or even vomit. This is a relatively common side effect, and usually occurs within

---

Glucagon

➠ Every person treated with insulin should have a glucagon kit and know how to use it.

➠ Give glucagon if a person with diabetes is unconscious, has seizures or cannot eat or drink.

➠ Dose: 0.1-0.2 mg per 10 kg (20 lb) body weight (1 mg/ml solution). If in doubt, give more rather than less. Glucagon is not dangerous if you accidentally overdose.

➠ Glucagon takes effect within 10-15 minutes.

➠ The effect lasts for 30-60 minutes.
Eat something when you are feeling better to keep your blood glucose level up until the next meal. But don't eat too much at once.

➠ Nausea is a common side effect.
Wait at least 30 minutes before you eat to avoid this problem.

➠ Do *not* repeat the dose! One injection gives a sufficient level of glucagon in the blood.

➠ Loss of effect can be caused by:

Store of glycogen already depleted by	Glucagon counteracted by
1) Exercise	1) Alcohol [365]
2) Recent hypoglycaemia	2) High dose of insulin
3) Reduced food intake, e.g. through illness	

➠ Always take glucagon with you, e.g. when going on a picnic, hiking trip, sailing trip or holiday abroad.

➠ Teach people close to you how to administer glucagon!

➠ Glucagon has the same effect whether injected into subcutaneous tissue or into muscle.

30-60 minutes. You will be more likely to suffer in this way if you eat large amounts of food. Don't repeat the glucagon injection either, as this will make sickness more likely without

Mini-dose glucagon

♠ A small dose of glucagon has been effective in treating mild or impending hypoglycaemia associated with gastroenteritis or refusal to eat.[466,472]

♠ In one study, children aged 2 years or under, received two "units" using a standard U-100 insulin syringe (= 20 µg), while those older than 2 years received one "unit" for each year of their life, up to 15 units (150 µg).[472] If, after 30 minutes, the blood glucose was essentially unchanged, the initial dose was doubled.

♠ The average increase in blood glucose was 3.3-5 mmol/l (60-90 mg/dl) within 30 minutes, and with a duration of effect of around 1 hour. Approximately 50% of the children needed more than one dose.

♠ Some children received up to five injections over a 25-hour period, without the glucagon losing its beneficial effect. They didn't suffer any more sickness or vomiting than before.

♠ In another study, 25 children were treated with mini-dose glucagon, half of them needing an additional dose.[466] The child needed continued treatment at hospital on only 16% of the occasions, none of them for hypoglycaemia.

Glucagon, fatty acids and ketones

♠ Glucagon stimulates the transformation of fatty acids to ketones in the liver (see illustration on page 25).

♠ The fatty acids are formed from the breakdown of fat in the starving cells, caused by a lack of food or not enough insulin.

♠ The ketones contribute to nausea as a side effect after a glucagon injection.

♠ Ketones can easily be detected in blood or urine by self-monitoring (see page 109). See also "After hypoglycaemia" on page 71.

raising the blood glucose level any further.[23] If your blood glucose level does not go back to normal after a glucagon injection, this suggests your glycogen store has been completely emptied out, for example by heavy exercise or a recent hypoglycaemic episode.

If you have to give glucagon, wait 10-15 minutes for the person to wake up. If they are still unconscious after this time, call an ambulance. However, if the person has revived, is feeling well and has a normal blood glucose when the ambulance arrives, they will not need to go to hospital.

Glucagon is counteracted by insulin. This is logical given that people who don't have diabetes will never have high concentrations of both hormones at the same time. Insulin is secreted when the blood glucose is high and glucagon when it is low. If hypoglycaemia is caused by too large a dose of insulin, glucagon will have less effect than if the low blood glucose is caused by not eating enough (see also "Too little food or too much insulin?" on page 55).

Some people with diabetes, especially children and adolescents, feel sick after a difficult hypoglycaemic episode, even if glucagon has not been injected. One explanation is that the production of glucagon from their own pancreas also can result in nausea as a side effect.

At present, glucagon can only be given as an injection, but recent experiments giving glucagon as a nasal spray have been encouraging.[994]

Adrenaline

Adrenaline is a stress hormone secreted by the adrenal glands. It raises the blood glucose primarily by breaking down the glycogen stores in the liver. The concentration of adrenaline rises when the body is exposed to stress, fever and acidosis (when the blood becomes acidic, for

Adrenaline and cortisol are produced in the adrenal glands.

Cross-section of the brain. Growth hormone is produced in the pituitary gland.

example in diabetic ketoacidosis).[637] Adrenaline also reduces the amount of glucose taken up by the cells of the body. This might strike you as odd until you remember that all bodily reactions during hypoglycaemia are aimed at reserving any available glucose for the brain.

The human body was originally designed for living in the Stone Age. If a person ran into a polar bear or a mammoth, the only alternatives were to fight or take flight. In both situations extra fuel, in the form of glucose, was needed by the body. The problem with our present way of life is that adrenaline is still secreted when we get excited or fearful, though this is more likely to be caused by a frightening TV programme than by an activity which actually calls for extra

strength. A healthy person, whose insulin production is working as it should, will not find this causes a problem. However, a person with diabetes will find their blood glucose level rises (see "Stress" on page 298).

When a person with diabetes becomes hypoglycaemic, secretion of adrenaline can raise the blood glucose by stimulating the breakdown of the glycogen stores in the liver [974] and at the same time causing shakiness, anxiety and a pounding heart. Adrenaline also stimulates the breakdown of body fat to fatty acids, which can be converted into ketones in the liver. See illustration on page 25.

Effects of adrenaline

⇒ Adrenaline is produced in the adrenal glands.

① Adrenaline raises blood glucose by:
 ⇒ Releasing glucose from the glycogen stores in the liver.
 ⇒ Activating the production of glucose from proteins.
 ⇒ Reducing uptake of glucose into the cells.
 ⇒ Reducing insulin production (in people who don't have diabetes).

② Adrenaline causes symptoms of hypoglycaemia, such as shakiness, rapid heartbeat and sweating.

③ It also stimulates the breakdown of body fat.

Effects of cortisol

⇒ Cortisol is produced in the adrenal glands.

① Cortisol raises blood glucose by:
 ⇒ Reducing cellular uptake of glucose.
 ⇒ Breaking down proteins that can be used to produce glucose in the liver.

② It also stimulates breakdown of body fat.

Cortisol

Cortisol is another important hormone which is released by the adrenal glands in response to stress and affects the body metabolism in many ways. It increases the amount of glucose in the blood by producing glucose from proteins (gluconeogenesis) and by decreasing the amount of glucose that is absorbed and used by the cells. Cortisol also promotes the breakdown of body fat into fatty acids that can be converted into ketones.

Growth hormone

Growth hormone is produced in the pituitary gland, which is found just below the brain. Some of the body's most important hormones are produced in this gland. The most important effect of growth hormone is to stimulate growth during childhood and adolescence. It has the effect of raising blood glucose by counteracting insulin on the cell surface, thereby reducing the uptake of glucose into the cells. Growth hormone increases muscle tissue and stimulates the breakdown of body fat.

During puberty, when a young person is growing quickly, large amounts of growth hormone are secreted. This results in the person needing more insulin.[307] Growth hormone is released in high concentrations during the night which explains why teenagers often need very high doses of bedtime insulin. The blood glucose-raising effect of growth hormone will start after 3-5 hours.[129] This contributes to the problem of high morning blood glucose that is common among teenagers, especially if their HbA$_{1c}$ level is high [129] (see "Dawn phenomenon" on page 58).

The effects of growth hormone

➠ Growth hormone is produced in the pituitary gland.

① It stimulates growth.

② It raises blood glucose by reducing the cellular uptake of glucose.

③ Growth hormone breaks down body fat.

④ It increases muscular mass.

Growth hormone also stimulates the production of ketones, thereby increasing the risk of ketoacidosis in adolescents.[307]

Teenagers with diabetes have higher levels of growth hormone than their peers without diabetes. Despite this, their growth can be slower than it should be if their glucose control is not adequate. This is because the effect of growth hormone in the body is partly dependent on the protein IGF-1 (insulin-like growth factor). IGF-1 is produced in the liver but insulin is necessary to stimulate this. Since the insulin concentration in the liver is lower in people with diabetes (see page 36) the levels of IGF-1 will also be lower.[307] IGF-1 has been given in a trial to children and adolescents with diabetes, and an improvement was seen in the levels of HbA$_{1c}$ (see page 117) in the blood. However, this improvement lasted for only 3 months.[2] A study of adults showed an improved HbA$_{1c}$ level, but also a worsening of retinopathy (eye damage), which has discouraged further research on IGF-1.[1040]

Hypoglycaemia

Hypoglycaemia means "low blood glucose". Sometimes symptoms of hypoglycaemia can be experienced when the blood glucose is not particularly low, or even when it is high (see "Blood glucose levels and symptoms of hypoglycaemia" on page 44). It may be appropriate to refer to the symptoms of hypoglycaemia as "sensations", warning of a particular blood glucose level, but not necessarily actually being proof of a low level.

The risk of hypoglycaemia is a part of everyday life with diabetes, and it is important to know that this is not something you should be afraid of. When aiming for a normal glucose level of 4-8 mmol/l in the treatment of diabetes, it is impossible not to have hypoglycaemia every now and then. Learn to treat it quickly and efficiently, and it as an indication that you are keeping your blood glucose control sufficiently low. Of course, if the hypoglycaemia is severe or troublesome, you need to take measures to keep your blood glucose level a little higher. But see mild hypoglycaemia as a sign that you are actually having glucose levels close to that of a person without diabetes. When asked, people with diabetes will most often say that it is easier to treat a low glucose level than a high.

The glucose level can be measured as whole blood glucose or plasma glucose. Most patient meters now display plasma glucose which is approximately 11% higher than whole blood glucose.[357] In this book the numbers refer mainly to plasma glucose, unless otherwise stated (in the first edition whole blood glucose was used so the numbers were slightly lower).

Not everyone will have the same symptoms when they develop hypoglycaemia. However, the symptoms usually follow the same pattern for each person.[218] You should check your blood glucose level whenever you have symptoms or simply feel strange. This is particularly important in the early days following diagnosis, when you are learning how to recognize your own individual reactions to hypoglycaemia. When your diabetes is newly diagnosed it is important that the diabetes team at your hospital or outpatient clinic help you to understand what your individual symptoms mean. It is important that all family members know how to treat hypoglycaemia in a safe and effective manner.

Usually symptoms of hypoglycaemia are divided into two categories: symptoms caused by the body attempting to raise the blood glucose level, by adrenaline for example (known as "autonomic" or "adrenergic" symptoms); and symptoms originating in the brain as a result of a deficiency of glucose in the central nervous system ("neuroglycopenic" symptoms). See the key fact boxes on page 42.

When a person with diabetes starts to become hypoglycaemic, he or she is likely to notice bodily symptoms (e.g. shakiness, heart pounding) at first. However, observers are more likely to be aware of symptoms such as irritability, and behavioural changes, which indicate the brain is

---

Hypoglycaemic reactions

Hypoglycaemic symptoms are usually divided into two types:

① Symptoms caused by the defence mechanisms in your body, such as adrenaline, attempting to raise the blood glucose (called adrenergic and autonomic symptoms).

② Symptoms from the brain due to low blood glucose (called neuroglycopenic symptoms).

Avoid situations where hypoglycaemia could have catastrophic consequences. This does not mean that it is impossible for people with diabetes to engage in risky sports such as mountain climbing, paragliding or scuba diving. What it does mean, however, is that they should prepare very carefully, think about the sorts of adverse situations that could arise, and not practise the activity alone. See the section on diving on page 295 for more information.

Symptoms of hypoglycaemia from the brain

The blood glucose concentration at which your brain begins to show symptoms of dysfunction (neuroglycopenic symptoms) is lower than that for bodily symptoms, and largely independent of your recent blood glucose levels. [36,218]

➠ Weakness, dizziness.

➠ Difficulty concentrating.

➠ Double or blurred vision.

➠ Disturbed colour vision (especially red-green colours).

➠ Difficulties with hearing.[340]

➠ Feeling warm or hot.

➠ Headache.

➠ Drowsiness.

➠ Odd behaviour, poor judgement.

➠ Confusion.

➠ Problems with short-term memory.

➠ Slurred speech.

➠ Unsteady walking, lack of coordination.

➠ Lapses in consciousness.

➠ Seizures.

being affected. The brain's reaction to hypoglycaemia is usually triggered at a slightly lower blood glucose level than the symptoms from the body.[40,218]

The brain is very sensitive to hypoglycaemia so the body automatically reacts in such a way as to help avoid this. Both children and adolescents will find that their mental agility and their ability to plan, make decisions and pay attention to detail will be affected, as will the speed of their reactions. This will be evident when the blood glucose concentration is no lower than 3.3-3.6 mmol/l (60-65 mg/dl).[914] Adults seem to adjust slightly better to low blood glucose concentrations as they experience neuroglycopenic symptoms (i.e. symptoms from the brain, see above) at lower blood glucose concentrations (2.8-3.0 mmol/l, 50-55 mg/dl).[206,218]

Hypoglycaemia is usually an unpleasant experience, involving loss of control over your body. This is indeed what happens as the brain cannot function normally without glucose. Some people become unusually irritable, while others may look pale, sick or sleepy. Fortunately, it is rare for people to do something uncharacteristically dangerous or stupid that may damage themselves or someone else. Traffic accidents on

a bicycle or in a car can sometimes be caused by hypoglycaemia (see page 334). Occasionally people do really strange things, for example one boy spread butter on a paper towel and tried to eat it. So it is very important that your family

The "glucostat"

mg/dl	mmol/l	
99	5.5	
90	5.0	High-level
81	4.5	hypoglycaemia
72	4.0	Normal-level hypoglycaemia
63	3.5	
54	3.0	Low-level
45	2.5	hypoglycaemia
36	2.0	

The blood glucose level at which you experience symptoms of hypoglycaemia functions like a thermostat (the "glucostat"). Unfortunately, this thermostat is adjusted up or down much too easily. When your blood glucose has been high for a couple of days you will have symptoms at a higher blood glucose level ("high-level hypoglycaemia") and when it has been low for several days you will experience symptoms at a lower blood glucose level ("low-level hypoglycaemia").

	Symptoms at mmol/l mg/dl	Measure
High-level hypoglycaemia	> 4.0-4.5 70-80	Wait before eating
Normal-level hypoglycaemia	3.5-4.0 65-70	Eat something sweet if your blood glucose is falling*
Low-level hypoglycaemia	< 3.5 < 65	Eat something with glucose

*A non-diabetic person often has a blood glucose of < 4 mmol (70 mg/dl) before a meal, so if you are going to eat within 30-60 minutes you will probably not need to attend to a blood glucose level of 3.5-4.0 mmol/l (65-70 mg/dl) if it is not falling further.

If you are not having symptoms until your blood glucose goes below 3.0-3.5 mmol/l (55-65 mg/dl) you are having unaware hypoglycaemia. If you avoid all blood glucose values below 3.5-4.0 mmol/l (65-70 mg/dl) for 2-3 weeks, you will experience symptoms at a normal level again (see page 52).

Research findings: Effects of low blood glucose

♠ In one study, tests involving associative learning, attention and mental flexibility were the aspects most affected at a blood glucose level of 2.2 mmol/l (40 mg/dl).[304]

♠ Women were less affected than men in this study. This may be explained by women having lower levels of adrenaline and less pronounced symptoms of hypoglycaemia than men.[38]

♠ Changes in EEG (brain wave) activity will occur when the blood glucose falls below 3.0 mmol/l (55 mg/dl) in children[99] and 2.2 mmol/l (40 mg/dl) in adults.[36]

♠ Unconsciousness occurs when the blood glucose level drops to approximately 1 mmol/l (20 mg/dl).[7]

♠ Symptoms of hypoglycaemia can change over time, depending on your average blood glucose levels (see page 44).

mg/dl). However, in a group of children and adolescents with an average HbA$_{1c}$ of 95 mmol/mol (10.8%), no symptoms of hypoglycaemia were noted when the blood glucose level was dropped from 21 mmol/l to 6 mmol/l (380 to 110 mg/dl).[425]

Blood glucose levels and symptoms of hypoglycaemia

Symptoms of hypoglycaemia may not be recognized by a person with diabetes, particularly when the focus of his or her attention is elsewhere. For example, some people report that they are less likely to recognize symptoms of hypoglycaemia at work than when relaxing at home. Children may notice symptoms more readily when there is little distraction, compared with when they are playing with friends.

Symptoms of hypoglycaemia in children and adolescents

Hypoglycaemic symptoms in children and adolescents differ slightly from those experienced by adults in that behaviour changes are more common. The table below is from a Scottish study in which parents were asked how often certain symptoms of hypoglycaemia occurred in their children and teenagers, aged from 18 months to 16 years.[735]

Pale skin	88%
Sweating	77%
Tearfulness	74%
Irritability	73%
Poor concentration	69%
Argumentativeness	69%
Hunger	69%
Tiredness	67%
Aggression	64%
Trembling	64%
Weakness	64%
Confusion	60%
Dizziness	51%
Headaches	47%
Abdominal / tummy pain	43%
Naughtiness	40%
Nausea	33%
Slurred speech	29%
Nightmares	20%
Blurred vision	19%
Seizures	16%
Double vision	11%
Bed-wetting	10%

What caused your hypoglycaemia?

➠ Too little to eat or a delayed meal?

➠ Skipped a meal?

➠ Neglecting to eat despite symptoms of hypoglycaemia.

➠ Physical exercise?
   Heavy physical exercise will increase the risk of hypoglycaemia for the rest of the day and the following night.

➠ Too large a dose of insulin?

➠ New site for the injection?
   e.g. from thigh to abdomen or to a site free of fatty lumps (lipohypertrophy).

➠ Recent hypoglycaemia?
   ➠ glucose stores in the liver depleted
   ➠ fewer warning symptoms of hypoglycaemia (hypoglycaemic unawareness).

➠ Very low HbA_{1c}? (increased risk of hypoglycaemia unawareness).

➠ Drinking alcohol?

➠ Not mixing the cloudy insulin thoroughly enough (see page 133)?

➠ Variable insulin absorption (see "How accurate is your insulin dose?" on page 88)?

➠ Gastroenteritis or tummy upset?

➠ Certain drugs used for the treatment of high blood pressure (so called non-selective beta-blockers) can increase the risk of hypoglycaemia (by diminishing the adrenergic symptoms of hypoglycaemia).[1028]

Your brain contains a kind of blood glucose meter that triggers defence reactions in your body and raises a low blood glucose level. It works in a similar way to a thermostat ("glucostat"), and is triggered at a certain blood glucose level. This reaction depends very much on where your blood glucose level has been during the last few days.[223,676] If your blood sugar has been high for some time, symptoms of hypoglycaemia and the release of counter-regulating hormones will appear at a higher blood glucose level than usual.[140,279] If your HbA_{1c} is high, you may start having symptoms of hypoglycaemia when your blood glucose level is 4-5 mmol/l (70-90 mg/dl).[140,508,574] However, this type of reaction seems to occur less frequently in adults.[74]

When the "glucostat" adjusts to another blood glucose level, the effect will be most pronounced on your bodily (autonomic) symptoms (mediated by adrenaline or the autonomic nervous system). The blood glucose level at which

Caffeine in coffee and cola can increase your awareness of hypoglycaemic symptoms.

The level at which you start experiencing symptoms of hypoglycaemia will change depending on how often your blood glucose level has been low in the last few days. Make it part of your routine to measure blood glucose as soon as you notice symptoms. If you usually become hypoglycaemic when the level is 3.7 mmol/l (67 mg/dl, "normal-level hypoglycaemia") and now have no symptoms until it falls to 3.2 mmol/l (58 mg/dl, "low-level hypoglycaemia") you have probably had too many low blood glucose values recently. On the other hand, if you start experiencing symptoms of hypoglycaemia with a blood glucose level of 4.0-4.5 mmol/l or higher (72-81 mg/dl, "high-level hypoglycaemia") you have had too many high blood glucose values and your HbA_{1c} is probably rising (see also page 62).

symptoms from the brain (neuroglycopenic symptoms) occur is influenced not so much by recent blood glucose levels as by the bodily symptoms.[36,37,39,218] This may be due to the way in which the body's cells adjust to preserve as much glucose as possible for use by the brain when blood glucose levels are low.[141] The function of the brain is affected when the blood glucose falls below approximately 2.8-3.0 mmol/l (50-55 mg/dl) in people who don't have diabetes.[1066] A study of people whose glucose control was poor and whose HbA_{1c} was high [77 mmol/mol (9.2%)] found their short-term memory was deteriorating by the time the blood glucose level had reached 3.9 mmol/l (70 mg/dl).[508] A more recent study of adults in better glucose control [HbA_{1c} around 64 mmol/mol (8%)], found that recalling a recently learnt task (shopping instructions) was more difficult during hypoglycaemia.[1091] Learning that took place during hypoglycaemia resulted in poorer results

on verbal tests, but not visual tests. See also page 63.

To decrease the blood glucose level at which symptoms of hypoglycaemia appear, you must keep yourself from eating until your blood glucose level has come down to 3.5-4.0 mmol/l (65-70 mg/dl), even though you will have symptoms of hypoglycaemia. Do everything you can to avoid high blood glucose levels during the 2 weeks that follow. The "glucostat" threshold will then automatically be lowered, until your symptoms of hypoglycaemia appear at the appropriate level (see also "Insulin sensitivity and resistance" on page 223).

The opposite applies if your blood glucose has been low for some time or you have had a lot of episodes of hypoglycaemia. The "glucostat" will then change so that the defence mechanisms of hypoglycaemia will not start until your blood glucose falls below 2.6 mmol/l (45 mg/dl).[36,507]

Coffee and cola contain caffeine which may cause the symptoms of hypoglycaemia to be noticed at a slightly higher blood glucose level than usual.[276] This may be useful for individuals with "hypoglycaemic unawareness" (see page 52) as caffeine enhances the intensity of the symptoms that warn of hypoglycaemia.[1094]

Some drugs used for treating high blood pressure (beta-blockers) can have the opposite effect and make symptoms of hypoglycaemia less obvious. If you have diabetes and are taking beta-blockers, you should always check your blood glucose level if you start to sweat for no obvious reason, as this may be the only symptom of a very low blood glucose, 3.3 mmol/l (60 mg/dl) or below.[508] Some drugs for treating depression (so called SSRIs, for example paroxetine/Paxil® and sertraline/Zoloft®, Lustral®) have caused the symptoms of hypoglycaemia to be lost in some people with diabetes.[940] Certain drugs (beta-stimulating agents) used to treat asthma increase the blood glucose level by stimulating adrenaline and have been successfully used to prevent night time hypoglycaemia.[923]

Symptoms of hypoglycaemia when the blood glucose level is high

Some children will experience the same symptoms when the blood glucose is high as when it is low. Younger children are particularly likely to find it difficult to differentiate between the two. They may feel hungry or hollow in the stomach when their blood glucose is high because the cells are starving due to a lack of insulin (see figure at the bottom of page 26 and "What to do if your blood glucose level is high" on page 147).

Severe hypoglycaemia

Severe hypoglycaemia is defined as a hypoglycaemic reaction with documented low blood glucose (< 3.1 mmol/l, 55 mg/dl) or reversal of symptoms after the intake of glucose, with symptoms sufficiently severe for the individual to need help from another person or even admission to hospital.[264] In many cases, the individual with diabetes will lose consciousness (either fully or partially) and may have seizures. Insulin coma involves severe hypoglycaemia with loss of consciousness. In a review, 10-25% of individuals with type 1 diabetes were found to experience a severe hypoglycaemic episode during a period of 1 year.[215] Severe hypoglycaemia was more common in adults with long-term complications, alcohol use, a threshold for hypoglycaemia symptoms of < 3 mmol/l (55 mg/dl) and use of certain medications (so called non-selective beta-blockers).[1028] Other factors

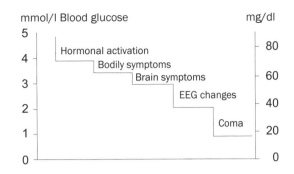

When your blood glucose is lowered, the reactions in your body and brain take place at different levels. These levels are in turn dependent on your recent blood glucose levels; i.e. if you have recently had higher blood glucose readings, the symptoms will occur at a slightly higher blood glucose level and if you have recently had lower blood glucose readings and hypoglycaemia, the symptoms will occur at a slightly lower blood glucose level. The graph is from reference [40].

that will increase your risk of severe hypoglycaemia include taking the wrong dose of insulin, missing a meal, or drinking alcohol after an unusual amount of activity such as energetic dancing. Some studies show severe hypoglycaemia to be more common in younger children.[257] Others, however, do not.[449,1051] It is rare in the first 12 months after diagnosis.[258] Some research from Sweden indicates that there may be a genetic explanation (high ACE activity, see glossary) for why some individuals are more susceptible to severe hypoglycaemia.[793] However, this does not seem to be the case in the Australian population.[158]

An international study involving participants from 18 countries found that 20-30% of primary school children and 15-20% of teenagers had severe hypoglycaemia with unconsciousness or seizures in a year.[762] In a large US study from 2013, 9.6% of children aged < 6 years (HbA$_{1c}$ 65 mmol/mol, 8.1%), and 5.2% aged 6-12 years (HbA$_{1c}$ 67 mmol/mol, 8.3%) had hypoglycaemia with unconsciousness or seizures in a year, but the risk was more associated with high than low HbA$_{1c}$.[181] However, a Swedish study from 2013 did not find any such episodes at all in children below the age of puberty,

Research findings:
Hypoglycaemic symptoms

♠ In one study the threshold for symptoms of hypoglycaemia changed, being 0.3 mmol/l (5 mg/dl) lower after only 4 days with low blood glucose values (2.3 mmol/l, 42 mg/dl) during one or a couple of hours per day.[1106]

♠ In another study, a single episode of afternoon hypoglycaemia (approximately 2.8 mmol/l, 50 mg/dl) caused fewer symptoms as well as a reduction of the hormonal defence when hypoglycaemia occurred again the following morning.[223] The participants were also more than usually sensitive to insulin, i.e. the blood glucose was lower than the day before although the insulin level in the blood was the same.

♠ However, 2 days after a hypoglycaemic episode (2 hours of 2.8 mmol/l, 50 mg/dl) the ability to recognize symptoms of hypoglycaemia was back to normal according to another study.[394]

♠ Night time hypoglycaemia with an average blood glucose of 2.7 mmol/l (48 mg/dl) over a 3-hour period resulted in fewer bodily (adrenergic) symptoms but no significant difference in brain (neuroglycopenic) symptoms when having a new hypoglycaemia with the same blood glucose level the next day.[344]

♠ However, the subjects in the study scored better during hypoglycaemia on tests that measured memory, attention, and recognition after a night with hypoglycaemia (compared with a control night with normal blood glucose). This indicates that the brain does have some ability to adjust to lower blood glucose levels, thereby preserving brain function.

from the time they were diagnosed, in spite of a low mean HbA_{1c} of 54 mmol/mol (7.1%) in the < 6 age group, and 51 mmol/mol (6.8%) in the 6-11 year olds.[459] A German/Austrian study found a mean HbA_{1c} of 57 mmol/mol (7.4%) in children below the age of 6 years, with only 1.9% having a severe hypoglycaemia (seizure or

unconsciousness) during the past year.[704] In contrast, children < 6 years in the US had an HbA_{1c} of 66 mmol/mol, 8.2% and a higher risk of severe hypoglycaemia, 2.8%.[704] There was no increased risk of severe hypoglycaemia with a lower HbA_{1c} in either country. The authors state that a contributing factor to the higher HbA_{1c} in the US may be that the HbA_{1c} goal in children below the age of 6 has been below 69 mmol/mol, 8.5%, while in Germany and most other countries it is below 58 mmol/mol (7.5%) in line with ISPAD's goal for all paediatric age groups. According to national data from the Swedish National Register SWEDIABKIDS for 2012, the mean HbA_{1c} was 63 mmol/mol (7.9%), with a risk of severe hypoglycaemia of 3.0%.[929] In the light of these findings, it seems unnecessary to aim for a higher HbA_{1c} in younger children just to avoid severe hypoglycaemia, and the American Diabetes Association recently lowered their targets to match ISPAD's. A careful adjustment of insulin doses, frequent blood glucose testing (or continuous glucose monitoring, CGM), and the use of insulin pumps are more important factors that can result in both a lower HbA_{1c} and avoidance of hypoglycaemia with unconsciousness or seizures.[459] One pump (Medtronic Veo) can shut off the basal rate for 2 hours if the CGM reading goes below the set threshold. It automatically restarts again, but can shut off a second time if there is continued hypoglycaemia. When this feature was used for 6 months, the number of episodes of severe hypoglycaemia with unconsciousness or seizures dropped from 6 in the preceding 6 months (in 41 patients aged 4-50 years) to zero.[702]

The anxiety over having a repeated episode of severe hypoglycaemia and not being able to trust one's body can be troublesome, and may result in the avoidance of any low glucose levels, resulting in a higher HbA_{1c}. If you or your child experience severe hypoglycaemia, you should immediately review your insulin doses with your diabetes team. Usually, you will be able to identify why it has happened, e.g. a dose of insulin that is too high, increased exercise, a missed meal, an incorrect dose administered,

Thresholds for reactions to hypoglycaemia

	Without diabetes	With diabetes	
mmol/l		HbA_{1c} 9.0%*	HbA_{1c} 5.2%*
Symptoms start at	2.9	3.7	2.2**
Adrenaline response	3.5	3.4	2.6
EEG changes	~2.2	~2.2	~2.2
mg/dl		9.0%	5.2%
Symptoms start at	52	67	40
Adrenaline response	63	61	46
EEG changes	~40	~40	~40

With a low HbA_{1c} you will get bodily (adrenergic) hypoglycaemic symptoms and adrenaline responses at much lower blood glucose values than if your HbA_{1c} is high.[36] However, the blood glucose level at which your brain starts showing symptoms is the same whether your HbA_{1c} is high or low.

* 9.0% equals 75 mmol/mol in IFCC units and 5.2% equals 33 mmol/mol

**Values have been recalculated to plasma glucose

alcohol drunk after a lot of dancing or other activity. If you cannot identify a clear reason, you should decrease the "responsible" dose of insulin (see table on page 146). Anxiety about having another episode of severe hypoglycaemia and the feeling of not being able to trust your body can be very frightening. If you have recurrent severe hypoglycaemia, you must discuss altering the insulin or food regimen with your diabetes team. Some people may find an insulin pump helpful in this situation.[509]

Seizures

A very low blood glucose, usually close to 1 mmol/l (20 mg/dl), can trigger seizures. Some very sensitive children may have muscle twitches when their blood glucose level is within the low-normal range.[694] These children are likely to be conscious when the twitching starts. Some will be able to talk, and even maintain eye contact at this time.

Seizures are not usually dangerous, but can be very alarming for those who witness them. The child may even appear to be dying. However, breathing is seldom affected. Turn the child onto his or her side (recovery position), after making sure that the airways are free. This is the safest position for someone who might be sick. Prepare glucagon and give an injection (for doses see page 37). Call an ambulance if the child does not wake up within 10-15 minutes.

Insulin doses should always be looked at again after hypoglycaemia with seizures, and the dose should be reduced if the cause of the blood glucose being so low cannot be identified. Anticonvulsive medicine can be considered for preventing repeated seizures, especially when these happen at a blood glucose level of 2.5-3.5 mmol/l (45-65 mg/dl), even if this is accompanied by a normal EEG (brain-wave trace).

We have seen several school children and teenagers who have had seizures when their blood glucose level has been around 2.5-3.5 mmol/l (45-65 mg/dl). After medication their blood glucose level can dip down to 2.0 mmol/l (35 mg/dl) without seizures, while they treat their hypoglycaemia by taking glucose.

The glucose level is often very low for several hours before the seizure occurs, as has been demonstrated by CGM (continuous glucose monitoring, see page 107).[155] This means that if a person is wearing a monitor with an alarm, which wakes them up, there will be time to take action to prevent the seizure. One pump (Medtronic Veo) can shut off the basal rate for 2 hours if the sensor detects a low glucose level, thereby hopefully preventing the seizure even if the person does not wake up.

Does severe hypoglycaemia damage the brain?

It is not clear how or whether repeated severe hypoglycaemia affects the physical or intellectual development of children with diabetes. Glucose is the most important source of energy for the brain. When the blood glucose is low, the blood flow to the brain can be increased to allow a larger supply of glucose.[316]

Small children (under the age of 5) are more vulnerable to severe hypoglycaemia with seizures because their nervous systems are still developing.[92] Children under the age of 2 are especially vulnerable. Severe hypoglycaemia should be avoided at all costs in this age group, even if it means having a higher HbA_{1c}.[691] However, severe hypoglycaemia is not very common in this age group: In a Swiss study, there were no episodes of severe hypoglycaemia with unconsciousness before the age of 6 years,[951] and a Swedish study from 2013 did not find any severe hypoglycaemia with unconsciousness or seizures below the age of 12 years.[459]

Permanent neurological damage and EEG (brain-wave) changes have been described in exceptional cases where children have had such severe hypoglycaemia that they have become unconscious, mostly with seizures.[985] One study of children and teenagers between the age of 10 and 19 years showed poorer results on neuropsychological tests for those who had developed diabetes before the age of 5, presumably having had more severe hypoglycaemia.[913] However, when the same individuals were tested again as adults, their performance was no different from that of the control group, made up of people without diabetes. This indicated there had been no permanent neurological damage.[915] Another explanation for the lower test results in the childhood age group may have been a long-standing poor diabetes control with high blood glucose levels. High blood glucose levels early in life will affect the brain's structure and development negatively (so called white matter dys-

> ## Research findings:
> ## Severe hypoglycaemia and HbA_{1c}
>
> ♠ The risk may be increased with lower HbA_{1c} values. In an Australian study of children and adolescents on two insulin injections per day and an HbA_{1c} of 76 mmol/mol (9.1%), the risk of having an episode of severe hypoglycaemia with unconsciousness or seizures was 4.8% per year.[258]
>
> ♠ In a Finnish paediatric study using 3-4 doses per day and an HbA_{1c} of 75 mmol/mol (9.0%) the risk was only 3.1%.[1051] However, in a Swedish study using mostly 4-5 injections per day and an HbA_{1c} of 65 mmol/mol (8.1%) the risk was 15%.[694] There was no correlation between HbA_{1c} and the risk of severe hypoglycaemia in this study. The HbA_{1c} of those that had had a severe hypoglycaemia with unconsciousness was between 44 and 77 mmol/mol (6.2 and 9.2%).
>
> ♠ Compare this figure with the DCCT study (see page 367) where the 13-17-year-olds had a risk of 26.7% of unconsciousness or seizures in the intensively treated group with HbA_{1c} of 65 mmol/mol (8.1%) and 9.7% risk in the conventionally treated group with HbA_{1c} of 84 mmol/mol (9.8%).[262]
>
> ♠ A Swedish study from 2013 did not find any severe hypoglycaemia with unconsciousness or seizures below the age of 12 years, in spite of low HbA_{1c} levels (a mean of 54 mmol/mol (7.1%) in the <6 age, and 51 mmol/mol (6.8%) in the 7-11 year old).[459]

function due to demyelination, i.e. less isolation of the nerve fibres).[58] This makes the brain more vulnerable to any subsequent insult (hypoglycaemia, head injury, alcoholism, other central nervous system conditions) that occurs later in the child's life.[918] One study found alterations in white matter structure being related to a recent HbA_{1c} level and CGM measures of hyperglycaemia and glucose variability but not for hypoglycaemia.[68]

Research findings: Severe hypoglycaemia and brain function

♠ An Australian study including 84 children looked at the effect of severe hypoglycaemia (defined as seizure or coma) in children with diabetes onset below the age of 6 years.[1001] They found no difference in intellectual, memory or behavioural measures when compared to diabetic children with no severe hypoglycaemia. Even children with their first episode of severe hypoglycaemia before age 6 did not score differently.

♠ A US study, also in children with diabetes onset below age 6, found that poor glucose control, i.e a higher HbA_{1c} at the time of testing, was related to lower general learning abilities, slower fine motor speed and lower understanding of language scores.[822] In contrast, a history of severe hypoglycaemia did not affect the scores. Even though a blood glucose outside 3.9-11.1 mmol/l (70-200 mg/dl) was corrected with food or insulin, children with a higher blood glucose performed less well on the understanding of language scores (but not on expressing language scores). This has clear implications for school performance (see page 330).

♠ A small Canadian study followed 16 children for 7 years from the onset of diabetes. They found a deterioration mainly in visual memory and attention in those that had had hypoglycaemic seizures.[910] However, 9 out of the 16 children in this study had seizures during the follow-up, which is not expected with modern intensive diabetes management. A Swedish study using intensive insulin therapy found severe hypoglycaemia with unconsciousness (with or without seizures) in only 10-16% of the patients, in spite of a decrease in HbA_{1c}.[791]

♠ A meta-analysis that looked at the results of 19 studies in children with 2,144 participants (1,393 had diabetes), found that the children with type 1 diabetes had slightly lower overall cognitive (knowing, understanding and learning) abilities, with small differences compared with control subjects across a broad range of tests.[392] However, learning and memory skills were similar for both groups. They did however find a significant impairment of learning and memory skills in children with early onset diabetes (before age 7), but no consistent relationships between cognitive performance and the occurrence of hypoglycaemic seizures.

♠ Parents of children with diabetes may find it difficult to interpret these somewhat contradicting study results. It doesn't make it easier when you learn that in some studies the children were tested at blood glucose levels in themselves high enough to cause impairment of mental function. For example, in one study the children had a mean blood glucose of 14 mmol/l at the time of testing.[798] However, the emerging evidence for the importance of avoidance of chronic high blood glucose levels to optimise brain development in young children should encourage parents to strive for equally low HbA_{1c} levels in all age groups (see page 119).

In an Austrian study of children and adolescents aged 4-18 years, neurophysiological studies (so called auditory and visually evoked potentials) showed poorer results in participants who had both severe hypoglycaemia (unconsciousness/seizures) and poor glucose control (HbA_{1c} > 86 mmol/mol, 10%) during the last two years.[958] In an Australian study, both recurrent severe hypoglycaemia and chronically elevated blood glucose levels were associated with reduced memory and learning capacity in children 2 years after the onset of diabetes.[797] A Swiss study of children diagnosed with diabetes before the age of 10 found a decline in intellectual performance only in boys diagnosed before the age of 6.[951] This was attributed to long-term high HbA_{1c} and ketoacidosis at the onset of diabetes, but not to severe hypoglycaemia. A US study from 2003 did not find that severe hypoglycaemia with seizures or coma in children aged 6-15 years had adverse effects on attention, planning or simultaneous processing when they were tested 18 months later.[1123]

It seems as if children are especially vulnerable to seizures in combination with severe hypoglycaemia. One study showed differences in the ability to concentrate in children who had experienced at least one severe hypoglycaemic episode with seizures.[909] However, parents did not report any difference in the children's ability to concentrate, and their school work did not appear to suffer either. In the same study, children with high blood glucose levels at the time of the test appeared to be more impulsive in their behaviour. An American study compared children with 1-2 vs. 3-4 injections per day.[497] The multiple injections group had more severe hypoglycaemia (0.80 vs. 0.24 episodes per person per year) and tests revealed them to have reduced ability to recall past events. However, the rate of severe hypoglycaemia when using multiple injections in this study was much higher than that reported from other centres.[449,791] Another study, of 55 children aged 5-10 years, found a significant reduction in memory scores but only in the group that had experienced unconsciousness with seizures while severely hypoglycaemic.[597]

Adults with diabetes seem to withstand severe hypoglycaemia very well, even if they have been unconscious. Episodes of hypoglycaemic coma were not found to be associated with any permanent brain damage in people who developed type 1 diabetes as adults.[636] Neither the DCCT[265] nor the Stockholm study[883] found any impairment in neuro-psychological testing in people who had experienced repeated severe hypoglycaemic episodes.

Hypoglycaemia unawareness

Hypoglycaemia unawareness is defined as a hypoglycaemic episode that comes on without the warning symptoms that are usually associated with decreasing blood glucose. If you have frequent hypoglycaemic episodes, the threshold at which you recognize symptoms will occur at a lower blood glucose level (see page 44). If the threshold for secreting counter-regulatory hor-

It is difficult to determine whether a child's development is affected by severe hypoglycaemia. Single episodes will probably have no effect, but if the child has recurrent severe hypoglycaemia with seizures during the first 2-3 years of life, some studies indicate that school performance will not be as good as it should be. If the child has been suffering from severe hypoglycaemia, the insulin doses should always be adjusted to avoid another such episode. With young children, it may sometimes be necessary to accept a higher HbA$_{1c}$ in order to avoid severe hypoglycaemia.

mones falls below the blood glucose level that provokes a reaction in the brain, you will not have any physical warning symptoms. Because of this, you will not react in time (by eating, for example) so your hypoglycaemia can rapidly become severe. Sometimes you will not even remember afterwards that you had hypoglycaemia. This is a common phenomenon. In one study of children and adolescents 37% were unaware of some or all episodes of hypoglycaemia.[67]

Hypoglycaemic unawareness will substantially increase the risk of severe hypoglycaemia in both children[67] and adults,[216] and is more common among those prone to severe hypoglycaemia.[217] It should be part of your routine always to check your blood glucose as soon as you start getting symptoms that might indicate hypoglycaemia. If your readings are below 3.5 mmol/l (65 mg/dl), this is a warning sign that your risk of becoming severely hypoglycaemic may increase considerably.[1028]

If you have hypoglycaemia unawareness, you should aim for a slightly higher average blood glucose. Above all, you should avoid a blood glucose level that is lower than 3.5-4.0 mmol/l (65-70 mg/dl).[39] Within a fortnight, you are likely to find you can recognize symptoms of hypoglycaemia more easily.[218,342] By training yourself to recognize subtle symptoms as your blood glucose is decreasing, you will increase your chances of treating your hypoglycaemia in time.[37] See also pages 63 and 122.

The reason that you have no symptoms although the blood glucose level is low is that there is an adaptation in your brain so that the blood circulation is changed and the central parts of the brain will get more of the small

Research findings: Hypoglycaemia unawareness

⇒ A single episode of afternoon hypoglycaemia can mean that your blood glucose must fall even lower the next morning before you will start having symptoms of hypoglycaemia and hormonal defence reactions.[223]

⇒ The same thing can happen after exercise: low or moderate exercise one day may result in fewer symptoms of hypoglycaemia and decreased hormonal reactions the next day.[931]

⇒ This reaction can be reversed by avoiding low blood glucose levels. In one study of adults, the ability to recognize symptoms of hypoglycaemia had improved after only 2 days of careful avoidance of blood glucose levels less than 3.6 mmol/l (65 mg/dl).[676]

⇒ In a group of adults with an HbA_{1c} of 45 mmol/mol (6.3%) and hypoglycaemia unawareness, low blood glucose readings were carefully avoided.[342] These patients aimed instead for a slightly higher average blood glucose. After just 2 weeks, the patients found it easier to recognize their hypoglycaemic episodes.

⇒ After 3 months, the threshold for triggering the counter-regulatory hormones (the defence against low blood glucose, see page 33) had changed from 2.3 to 3.1 mmol/l (42 to 56 mg/dl). At the same time HbA_{1c} was raised to 57 mmol/mol (7.4%).

A British study compared individuals who did not have diabetes with two groups of people with type 1 diabetes who had an HbA_{1c} of 87 mmol/mol (10.1%) and 61 mmol/mol (7.7%) respectively.[716] Both diabetes groups had the same number of symptomatic hypoglycaemic episodes while in the group with lower HbA_{1c} all had recorded at least three blood glucose readings of less than 3.0 mmol/l (54 mg/dl) without symptoms of hypoglycaemia (hypoglycaemia unawareness) during the past 2 months. Most of them also had experienced one or more severe hypoglycaemic episodes (where they needed help from another person) during the previous 6 months.

In the group with hypoglycaemia unawareness, people had no symptoms of hypoglycaemia until their blood glucose went down to 2.3 mmol/l (41 mg/dl). Despite this, their reaction times deteriorated at the same blood glucose level (2.9 mmol/l, 52 mg/dl) as those of the other groups. This means that if you have experienced hypoglycaemia unawareness and drive a car with a blood glucose of 2.8 mmol/l (50 mg/dl), you may feel quite well but your reaction times will be slow, making you a danger on the roads. However, a recent study by the same group indicates that the reaction time is not delayed in people with hypoglycaemic unawareness (see page 71).

amount of glucose that is available in the blood.[95] Thus, the part of the brain that triggers hypoglycaemic symptoms is satisfied with the amount of glucose delivered by the blood, and will not raise the alert.

Many people with long-standing diabetes will have a reduced adrenaline response to low blood glucose, which will mean they have fewer warning symptoms from their autonomic nervous system. This contributes both to diminished symptoms and to less effective counter-regulation when the blood glucose is decreasing.[37] The change from porcine (pork) and bovine (beef) insulin to human insulin has been associated with an increase in hypoglycaemia unawareness. Although several studies have looked at this issue, there has been no scientific evidence of such an increase.[37]

Rebound phenomenon

Your body will try to reverse hypoglycaemia by using counter-regulatory responses (see "Regulation of blood glucose" on page 33). Sometimes this counter-regulation will be too effective and the blood glucose will rise to high levels during the hours following hypoglycaemia. This is called the "rebound phenomenon". During the hours when the levels of the counter-regulatory hormones are increased, your body will be resistant to insulin (see page 223), i.e. higher doses of insulin than usual are needed to lower the blood glucose to normal levels (for example when taking an injection before eating).

Many people, when experiencing hypoglycaemia, have a tendency to eat too much to compensate for the effect of low blood glucose. They are also likely to decrease the next insulin dose in order to avoid further hypoglycaemia. Both these factors contribute to the rebound phenomenon, resulting in an even higher blood glucose level.

The rebound phenomenon will only develop if the insulin level in the blood is low during the hours following a hypoglycaemic episode.[129] For example, it may occur if your hypoglycaemia has been caused by exercise or skipping a snack. Your insulin level after night time hypoglycaemia decreases as the night goes on if you are using NPH as your bedtime insulin. If

> ## Two situations of hypoglycaemia
>
> ⟱ **Not enough food:**
> Typical of this type is hypoglycaemia before a meal. If you use premeal injections you will not yet have taken the insulin, and the insulin level in the blood will not be so high. Adrenaline and glucagon, therefore, can easily release glucose from the liver and you may very well get a rebound effect with high blood glucose lasting several hours after hypoglycaemia.
>
> ⟱ **Too much insulin:**
> Typical of this type is taking the insulin as usual but not eating enough (e.g. if you don't like the food). The blood glucose is low at the same time as the insulin level increases. The insulin then counteracts the production of glucose from the liver, resulting in more severe hypoglycaemia. The high insulin level prevents the rebound phenomenon.

hypoglycaemia is caused by too large a dose of insulin, however, the high level of insulin will cause a smaller amount of the counter-regulating hormones to be secreted, making the rebound phenomenon much less likely to occur.

Children are more likely to experience rebound phenomenon, because their hormones react more strongly to hypoglycaemia than those of adults.[37,574] The defence mechanisms are also triggered at higher blood glucose levels than those of adults.[574] The rebound phenomenon often lasts 12 hours or more in adults,[8] whereas in children the high blood glucose level usually lasts a few hours only (see the blood glucose graph on page 55). Sometimes a rebound phenomenon can keep the blood glucose level high for more than 24 hours.[903] As the hormone levels return to normal, so the blood glucose level too will gradually normalize.

If you take an extra insulin injection when your blood glucose is high due to a rebound phenomenon, your blood glucose may fall rapidly, causing you to become hypoglycaemic again. The more sensitive your body is to insulin, the more likely this is to happen. You should therefore be careful about taking extra insulin after a rebound phenomenon. There are large individual differences in the tendency to develop rebound phenomena. If you are likely to have long-lasting rebound effects, you can try increasing your insulin injection at the meal following the hypoglycaemic episode.[8]

Too little food or too much insulin?

Both can result in a low blood glucose level, but the body's way of handling the situation is different. The effect of glucagon in breaking down the stored glucose (glycogen) is counteracted by insulin. Insulin acts in the opposite direction, by transporting glucose into the liver cells to be stored as glycogen. From this it follows that the more insulin you have injected (resulting in a higher insulin level in the blood), the more difficult it will be to release glucose from the liver.

This means that a low blood glucose caused by a large insulin dose (e.g. if you have taken extra insulin) will be more difficult to reverse than a low blood glucose due to inadequate food intake.

Night time hypoglycaemia

Night time hypoglycaemia is more common than most people tend to believe. A number of studies have shown that as many as 30-40% of both children and adults have night time hypoglycaemia.[707,728,859] Adrenaline responses

r-a = rapid-acting insulin.

This 5-year-old girl has recently been diagnosed with diabetes. She has a pronounced rebound phenomenon in the evening. Note the ketones in the urine after the hypoglycaemic episode, which are caused by her own production of glucagon (see also "Ketones" on page 109). The blood glucose may have followed the dashed line instead, if she had not experienced hypoglycaemia and the resulting rebound effect.

CGMS (Continuous Glucose Monitoring System, see page 107) chart showing two rebound phenomena in the same day in a 9-year-old girl (arrows).

are reduced during deep sleep which may contribute to the failure to wake up.[575] Symptoms
of hypoglycaemia may also be more difficult to
recognize when you are lying down than when
you are standing up.[510]

As many as 45% of children and adolescents
using twice-daily injections had night time
hypoglycaemia with blood glucose below 3.5-
3.9 mmol/l (60-70 mg/dl) in two studies.[83,728]
Half of the children did not show any symptoms of low blood glucose during the night. A
negative effect on mood in the morning was
observed in one of the studies.[728] When children
using multiple injections or insulin pumps were
studied on repeated occasions over a 6-month
period, using continuous subcutaneous glucose
monitoring (CGMS), every participant had at
least one instance of a night time glucose level
below 3.5 mmol/l (65 mg/dl).[697]

Often, a young person will not be woken by
mild symptoms of hypoglycaemia, and this provides the opportunity for the blood glucose
level to drop even further. The only way to be
certain whether your blood glucose level is low
is to get up in the night (02-03AM with NPH

and 04-05AM with Levemir or Lantus) and test
it. It is a good idea to do this at least every second week. Sometimes children with diabetes
wake up in the night on account of becoming
hypoglycaemic, and tell their parents. In other
cases a parent will wake up to strange or unusual sounds. If your child has recently been
diagnosed with diabetes, or if you have changed
your bedtime insulin treatment, it would be a
good idea to check the blood glucose once or
twice during the night. A baby alarm may be
helpful for some families with young children.
See pages 100 and 174 for recommendations on
when to test at night, depending on which bedtime insulin you use.

Night time hypoglycaemia can be caused by too
large a dose of bedtime insulin. Another cause
can be too high a dose of short-acting insulin
just before your evening snack which will result
in hypoglycaemia early in the night. There are
several studies with NovoRapid and Humalog
insulins which suggest that reducing the action

CGMS chart from a 13-year-old boy, showing low glucose
readings during the night. After breakfast there is a
sharp rise in the glucose level, indicating that the insulin
dose before breakfast needs to be increased. The glucose level falls again during the following night.

**Night time hypoglycaemia may
be caused by:**

→ The dose of short-acting insulin before the evening snack being too high (hypoglycaemia early in the night).

→ The dose of bedtime or basal insulin being too high.

→ The action profile of your bedtime or basal insulin does not fit you. Changing to Levemir or Lantus may improve the situation.

→ Short-acting insulin before dinner/tea or the evening snack being given in the thigh (hypoglycaemia in the middle of the night is caused by a slower absorption from the thigh).

→ Not enough to eat in the evening or an evening snack containing mostly "short-acting" foods being absorbed too quickly.

→ Exercise in the afternoon or evening without decreasing the dose of bedtime insulin.

→ Alcohol consumption in the evening.

time of the short-acting insulin (by the use of rapid-acting insulin) helps to decrease night time hypoglycaemia.[528,845] Night time hypogly-caemia can also be caused by vigorous after-noon or evening exercise (see page 284).

If you are injecting regular short-acting insulin in your thigh before the evening snack, the slow absorption of insulin can result in night time hypoglycaemia.[489] If you inject your bedtime insulin holding the needle at right angles to the skin, or without lifting a skinfold, you might be injecting intramuscularly. The insulin will then be absorbed more quickly, putting you at risk of low blood glucose early in the night. [490]

A good basic rule for avoiding night time hypoglycaemia is always to have something extra to eat if your blood glucose is below approximately 7 mmol/l (120-130 mg/dl) before going to bed.[83,947] See also "Basal insulin" on page 166. Remember that an extra sandwich before going to bed is never a guarantee that you will avoid night time hypoglycaemia. If in doubt, the only way to be certain is to get up in the middle of the night to check your blood glu-cose level.

You can also experiment with the evening snack to find something that gives a slower rise in blood glucose over a longer period of time. Try, for instance, bread with margarine and cheese on it. Your stomach will empty more slowly, resulting in sustained glucose absorption. High-fat ice cream may have the same effect. How-ever, extra fat will not be a good idea if you are prone to weight problems.

The most "long-acting" carbohydrate available for an evening snack is raw corn starch, which gives a rise in blood glucose over about 6 hours and is effective in preventing night time hypoglycaemia. It is given to children with dis-eases other than diabetes who experience prob-lems maintaining their blood glucose during the night. However, one drawback is the taste. It cannot be heated or prepared in any way or the carbohydrates will become more "short-act-ing". Younger children can usually get used to the taste of corn starch formula. Older individ-uals may find the taste of a corn starch bar (Z-bar) more acceptable.

Another possibility worth trying, if you are hav-ing problems with night time hypoglycaemias,

---

Symptoms indicating night time hypoglycaemia

➠ Nightmares.

➠ Sweating (damp sheets).

➠ Headache in the morning.

➠ Tiredness on waking.

➠ Bed-wetting (can also be caused by high blood glucose during the night).

Research findings: Corn starch and hypoglycaemia

♠ In a study of children and adolescents, the number of hypoglycaemic episodes (< 3.6 mmol/l, 65 mg/dl) at 2 AM and before break-fast were reduced from approximately one per week to 0.3 per week when 25-50% of the carbohydrate in the evening snack was given as uncooked corn starch in milk.[596]

♠ In children aged 2.5-6 years, 0.3 g/kg (0.6 g/lb) of corn starch reduced the number of night time blood glucose readings < 5.6 mmol/l (100 mg/dl) by 64%.[288] Extra pancre-atic enzymes were not being given.

♠ Unheated corn starch (0.3 g/kg, 0.6 g/lb) given to adults at the time of the bedtime injection over a 4-week period increased the blood glucose level at 3 AM by, on average, 2 mmol/l (35 mg/dl) in adults with diabetes.[57]

♠ The number of night time hypoglycaemic epi-sodes < 3.4 mmol/l (60 mg/dl) were reduced by 70% without changing the HbA_{1c}.

In these studies, patient meters showing whole blood glucose readings were used. Values have been recalculated to plasma glucose.

is to eat ordinary (not "light") potato crisps as an extra late snack before going to sleep (unless you have weight problems). The manufacturing process and the high fat content result in the glucose from potato crisps being absorbed very slowly. The blood glucose will still not have reached its peak after 3 hours (see graph on page 270).[177] Twenty-five grams of potato crisps have the same content of both fat (8 g, 1/3 ounces) and carbohydrates (15 g, ½ ounces) as an open cheese sandwich. This is often an attractive alternative to minimize the risk of night time hypoglycaemia for youngsters and teenagers who play demanding sports.

A late evening snack with high protein content has been recommended to avoid night time hypoglycaemia. However, according to one study the addition of protein (bread with meat) did not give better protection against hypoglycaemia 3 hours after the snack.[415] A fibre-enriched bedtime snack (with beta-glucan) did not help to prevent children developing hypoglycaemia at around 2 AM.[869]

Dawn phenomenon

Blood glucose levels rise early in the morning because of the so called "dawn phenomenon" which occurs in 80-100% of adults with type 1 diabetes.[129] This effect is caused by an increased secretion of growth hormone raising the blood glucose late in the night and early in the morning.[8,128,307] The dawn phenomenon increases the morning blood glucose by approximately 1.5-2 mmol/l (25-35 mg/dl) compared with the blood glucose levels at midnight when adequate

Corn flour mix when going to bed

Mix 2 tablespoons of corn flour with 100 ml (around 0.5 cup) of water. This mixture contains 14 g of very slow-acting carbohydrates. It should be mixed cold and heated up as little as possible. Heat breaks down the cells of the corn flour making the carbohydrates faster-acting.

If the child has a meal of formula at bedtime you can replace parts of it with corn flour mix. Begin with a small part and increase it gradually as the child accepts it. Try to lower the temperature a little each day so that the child comes to accept drinking the mixture at room temperature.

If the child is less than 3 years old, it might be necessary to add pancreatic enzymes for breaking down the corn starch. Ask your paediatrician about this.

Some older children and adults find the taste of corn starch bars acceptable, so these may be useful.

r-a = rapid-acting insulin

Night time hypoglycaemia with rebound phenomenon. Without a blood glucose test at 1 AM, this 6-year-old girl would appear to have had a high blood glucose all night long. An increase in her bedtime insulin would have led to an even lower blood glucose the following night (the Somogyi phenomenon). Note the presence of both ketones and glucose in the morning urine. Without the night time hypoglycaemia, her blood glucose may have followed the dashed line.

amounts of insulin are supplied throughout the night.[129] A high morning blood glucose is a common problem for growing children, especially during the later part of puberty when the growth spurt is at its peak.[307] It may be difficult to tailor the insulin regimen to match an increasing insulin blood glucose level in the morning. Lantus or an insulin pump can be good alternatives in this case. Younger children (who go to bed early) tend to have their highest need for basal insulin earlier in the night (often before midnight).[205]

Somogyi phenomenon

If your blood glucose level is low at night, you are likely to continue sleeping without noticing it. However, the secretion of counter-regulating hormones in your body can result in a rebound phenomenon with a rise in blood glucose to high levels in the morning if the level of insulin in the blood is low. If you haven't recorded a low blood glucose value in the middle of the night, you may believe that your bedtime insu-

lin needs to be increased. A higher dose of bedtime insulin the next night will give an even lower blood glucose level and a more intense rebound effect, resulting in an even higher blood glucose level the following morning. You can easily end up in a vicious cycle. This type of night time rebound phenomenon is called the Somogyi phenomenon after the chemist who first described it.[629,986]

If your morning blood glucose is sometimes low and sometimes high, it may be because you have problems with the Somogyi phenomenon. Some nights your blood glucose might be low enough to start the rebound phenomenon, causing the morning blood glucose to be high. On other nights, the blood glucose will not be low enough to trigger the rebound phenomenon and the morning blood glucose will subsequently be lower.

The Somogyi phenomenon has been questioned over the years, but consensus today is that it is mainly seen in individuals using less intermediate-acting insulin (such as multiple injection therapy) resulting in a lower level of insulin in the blood in the morning before waking

CGMS chart from a 17-year-old boy, showing a pronounced Somogyi phenomenon with high glucose level early in the night, very low readings in the middle of the night, and further high levels on waking. Had he relied on his high morning reading alone, he might very well have increased his bedtime dose, resulting in even lower night time levels.

CGMS chart from a 16-year-old girl, showing a dawn phenomenon with considerable increase in glucose levels from the middle of the night until waking-up time.

up.[129,214] These people also have a higher than normal rise in blood glucose after breakfast following night time hypoglycaemia.[629] In a study using continuous glucose monitoring (CGMS) in children and adolescents, Somogyi phenomenons were seen more often in those using multiple daily injections compared to those with insulin pumps.[697]

If you are using twice-daily injections, the proportion of intermediate-acting insulin is higher, and the amount of insulin your body will be able to store is larger (see page 86). Insulin can be released from this store (or "depot") during the night, resulting in a level of insulin that is unlikely to be low enough to allow a night time rebound phenomenon.[129]

A urine test in the morning may be difficult to interpret in this situation. It can show both ketones (caused by a low blood glucose in the middle of the night or by insulin deficiency later in the night when the blood glucose was high) and glucose (from the later part of the night). You can have the same urine test result (ketones and glucose) if your blood glucose has been high all night without hypoglycaemia (see page 171).

Will low blood glucose levels return to normal if the child doesn't wake up?

The intermediate-acting insulin that was given during the afternoon or at bedtime will have lost most of its action by morning, and blood glucose levels will rise even if a hypoglycaemic child does not wake up. Long-acting insulin will still be having effect in the morning but the body will then try to raise the blood glucose level by different defence mechanisms (see "Regulation of blood glucose" on page 33).

Can you die from hypoglycaemia?

All parents are worried about night time hypoglycaemia and wonder if their child might die from this. However, this almost never happens and we always try to prevent night time hypoglycaemia by advising an evening or bedtime snack. On very rare occasions, otherwise healthy individuals with type 1 diabetes have been found dead in their bed in the morning. This uncommon phenomenon has been called the "Dead-in-bed" syndrome.[1023] It is believed to be caused by a disturbed cardiac rhythm and can happen also in individuals without diabetes,

Different factors influence the blood glucose level during the night and in the morning. The dawn phenomenon depends on the night time secretion of growth hormone, and the Somogyi phenomenon is a night time rebound phenomenon. The insulin waning effect depends on the pharmacological properties of the intermediate-acting NPH insulin used for bedtime injections. Basal analogues (Levemir, Lantus) do not have this disadvantage. In studies looking at children and adolescents, the risk of night time hypoglycaemia decreased by 43% after switching to Lantus [770] and by 36% with Levemir.[894]

Taking the wrong type of insulin

☞ Be careful not to mix up different bottles or types of insulin when using syringes.

☞ Make sure that the pens you use for day time and night time insulin are so different that you cannot accidentally use the wrong pen, even if it is completely dark.

☞ Often only the colour coding will differ between pens from the same company. You may want to consider using disposable pens for one type of insulin and a regular pen for the other or use pens from two different manufacturers.

Research findings: Hypoglycaemia and death

♠ A follow-up was published in 2005 of the 10,200 children aged up to 15 years who were diagnosed with diabetes in Sweden in the years 1977-2000. The total risk of dying was increased twofold for this group of young people with diabetes compared with their peers without diabetes.[238]

♠ Seventeen of them (aged 11-25) were found dead in their beds. None had signs of alcohol in their blood.[238] Hypoglycaemia may be a possible cause as a history of night time hypoglycaemia has been noted in most cases.[989]

♠ During the same period, 20 individuals died (six of them at the onset of diabetes) because of ketoacidosis. Ten of these were young adults who had had diabetes for a considerable number of years, all living alone. They were found at home, and in these cases death would certainly have been preventable, unless they were intended as suicide. One person died of severe alcohol intoxication with strong suspicion of hypoglycaemia and two died from acute heart attack related to late diabetes complications.

♠ In 1989, 22 cases of "dead-in-bed" in individuals with diabetes (aged 12-43 years) were recorded in England.[1023]

♠ In another British study all deaths under 20 years of age were recorded from 1990 to 1996.[320] Ketoacidosis caused 69 deaths and hypoglycaemia seven. In three cases there was no evident explanation for the deaths, defining them as "dead-in-bed".

Hypoglycaemia and other diseases

People with diabetes are at increased risk of other autoimmune diseases (see page 350). If you encounter an increased number of hypoglycaemic episodes, in spite of lowering your insulin doses, you may need to be investigated for the following diseases:

⇒ Coeliac disease.

⇒ Hypothyroidism (underactive thyroid gland).

⇒ Adrenal insufficiency (deficiency of cortisol, Addison's disease).

A possible explanation for such night time deaths could be an erroneous injection of short- or rapid-acting insulin at bedtime instead of the usual intermediate- or long-acting insulin.[446] Teenagers and young adults often have high doses of bedtime insulin and it is not uncommon to take insulin from the wrong vial or pen when administering the bedtime insulin. For example, this happened twice to the same 13-year-old during one of our diabetes summer camps. Lantus and Levemir can be confused with rapid-acting insulin if syringes are used for injections, as both are clear solutions. In one case, this resulted in hypoglycaemia that needed treatment with intravenous fluids containing glucose.[9]

Another explanation is that nerve damage after many years of diabetes can result in the body's response to hypoglycaemia being blunted or absent. This is more likely to be the case in people who have had diabetes for more than 20-30 years.

Adults with type 1 diabetes have died from hypoglycaemia after drinking alcohol (which prevents the liver from producing glucose).[802,1023,1036]

although this is even more infrequent.[5] In an individual with diabetes, severe hypoglycaemia may, in rare cases, trigger cardiac arrhythmia.[488] It may be possible to find individuals at risk to this by using DNA tests, and preventative treatment could then be given.[5,488]

Why does awareness of hypoglycaemia occur at different levels of blood glucose?

The hot air balloon

A hot air balloon can be used to illustrate the variations in the level where hypoglycaemia is first noticed. The height of the balloon corresponds to your average blood glucose level during the day. The basket under the balloon corresponds to the blood glucose level where you first notice symptoms of hypoglycaemia. With an average glucose level of 9-10 mmol/l (160-180 mg/dl) symptoms are usually noticed when the level is around 3.5 mmol/l (65 mg/dl).

The HbA$_{1c}$ scale on the right corresponds to the average blood glucose level over a 2-3 month period, which is presented on the left side of the scale. An average blood glucose of 10 mmol/l (180 mg/dl) will give an HbA$_{1c}$ of approximately 65 mmol/mol in IFCC numbers (8% in DCCT numbers) (see page 118 for information on the two different units and conversion tables). The illustrations on the next page show what will happen when the blood glucose level changes. However, illustrating the level of hypoglycaemia with only one basket is really a simplification. The level at which you recognize hypoglycaemia will change depending on your recent blood glucose levels, but the level where clear thinking and reaction times are impaired is less dependent on these levels.[39,716] This implies that while the body can adjust to a low blood glucose level, brain function cannot adjust as much. See also page 44.

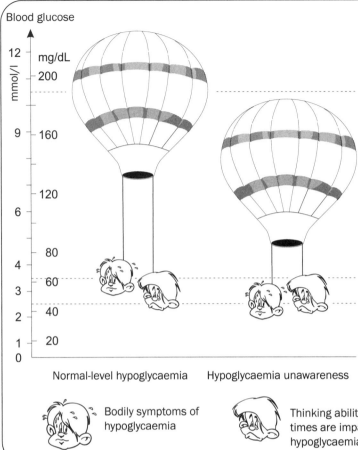

Normal-level hypoglycaemia   Hypoglycaemia unawareness

Normally you will notice bodily symptoms (such as shaking and cold sweats) at slightly higher blood glucose levels than symptoms from the brain (such as difficulty in concentrating). This enables you to continue to think clearly and to take appropriate action promptly.

If you have many low blood glucose readings (less than 2.5-3.0 mmol/l, 45-55 mg/dl) you will risk having hypoglycaemic unawareness (see page 52). The hypoglycaemia may then go unnoticed until the blood glucose level is so low that it affects the brain. By then, you will find it difficult to think clearly and your reaction times will have slowed down. Bodily symptoms begin to occur when your blood glucose level drops even lower, but by this time you will have problems taking appropriate action because you will be unable to think rationally.

It would be much better if your bodily symptoms could appear before the symptoms from the brain, warning you in time to do something about your low blood glucose level in an effective way.

Bodily symptoms of hypoglycaemia

Thinking ability and reaction times are impaired due to hypoglycaemia in the brain

Increased doses to bring blood glucose down

"High-hypo"

"Normal-hypo"

Insulin resistance due to high blood glucose for a period of time

Normal sensitivity to insulin

High blood glucose levels

If your blood glucose has been high for a period of time the "glucostat" (see page 44) in your body will readjust and you will notice symptoms of hypoglycaemia at higher blood glucose levels ("high-level hypoglycaemia"). If you have had an average blood glucose level of 15 mmol/l (270 mg/dl) for a week or two (sometimes even less) you may even find you notice symptoms of hypoglycaemia when your blood glucose is 4.5-5.5 mmol/l (80-100 mg/dl). When you tighten your blood glucose levels the level at which you will notice hypoglycaemic symptoms will fall. It will then be very important to measure your blood glucose when you experience symptoms of hypoglycaemia and not to eat until it comes close to 3.5-4 mmol/l (65-70 mg/dl). After 1-2 weeks of "suffering", your sensitivity to insulin will again be normal, and you will recognize symptoms of hypoglycaemia at a lower glucose level ("normal-level hypoglycaemia").

Low blood glucose levels

If you continue with the increased insulin doses, your blood glucose level will fall even more after a week or two since your sensitivity to insulin now increases (less insulin resistance). With a lower average blood glucose, the level where bodily symptoms of hypoglycaemia appear will also go down. If your average blood glucose level is 7-8 mmol/l (125-145 mg/dl) you will probably not notice symptoms of hypoglycaemia until your glucose level falls below 3.0-3.5 mmol/l (55-65 mg/dl) ("low-level hypoglycaemia"). The risk of having hypoglycaemia unawareness will increase.

When your average blood glucose level decreases, your sensitivity to insulin will increase, so you will need to lower your insulin doses to avoid hypoglycaemia. See the graphs on pages 226 and 227 for further explanation of how the insulin resistance is affected by your recent blood glucose level.

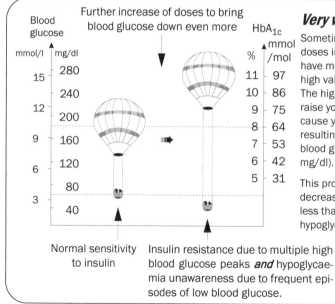

Very variable blood glucose levels

Sometimes it may be difficult to manage your insulin doses in that when you increase them you will indeed have many low blood glucose readings but also many high values (often caused by rebound phenomena). The high values will make you resistant to insulin and raise your HbA_{1c}. At the same time, these low values cause your body to adapt to low blood glucose levels, resulting in a loss of warning symptoms until your blood glucose drops below 3.0-3.5 mmol/l (55-65 mg/dl).

This problem can be difficult to resolve. Start by decreasing insulin doses to avoid blood glucose levels less than 3.5-4 mmol/l (65-70 mg/dl). When your hypoglycaemic symptoms start coming at levels of 3.5-4 mmol/l (65-70 mg/dl) again, you can carefully increase those doses that are needed to cut off the high blood glucose peaks.

Treating hypoglycaemia

Although giving pure glucose may be the preferred treatment for hypoglycaemia, any form of carbohydrate that contains glucose will raise blood glucose levels.[365] Ten grams of glucose will raise the blood glucose of an adult by about 2 mmol/l (35 mg/dl) after 15 minutes.[148,218] The blood glucose will rise over 45-60 minutes and then start to fall. Smaller children can be given a smaller amount of glucose. For instance, 1.5 g of glucose/10 kg (1.5 g/20 lb) body weight will raise the blood glucose by approximately 2 mmol/l (35 mg/dl) (see table on page 66). It is important not to take too much glucose "just to be on the safe side" since the blood glucose will then rise too steeply. If you tend to eat too much when your blood sugar is low, you will put on weight.

The glucose from food can only be absorbed into the blood after it has passed from the stomach into the intestine. Glucose can not be absorbed from inside of the mouth[430] or the stomach.[368] Glucose given rectally (as a suppository) will not raise blood glucose levels in children[21] or adults.[52]

Always take glucose tablets or some other source of sugar or sugary drink like Lucozade or Gatorade with you wherever you go. Older children can keep glucose tablets in their pockets. Younger children may find some kind of small bag that can be attached to their wrist or belt useful. Make sure that your friends know where you keep your glucose tablets in case you need help finding them after becoming hypoglycaemic. It may also be useful to ensure you always have a small amount of cash available in case you need to buy yourself something to eat.

Practical instructions

① Test your blood glucose. The sensations of a hypoglycaemic reaction do not necessarily imply that your blood glucose is actually low. If your symptoms are so intense that it is difficult to measure the blood glucose you should of course eat something containing glucose or sugar as soon as possible. If your blood glucose happens to be high, a little extra glucose will not make much difference. This will outweigh the risk of having a more severe hypoglycaemia if you had not started reversing it straight away.

② If your blood glucose is low (less than 3.5 mmol/l, 65 mg/dl), have something sweet to eat, preferably glucose tablets. Start with a lower dose according to the table on next page and wait 10-15 minutes for the glucose to take effect. Give enough glucose to have a normal glucose level again, i.e. above 4 mmol/l, 70 mg/dl. If you eat something after that, you will need to take insulin to decrease the risk of a following rebound effect.[1006] If you don't feel better after 15-20 minutes and your blood glucose has not risen, you can take a repeat dose of the same amount of glucose.

Which dose of insulin contributed to your hypoglycaemia?

① *Multiple injection therapy*

Premeal *rapid-acting* insulin (NovoRapid, Humalog, Apidra) and two doses of basal insulin per day

Time of hypoglycaemia	"Responsible" insulin dose Time of inj.	Type
After breakfast	Breakfast	Rapid-acting
Before lunch	Breakfast	Basal insulin
After lunch	Lunch	Rapid-acting*
After dinner/tea	Dinner/tea	Rapid-acting
After evening snack	Evening snack	Rapid-acting
Before midnight	Evening snack	Rapid-acting
After midnight	Bedtime	Basal insulin

Basal insulin can be intermediate-acting (NPH) or long-acting (Lantus, Levemir).

With rapid-acting insulin the premeal dose will be "responsible" for hypoglycaemia for 2-3 hours after the injection. After that, the basal insulin is more likely to contribute to hypoglycaemia.

* NPH for breakfast can contribute to hypoglycaemia after lunch.

Premeal *short-acting* insulin and NPH-insulin at bedtime

Before lunch	Breakfast	Short-acting
In the afternoon	Lunch	Short-acting
In the evening	Dinner/tea	Short-acting
After evening snack/ Before midnight	Evening snack	Short-acting
After midnight	Bedtime	NPH insulin

② *Two-dose treatment*

Short-acting and NPH-insulin before both breakfast and dinner/tea

Time of hypoglycaemia	"Responsible" insulin dose Time of inj.	Type
Before lunch	Breakfast	Short-acting
In the afternoon	Breakfast	NPH insulin
Early evening	Dinner/tea	Short-acting
After evening snack/ Before midnight	Dinner/tea	NPH insulin
After midnight	Dinner/tea	NPH insulin

How many glucose tablets (3 g) are needed to treat hypoglycaemia? [218]

Body weight		Rise in blood glucose	
		1.5-2 mmol/l	3-4 mmol/l
Kg	lb	27-35 mg/dl	55-70 mg/dl
10	22	½ tablet	1 tablet (3 g)
20	45	1 tablet (3 g)	2 tablets
30	65	1½ tablet	3 tablets
40	90	2 tablets	4 tablets
50	110	2½ tablets	5 tablets
60	125	3 tablets	6 tablets
70	155	3½ tablets	7 tablets
Glucose /10 kg		1.5 g	3 g
" /10 lb		0.75 g	1.5 g

"Rule of thumb"

1 tablet (3 g) of glucose/10 kg (0.5 tablet/10 lb) body weight will raise the blood glucose approximately 3-4 mmol/l (55-70 mg/dl),[148,200,395,1108] i.e. your blood glucose will be approximately 3-4 mmol/l (55-70 mg/dl) higher after 15-30 minutes than it would be without extra glucose. Usually, an increase of 2 mmol/l (35 mg/dl) will be enough, but if you have recently taken insulin or exercised and your blood glucose level is falling, you may need more glucose. Check the type of glucose tablets you use as they are likely to contain 3-4 g of glucose.

Glucose will give a quicker rise in blood glucose than other types of carbohydrate.[148] Avoid food and drink containing fat (e.g. chocolate, biscuits, milk or chocolate milk) if you want a quick increase in blood glucose. Fat causes the stomach to empty more slowly, so that the glucose reaches the bloodstream later (see page 234).

A blood glucose level of 3.5-4.5 mmol/l (65-80 mg/dl) may require a management decision such as eating some carbohydrate, or postponing exercise. In this situation, a piece of fruit may be appropriate.

③ Do *not* lower the insulin dose for the meal if you have had a hypoglycaemia just recently. You will then risk having a rebound phenomenon with high blood glucose (see page 54). Taking glucose tablets will bring your blood glucose level up to normal within 10-15 minutes, and you will then need to take a normal insulin dose *before* the meal. If you take it after the meal to be on the safe side, you will also risk having a rebound phenomenon as the insulin will take effect too late to cover the rise in blood glucose that the meal causes.

④ If the person is conscious but has difficulty in chewing, give glucose gel (Hypostop®) or honey. Gels are very useful for infants and toddlers since no chewing is required.

⑤ If the person is unconscious or has seizures, give a glucagon injection (for dosage, see page 37). Never give an unconscious person food or drink because it might be accidentally inhaled and cause suffocation or subsequent pneumonia.

⑥ Don't take any physical exercise until all symptoms of hypoglycaemia have vanished. Wait at least 15 minutes before you

A carton of juice can come in handy when the blood glucose is low. It is easy to carry with you and if a child does not want to eat anything it is often easier to give a sip of juice than to use glucose tablets or gel.

do anything that demands your full attention or quick understanding, such as driving, operating a machine or taking an exam in school.

⑦ Don't leave a child alone after a hypoglycaemic reaction. If this happens in school, make sure someone who knows how to cope with the situation will be able to look after the child at home. Smaller children need someone to take them home if their parents cannot come to the school.

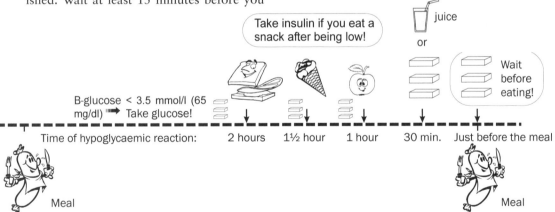

Take insulin if you eat a snack after being low!

juice or

Wait before eating!

B-glucose < 3.5 mmol/l (65 mg/dl) ⟶ Take glucose!

Time of hypoglycaemic reaction: 2 hours 1½ hour 1 hour 30 min. Just before the meal

Meal   Meal

It is important to consider how much time there is before your next meal when you have hypoglycaemia. Don't eat more than you will need to get you through to your next meal. It is all too easy to have too much to eat since it takes a while before the blood glucose rises and makes you feel better. If your blood glucose is below 3.5 mmol/l (65 mg/dl) or the symptoms of hypoglycaemia are troublesome, it is best to take only glucose; then wait 10-15 minutes to cure the hypoglycaemia as quickly as possible. If you feel that you need to eat a snack before the next meal, you will probably need a dose of insulin with it, since the rescue glucose now has raised your blood glucose to a normal level. If you become hypoglycaemic while sitting with a meal in front of you, it may be quite a while before you feel better again if you eat immediately. It is better to eat something with a higher sugar/glucose content (e.g. glucose tablets), wait 10-15 minutes or until you feel better, and then take your insulin dose before enjoying your meal.

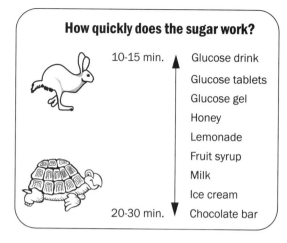

How quickly does the sugar work?

10-15 min.

- Glucose drink
- Glucose tablets
- Glucose gel
- Honey
- Lemonade
- Fruit syrup
- Milk
- Ice cream
- Chocolate bar

20-30 min.

food will mix with the glucose in your stomach. Since it normally takes about 20 minutes for solid food to be digested (sufficiently to be emptied into the intestines) an increase in your blood glucose will take at least this long. Remember that glucose from the food must reach the intestines before it can be absorbed into the blood.

Give a normal dose for the meal even if the child has just had a hypoglycaemia since the glucose has caused the blood sugar to rise to a normal level. Give the dose before, not after the meal! If you give it after the meal, there will be a high risk of a rebound phenomenon.

⑧ If eating something containing glucose or sugar doesn't bring the blood glucose level back to normal, it may be because the stomach isn't emptying its contents into the intestine (where the glucose is absorbed). Occasionally, there may be additional problems and hypoglycaemia will carry on for hours unless some other measure is taken (for example, if you have gastroenteritis). The most effective of these is likely to be injecting a small dose of glucagon, which may need to be repeated (see page 38).

⑨ If there is no apparent explanation why the hypoglycaemia occurred, you should decrease the "responsible" dose of insulin the next day. For more information, see the chapter on adjusting insulin, page 146.

Timing and hypoglycaemia

The time interval between the bout of hypoglycaemia and your next meal will determine which response is appropriate.

Hypoglycaemia just before you eat

Take glucose and wait 10-15 minutes before starting to eat. If you eat straight away, your

Hypoglycaemia 45-60 minutes before your next meal

The same advice applies as in the example above for a rapid reversal of your hypoglycaemia. Glucose will keep up your blood sugar level up for 30-45 minutes, so you can easily wait for this period of time without eating something more if you are due to have a meal. However, you may need something to eat (like a piece of fruit) to keep your blood glucose level up until the next meal if you have been exercising, for example.

Hypoglycaemia 1-2 hours before your next meal

Take glucose and wait 10-15 minutes to reverse your hypoglycaemia quickly. This should have brought up your blood glucose to normal levels. Since it will be a while until your next meal, it is important to consider eating something that will keep your blood sugar up until then (see illustration on page 67). You will then probably need some insulin for this snack unless you have been exercising. An alternative approach is to take fast-acting sugar only, and repeat if necessary. This has the advantage of helping to avoid unwanted weight gain. Try to find out what works best for you and discuss with your diabetes team. If the hypoglycaemia develops slowly,

Should you always eat when you feel hypoglycaemic?

① Measure your blood glucose.

② If it is < 3.5 mmol/l (65 mg/dl), treat quickly! Eat something sweet, preferably glucose tablets.

③ If it is 3.5-4 mmol/l (65-70 mg/dl), no such hurry! Eat something if your next meal is more than 0.5-1 hour off or if you know that your blood glucose is decreasing, e.g. after physical exercise.
If you have symptoms of hypoglycaemia, take glucose.

④ If it is > 4.0-4.5 mmol/l (70-80 mg/dl), you may be having hypoglycaemic symptoms at too high a blood glucose level. Wait a short while and test yourself again. Don't eat until the blood glucose has fallen below 4.0 mmol/l (70 mg/dl), see point ③. See also the text on pages 46 and 62.

Younger children often run around a lot while playing and so get a certain degree of exercise in a natural way. Glucose gel may come in handy if a child develops hypoglycaemia while at the park or the beach. Glucose tablets will easily become wet and sticky.

you can skip the glucose and have some fruit instead.

Helping someone with diabetes who is not feeling well

If you find yourself in the situation of helping someone else with hypoglycaemia, it is very unlikely you will know what the individual's blood glucose level is, and you may lose precious time trying to measure it. The best course of action is to give something containing sugar as quickly as possible and then call for help. Make sure that people (e.g. teachers, sports coaches etc.) who may need to help, know this simple advice.

Remember that the little packets of sugar available in cafes and fast food restaurants will be very effective in this situation, as will fruit juice or fizzy drinks such as lemonade or cola (as long as they are not the "diet" variety).

If a high blood glucose is making the person feel ill, the extra glucose will not have any adverse effects. It is not the high blood glucose as such that causes the unpleasant sensation, but the lack of insulin, which also causes the high blood glucose. If the blood glucose is low, it is essential the person in question gets sugar as quickly as possible.

Glucose

Pure glucose has the quickest effect when correcting hypoglycaemia.[148] Emergency glucose is available in tablets and gel form (for example Hypostop®). It is important to think of glucose as a medicine for hypoglycaemia and not as a "sweet". Everyone with diabetes should always have glucose handy and must know when they need to take it. Friends must also know in which pocket the glucose tablets are kept. A wrist bag or waist bag for carrying glucose is useful.

Sports drinks contain different mixtures of sugars and give a quick increase in blood glucose. Pure fruit juice contains mostly fructose, which gives a slower increase in blood glucose. A glass of juice containing 20 g (2/3 ounce) of carbohydrate gives a slower increase in blood glucose than glucose tablets containing the same amount of carbohydrate.[148] Ordinary sugar consists of sucrose (also called saccharose) which is composed of both glucose and fructose (see illustration on page 232). It will therefore not give the same increase in blood glucose as an equal amount of pure glucose,[395] but it is useful if glucose is not available. It seems as if glucose gives a quicker rise after 5 minutes,[395] but after 15 minutes the rise from glucose tablets or sucrose sweets (10 g for a child 10 years or younger, 15 g if older) was similar, approximately 2.5 mmol/l (45 mg/dl) in both age groups.[542]

It is extremely important that everyone understands why children with diabetes must carry glucose tablets with them everywhere they go. Those who do not understand might otherwise think that the child is "cheating", eating the tablets as sweets instead of taking them as a medication for hypoglycaemia.

Fructose

Fructose has a sweeter taste than ordinary sugar. Fructose is absorbed more slowly from the intestine and is not as effective as glucose in raising the blood glucose level.[349,542] Fructose does not affect the blood glucose directly. It is mainly taken up by the liver cells (without the help of insulin) where it is converted into glucose or triglycerides. A high intake of fructose will increase the body fat.[349] Fructose can also raise the blood glucose by stimulating glucose production in the liver.[349] Honey contains 35-40% glucose and the same amount of fructose. Sorbitol, found in many sweets, is converted in the liver to fructose (see also page 261).

Sweets and hypoglycaemia

Sweets containing only pure sugar (caramels, boiled sweets) will raise the blood glucose quickly. However, it is not a good idea to reserve sweets so you only give them to children when they are hypoglycaemic. This strategy can encourage children to try to make themselves

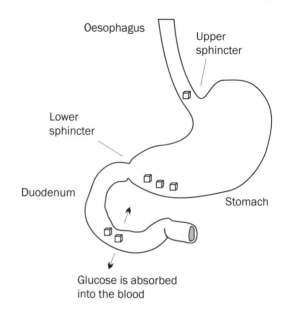

Oesophagus
Upper sphincter
Lower sphincter
Duodenum
Stomach
Glucose is absorbed into the blood

Sugar must reach the intestine to be able to be absorbed into the bloodstream so that it can raise the blood glucose level. Glucose cannot be absorbed through the lining of the mouth (oral mucosa),[430] or from the stomach.[368] The lower sphincter (pylorus) regulates the emptying of the stomach. Different factors influence how quickly the stomach empties (see page 231) and this will have a direct effect on the speed with which glucose can be absorbed into the blood to correct hypoglycaemia.

hypoglycaemic so that they will get sweets. It is best to reserve glucose tablets as "medicine" for low blood glucose. Medicine is not for treating your friends so glucose tablets will not be regarded as sweets. Giving a child sweets for treating hypoglycaemia involves a risk of them being shared out among friends, leaving none for when they are really needed. Another advantage with emergency glucose tablets is that they deliver a precise dose, allowing better control when it is most needed. If your child has hypoglycaemia at school, this will also make it easier for the teacher to know how much to treat with. An alternative may be to give sweets for hypoglycaemia only when the child is engaged in sports, for example swimming or football.

Sweets containing chocolate and chocolate bars raise the blood glucose very slowly and should not be used to treat hypoglycaemia (see graph on page 270). This is particularly important when blood glucose levels are below 3.5 mmol/l (65 mg/dl) as you then will risk a rebound phenomenon (see page 54).

After hypoglycaemia

Usually you will feel better within 10-15 minutes after you have eaten something containing glucose. However, it will often take 1 or 2 hours after the blood glucose has normalized before returning to a level of maximum performance again, necessary for example for an exam at school. It is difficult to state a time limit, but full recovery will not have taken place until after 40-90 minutes, according to a review.[377] One study tested children at a diabetes camp following recovery from hypoglycaemia (the time intervals varied between 10 and 45 minutes). These children were found to score less well on neuro-psychological tests that measured memory and concentration.[863] A study of adults with diabetes, however, found that reaction times returned to normal 10-40 minutes after the blood glucose had risen to a level above 3.3 mmol/l (60 mg/dl).[495]

It appears that individuals with hypoglycaemic unawareness (see page 52) do not have any deterioration on test results when the blood glucose is low (2.5 mmol/l (45 mg/dl) for 1 hour), and they did not have any concentration difficulties during the recovery from hypoglycaemic levels of blood glucose.[1130] So in this sense, you will only have difficulties concentrating when you are low and during the recovery time, if you have symptoms of the low blood glucose level. In this study, the reaction time was delayed for up to 75 minutes after the hypoglycaemia event in people with symptoms of hypoglycaemia at 2.5 mmol/l (45 mg/dl), while those who did not have symptoms due to hypoglycaemia unawareness had a normal reaction time.[1130]

Headaches are common after recovering from hypoglycaemia, particularly if your blood glu-

The graph shows results from a study where 13 adults with type 1 diabetes were given different types of sugar to reverse hypoglycaemia.[148] Four hundred ml (2/3 pint) of water was given with the glucose tablets. Milk contains fat and gives a slower rise in blood glucose, as fat leads to a slower emptying of the stomach.

cose level was very low. Although they are less common, you may also experience transient neurological symptoms such as a temporary paralysis or difficulties of speech caused by some degree of brain oedema (swelling).[854,965] If you find yourself suffering from any of these, you should contact your doctor.

If you are caring for a child with diabetes who doesn't wake up or return to full consciousness within 15-30 minutes after being severely hypoglycaemic, even though his or her blood glucose has returned to normal, this may indicate swelling of the brain (brain oedema).[705] It may take many hours before the child is awake and behaving in the usual way again.

➠ *This is an acute condition that requires immediate treatment in hospital!*

Sometimes people feel sick or vomit after hypoglycaemia, especially if the blood glucose has been low for some time. This seems to be particularly common during pregnancy when women are trying very hard to keep their blood glucose levels low, and will often be associated

It will be difficult to achieve top results in an examination if you have hypoglycaemia, or have had it recently. Usually it will take a couple of hours after a difficult hypoglycaemic episode before you are back on top form.

with raised levels of ketones in the blood and urine. Both ketones and nausea are caused by the hormone glucagon, which is secreted from the pancreas during hypoglycaemia. This is the same type of side effect that can be experienced after a glucagon injection. If the vomiting continues you should contact the hospital. Since the glucagon secretion from a person's body usually decreases after several years with diabetes, this reaction is more common in people who have had diabetes for a few years only.

Learning to recognize the symptoms of hypoglycaemia

Every time your blood glucose measures less than 3.5-4.0 mmol/l (65-70 mg/dl) you should ask yourself: "Exactly what symptoms caused me to take the blood test now? Did I experience any symptoms 10 or 20 minutes earlier that might have warned me my blood glucose was falling?" If your blood glucose is below 3.0-3.5 mmol/l (55-65 mg/dl) and you have not experienced any symptoms, you should always ask yourself: "Were there really no symptoms at all warning me that my blood glucose was low?" Ask your friends if they have noticed any change in your behaviour that could have been caused by a drop in your blood glucose.

There are now programmes that train people with diabetes to recognize subtle and variable changes in their behaviour and how they feel

Research findings: Recovery from hypoglycaemia

♠ In one study of adults without diabetes, hypoglycaemia was induced using insulin (blood glucose 2.7 mmol/l, 50 mg/dl, for 70 minutes). The reaction time was decreased for 1.5 hours and only returned to normal 4 hours after the blood glucose had normalized.[317]

♠ Another study of adults found cognitive functions (short-term memory, attention and concentration) to be normal in the morning after a night with hypoglycaemia (blood glucose < 2.2 mmol/l, < 40 mg/dl, for 1 hour).[80]

♠ A British study of adults shows their capacity for exercise was unchanged after an episode of night time hypoglycaemia (2.6-3.0 mmol/l, 45-55 mg/dl for 1 hour) even though participants complained of more fatigue and less well-being, and felt that they had experienced a bad night's sleep.[614]

♠ In children, cognitive testing (coordination, memory, attention and creative thinking) was not affected after night time hypoglycaemia (< 3.9 mmol/l, 70 mg/dl) but their mood was influenced negatively.[728]

In these studies, patient meters showing whole blood glucose readings were used. Values have been recalculated to plasma glucose.

while hypoglycaemia is developing. Such programmes include the use of simple cognitive tests, and their success has been demonstrated.[210] To test for bodily symptoms, stand up and walk around. Move your outstretched arm in a circle or hold a pen between your fingers to test for shakiness. To test for symptoms from your brain, repeat your mother's or brother's age and birthday, your friends' phone numbers or the combination for your locker or bike key. Younger children may try counting backwards from 100. Whatever test you set yourself should be sufficiently difficult when your blood glucose level is normal, for you to notice the difference when doing the same thing while your blood glucose is low.

Insulin treatment

The pancreas of a person without diabetes will always be secreting a small amount of insulin into the bloodstream, constantly throughout the day and night (called basal secretion). After a meal, a larger amount of insulin is secreted to deal with the glucose coming from the food (called bolus secretion, see graphs on page 23). The goal of all insulin treatment is to mimic this function and provide insulin to the bloodstream.

In the past, bovine (beef) and porcine (pork) insulin were used for all people with diabetes. Nowadays, mostly human insulin is used, i.e. insulin with a chemical structure identical to the insulin produced by the human pancreas. Human insulin is produced using gene technology or by semi-synthetic methods. Genetic engineering involves the insertion of human insulin-producing genes into a yeast cell or bacteria. In this way yeast cells or bacteria are tricked into producing insulin instead of their own proteins. By changing specific building blocks (amino acids) in the insulin molecule, the action time can be modified. These insulins are called insulin analogues, and can have both a quicker action (rapid-acting insulin) and a slower action (basal insulin analogues).

Short- and rapid-acting insulins are pure insulin without any additives. They are in the form of a clear liquid and don't require stirring or mixing before use. Different additives are used to make the insulin longer-acting, and these are what make it cloudy. The cloudy part of the contents will collect as sediment at the bottom of the bottle or cartridge. This sediment must be mixed again with the rest of the contents by turning over or rolling (but not shaking) the cartridge 20 times before use.[559]

The newer basal insulins such as Lantus and Levemir are clear because they are both solutions rather than suspensions. These types of insulin have an extended effect because of changes to the molecular structure which slow down their absorption, rather than added molecules such as zinc or protamine.

Production of human insulin

① **Semi-synthetic method:**

Porcine insulin is engineered enzymatically	Older method of making human insulin.

② **Biosynthetic DNA-technology method:**

Production from baker's yeast	Novo Nordisk insulins.
Production from coli-bacteria	Eli Lilly insulins. Sanofi-Aventis insulins.

Methods of postponing the action of insulin

①	NPH insulin	Binds to a protein from salmon (protamine).
②	Lente insulin	Excess of free zinc.
③	Lantus	Clear solution but precipitates (gets cloudy) after injection due to a higher pH in the subcutaneous tissue.
④	Levemir	Binds to a protein (albumin).
⑤	Tresiba	Formation of multihexamers

Regular short-acting insulin

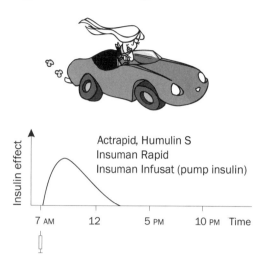

Actrapid, Humulin S
Insuman Rapid
Insuman Infusat (pump insulin)

Regular short-acting insulin (also called soluble insulin) is given as a bolus injection before meals. The listed brand names are examples of insulins. Ask your diabetes healthcare team to find out which insulins are available where you live.

Basal insulin analogues

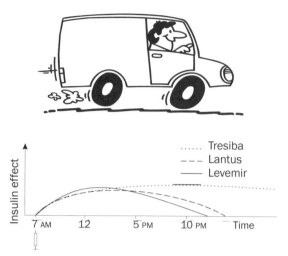

...... Tresiba
– – – Lantus
——— Levemir

Basal insulin analogues have effect over up to 24 hours. Levemir is usually injected twice daily to give a basal insulin level between meals and during the night. Lantus gives a slightly longer insulin effect and is injected once or twice-daily. Ultratard and Humulin Zn are older types of long-acting basal insulins are no longer available in many countries.

Intermediate-acting insulin

NPH type (isophane):
Insulatard, Humulin I
Insuman Basal

Lente type:
Monotard
Humulin L

Intermediate-acting insulin is used as basal (background) insulin when injecting twice daily and once or more daily in a multiple daily injection regimen. There are different types: NPH insulin (——) and lente (zinc-depot) insulin (– – –).

Intravenous insulin

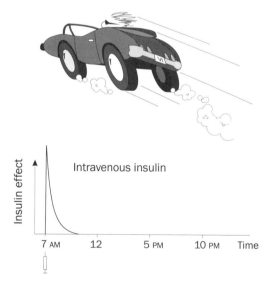

Intravenous insulin

Short-acting insulin given intravenously has an extremely rapid action with a half-life (length of time when half of the insulin is broken down) of only 3-5 minutes.[988]

The rapid-acting insulin analogues (NovoRapid, Huma-log, Apidra) have a much more rapid action than regular short-acting insulin. You can inject them just before a meal and still get a good insulin effect at the time when the glucose from the food reaches the bloodstream. However, the insulin will have less effect after 2-3 hours,[522] so the blood glucose may rise before the next meal. Because of this, a basal insulin that takes effect during the day is usually given (see page 144).

Regular short-acting insulin

This is the same molecule that is secreted in the normal pancreas (it is also called soluble insulin). Normally, insulin molecules stick together in groups of six (so called hexamer formation, see illustration). These groups must be broken up before the insulin can be absorbed into the blood.

Short-acting regular insulin (Actrapid, Humulin S, Insuman Rapid) begins to act 20-30 minutes after a subcutaneous injection and begins its maximal effect after 1.5-2 hours. The blood glucose-lowering effect lasts for about 5 hours.

In intravenous insulin therapy, insulin (usually short-acting) is given directly into the bloodstream. This is the most effective way to treat diabetic ketoacidosis. It is given only in hospitals as an intravenous drip or in a motorized syringe. Both short- and rapid acting insulins can be used for intravenous therapy, but there is no difference in the onset of effect (see below). Since the half-life of insulin is very short, only about 4 minutes,[358] the blood glucose will increase sharply if intravenous insulin is stopped. If intravenous insulin is being used, the blood glucose must be checked every hour (even during the night) to monitor the correct dosage.

Intravenous insulin is often used during surgery or if a patient is suffering for any length of time from diarrhoea and vomiting. It also gives us a practical way of working out how much insulin the patient needs over a 24-hour period, for example when starting treatment with an insulin pump.

Rapid-acting insulin

Regular short-acting insulin is actually a bit too slow in action. The insulin level in your blood is not high enough during the meal. Rather, it is higher than necessary a couple of hours later, which is what causes you to need a snack. If the

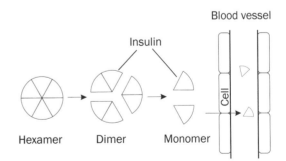

Insulin is always in a so called hexamer form when it is injected. It must then divide into dimers and monomers before it can pass between the cells of the blood vessel to enter the bloodstream. The new rapid-acting insulin analogues (NovoRapid or Humalog) dissolve much faster than regular short-acting insulin, thus making the time of action much faster.[540] Massage of the injection site can also enhance the dissociation into monomers, causing a faster absorption of the injected insulin.[674]

Different types of insulin

Rapid-acting meal insulin	Humalog
	NovoRapid
	Apidra
Basal insulin	Lantus
	Levemir
Very long-acting insulin	Tresiba
Older basal insulin (cloudy) (intermediate-acting insulin)	NPH
Older mealtime insulin (short-acting insulin)	Regular

---

insulin molecules could be injected in a solution of single molecules (monomeric insulin), the action would be much quicker, as there would be no need to break up the hexameric group. Due to the shorter action span, it would also be possible to achieve more normal insulin levels between meals, lessening the need for snacks.[336]

By changing the amino acid building blocks in the insulin molecule, the problems of hexamer formation are considerably reduced. Rapid-acting insulin begins to act after 10 minutes and is at its most effective after just 1 hour. Although rapid-acting insulin can be given intravenously, there is no advantage in giving rapid-acting insulin intravenously, since the blood glucose-lowering effect is no quicker than that of regular short-acting insulin.[998] This is because when insulin is given directly into the bloodstream, there is no need to break the hexamer groups.

The rapid-acting insulin analogue (Lispro or Humalog), which was introduced to the market around the world in 1996, takes effect very quickly.[540] Today, it is used by many children and adults with diabetes.

Another rapid-acting insulin analogue that is being used successfully both in adults[527] and children[763] was introduced in 1999 (aspart or NovoRapid, NovoLog in some countries). A double-blind study of people with type 1 diabe-

tes showed that the two analogues, Humalog and NovoRapid, gave very similar levels of insulin in the blood and had identical action on the blood glucose profiles.[852] A third rapid-acting insulin analogue called Apidra (glulisine) was introduced in 2005. The Apidra preparation differs from the other insulins in that it does not contain any zinc. The effect was similar to that of Humalog in one study,[75] while another found a slightly faster onset of action for Apidra.[484] The action profile is the same for children and adolescents as for adults.[250]

Basal insulin

People without diabetes always have a low level of insulin in their body between meals and even during the night (see graphs on page 23). This steady release of insulin from the pancreas takes care of the glucose that is released between meals from the store in the liver. This constant

---

Research findings: Lantus

♠ Lantus has been shown to give similar levels of basal insulin over 24 hours as an insulin pump.[664]

♠ In one study, researchers found both lower morning blood glucose and less night time hypoglycaemia.[848]

♠ In another study, adults compared Lantus (given once at bedtime) with NPH (given once or twice daily).[907] Fasting glucose was 2.2 mmol/l (40 mg/dl) lower when using Lantus.

♠ In the group using NPH once a day, the doses of Lantus were similar. But Lantus doses for the group using NPH twice daily were 6-7 units lower than the sum of the NPH doses.

♠ Even though Lantus can have an effect for a period of up to 24 hours or more, there is no evidence of the effect of the insulin increasing when it is given for several days in a row.[481]

low level of insulin is known as basal insulin or background insulin. The basal insulin dose given to people with diabetes in whom this natural supply is not available, will be either intermediate-acting or long-acting. A new insulin (Tresiba) is extremely long-acting with an effect up to 42 hours in children and adolescents.[93] Because of high growth hormone levels, adolescents often need high doses of basal insulin.

Traditional basal insulins

Before the appearance of the new long-acting analogues, the only insulins used as basal insulin were two types of intermediate-acting insulins (NPH and lente insulin) and lente type long-acting insulin (Ultratard, Humulin Zn).

NPH insulin

The prolonged effect of this insulin is attained by the addition of protamine to the molecule of short-acting insulin. The dose of NPH insulin (Insulatard, Humulin I, Insuman Basal) taken in the evening will take effect after 2-4 hours, has its peak action after 4-6 hours, and will usually give an effect on your blood glucose for a good 8-9 hours of sleep.

Lente insulin

The effect of "Lente" insulins is made longer by binding the insulin monomers into large crystals in the presence of an excess of free zinc. Lente insulins are not available in cartridges for insulin pens. The reason for this is that the insulin is in crystal form and the crystals will break if a glass ball is used in the cartridge for mixing.

Lente insulins (Monotard, Humutard) are a bit more long-acting and at their most effective after the first 4 or 5 hours.

Ultratard

The older long-acting ultralente type insulins (Ultratard, Humulin Zn) begin to take effect 2-4 hours after the injection, are at their most powerful between 6 and 12 hours and may still be having some effect after 24 hours.[370]

Ultratard and Monotard have been withdrawn from the UK market but these insulins may still be in use in other parts of the world so some advice on their use is included in this book.

Analogue basal insulins

NPL

NPL is an intermediate-acting insulin originating from Humalog. The longer effect is achieved by adding protamine, in the same way as for ordinary NPH insulin. NPL has the advantage of being stable for at least a year if mixed with Humalog. It has the same action profile as ordinary NPH insulin.[555]

Lantus (Glargine)

Once a day injections of traditional intermediate- or long-acting insulin preparations do not provide an appropriate 24-hour basal insulin level (between meals and during the night) in most people with diabetes.[908] The long-acting analogue Lantus (glargine) was introduced in 2000. By altering the insulin molecule, the blood glucose-lowering effect has been spread more evenly over up to 24 hours,[813] resembling the background insulin secretion in a healthy person. The subcutaneous uptake of insulin is more stable from day to day with Lantus, compared with NPH insulin.[664]

Occasionally, people report a stinging sensation when injecting Lantus,[873] which may be a disadvantage for children in particular. This is due to the acidity of the insulin. However, this seems to be a minor problem, as the vast majority of children for whom Lantus is prescribed feel no pain when injecting.

Levemir (Detemir)

Levemir (detemir) is another basal insulin which was introduced in 2004. A 6-month study of adults using NovoRapid as premeal insulin showed that the same HbA_{1c} level [61 mmol/mol (7.7%)] was obtained with Levemir as with NPH insulin (Insulatard, Humulin I, Insuman Basal), but with a lower risk of hypoglycaemia, especially during the night.[1061] Overnight glucose profiles were more even with Levemir, and body weight was significantly lower after 6 months in the Levemir group.

Lantus and Levemir are clear solutions and are usually given with a pen injector but can also be given with a syringe.

Pre-mixed insulin

The cartridges of pre-mixed insulin that are available for insulin pens contain different pro-

portions of rapid-acting and intermediate-acting insulin of NPH type. You can also find cartridges containing mixtures of short-acting and intermediate-acting insulins. With pre-mixed insulins the proportions of the two insulins cannot be adjusted. If you change the dose you will get more or less of both types of insulin. It is important to assess the use of different mixtures depending on your meal schedule. For example, the prolonged effect of the intermediate-acting part in a 30-50% mix with rapid-acting may be useful if you have a long wait between lunch and dinner/tea.

A larger dose lasts longer

A larger insulin dose will give a stronger insulin effect which also lasts a longer time.[470,656] An exception to this rule seems to be the rapid-acting insulins NovoRapid[799] and Humalog,[1117] which last for the same period of time even when the dose is increased. Later and more thorough studies of the rapid-acting analogue Apdra has shown a clear dose-dependent effect,[76] which makes it probable that this applies to all rapid-acting insulins.[615]

Units and insulin concentrations

Insulin is measured in units, abbreviated U (international units, previously abbreviated IU). One unit of insulin was defined as the amount

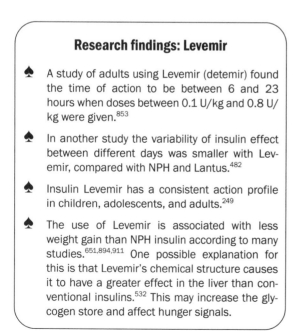

Research findings: Levemir

♠ A study of adults using Levemir (detemir) found the time of action to be between 6 and 23 hours when doses between 0.1 U/kg and 0.8 U/kg were given.[853]

♠ In another study the variability of insulin effect between different days was smaller with Levemir, compared with NPH and Lantus.[482]

♠ Insulin Levemir has a consistent action profile in children, adolescents, and adults.[249]

♠ The use of Levemir is associated with less weight gain than NPH insulin according to many studies.[651,894,911] One possible explanation for this is that Levemir's chemical structure causes it to have a greater effect in the liver than conventional insulins.[532] This may increase the glycogen store and affect hunger signals.

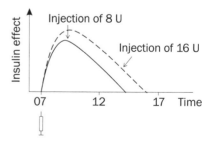

A larger insulin dose (dashed line) gives both a stronger and longer-lasting insulin effect.

of insulin that will lower the blood glucose of a healthy 2 kg (4.4 lb) rabbit that has fasted for 24 hours to 2.5 mmol/l (45 mg/dl) within 2.5 hours.[1058] Quite a complicated definition, don't you think? With better analytical methods, one unit has been defined as 6 nmol of insulin and 1 mg of insulin equals 29 units.[526] See also "How much does insulin lower the blood glucose level?" on page 146.

Today, the most common insulin concentration around the world is 100 units/ml (U-100). In some countries other concentrations are used, mostly 40 U/ml (U-40).

Some standard pens for insulin 100 U/ml can be used for giving half-units and there are pens that have half-unit increments on the scale (NovoPen Echo®, NovoPen 5®, Humapen Luxura HD®). Insulin 40 U/ml or 50 U/ml can be used for low doses (less than 2-3 units) when

---

Disposable syringes

♠ Disposable syringes can be practical to use if you need to change the insulin dose in very small increments.

♠ In one study, syringes for 30 units (100 U/ml) were found to be accurate for adjusting doses of ± 0.25 units in the interval between 2.5 and 3.5 units.[969] However, they may be difficult to use for very small doses of only 0.5-1 unit.

♠ Another study found an error rate of 10% when doses of less than 5 units were given by syringe.[687] When a pen injector was used, the error was only 5%.

♠ In a study where parents were supposed to deliver 1.0 units of insulin, the actual dose varied between 0.6 and 1.3 units.[174] The variability was even greater when the dose was administered by paediatric nurses.

♠ Syringes for U-100 insulin must not be used with U-40 insulin (risk of under-dosage), nor should syringes for U-40 insulin be used with U-100 insulin (risk of over-dosage).

---

giving insulin to young children. For the very youngest children, insulin can be diluted to 10 U/ml (U-10) to make small insulin dose adjustments possible.

Insulin units are counted in the same way, regardless of the concentration. A weaker insulin will be absorbed more quickly.[373] Insulin of 40 U/ml gives approximately 20% higher insulin levels 30-40 minutes after injection compared with the same number of units of 100 U/ml.[971] People taking insulin need to be aware that it will take effect more quickly if they switch from 100 U/ml to 40 U/ml.

Twice-daily treatment

Twice-daily injections are still the standard treatment for many people with type 1 diabetes today. This may be advantageous when the person has a low total daily insulin requirement, for example during the honeymoon phase (remission phase). It is also useful if the person, for whatever reason, finds it difficult to take multiple injections. A twice-daily injection regimen usually means that there is less flexibility for planning mealtimes. The afternoon dose of intermediate-acting insulin may not last long enough, especially in adolescents, to cover insulin requirements during the night, so morning hyperglycaemia may result. A large amount of intermediate-acting insulin during the day will increase the need for snacks between meals.

Three-dose treatment

If the insulin given with dinner/tea with a two-dose treatment does not last until morning, you can take only the rapid- or short-acting component for dinner/tea and postpone the injection

Rapid-acting
insulin

GOAL

Short-acting
insulin

20-30 min.

The rapid-acting insulins (NovoRapid and Humalog) are much quicker to take effect than regular short-acting insulin (Actrapid, Humulin S, Insuman Rapid) that needs to be given 20-30 minutes before the meal for the insulin to take a head start or the race will be very uneven.[920] The carbohydrates from your meal will enter the bloodstream first and raise your blood glucose level. The insulin will enter your bloodstream later, putting you at risk of a low blood glucose before your next meal.

By using continuous glucose monitoring (see page 107), we have seen that the blood glucose rises quickly even when the dose is given immediately before the meal. It is therefore a good idea to take it 15-20 min. before the meal, especially at breakfast.

Multiple daily injections

Multiple daily injections (MDI) aim at mimicking the normal secretion of the pancreas that provides a basal insulin level for the night and the hours between meals, and insulin peaks for each meal.

MDI is an intensive insulin treatment. It is also called multiple injection treatment or basal-bolus treatment. It has been used since 1984 and the first insulin pen was introduced in 1985. Studies in both children [949,1044] and

---

Research findings:
Multiple injections

♠ Studies indicate that more than 90% of participants have found multiple injections acceptable.[539]

♠ In a French paediatric study of 5-19-year-olds, 77% experienced an improvement in their quality of life when switching from a 2-3 dose regimen with syringes to a 4-5 dose regimen with pen injectors.[1044] No significant change in glucose control was observed in the group as a whole, but the sub-group with poor control improved their HbA$_{1c}$ significantly.

♠ In the DCCT study (see page 367), the majority of participants on intensive treatment used multiple injections with syringes if they were not on insulin pumps.

♠ Results from the DCCT study show that starting an intensive treatment regimen at an early stage sustains the insulin production in your own pancreas, reducing the risk both of severe hypoglycaemia and the development of diabetic complications.[269]

♠ In 1987 we switched all patients in our clinic (aged 2-20 years) from twice-daily injections with syringes to multiple injection treatment with insulin pens. Only one person was dissatisfied with this new regimen and switched back to twice-daily injections.

♠ Since then our policy has been to use multiple injections from the onset of diabetes. Children are started on rapid-acting insulin and take 1 or 2 injections of basal insulin per day. This regimen mimics the insulin secretion of the pancreas better than a twice-daily regimen (see graphs on pages 23, 143 and 144). All are taught carbohydrate counting from the onset of diabetes. Young children below age 6-7 are started on an insulin pump within a few weeks of diagnosis.

---

of intermediate-acting NPH (Insulatard, Humulin I, Insuman Basal) or Lente insulin until bedtime. This regimen decreases the risk of night time hypoglycaemia compared with a two-dose treatment.

adults [261,463,946] have shown that it is possible to improve glucose control with this regimen. Using multiple injection treatment will not necessarily give you a better HbA_{1c},[300,537] but you may well find you are happier and have a better quality of life [538] as well as more freedom to choose a lifestyle you enjoy and greater flexibility over meal planning.[1017]

With multiple injection treatment it is fairly easy for people with diabetes, along with the rest of their family, to understand how their insulin affects blood glucose at any given time of day. This is particularly important as the goal of diabetes education is to enable the person with diabetes (and where appropriate, the family) to take an increasing responsibility for their treatment, so that they eventually become experts on their own diabetes.

Injections before meals (bolus insulin)

Bolus insulin is the rapid- or short-acting insulin that you take before a meal. If you are using short-acting insulin, you must remember that the blood glucose-lowering effect of each bolus lasts for about 5 hours. This means that with a multiple injection regimen there should not be more than 5 hours between your main meals and injections of regular short-acting insulin (if you use only 1 dose of NPH as basal dose for the night).

If you are using rapid-acting insulin, you will not have to be as strict about mealtimes if you have enough basal insulin during the day (see page 156).

One big difference between rapid- and short-acting insulins for multiple injections is that with rapid-acting insulin you will often need another injection of rapid-acting insulin if you eat a large afternoon snack, unless you are playing a vigorous sport or being otherwise very

active. With short-acting insulin, the opposite is the case as you will need to take snacks between main meals to avoid hypoglycaemia. Check your blood glucose level to help you decide what dose you need.

When should you take your premeal dose?

The abdomen or tummy is the most common injection site for premeal injections (see page 127). See the table on page 154 for recommended times of injections at breakfast. The time limits given in this chapter refer to abdominal injections of regular short-acting insulin if not otherwise stated. If you take regular premeal insulin in the thigh (or buttocks) you will probably need to add another 15-30 minutes to these time limits.

Rapid-acting insulin

The rapid-acting insulin analogues (Novo-Rapid, Humalog and Apidra) start working sooner than regular short-acting insulin. They can be injected just before a meal and still give a good insulin effect at the time when glucose from the meal enters the bloodstream. If your blood glucose is high before the meal, you can try waiting 15-30 minutes before eating.[871] NovoRapid [152,248] and Humalog [943,278] can be given after the meal with a relatively good effect if you are not sure exactly how much you or your child are going to eat when you start the meal. However, clinical practice shows that this routine often contributes to a higher HbA_{1c} by resulting in a higher glucose level after meals and forgetting meal doses. We therefore recommend all children and adolescents to always take insulin before meals. If this is difficult, it is better to divide the dose into one part taken before the meal and one when it is apparent how much the child has eaten. This causes no problems if the child is using a pump or an injection aid (i-Port or Insuflon). From the moment that type 1 diabetes is diagnosed, it is a good idea for older children and adolescents to learn to make decisions about how much they will eat in advance, so that they can take their insulin before the meal.

One of the most important tasks of the insulin dose taken before eating is to shut off the glucose production in the liver, which is caused by an elevation of glucagon. In a person without diabetes, the rapid release of insulin into the blood stream at the start of the meal suppresses the glucagon level. This stops the production of glucose which is kept at a steady level between meals. The insulin that you give for a meal will suppress glucagon, but only if you give it early, before the meal and in a large enough dose.[615]

It is usually best to give the insulin before the meal even in case of hypoglycaemia. When the hypoglycaemia has been cured with extra glucose or sugar, the glucose level will be in the normal range within 10-15 minutes, and it is then better to take your insulin before beginning to eat. You otherwise risk a rebound phenomenon with high blood glucose after the meal.

Short-acting insulin

There is no difference in effect between different brands of regular short-acting insulin. Your insulin depot (store) from the bedtime injection will be almost gone by the morning. You should therefore have your morning injection of regular insulin at least 30 minutes before breakfast. Wait if possible for even longer if your blood glucose is high, up to 45-60 minutes before eating. See also the table on page 151. If you inject regular insulin in the thigh or buttocks, you will probably have to add an additional 15-30 minutes to the above intervals.

When should I take my premeal insulin? (abdominal injections)

Meal	Rapid-acting insulins*	Regular short-acting insulin
Breakfast	20 min. before	At least 30 min. before
Other meals	Just before the meal	0-30 min. before (see text)
Hypoglycaemia at mealtime	Take glucose, wait 10 min., take insulin and then eat	Just before you eat
High blood glucose at mealtime	15-30 min. before eating	30-60 min. before eating

*NovoRapid, Humalog, Apidra

You should always take the dose before the meal! If you take it after the meal, your glucose level will have risen before it begins to take effect. This is the case even if you have hypoglycaemia before the meal. You will then easily get a rebound effect if you do not take a full insulin dose for the meal, as you probably have corrected the hypoglycaemia by taking some glucose tablets.

Can regular insulin injections be taken just before a meal?

To find out, take the injection just before your meal and measure your blood glucose before and 1.5-2 hours after the meal. The blood glucose should have risen 3.0-4.0 mmol/l (55-70 mg/dl) at the most. If it has risen more, the effect of your regular insulin is too slow.

Try the same thing when you take your insulin 15 and 30 minutes before eating, to find out which suits you the best. If the blood glucose is too high, even when you have taken the insulin 30 minutes before the meal, you will probably need a higher dose.

If you use rapid-acting insulin (NovoRapid or Humalog) it should normally be injected just before the meal.

Ideally, regular short-acting insulin should be administered 20-30 minutes before all meals since the blood glucose is not affected immediately.[943] However, at lunchtime some of the short-acting breakfast insulin still remains in your body and the same holds true for the other meals. On the contrary, the insulin depot (store) from the bedtime injection will be almost gone by the morning. Because of this, the 30 minute insulin "head start" is not as essential with other meals as it is with breakfast.

Children using small doses will absorb the insulin faster than adults, especially if they do not have much subcutaneous fat. Because of this, they rarely need to wait 30 minutes before they eat [691] (provided the premeal blood glucose isn't high). Taking insulin 30 minutes before each meal can be very difficult for younger children as it causes so many interruptions to their daily routine. So younger children are recommended to take their regular insulin just before meals (except breakfast). Some children, however, will absorb the insulin slowly and individual advice on this point is necessary. Older children and teenagers are unlikely to experience problems taking the insulin 30 minutes before meals.

If you inject regular insulin just before your meal, it is important that the food is not absorbed too quickly from the intestine. Other-

wise, the blood glucose will increase before the insulin reaches the bloodstream. Any fat content of the meal will slow down the gastric emptying rate. For example, ice cream made with milk products has a higher fat content and will therefore give a slower rise in blood glucose than water ice. See the nutrition chapter, page 228.

Combining boluses and basal insulin

Multiple injection treatment implies taking rapid-acting insulin (NovoRapid, Humalog, Apidra) or short-acting (Actrapid, Humulin S, Insuman Rapid) before each main meal, and one or two doses of intermediate-acting (Insulatard, Humulin I, Insuman Basal) or long-acting insulin (Lantus, Levemir) to cover the need for insulin between meals and during the night. Usually 4 short-acting insulin premeal doses are combined with a single bedtime basal dose. When using rapid acting insulin you usually combine 3-4 pre-meal bolus with once or twice-daily injections of basal insulin (intermediate- or long-acting, see page 145).

The basal insulin is often given as separate injections if you use insulin pens. If you use syringes, and you prefer to take only 4 injections, you can mix the basal insulin with the rapid-acting insulin in the same syringe if you use NPH. There are also some successful reports of mixing Lantus with rapid-acting insulin,[352,588] although this is not recommended by the manufacturer. Mixing these insulins in one syringe or taking them as pre-mixed insulin is not an ideal method however. If you inject yourself in the thigh, there is a risk of hypoglycaemia early in the night from the short-acting component. But if you inject yourself in the abdomen, there is a risk that the intermediate-acting insulin will not last until morning.

Remember that it takes at least 2 hours for the bedtime injection of NPH type insulin to have any significant effect (even longer in the case of Lantus). This means that the time span between the last dose of regular insulin and the bedtime

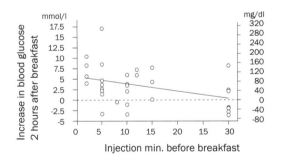

It is important to give regular short-acting insulin 30 minutes before breakfast. In this study, the blood glucose increased about 5 mmol/l (90 mg/dl) when the children took their insulin immediately before breakfast, compared with less than 1 mmol/l (20 mg/dl) when taking insulin 30 minutes before the meal.[920]

injection should not be more than 3-4 hours. With rapid-acting insulins, this interval should be shorter since there is a risk of a rise in blood glucose and ketones if the interval is longer than 2-3 hours.[14]

Younger children often need a higher level of basal insulin after they fall asleep. This is often seen as a rise in blood glucose before midnight when using long-acting basal insulin (Lantus, Levemir). It may then be a good idea to use regular short-acting insulin (Actrapid, Humulin S, Insuman Rapid) instead of rapid-acting insulin for the evening snack, to get a longer basal insulin effect that lasts until the bedtime insulin effect can take over. This also applies to younger children who get their bedtime NPH dose while asleep, since usually the bolus dose given with last meal will not last until when NPH starts having its effect. However, if the last dose of NPH is given at dinner/tea time, this advice will not apply.

Can I skip a meal?

Your body needs to have some insulin in the blood, even between meals, to take care of the glucose produced by the liver. If you use Novo-Rapid or Humalog and take basal insulin as well in the morning (or one daily dose of Lantus), you may try to skip both the meal and the corresponding NovoRapid or Humalog dose. If your blood glucose is high, you may need a corrective dose of a few units of rapid-acting insulin. Increase the dose of NovoRapid or Humalog, if necessary, the next time you eat.

If your blood glucose is above around 15 mmol/l (270 mg/dl) and you want to skip a meal, you still need to take some insulin to bring your blood glucose level down. Use the correction factor on page 146 to find a suitable dose. See also "Changing the content of the meal to affect blood glucose" on page 150.

If you are using multiple injection treatment with regular short-acting insulin (Actrapid, Humulin S, Insuman Rapid), and only one bedtime dose of NPH, you must take a low dose of insulin even if you skip a meal as the mealtime dose of short-acting insulin also covers the need for basal insulin between meals. Half the ordinary insulin dose will usually be enough, but you will need to try this out yourself. Intervals between meals and injections of regular insulin should not exceed 5 hours. Listen to your hunger signals and you will know when you must eat. You cannot skip a meal and also skip the snack a couple of hours later. And if your blood glucose is low, you must eat something immediately.

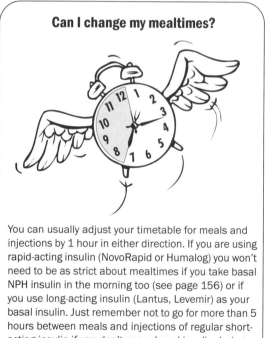

Can I change my mealtimes?

You can usually adjust your timetable for meals and injections by 1 hour in either direction. If you are using rapid-acting insulin (NovoRapid or Humalog) you won't need to be as strict about mealtimes if you take basal NPH insulin in the morning too (see page 156) or if you use long-acting insulin (Lantus, Levemir) as your basal insulin. Just remember not to go for more than 5 hours between meals and injections of regular short-acting insulin if you don't use a basal insulin during the day. If you wait more than 5 hours between injections of regular insulin, you will be at risk of insulin deficiency.

Basal/bedtime insulin

The bedtime insulin injection is the most diffi-cult dose to adjust. Although we do not eat dur-ing the night, our bodies need a continuous low level of insulin to take care of the glucose being produced by the liver. The most common bed-time insulin with multiple injection treatment used to be intermediate-acting insulin of NPH type. An insulin with longer effect (Lantus or Levemir) may be a better alternative for many people. The use of Lantus and Levemir is increasing, in children as well as in adults. Both have a more even effect compared with NPH insulin.

The bedtime insulin covers one third of a 24-hour day, so is likely to be the dose that has the greatest effect on your HbA_{1c} (see page 117). High blood glucose readings during the night can give you a high HbA_{1c} even if your glucose level during the daytime is normal.

When should the injection of basal insulin be taken?

It is important to take your injection of basal insulin at the same time every night on week days. If you change the time from one day to another, it will be difficult to see a pattern in your blood glucose readings.

NPH insulin

Since the most important thing with this type of insulin is to get the bedtime insulin to last until morning (see graphs on page 174), it is a good idea to take your bedtime injection as late as possible, i.e. shortly before your usual bedtime. There is no point your sitting up late, waiting to take your injection. While 11 PM might be fine

for adults, older children will usually find 10 PM more appropriate. Parents should be aware that many young children will sleep through a late night injection with only the smallest disturbance, if they give this just before they themselves go to bed at around 11 PM. An indwelling catheter (Insuflon or i-Port, see page 137) can make this easier if the child wakes up when the parents use regular syringes or pens.

If you use pen injectors, it is very important to turn over or roll the NPH pen cartridge care-fully at least 20 times before injecting for thor-ough mixing.[559] The cartridge with NPH insulin contains a small glass or steel ball that will help to mix the insulin with the clear liquid.

Long-acting basal insulins

The long-acting insulin analogue Lantus can be taken at the evening snack, at bedtime or even in the morning. The injection of Lantus will be effective after 3-4 hours so if you need more insulin effect around midnight, it may be best to take it at the time of the evening meal (7-8 PM). Most people find one daily dose of Lantus is sufficient, but some may need to split the dose and give part of it in the morning (see page 174). You should take at least 40-50% of the total 24-hour insulin dose as long-acting insulin to get a good basal insulin effect (30-40% if you are using short-acting insulin for meals). Remember that these long-acting insulins con-tinue to have an effect even into the next day.

The basal insulin Levemir has a longer action than NPH insulin, but usually not long enough to be given only once daily. In practice, most children will take one dose in the morning and one at bedtime, i.e. approximately the same times as with NPH insulin.

Since long-acting insulins act for up to 24 hours, sometimes even longer, it is important not to change the dose more often than two or three times per week.

Ultratard

Before Lantus and Levemir appeared, the only long-acting insulin available was ultralente insulin from the "lente" type group. Because of the very long action of Ultratard you should take the injection earlier in the evening, e.g. at the evening snack or even at tea-time (if you eat four meals a day, see graph on page 143). The timing is very individual and you will need to experiment to find out what suits you best so that you wake up with a good blood glucose level before breakfast.

With high doses of long-acting ultralente insulin, it is often advisable to divide the dose and take half in the morning and half before dinner/tea, the evening or bedtime meal. If you use rapid-acting insulin (NovoRapid or Humalog) for premeal injections, you will probably need to divide the long-acting basal insulin into two daily injections. Ultratard is not available any more in most countries.

Insulin pump

If you are using an insulin pump, you will take the premeal doses (called bolus doses) by pressing some buttons on the pump. In addition to

Camilla C

this, the pump will deliver small doses of rapid-acting insulin continuously instead of the basal insulin injection, to cover your body's need for a low insulin level in the blood between meals and during the night. See the pump chapter on page 181.

Mixing insulins

Insulin of NPH type (Insulatard, Humulin I, Insuman Basal) can be mixed with both rapid-acting NovoRapid [434] and Humalog [578] and regular short-acting insulin.[476] If, however, you mix insulin of lente type (Monotard, Humulin L, Humulin Zn, Ultratard or similar) with short-acting insulin, you will lose part of the short-acting effect. This is due to an excess of zinc in the Lente insulin that binds to the short-acting insulin and flattens the peak of action, making it more long-acting.[94,476] If you prepare the mixture from vials stored in the refrigerator and inject immediately after mixing in the syringe, this problem seems to be less pronounced.[830] If you use long-acting lente insulins (Ultratard, Humulin Zn) together with short-acting insulin in a multiple injection treatment these should preferably be taken as separate injections.

It is also not a good idea to use lente insulins in indwelling catheters (Insuflon) for the same reason. However, rapid-acting Humalog seems to be an exception to this rule. Mixing Humalog and Ultralente did not change the peak action when injected within 5 minutes of mixing.[70] Mixing the basal insulin analogues Levemir and Lantus with any other insulin is not recommended.[130] However, studies show that Lantus can be mixed with either NovoRapid or Humalog without any negative effect on blood glucose [588] or HbA_{1c} after 3 months.[352]

Depot effect

If only intermediate- or long-acting insulin is used, a depot (store) of insulin is formed in the subcutaneous fat tissue, corresponding to about 24 hours of insulin requirements.[103] The smaller

Jacuzzi pool. Not for people with diabetes!

You may feel sad and disappointed when you see a sign like this, maybe even feel as if you have the plague. The reason for the warning is that insulin will be absorbed faster when the skin is heated by the hot water. This might cause hypoglycaemia. If you are aware of this phenomenon and have taken proper precautions, you can spend time in a spa bath or jacuzzi without worrying. When using rapid-acting insulin (NovoRapid, Humalog) the absorption will be less affected by the skin temperature.

Adults with diabetic foot ulcers or nerve damage have to talk this over with their doctor or chiropodist before using a spa bath, since hot water softens the skin on the feet and increases the risk of infection.

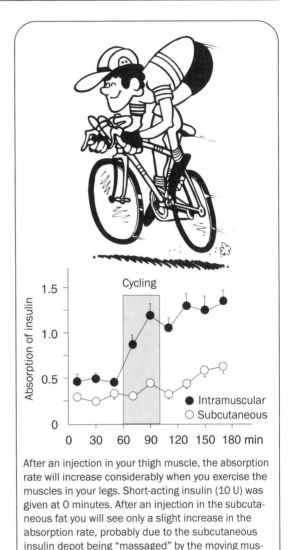

After an injection in your thigh muscle, the absorption rate will increase considerably when you exercise the muscles in your legs. Short-acting insulin (10 U) was given at 0 minutes. After an injection in the subcutaneous fat you will see only a slight increase in the absorption rate, probably due to the subcutaneous insulin depot being "massaged" by the moving muscles.[372]

the share of intermediate- or long-acting insulin you use, the smaller the depot will be. If you are using a multiple injection treatment you will be using less intermediate- or long-acting insulin and the depot will correspond to only about 12 hours of insulin requirements.[103] If the dose of bedtime insulin is changed, the size of the insulin depot makes it necessary to allow 2-3 days for your body to adjust until you see the full effect of the change (see "Basic rules" on page 152).

The disadvantage of a large insulin depot is that the insulin effect will vary from day to day. The disadvantage of a small insulin depot is that little or no extra insulin is stored in your body. The depot functions like a "spare tank" in that the extra insulin stored in your body can be

used if you run short of insulin, for example if you forget an injection. If your insulin needs are increased (e.g. when you get an infection) or if you forget an insulin injection, you are more susceptible to insulin deficiency (elevated levels of ketones, nausea or vomiting). With pump therapy only rapid- or short-acting insulin is used, resulting in a very small depot of insulin. If the insulin supply is stopped or blocked,

Massaging the injection site will increase the absorption of insulin considerably.[674] Short-acting insulin (10 U) was given at 0 minutes. You can do this if you want your short-acting insulin to take particularly rapid effect, for example if you have a high blood glucose level and increased levels of ketones in blood or urine. Give the injection site a thorough rubbing for 15-30 minutes and you will find that the insulin takes effect much faster.

symptoms of insulin deficiency will develop within as little as 4-6 hours (see page 197).

How accurate is your insulin dose?

A correctly used insulin pen will give a very accurate insulin dose with an error of only a few per cent. However, the effect of a given insulin dose also depends on a number of other factors. The effect of an identical dose of insu-

lin, given to an individual at the same site, can vary by as much as 25%. It can vary by nearly 50% when the same dose is given to two different individuals.[470,507] This explains the often very frustrating fact that you can eat the same food, do exactly the same things and give identical doses of insulin for two days in a row, but may get quite different blood glucose results. However, there is less variation with the new basal insulin analogues Lantus and Levemir compared to NPH insulin.

Insulin absorption

The absorption of insulin from the injection site can be influenced by a number of factors. Heat will increase the absorption. If the room temperature increases from 20° to 35° C (68-95° F), the speed of absorption of short-acting insulin will increase by 50-60%.[626] Taking a bath or a sauna at a temperature of 85° C (185° F) may increase the absorption by as much as 110%! In other words, you could be at risk of hypoglycaemia if you inject a bolus of insulin shortly before taking a hot bath. A temperature of just 42° C (108° F) in a shower, spa bath or jacuzzi may double the insulin level in your blood, while a cold bath (22° C, 72° F) will decrease the absorption of insulin.[87] Massage of the injection site for 30 minutes has been found to give higher insulin levels and lower blood glucose, with both short-acting [674] and long-acting insulins.[87]

The skin temperature is also important. In one study, the same insulin injection gave twice the concentration in the blood after 45 minutes when a skin temperature of 37° C was compared with that of 30° C (same room temperature).[971] In the same study, individuals with a thicker subcutaneous fat layer (10 mm) had lower insulin levels than those with a thin subcutaneous fat layer (2 mm).

The absorption of the rapid-acting insulin analogues is less affected by the above mentioned factors, but heating the infusion site of an insulin pump needle can increase the rate of absorption of Humalog and NovoRapid.[877] See also "Where do I inject the insulin?" on page 125.

What happens if a child won't finish a meal?

If it is your child who has diabetes, you will be only too aware as a parent how much your child will eat of any particular dish. If lunch is served at school, it may be helpful, if possible, to read through the school menu in advance and discuss what your child does and doesn't like, and what can be eaten instead. Smaller children are especially unpredictable as to how much they will eat at the time when the insulin is given. If the child eats less than anticipated there will be a risk of hypoglycaemia. It is not ideal to give insulin after the meal, but in exceptional cases it might be the best alternative if you use rapid-acting insulin (NovoRapid [248] or Humalog [278]). Better still try giving insulin corresponding to a smaller meal first and then give the rest of the insulin if the child eats a normal-sized meal after all. If the child uses pump or indwelling catheters (Insuflon or i-Port), the extra dose will not create a problem. We should try to train children to estimate how much food they will eat, and then take the insulin dose before the meal. Otherwise there is a risk that the habit of taking insulin after the meal will carry on until the teenage years, and it is then very easy to forget completely to take the dose.

A child with good glucose control will often have a well-balanced opinion of how much he or she needs to eat. If the blood glucose is high, the child will often not be as hungry as usual and will not need to eat as much but may need a bigger snack later on to balance the insulin level. (see "Hungry or full?" on page 244). Even adults often feel more fullness when the blood glucose level is high.[571]

A practical rule is to always offer bread to eat after a cooked meal so that the child can eat

Sometimes it is difficult to know if a small child will finish a meal. It may then be better to give a smaller insulin dose before the meal to avoid the situation where you will have given a full dose of insulin and the child refuses to eat. If the child has a pump or an indwelling catheter (Insuflon) it is easy to give half the insulin dose before the meal and then add a few units afterwards, depending on how much the child eats (or give a combined bolus with the pump).

enough even if he or she does not like the food that has been served.

If a child has more or less than usual to eat, you can compensate when it is time for the next snack. If the child has had a small lunch, schedule the snack a bit earlier and give him or her a little more at this time, perhaps something extra tasty if appetite has been a problem. If you use rapid-acting insulin (NovoRapid, Humalog, Apidra), you will need to give extra insulin for a snack.

If the child eats less while using twice-daily injections, it may be possible to decrease the dose of rapid-acting (NovoRapid Humalog, Apidra) or short-acting (Actrapid, Humulin S, Insuman Rapid) insulin but give the same dose of intermediate-acting insulin (Insulatard, Humulin I, Insuman Basal).

Factors influencing the insulin effect

① Subcutaneous blood flow
(increased blood flow will give a faster insulin absorption).

Increased by	Heat, e.g. sauna, jacuzzi, hot shower, hot bath or fever.[470,1037] Electrical heating around the pump needle has been tried successfully.[180]
Decreased by	Cold, e.g. a cold bath.[87] Smoking (constriction of the blood vessels).[621,626] Dehydration.[470]
② Injection depth	Faster absorption after an intramuscular injection.[373,1059]
③ Injection site See page 127	An abdominal injection of short-acting insulin will be absorbed faster than a thigh injection. The absorption from the buttocks is slower than from the abdomen but slightly faster than from the thigh.
④ Insulin antibodies	Can bind the insulin resulting in a slower and less predictable effect.
⑤ Exercise	Increases the absorption of short-acting insulin even after you have finished exercising, particularly if the injection is given intramuscularly.[371,626]
⑥ Massage of the injection site	Increased absorption of short-acting insulin, probably due to a faster breakdown of the insulin.[674]
⑦ Subcutaneous fat thickness	A thicker layer of subcutaneous fat gives a slower absorption of insulin.[500,971]
⑧ Injection in fatty lumps (lipohypertrophies)	Slower[1128] and more erratic absorption of insulin.
⑨ Concentration of the insulin	40 U/ml is absorbed faster than 100 U/ml.[373]

What if you forget to take your insulin?

You can try the following suggestions if you have had diabetes for some time and are confident about how the insulin you inject works. *If you are even slightly unsure you should contact the hospital or diabetes clinic.*

Forgotten premeal injection (multiple injection treatment)

Take the same dose of insulin if you remember immediately after you have eaten or within one hour. If 2 or 3 hours have passed, measure your blood glucose level and give a dose corresponding to ½ the meal bolus and if needed correct according to the correction factor. If you remember first at the next meal, give extra insulin according to the correction factor along with that meal bolus.

If you are out clubbing, remember that dancing is exercise too. Don't forget to eat something during the evening. Because of the exercise you will probably not need an extra meal injection, that is if you are not planning on staying up very late. You may also need to decrease your bedtime injection by 2-4 units (decrease by 10-20% using the temporary basal rate if on a pump) to avoid hypoglycaemia if you have been dancing a great deal.

Forgotten bedtime injection (multiple injection treatment)

If you are using NPH at bedtime (9-11 PM) and you wake up before 2 AM you can still take your forgotten bedtime insulin (of NPH type), but you should decrease the dose by 25-30% or 1-2 units for every hour that has passed since the normal time of injection. If there are less than 5 hours before your usual waking time, measure your blood glucose and take an injection of regular short-acting insulin if you have this. You can try a dose with one third or a quarter of the number of units of your normal bedtime injection of intermediate-acting insulin. However, never inject more than 0.1 U/kg (0.5 U/10 lb) of body weight at one time. Novo-Rapid or Humalog will have too short an insulin action in this situation.

If you have forgotten your evening or bedtime Lantus or Levemir dose you can take the same number of units when you remember it, as long as only a few hours have passed. You may need a small dose of NovoRapid or Humalog if your blood glucose has already risen. If you only take basal insulin in the evening and remember in the morning, try taking approximately half of the Lantus or Levemir dose you should have taken in the evening. If you take Lantus or Levemir twice daily, take the morning dose as usual. If your blood glucose is high, take some extra mealtime insulin for breakfast according to the correction factor.

If you wake up with high blood sugar, nausea and elevated levels of ketones in your blood or urine, you have symptoms of insulin deficiency. Take 0.1 U/kg (0.5 U/10 lb) body weight of insulin (preferably rapid-acting NovoRapid or Humalog) and measure your blood glucose again after 1-2 hours. If your glucose level has not decreased after 2 hours, take another dose of 0.1 U/kg (0.5 U/10 lb) body weight. *If you are still feeling sick or if you vomit, you should contact your doctor immediately.*

Forgotten injection with twice-daily treatment

If, for example, you forget the morning dose, take the same dose or decrease the regular short-acting (or rapid-acting) part by 1 or 2 units if you remember immediately after having eaten (but take the same NPH dose). If you remember after an hour or two, you can try decreasing the rapid- or short-acting part by about half and the intermediate part by about 25%. If you remember your injection even later, measure your blood glucose before the next meal and take only rapid- or short-acting insulin at this meal. If you are using pre-mixed insulin, it won't be possible to decrease only one of the components. Give a smaller dose of this insulin when you remember, or use only rapid- or short-acting insulin until it is time for the afternoon injection.

If you have forgotten your dinner/tea injection and remembered in the evening (three or more hours after dinner), you must take a smaller dose of intermediate-acting insulin before going to bed. A little more than half should be enough but you must test this with blood glucose controls. You will probably also need an injection of rapid- or short-acting insulin at your evening snack. Try the same dose (or a few units less) than the rapid- or short-acting part of your afternoon injection. You should check your blood glucose at night to avoid hypoglycaemia.

What if you take the wrong type of insulin?

At bedtime

Taking your premeal insulin instead of the bedtime insulin by mistake when going to bed is not uncommon. This may happen if your day and night pen injectors are very similar. Long-acting Lantus insulin is a clear solution so it can be easy to mistake short-acting or rapid-acting insulin for the long-acting variety if both are drawn from vials and given with syringes.[9]

This can be frightening, but it is not a catastrophe! However, you may have problems with low blood glucose for a couple of hours and you will have a rather sleepless night as you will need to check your blood glucose levels at frequent intervals during it. Make sure you are not alone at home, as you will need somebody awake and ready to help you throughout the night. If you are alone in this situation, you would be best off going to hospital.

You need to have glucose and food close at hand. Start by checking your blood glucose values at least every hour, and more frequently if your blood glucose falls below 6 mmol/l (110 mg/dl). Eat extra meals during the night, preferably food that is rich in carbohydrates but contains as little fat as possible. If you need to take glucose to counter hypoglycaemia, the effect will be much slower if you have a fat-rich meal in your stomach. If you happen to take a large dose of NovoRapid or Humalog instead of bedtime insulin, you should expect a very rapid insulin effect. In this situation, it is even more important that what you eat is rich in carbohydrates and low in fat.

If you practise carbohydrate counting, you can count backwards to find out how much carbohydrate you need to eat to match the extra amount of premeal insulin. For example, if you have taken 20 U of Lantus and your carbohydrate ratio is 12 (1 unit of insulin takes care of 12 g of carbohydrates), multiply 20 with 12 = 240 g carbohydrates. This means you will need to eat approximately 240 g carbohydrate to avoid a low blood glucose. Begin by drinking something sweet, then top up with some sweets, for example.

What if I do not have a carbohydrate ratio?

Well, then you can use the 500-rule: Divide 500 by your total daily insulin dose (including basal insulin and mealtime insulin). If, for example, you take 50U in total per day, the ratio will be 500/50 = 10, i.e. one unit of insulin takes care of 10 g of carbohydrates. See also the calculations on page 248 about a child who had taken too large a dose of insulin.

Taking the wrong type of insulin will only be dangerous if you take short- or rapid-acting insulin at bedtime without noticing it. If you are used to low blood glucose levels, your body might not give any warning symptoms until the blood glucose is dangerously low (see "Hypoglycaemia unawareness" on page 52). See also page 61.

Remember that the effect of rapid-acting insulin usually diminishes after 4-5 hours. Short-acting insulin will last a little longer, especially if you have taken a dose larger than 10 units. Because of this, you need to take your bedtime dose of intermediate- or long-acting insulin as well, but lower it to approximately half the dose, and wait until a few hours after taking the accidental injection before giving it. In the morning you can take your breakfast insulin as usual, adjusting it according to your morning blood glucose reading. If you take basal insulin twice daily, you might as well omit the bedtime dose in this situation and check your blood glucose during the night. Give some extra rapid- or short-acting insulin if and when your blood glucose starts rising in the morning hours.

During the day

If you happen to take a dose of intermediate-acting or long-acting analogue insulin instead of your mealtime rapid- or short-acting insulin during the day, it will not give you much of a blood glucose-lowering effect for that meal. The effect will come some hours later. If, for example, you have taken the wrong type of insulin for breakfast (on a multiple injection treatment), you can try taking a small dose (roughly 3/4 of your ordinary dose of rapid-acting insulin, half of short-acting regular insulin) of your ordinary premeal insulin as well, to help take care of your breakfast. Measure your blood glucose before the next meal. Here the extra basal insulin begins to kick in, so half your ordinary dose might be appropriate. Continue with lower mealtime doses during the day depending on your blood glucose levels.

Having a lie in at weekends

You can sleep a little longer at weekends without problems. One hour more is rarely a problem and usually you can even extend your lie in for 2 hours. When using one of the long-acting Lantus or Levemir insulins, having a lie in is usually not a problem. Take the injection at the usual time even if you are staying up late. If you take the basal insulin twice daily, you can probably give the morning injection when you wake up if it is not too late. Check your blood glucose level to find out if this works for you. If you use an insulin pump, having a lie in will not cause a problem as long as you have adjusted the basal rate to keep your blood glucose levels at the same level in the morning even if you don't have breakfast (see page 212).

Some people with diabetes experience problems with high morning blood glucose (see page 170), and they will find it difficult to sleep longer since their glucose level can rise rapidly during the early hours. This is more common when using NPH insulin as your basal insulin. In some families this may be solved by parents giving an early morning injection. The child or teenager can then sleep in for an hour while

their blood glucose starts to decrease before having breakfast.

If you stay up late at night and plan to sleep in late in the morning, you should take your bedtime NPH insulin when you go to bed. It will then last the duration of a normal night's sleep, including the extra hours in the morning. Your blood glucose may rise after midnight when the morning dose of NPH is no longer effective, but this can be solved by an extra night meal and an insulin dose.

If you are planning on having an early breakfast, however, you should decrease the bedtime NPH dose as the night will then be shorter than usual. Otherwise there is a risk of hypoglycaemia when your breakfast insulin starts working.

If you have a late breakfast, your lunch will usually be a little late too, since you will not be as hungry by your normal lunchtime. In this way your whole day will be shifted and you will usually have no problem spreading your meals evenly over the day. Just remember that the time between the injections of regular short-acting insulin should not exceed 5 hours. With rapid-acting insulin analogues, this time interval is less important since the need for insulin between the meals is covered by the basal insulin.

If you stay awake very late (2-3 AM), you will probably want to eat a night meal and should then take insulin along with it.

When switching time with daylight savings at summertime and wintertime, you need only adjust your watch. You do not need to gradually adjust the time for meals and insulin injections.

Staying awake all night

Being up all night is not common practice, but it is sometimes unavoidable for teenagers or young adults. One of our patients, an 18-year-old boy, worked as a travel guide and was required to stay awake all night in the bus on the way to a ski resort. During intercontinental flights, people often have to stay awake for long periods (see "Passing through time zones" on page 346).

If you stay awake all night you can take the dose of long-acting analogues as usual. Take a meal bolus when you eat, for example during a long flight. If there is a time shift towards a shorter day, decrease the basal insulin. If the day gets longer, the easiest way is to take a small dose of long-acting insulin to cover this. If, for example, you travel from Europe to USA (6-8 hours of time difference), you can take extra basal insulin approximately 12 hours (when taking basal insulin twice daily) or 24 hours (when taking basal insulin once daily) after your latest basal dose before leaving home.

If you use regular short-acting insulin for meals and one bedtime injection of NPH, you should not take your bedtime insulin when awake at night. Instead, inject your premeal regular insulin when you eat every fourth or fifth hour as this will give you a good basal effect as well.

Adjust the dose according to how much you eat (compare the carbohydrate content of your meal with your usual lunch, dinner/tea or evening snack). You should not use the amount of insulin taken at breakfast for comparison because more insulin is commonly needed for breakfast (see "Starting insulin treatment" on page 142). If you use rapid-acting insulin (NovoRapid or Humalog), and twice-daily intermediate-acting basal insulin (Insulatard, Humulin I, Insuman Basal), you may need to take half the night time dose to cover your basal need for insulin during a long-distance flight.

Shift work

It may be difficult to combine diabetes with shift work. When you come back home after a night shift you will need to take insulin to cover both the meal you will eat and the background insulin you will need while you sleep during the day. Long-acting analogues (Lantus or Levemir) together with rapid-acting insulin as mealtime insulin will probably be a better solution in this situation as its effect will have declined before the basal insulin has reached a higher effect. You can try giving Lantus or Levemir at the same time points every day.

With regular short-acting insulin there will be a risk of overlapping effects, which could cause hypoglycaemia after 3-4 hours, especially if you use NPH as your basal insulin. You will then probably need to lower the morning NPH dose before going to sleep. An insulin pump may be easier to use in this situation, since you can easily adapt the basal rates to your shift hours.

Birthday parties

It is very important for children with diabetes to be able to take part in birthday parties or school parties without being embarrassed about having diabetes. We believe people with diabetes should learn how to handle whatever food is served at a party instead of bringing their own "diabetes food". It is often a good idea to call the parents giving the party beforehand and ask them to provide drinks containing artificial sweeteners (preferably the same for all children so that a child with diabetes will not feel singled out). You can also request that not too many "goodies" be served. Older children will learn to ask for non-sugary drinks. At many parties, the children receive a bag of sweets at the end to take home rather than eating sweet things all through the party, which works particularly well for a child with diabetes.

Food served at birthday parties these days tends not to be as sweet as it used to be. There may be cake or ice cream on the menu, but preceded by pizza, hamburgers or hot dogs. Try giving an extra unit of insulin with the birthday cake, depending on the size of the cake slices and also on the amount of activity (running around, dancing and so on) that is likely to happen at the party. If the party is a very active one, the child may not need any extra insulin at all! It is a good idea to check your child's blood glucose level once the party is over and make a note of the result in your logbook. This will help you plan ahead for the next party.

If your child is at nursery or playgroup, the best time to celebrate a birthday may well be during break time. Make sure that all drinks for your child (and preferably for the other children as well) contain artificial sweeteners. Staff are usually very obliging for the small extra arrangements needed to accommodate a child with diabetes. Depending on the activity, you might need to give an extra unit of insulin if birthday cake or other sweet foods are served. Use the carbohydrate ratio or "measurement by eye" for dosing.

If you are taking your child to an adult tea party, you are likely to find biscuits, cakes and other sweet things being served. Your child will need extra insulin to be able to pick and choose from all that is on offer. Try to find some kind of compromise here, for example only a few biscuits or a small piece of cake (and 1 or 2 extra units of insulin or according to the carbohydrate ratio). It is generally not a good idea to eat too much of everything offered at a party. And do tell grandparents (who have only their grandchild's best interests at heart) that so called "sugar-free" biscuits or "diabetes cookies" are not a very good alternative. They are often not sugar-free at all and, anyway, many children find their taste disgusting.

Of course, how you manage will depend on how often you or your child go to parties. Once in a while, a person with diabetes can certainly make an exception and accept some sweets or a piece of cake if it is offered. But if exceptions are being made every week, they cease to be exceptions. Eating too many sweet things too often will affect both your weight and your long-term blood glucose levels.

Insulin at school and day nurseries

Sometimes it is difficult to get help with insulin injections at a day care centre or nursery, or to get the teacher to remind the child to take their insulin at school. The staff have no formal obligation to give injections when needed, but some schools have a nurse or teaching assistant who will help. At some larger schools where several pupils have diabetes, they might meet at lunch-time to eat together, and a staff member may be able to be on hand to help them if necessary. If food is served at the school, the cafeteria staff might be able to help with the carbohydrate counting. See also page 328.

Sleeping away from home

Many children thoroughly enjoy having "sleepovers" at friends' homes. This often means late night talking or playing games. It is advisable for the child to have a "midnight snack" to prevent hypoglycaemia. However, it is quite natural for parents of children with diabetes to be worried when faced with this situation. It is easy to be overprotective if you don't feel confident about how to deal with it. It is important that the friend's parents are familiar with how and when a child should take his or her insulin, and what to do if the child develops hypoglycaemia. A good idea is to write down a list of instructions for the child with when and how much insulin should be taken depending on the food eaten and blood glucose measurements. Don't forget to leave your telephone number if you will be out for the night, or have your mobile phone available.

Monitoring

"Everyone is like a child when starting something new." This saying is particularly relevant to the adjusting of insulin dosages. It is difficult, if not impossible, to manage your diabetes without monitoring it at home. Trying to manage your diabetes without home monitoring is like driving a car without a milometer, fuel gauge, or temperature gauge. Without these instruments, your car may run for a little while, but you will probably end up in the wrong place or have a breakdown.

Measuring your blood glucose level is like checking the fuel gauge in your car. The difference is that you don't just need to be careful to avoid running out of petrol (sugar) but you need to make sure the level doesn't go too high either.

Glucose monitoring can be divided into:

①	Immediate tests	Tests that you can perform at any given moment, in order to find out what your blood glucose level is, or whether your ketone level is raised.
②	Routine tests	Tests that you perform regularly, and which help you to make long-term adjustments in your insulin doses, eating habits and other activities.
③	Continuous glucose monitoring	A subcutaneous sensor gives continuous glucose readings for several days. These can be displayed on a monitor or downloaded to a computer.
④	Long-range tests	Tests that reflect your diabetes control over a long period of time. These include such tests as fructosamine and HbA$_{1c}$.

How many tests should I take?

Blood tests

It is recommended practice to take a 24-hour glucose profile at least every other week, even for very young children.[695] This means measuring your blood glucose before and 1.5-2 hours after each meal (including the evening snack) as well as once during the night, preferably between 2 and 3 AM. It is also a good idea to

Timetable of monitoring

Test	Reflects the blood glucose levels over:
Blood glucose	Minutes
Urine glucose	Hours
Fructosamine	2-3 weeks
HbA$_{1c}$	2-3 months

Symptoms of hypoglycaemia from the body

Bodily symptoms (autonomic and adrenergic symptoms) are the result of both adrenaline secretion and the autonomic nervous system. They usually start when the blood glucose concentration dips below 3.5-4 mmol/l (65-70 mg/dl). The threshold for triggering these symptoms will change depending on the person's recent blood glucose concentrations (the "blood glucose thermostat", see page 44). In very young children, bodily symptoms of hypoglycaemia are reported less frequently, if at all.[1052]

⟹ Irritability.

⟹ Hunger, feeling sick.

⟹ Trembling.

⟹ Anxiety.

⟹ Heart palpitations.

⟹ Throbbing pulse in the chest and abdomen.

⟹ Numbness in the lips, fingers and tongue.

⟹ Looking pale.

⟹ Cold sweats.

Different types of hypoglycaemia

⟹ **Mild hypoglycaemia**
Self-treatment is possible and blood glucose levels are easily restored.

⟹ **Moderate hypoglycaemia**
Your body reacts with warning symptoms of hypoglycaemia (autonomic symptoms) and you can take appropriate action. Self-treatment is possible.

⟹ **Hypoglycaemia unawareness**
You experience symptoms from the brain (neuroglycopenic symptoms) without having had any bodily (autonomic) warning symptoms beforehand. However, it is obvious to people observing you that you are having symptoms.

⟹ **Severe hypoglycaemia**
Severe symptoms of hypoglycaemia disable you temporarily, requiring the assistance of another person to give you something to eat or a glucagon injection. Severe hypoglycaemia can cause you to lose consciousness and have seizures.

and friends understand that when you are having a hypoglycaemic reaction you are not quite in control of yourself, and cannot help what you are doing.

Even if individuals with diabetes are aware of having symptoms of hypoglycaemia, they may find it difficult to eat or drink. This can still be a problem if food is right in front of them. It

might be difficult for parents to understand that their child can react so oddly, but adults with diabetes have described the feeling as follows: "You know you should drink the juice, but your body just does not obey the orders from the brain".

If the blood glucose is lowered quickly, even if it stays within the normal range, symptoms of hypoglycaemia can be provoked in certain people. This type of reaction is more common in people with a high HbA_{1c}[749] (see page 119) but there may be a difference between children and adults. In one study, the blood glucose level in a group of adults with diabetes with an HbA_{1c} of 97 mmol/mol (11%) went down from 20 to 10 mmol/l (360 to 180 mg/dl) using intravenous insulin.[316] These subjects showed the same type of increased blood flow to the brain that both people in good control and people without diabetes had at a blood glucose of 2.2 mmol/l (40

r-a = rapid-acting insulin, LA = Lantus

A 24-hour glucose profile can look like this when you take blood glucose tests before and 1.5 hours after meals. It is a good idea to combine the individual readings by drawing a line to link them if the readings are not more than 3-4 hours apart, which also makes it easier to read the chart. You will gather more information if you frequently test the urine passed first thing in the morning for glucose and ketones on the same day you perform the 24-hour glucose profile. Today, most blood glucose meters have a memory but it is still very valuable to record every test and insulin dose in a logbook to be able to recognize patterns after meals and other daily events.

Remember that you will not know anything about your blood glucose levels in between the times when you have performed tests. From the test results this chart may appear reassuring, but it covers the same day as the chart on the left, except with fewer readings. It is easy to fool yourself into believing that the lines also reflect the blood glucose levels in between the individual readings. But look at the urine test results. They show that glucose has been excreted into the urine, which indicates that the blood glucose must have been high somewhere in between the blood glucose measuring tests.

take a test before every meal, as a matter of daily routine, to help you adjust your dosages. Monitoring on other occasions should serve to answer a specific question such as: "Is this the beginning of a hypoglycaemic reaction?", "Can I get through the night without eating something extra?", or "How much insulin should I take in the morning?" There is no point in taking tests unless you are going to respond to the results.

Four or more blood glucose tests per day (before each main meal and before going to bed) are necessary to give the information needed to adjust your insulin doses from day to day in order to give you an acceptable level of control over your diabetes.[970] More frequent monitoring is needed in situations when you change your diet or other habits. After a while you will be more familiar with how much insulin is needed in different situations and you will then be able to get away with fewer tests.

You will need to test more frequently at times when your insulin requirements are changing. These include, for example, periods when you are under stress, if you have an infection, when you are exercising vigorously or playing sports, or if you are eating out or going to a party. At such times, it is a good idea to take a blood glucose test before and 1.5-2 hours after each meal and, if necessary, to change the dose accordingly. If you want to see what effect "quick-act-ing" carbohydrates (like sweets) have on your blood glucose, you should test this about 30 minutes after eating them. With slower carbo-hydrates, like chocolate or ice cream, measure your blood glucose level after 1-1.5 hours.

Urine tests

Although urine glucose monitoring is no longer recommended as the primary method of glucose monitoring,[31] it does have its advantages. Urine glucose monitoring can be particularly useful in situations where blood glucose monitoring is difficult or impractical, provided that the level of renal threshold is known. In the case of a small child who is still in nappies, it will usually be possible to squeeze a drop of urine out of the nappy for testing.

Measuring urine glucose is a "screening method" in that it enables you to determine when during the day glucose is excreted. When you have established this, you can follow up with blood glucose tests. This can be practical in periods when your diabetes is very stable, for example during the "honeymoon" phase. A urine glucose test can add information to the blood glucose test in the morning about the night time glucose levels (see page 171).

mmol/l and mg/dl			
mmol/l	mg/dl	mg/dl	mmol/l
1	18	20	1.1
2	36	40	2.2
3	54	60	3.3
4	72	80	4.4
5	90	100	5.6
6	108	120	6.7
7	126	140	7.8
8	144	160	8.9
9	162	180	10.0
10	180	200	11.1
12	216	220	12.2
14	252	250	13.9
16	288	300	16.7
18	324	350	19.4
20	360	400	22.2
22	396	450	25.0

The numbers in this book refer to plasma glucose unless otherwise stated, as this is what most new patient meters display. Plasma glucose levels are also used by doctors to diagnose diabetes, and in most studies. Plasma glucose is approximately 11% higher than whole blood glucose.[357]

It is a good idea for younger children to get into the habit of taking a urine test every time they go to the toilet, or in the morning if no tests were taken during the night.

Ketones could earlier only be measured in urine tests but there are now good methods available for measuring ketones in the blood at home. The blood strips for ketones are much more expensive in many countries, however, and this can make using urine strips more practical. Urine strips may be better to use for screening for ketones, but once detected, following the blood ketones gives you more accurate guid-ance (see page 115).

"Good" or "bad" tests?

It is common to refer to normal blood glucose readings as "good" and high readings as "bad". A young person who hears these terms used fre-quently may begin to look upon him or herself as "bad". "High blood glucose" sounds more neutral and is a more appropriate term. Test

Send your blood glucose charts by email or fax to your diabetes healthcare team and you can discuss them over the telephone. It may even be possible to send them by e-mail. Check this with your clinic.

24-hour profile tests

Blood tests:

① Before each meal.

② 1.5-2 hours after each meal.

③ One test during the night depending on which bedtime insulin you use:
2-3 AM: NPH insulin
(Insulatard, Humulin I, Insuman Basal)
3-4 AM: Lente insulin (Monotard, Humutard)
3-5 AM: Long-acting insulin
(Lantus, Levemir, Ultratard, Humulin Zn).

④ In many cases more intensive monitoring may be needed at times, with premeal and pre-snack blood glucose values along with tests every 2-3 hours during the night.

results are just pieces of information, and do not reflect on the quality of the person with diabetes.

Diabetes or not?

In a person who does not have diabetes, the blood glucose level will be regulated within close limits (normally between 3.3 and 7 mmol/l, 60-125 mg/dl). This is despite the fact that the intake and expenditure of food vary enormously throughout the day from one person to another. In the fasting state, the blood glucose level is normally below 5.6 mmol/l (100 mg/dl). Higher values indicate that the person's body is not able to handle glucose in the way that it should (impaired glucose tolerance). A fasting plasma glucose level greater than 7.0 mmol/l (126 mg/dl), or a non-fasting casual plasma glucose level higher than 11.1 mmol/l (200 mg/dl) with symptoms of diabetes (thirst, unexplained weight loss and needing to go to the toilet a lot more than usual), indicates that a person has diabetes.[27] The diagnosis should be confirmed by repeat testing on a different day unless the blood glucose is very high or ketones are present.

You should not rely on home blood glucose meters in order to diagnose diabetes. If an adult person without diabetes has recorded a high reading, you should never announce to the person "you probably have diabetes". Instead, ask them to check their fasting blood glucose with their doctor. If you are measuring an elevated value in a child, take the child to the doctor the same day.

Are some things forbidden?

We are often asked whether you are allowed to do this or that when you have diabetes. The best answer is that nothing is totally forbidden (except smoking!). It is important, however, to experiment in order to find out what you as an individual can and cannot do. It is a good idea to experiment with both food and insulin, provided this is done in conjunction with blood glucose monitoring. The only risk you are running is of having a temporarily high or low blood glucose.

Always write in your logbook the results of your tests along with details of the activity you were participating in. Next time you play rugby, or go for a pizza or to a party, you will find your notes really valuable.

Urine glucose

All the urine produced by your kidneys is collected in your bladder. This means that when you measure urine glucose, it will reflect an average blood glucose level since the last time you passed urine. It is also important to remember that urine glucose concentration is measured as a percentage. This means that 5% will represent much less glucose when you have small amounts of urine than if you have large amounts of urine with 5% glucose. A negative glucose reading says nothing about how low the blood glucose is or has been, only that is has not been above the renal threshold since the last time you went to the toilet.

You can determine your renal threshold by checking your blood glucose every 30 minutes, while watching for glucose to be shown in the urine. You can test this either as the blood glucose is going up or as it is going down. In this chart, the test taken in the morning contained glucose until the blood glucose dropped to between 11 and 9 mmol/l (200 and 160 mg/dl). In the afternoon, glucose was noted in the urine when the blood glucose rose from 9 to 10 mmol/l (160 to 180 mg/dl). This implies the person's renal threshold is between 9 and 10 mmol/l (160 and 180 mg/dl).

Renal threshold

The kidneys produce urine. They also try to reabsorb as much glucose as possible, so there is normally no glucose in the urine. When the blood glucose is above a certain level, the kidneys' "glucose absorption pump" becomes saturated and glucose will be passed out with the urine instead. The level where this happens is called the renal threshold and is usually 8-10 mmol/l (145-180 mg/dl) in children,[691] and 7-12 mmol/l (125-215 mg/dl) in adults. The renal

It may be difficult to attain urine samples from modern nappies, which often absorb urine very effectively. Try putting a piece of cloth inside the nappy to absorb some urine. It is easier to squeeze a couple of drops of urine out of an older-style disposable nappy (with a plastic covering), or a towelling nappy.

	Urine tests	
Glucose	Ketones	Interpretation
0	0	OK (can have been low).
+	0	Too much glucose (or more insulin needed).
+	+	Not enough insulin ("diabetes ketones").
0	+	Not enough food ("starvation ketones").

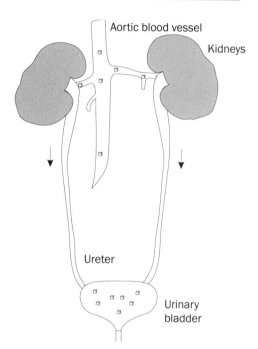

When the blood glucose level is higher than the renal threshold (usually 8-10 mmol/l, 145-180 mg/dl) glucose will appear in the urine. The urine from the kidneys collects in the bladder before urination.

When the blood glucose level has returned to normal values, glucose will stop leaking from the kidneys. However, there will still be glucose from the urine held in the bladder, as the fresh urine takes some time to clear from the body. So, when you take your next urine test you will find a high urine glucose, although by this time your blood glucose level will be registering as normal (see also the charts on page 171).

threshold usually increases with age. Certain individuals have a very low renal threshold, down to 5 mmol/l (90 mg/dl), while others have a high threshold of up to 15 mmol/l (270 mg/dl). It is important to know your renal threshold when interpreting urine tests.

You can determine your renal threshold by checking your blood glucose and passing urine once every 30 minutes. If there is glucose in the urine and your blood glucose is decreasing, your renal threshold will be the level at which

the urine is negative for glucose. If the blood glucose is increasing and your urine tests are negative for glucose, the renal threshold will be at a level where glucose is first noted in the urine (see chart on page 101). The renal threshold does not affect kidney function, but if your renal threshold is either very high or very low, you will find urine tests less reliable.

Blood glucose

When you take a blood test it will reflect your blood glucose level at that moment. However, the blood glucose can go up or down very quickly, and you may have quite a different reading 15 or 30 minutes later. Always check your blood glucose level when you are not feeling well so that you can avoid eating extra just to be on the safe side when you suspect hypoglycaemia. This is especially important in the early days of being diagnosed with diabetes, when you are not yet fully familiar with all the symptoms of hypoglycaemia. Later on, you will become more confident about these. (See also "Symptoms of hypoglycaemia when the blood glucose level is high" on page 47.)

Recognizing symptoms of high blood glucose is usually more difficult. However, teenagers often seem to learn how their body reacts when their blood glucose is high. Some develop a kind of "auto-pilot" which enables them to adjust insulin doses and food portions without as many blood tests as might be expected. Always try to guess your blood glucose level before checking it, and you will eventually become familiar with the way your body reacts when your blood glucose level is low or high.

How do I take blood tests?

Wash your hands with soap and water before taking a blood test. This is not just to ensure hygiene (though of course that is important), but to ensure there is no sugar on your fingers giving a false high reading, for example from glucose tablets, sweets or fruit. Use warm water if your fingers are cold. Do not use alcohol for cleaning your hands as this will make your skin dry. The risk of an infection from a finger prick is minimal.

There are a variety of different finger-pricking devices for taking blood glucose tests. With

It is easier to estimate low blood glucose values than high ones. In an American study of adults with diabetes, individuals were asked to estimate their blood glucose values.[1095] Potentially serious errors (dangerous failure to treat high/low blood glucose or erroneous treatment) were made by 17% when their blood glucose was 1.9 mmol/l (34 mg/dl) but by as many as 66% when the blood glucose was 18.4 mmol/l (330 mg/dl).

some you can adjust the pricking depth. Pricking devices and lancets can vary considerably in size and the way they puncture the skin. Try different types to find out which suits you best. From the point of view of hygiene, you can use the same lancet for a day's blood tests assuming that your fingers are clean. However, the lancet will be very slightly blunted every time you use it, so the pricks might become more painful with repeated usage.

If you prick the sides of your fingertips, your sensitivity will be less affected, which may be important if you play the piano or guitar, for example. Don't use your thumbs and right index finger (or left if you are left-handed) for finger-pricking. You need the sensation of touch most in these places and sometimes you will even feel pain the day after a finger prick.

Most blood glucose meters have memories for storing test results and can show the average of your readings over 1-4 weeks, which will give you a good picture of how your blood glucose levels have been during this time. The stored information can be transferred to a computer to view, analyse and print. This may be a very useful tool for young people with diabetes who may be interested, as well as for their parents and members of the diabetes team. Some newer meters have built-in blood glucose graphing programmes for summarizing patterns of blood glucose control.

Borrowing someone else's finger-pricking device

Borrowing another person's device for pricking your fingers is not a good idea. This is because one small drop of blood left on the device can cause contamination if it is infected. For example, an epidemic of hepatitis B in a hospital ward was caused by using the same pricking device (Autolet®) despite switching lancets between each test.[302]

Does the meter show the correct value?

The margin of error in a correctly used blood glucose meter should not be larger than ±20% for 95% of the tests. This means that with a blood glucose level of 20 mmol/l (360 mg/dl), the meter can show 4 mmol/l, 72 mg/dl above or below the correct value. However, at a blood glucose of 3 mmol/l (55 mg/dl) the error should not exceed 0.6 mmol/l (10 mg/dl). A new standard that states a maximum of ±15% for 99% of the tests is being implemented. Some meters on the market already perform within ±15%. It is very important to apply enough blood to the strip. Too small a drop may give a false low reading. Don't rub the blood onto the strip. If you have sugar on your fingers when you take the test, this will cause a false high reading.

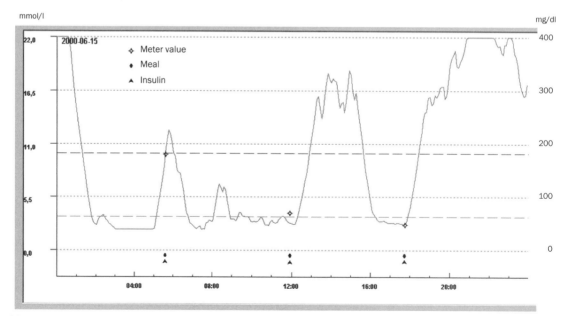

MiniMed Medtronic CGMS (Continuous Glucose Monitoring System) chart showing wide fluctuations of glucose levels during the day and night in a 16-year-old boy with an HbA$_{1c}$ of 55 mmol/mol (7.2%). The three tests that the boy took (¤) are not sufficient to detect patterns that can lead to appropriate changes in insulin dosages. The dashed lines represent 3.0 and 10 mmol/l (55 and 180mg/dl).

Why take blood tests?

☞ *Advantages*

➤ You can take a test instead of eating "just to be on the safe side".

➤ Helps you learn about hypoglycaemia and its symptoms.

➤ Lets you know when you need to change insulin doses, e.g. with infections, stress, physical exercise or going to a party.

➤ The only way to find out if you have night time hypoglycaemia.

➤ Blood glucose monitoring is necessary to get good glucose control and in the long run lessen the risk of complications as much as possible.

☞ *Disadvantages*

➤ Pricking your finger can be painful.

➤ Monitoring takes time and extra effort.

Sources of error when measuring blood glucose

False high reading	False low reading
Glucose on fingers	Drop applied too late
	Finger removed too quickly
	Not enough blood on the strip
	Water or saliva on finger

Regular use of the control strip or control solution provided with your meter for calibration is very important to get and maintain reliable values.

Ask your diabetes nurse for advice about the available meters and their prices. You can often can get a discount on the cost of a new meter if you hand in your old one at the time of purchase.

Comparing different meters can be confusing as they often show different readings. For example, one may show a blood glucose level of 12 mmol/l (215 mg/dl), while another (used at the same time on the same patient) shows a level of 14 mmol/l (250 mg/dl). However, this difference is well within the error margins stated by the manufacturers of the meters. It is advisable to stick to one meter that works well, as the difference of 1 or 2 mmol/l is not particularly significant at high readings. Bring the meter with you when you come to clinic, and ask your diabetes nurse to check your meter with glucose control solution at regular intervals.

In hospital, blood for glucose monitoring is often taken through an intravenous needle to lessen the pain. In people without diabetes, venous blood tested after a meal has about 10% less glucose than capillary blood. This is logical if you remember that venous blood has already delivered some of the glucose it contains to the body tissues. However, in people with diabetes, the difference was only 0.1 mmol/l (2 mg/dl).[649] This can probably be explained by the lack of fine-tuned insulin release in response to the blood glucose level.

Some meters based on a new technology (glucose dehydrogenase), for example Ascensia Contour, Accu-check Compact and Freestyle, gave more accurate readings at high altitude when tested in a hypobaric pressure chamber at 2,500 and 4,500 metres above sea level.[804] However, when tested at low temperature of 8° C (46° F) at ground level, some meters overestimated and some underestimated by approximately 8 mmol/l (145 mg/dl). When tested at the summit of Mount Kilimanjaro (5,895 m above sea level), results varied between 2.8 and 21 mmol/l (50 and 380 mg/dl) between the meters. From this follows that you must be aware that if you participate in activities at high altitude or, in particular, low temperature,

You can try to anaesthetize the fingertip with a piece of ice before pricking it. A topical anaesthetic cream (EMLA®, Ametop®) will not work on your fingertips as the skin is too thick. Pricking slightly on the side of the fingertip is preferable since it bleeds well and hurts less.

blood glucose meters may give totally unreliable false low or high readings.

Children and blood glucose tests

Small children think of their body as a balloon. If you puncture a balloon it will burst and the contents will pour out. A child may think, quite logically, "If I have a lot of jabs for blood tests, won't all the blood go out of my body?" The sticking plaster that is put over the puncture wound has an added significance: it can be seen as stopping the body contents from being poured out. Even those children who don't ask what will happen to their body need to be reassured that the doctors and nurses will take only a tiny amount of blood for the test and the body will quickly produce new blood again. The red blood cells are produced in the bone marrow, and live for only about 120 days. This means that there is a continuous production of new red blood cells going on in the body.

At times, it may be difficult to make your own child agree to giving a drop of blood for monitoring if the pricking hurts. If a small child struggles, the whole procedure will be more painful for everyone involved. Child psychologists recommend that, in this situation, the par-

ents (preferably both together) hold the child tightly in order to get the pricking done as quickly and efficiently as possible. After it is done, it is important to comfort the child. Remind the child that struggling makes the test more painful, especially as they are likely to need several jabs rather than just one if they are wriggling and fighting. It is also a good idea to let young children watch their parents and members of the diabetes team take blood tests from themselves, so they can see that is doesn't hurt too much if they remain calm. Remember that the goal is to get your child to accept blood glucose monitoring in the long run, not only for the time being.

If the child is feeling unwell it is important to emphasize that after taking a blood glucose test you will be able to do something to make the symptoms better. When children have experienced actually feeling better after testing and taking the necessary measures, they are often more willing to take the test the next time it is necessary.

Some young children are upset by the sight of blood coming from their fingers. If this applies to your child, you can try pricking the ear lobe instead.

Taking blood glucose tests from your toes in the evening, during the night or in the morning will spare your fingertips. Young people with healthy feet can usually do this without problems.[47] However, if you have reduced feeling in your feet, or any type of sores on them, you should avoid taking blood from the toes.

Alternative site testing

♠ Many meters are used for testing blood glucose at alternative sites. This usually hurts less, and may be helpful if you play the piano, for example, and do not want to keep pricking your fingers.

♠ In the fasting state, the glucose readings from the forearm are similar to the fingertip.[580]

♠ After an intake of 75 g of glucose, the rise in blood glucose in adults was 2.6-7.6 mmol/l (47-137 mg/dl) lower on samples taken from the forearm compared with the fingertip.[580]

♠ When blood glucose fell quickly after an insulin injection, the values from the fingertip were 3.4-6.6 mmol/l (61-119 mg/dl) lower than the forearm.[580]

♠ Blood glucose changes appeared on average 35 minutes later in forearm tests compared with the fingertip. By rubbing the skin vigorously for 5-10 seconds before pricking, the accuracy from a forearm test was improved considerably, but with large individual differences.[580]

♠ In another study of adults, where tests were taken after a meal, lower glucose readings were produced from the forearm and thigh compared with the fingertip, in spite of vigorous skin rubbing.[331]

♠ In a study of children and adolescents, testing at the arm and base of thumb was clinically reliable both before and after meals, giving the same results as fingertip testing.[688] However, during hypoglycaemic episodes, there were major differences between the arm and fingertip (on average 0.5 mmol/l, 10 mg/dl lower on the fingertip). Interestingly, in this study the base of the thumb gave accurate readings during hypoglycaemia.

♠ The differences are caused by a greatly increased blood flow in the fingertip. To be on the safe side, it is advisable to rely on fingertip tests when checking for hypoglycaemia (for example when driving a car or after exercise), or in individuals with hypoglycaemia unawareness (see page 52).

Is it worth taking tests?

A Belgian study of children and young adults with an average HbA$_{1c}$ of 52 mmol/mol (6.9%) found that HbA$_{1c}$ was affected both by the actual number of tests taken (on average up to 77 blood glucose tests per month) and the number of visits to the diabetes healthcare team (on average 6.6 visits per patient per year).[300]

It is important to reflect on the reasons for your blood glucose values and, if necessary, to take action and change your insulin doses after having evaluated the tests. The blood glucose level will not improve by merely measuring it. Remember that the tests are for your own sake, not just to show your diabetes nurse or doctor. (See also "Lowering the risk of complications" on page 366.)

Does continuous finger-pricking cause loss of feeling?

A lot of people are afraid that constantly pricking their fingers to test blood will cause them to lose all feeling in them. Fortunately, all the evidence suggests that this won't happen. When fingers that had been pricked an average of 1,000 times were compared with control fingers not used for pricking, it was only pressure sensitivity that was affected (due to an increased skin thickness). There were no signs of decreased sensitivity to heat or touch.[381]

Continuous glucose monitoring (CGM)

The Medtronic MiniMed CGMS (Continuous Glucose Monitoring System®) is a device that monitors glucose levels (2.2-22 mmol/l, 40-400 mg/dl) every 10 seconds and records an average value every 5 minutes. It measures through a thin plastic tube in the subcutaneous tissue, and

How to use CGM when taking a meal bolus

⟹ Decide on the bolus dose as usual and correct for premeal blood glucose level. Use the bolus calculator if you have a pump.

⟹ Look at the trend arrows on the sensor:

Navigator	Medtronic Dexcom	Measure [156]
↑	↑↑	Increase bolus by 20%
↗	↑	Increase bolus by 10%
→		No change of bolus
↘	↓	Decrease bolus by 10%
↓	↓↓	Decrease bolus by 20%

"Do you take the tests for your own sake or do you take them to have something to show your doctor or diabetes nurse / educator when you come to the clinic?"

can be worn for up to 3 days. When the monitor is connected to a computer, the data can be downloaded and viewed on screen. Using this method has made it easier to see patterns of glucose fluctuation, which has in turn led to changes in treatment and improved glucose control, in children [600,697] and in adults.[113] iPro™2 is a professional CGM device designed to collect blinded glucose data that can be viewed together with your doctor or diabetes nurse to provide you with a more complete picture of your glucose levels.

Real-time readings

In the later generation Guardian RT®, data is transmitted wirelessly to the monitor and glucose values can be viewed in real time, with alarms for high and low levels. When adults used this device with the hypoglycaemia alarm set to 3.9 mmol/l (70 mg/dl), the sensor detected 67% of glucose values < 3.9 mmol/l (70 mg/dl) but as many as 47% were false positive.[118] The duration of the low-glucose events was 50% shorter when the alarm was activated. When using the Guardian RT continuously for 3 months, HbA_{1c} decreased 7 mmol/mol (0.6%) lower than the control group.[281] The next step is to transmit the data to an insulin pump where

the glucose level also can be viewed graphically. The Paradigm REAL-Time Pump provides 3- and 24-hour glucose trend graphs. When adults used this system for up to 20 months, HbA_{1c} dropped by an average of 12 mmol/mol (1.1%).[725] The Medtronic Veo pump can shut off the basal rate for 2 hours if the sensor detects hypoglycaemia. The pump will automatically restart, but will shut off again after another 4 hours if the glucose level still is low. When used in children and adolescents, the time spent in hypoglycaemia (4.2 mmol/l, 70 mg/dl) decreased by 40% without affecting the overall mean glucose levels, indicating that high blood glucose values were reduced.[253]

Another continuous meter is the Abbot FreeStyle Navigator®.[1110] It shows real-time blood glucose levels, including the rate and direction of glucose change, and gives predicted low and high alarms, i.e. if the blood glucose will be high or low if the current rate of change continues. In one paediatric study, HbA_{1c} decreased from 54 mmol/mol (7.1%) to 51 mmol/mol (6.8%) after 13 weeks of use, and the percentage of glucose values between 71 and 180 mg/dl increased from 52 to 60%.[154] Promising results have been reported with the DexCom® STS sensor device, which shows real-time readings and displays glucose trend graphs. When using it for 72 hours, 21% less time was spent in hypoglycaemia (< 3.0 mmol/l, < 55 mg/dl), 23% less time in hyperglycaemia (> 13.3 mmol/l, < 240

Skin care with CGM

⟹ **Your skin**
    The sensor will be inserted under your skin
    for up to seven days, sometime even longer if
    you restart it. It s therefore very important
    with good skin care.

⟹ Apply a skin softener as a prophylactic meas-
    ure for a couple of days to prepare your next
    insertion site, or use a cream that contains
    carbamide that binds water to the skin twice
    daily as a protective measure, especially dur-
    ing wintertime. See page 194 for advice if
    you have problems with a sensitive skin.

Ketones

⟹ Can be measured with both urine and blood
    tests.

⟹ Common symptoms: Hunger (!)
                     Nausea
                     Vomiting.

☞ *Always check for ketones when you are feeling unwell!*

---

mg/dl), and 26% more time in the target range
of 4.5-7.8 mmol/l (81-140 mg/dl).[391]

In the JDRF (Juvenile Diabetes Research Foundation) study, all 3 above mentioned systems
were used together with pumps over a 6-month
period.[73] The results showed a decrease in
HbA_{1c} of 6 mmol/mol (0.5%) for adults and
adolescents, and 8 mmol/mol (0.7%) for children aged 8-14 years if the device was used 6
days or more per week. With 4-6 days' use, only
the adults showed a significant decrease in
HbA_{1c} of 4 mmol/mol (0.4%).

The GlucoWatch Biographer® looks like a
watch and monitors blood glucose through the
skin on the wrist three times per hour for 12
hours (after a 2-hour warm-up) using a method
called iontophoresis.[313,191] However, skin irritation has limited its use in clinical practice, and it
is no longer for sale.

Ketones

Ketones are produced by the body when the
cells do not have enough glucose energy. The
body then breaks down fat to produce energy,
and the breakdown products are called ketones.
Ketones can be used as fuel by the muscles,
heart, kidneys and brain. An excess of ketones
will be excreted in the urine. There will also be
a production of acetone which will give the
odor a somewhat sour breath. However, many
people cannot recognize this smell.

Ketones can be measured both in blood and
urine. Blood ketone monitoring (see page 113)
for home use is a new method. It is not available everywhere, however, so some people have
to rely on urine tests to find out how high their
body's ketone levels are. Positive urine ketone
readings are found in anyone who is fasting
(regardless of whether or not they have diabetes) and in up to 30% of early morning urine
samples from pregnant women.[31]

Ketones in the blood or urine indicate that the
cells are starving. Check the key fact box on
page 101 for information on how to interpret
urine tests. The ketones produced when the
body is starving, or when there is a deficiency of
insulin, are chemically the same. But they are
often described differently as "starvation
ketones" or "diabetes ketones" respectively,
since they are produced in different situations.
(See also the section on "Cellular metabolism"
on page 25.)

If possible, children and adolescents with diabetes should have the facility to monitor blood

Tips and tricks with CGM

➤ A CGM monitor is an extra device to insert and wear. You have to be motivated to put up with the extra hassle, or you will end up not wanting to continue, thereby missing the great opportunities of the system.

➤ You should be prepared to use the device for at least 2-4 weeks when starting it up. Do not give up just because you have problems with the first few sensors!

➤ **Alarms:**
Begin by setting only the low and high alarms. Set the high alarm at a realistic level depending on your current readings (for example 14 mmol/l (250 mg/dl) if you have high peaks like this daily), and the low alarm at a level where you will be warned before having difficult symptoms (usually around 4.5 mmol (80 mg/dl) to begin with).

➤ Older children and teenagers who are going to wear the system at school may benefit from shutting off as many alarms as possible (the low alarm may often not be possible to shut off). Instead encourage them to look at the glucose curve often during the day (i.e. not wait for the high alarm to go off before checking).

➤ Have an appointment after 1-2 weeks to discuss the alarm settings when you have had some experience of the system.

➤ As you begin to take care of the high glucose levels, you will be able to lower the high alarm level gradually towards 10 mmol/l (180 mg/dl) or perhaps even lower.

➤ Set the alarms so you will get no more than 2-3 alarms per day. It is easy to get alarm fatigue if it goes off every now and then.

➤ Remember to silence the alarms when you don't want to be disturbed, for example at an important test at school or a job interview.

➤ **High alarm - think!** [156]
Missed bolus? ➔ Take the bolus
Taken the bolus? ➔ Wait at least 2 hours after the previous bolus before you take a correction bolus (according to correction factor).

➤ **Low alarm - think!** [156]
Check blood glucose
➔ Security measure first 2 weeks.

When you are used to the system
➔ Take glucose without a blood test (see page 65 for hypoglycaemia treatment).
Predicted low alarm ➔ Take 2/3 of glucose dose.

➤ **Calibration:**
The calibration is very important, so wash your hands carefully and let them dry before taking the test.

➤ Some systems need to be calibrated when the blood glucose level is stable, i.e. before meals. Spread out your calibrations over the day and try to calibrate at different blood glucose levels.

➤ If you often get calibration errors, you can try measuring your blood glucose 2 or 3 times and use the average for calibration (can only be done with some systems).

➤ You can often restart the sensor to get a second set of readings from it. Beware of when the performance deteriorates so you can change it in time to get the most out of it.

➤ **Trusting CGM readings**
Remember that there is a lag time between capillary blood glucose and subcutaneous glucose of 10-15 minutes, i.e. you will see a change in glucose level 10-15 minutes earlier on a blood test compared to the CGM reading. If you forget this, you are likely to become frustrated and draw the conclusion that the CGM reading is incorrect,

➤ There can be a poor correlation between the sensor readings and blood glucose results during the first few hours after insertion due to an initial tissue reaction.[615]

➤ CGM will give you a lot of readings, but they may not be as accurate as your blood glucose readings due to the lag time. However, if you use it as a trend instrument and watch the direction of the arrows, you will get very valuable information. See the key fact frame on page 108 regarding how you can use the arrows when taking a meal bolus.

➤ Always check a blood test before giving yourself a meal or correction bolus when you are new to the system. However, many families find that after some months they can trust it so well that they do not need to double-check with a blood test before giving a bolus.

ketones, especially if they are using an insulin pump.

If a person has diabetes, ketones are produced in excess when there is a lack of insulin and the blood glucose levels are usually high. Diabetes ketones therefore indicate high blood glucose levels and the need for extra doses of insulin (see page 148).

It is particularly important to check for ketones if you are ill, if you are under a lot of stress, or if you are feeling sick or vomiting, as well as when your blood glucose level is consistently high (above 16 mmol/l, 300 mg/dl).[31] Ask your diabetes team if blood ketone testing is available, since they give much more reliable information compared to urine ketones.

Starvation ketones

Starvation ketones are produced when the blood glucose level is low. The urine glucose concentration will then be low too. The reason the cells are starving is because there is not enough food and glucose in the blood, which happens when you haven't been eating enough, when you have been vomiting, or if you have gastroenteritis. If low blood glucose is caused by a high dose of insulin, the production of ketones will be stopped as insulin counteracts the transformation of fat and fatty acids to ketones.

Diabetes ketones

If you are deficient in insulin, the available glucose will be in the wrong place, i.e. in the bloodstream outside the cell instead of inside the cell. Both the blood glucose level and the urine glucose concentration will then be high.

If your body is producing a lot of ketones, your blood will become acidic and you will be at risk of developing ketoacidosis (see page 29). Pass-

---

When to check for ketones

➠ When you are acutely ill, for example suffering from a common cold with fever.

➠ When your blood glucose has been higher than 14-15 mmol/l (250-270 mg/dl) for more than a couple of hours.

➠ If you are having symptoms of insulin deficiency (nausea, vomiting, abdominal pain, rapid breathing, fruity smell on your breath).

➠ Regularly during pregnancy (see page 320).

---

ing ketones into the urine is the body's way of getting rid of these excess ketones. A high blood glucose level at the same time as elevated ketones always suggests a shortage of insulin, as long as the ketone test is taken during the day and you have not recently suffered from hypoglycaemia (see the blood glucose chart on page 55).

Ketones in the morning urine

When you wake up in the morning, urine has been in your bladder for so long that it is difficult to say exactly when during the night the glucose or ketones entered the urine. A urine test might show both glucose and ketones if you had hypoglycaemia in the middle of the night, followed by a rebound effect in the morning (see page 54) with high blood glucose resulting in both glucose and ketones in the urine. The same results will be seen if your blood glucose has been high all night and the cells have been starved of sugar by a shortage of insulin (see chart on page 58). In this case, the ketones may make you feel sick when you wake up in the morning. Ketones without glucose in the urine indicate that you did not eat enough before going to bed (see page 171). Blood ketones are much easier to interpret, since they reflect the situation as it is right now.

Possible errors when measuring ketones in the urine

False positive
(looks like ketones but there are none)

⟹ If you take certain drugs
(e.g. captopril, valproate).

Acetone will also show on urine strips. Acetone may be present in the blood for many hours although no new ketones are formed after extra insulin has been taken. Because of this, urine strips may continue to be positive for ketones although blood ketone strips are normal.

False negative
(ketones don't show but they are there)

⟹ The lid of the jar has been off too long.

⟹ The strips are too old (discard the jar when the expiry date is passed).

⟹ If you have eaten too much vitamin C (ascorbic acid) or salicylic acid (common in pain killers such as aspirin).

Comparison of blood and urine ketone readings [645]

Blood ketones (mmol/l)	Urine ketones
0-0.5	Negative - trace
0.6-1.0	Trace - low
1.1-1.5	Moderate - large
1.5-3.0	Large

If blood ketones are 3.0 mmol/l or above, you should contact your doctor or go directly to the Accident and Emergency Department.

If your blood glucose level is normally below 10 mmol/l (180 mg/dl), you will be more likely to notice an increase. Even if you don't recognize this clearly yourself, somebody else (such as a teacher, parent or friend) will certainly notice that you are tired and irritable when your blood glucose level is high.

Vomiting and ketones

If you are the parent of a child with diabetes, you should always suspect an insulin deficiency if your child starts being sick. Keep suspecting this until the opposite has been proved! *Vomiting and diarrhoea may be caused by gastroenteritis, but vomiting alone is very likely to be caused by ketones produced as a result of insulin deficiency.* The blood glucose level will then be high and you will find that ketone levels are raised. It is important to stress this point firmly if, for example, you need to contact a doctor while on holiday. It is all too easy for vomiting to be misinterpreted as gastroenteritis by non-specialist doctors or those who are unfamiliar with a particular patient. If this happens, they are then likely to advise, wrongly, that you lower the insulin dose. In fact, a child or young person in this situation needs more insulin, not less. Children have died because of this type of incorrect advice! (See also "Nausea and vomiting" on page 303.)

Will ketones make you feel ill?

It is the increased level of ketones, rather than the high blood glucose level, that makes you feel ill. If you have a high blood glucose and ketones in your blood or urine, it is a sign of insulin deficiency. You are then likely to feel sick and generally unwell (see "Symptoms of insulin deficiency" on page 28). However, if your blood glucose level is temporarily high, but without raised ketone levels, you will often feel fine. You may not even notice your body isn't working as well as it should if you have had high blood glucose levels for some time and a high HbA$_{1c}$. But when your blood glucose has returned to normal levels again, you will almost certainly be aware of the difference. "Is this how alert I should really feel?" is a frequent comment.

Elevated ketone levels

Type of ketones	Treatment
Starvation ketones? (high ketones, low glucose)	Eat extra food that contains carbohydrates

If you have ketones in the morning urine, low glucose indicates that you have starvation ketones. You will then need to check blood glucose during the next night to find out if there is overnight hypoglycaemia. High urine glucose indicates that your blood glucose has been high during the night although it is low in the morning.

Diabetes ketones? (high ketones, high glucose)	Take extra insulin (see page 148). Drink extra fluid. If you feel sick, you may need to have a drink that is high in glucose to avoid hypoglycaemia later on. Contact your diabetes team or doctor if you are actually being sick.

In some countries, the strips used to test urine for ketones are much cheaper than the strips used for testing blood. They may therefore be more suitable for initial testing if you suspect an increased level of ketones. This may be if you feel sick or vomit, for example, or after your blood glucose has been high for more than a couple of hours. If you find ketones in your urine it is a good idea to use blood ketone strips for follow-up.

If the level of ketones is rising or above 0.5 mmol/l, you should take extra insulin (0.05-0.1 U/kg or 0.025-0.5 U/10 lb). See table on page 115 and page 149 if you are using two doses per day. Insulin will convert blood ketones (beta-hydroxybutyric acid, see also page 29) to urine ketones (acetoacetate).[30] Check for ketones in the blood every 1-2 hours. The level may increase the first hour,[618] but after that, should go down as the insulin takes effect, while the level of urine ketones may continue to be high for several hours.

Blood ketones

Meters for measuring the levels of ketones in the blood have been available since 2001 (Optium Xtra, Precision Xtra, Nova MAX Plus, GlucoMen LX Plus).[164] These measure a different type of ketone (beta-hydroxybutyric acid) from that measured by the urine strips (acetoacetate). In a US study of young people aged between 3 and 23 years, there was a 60% reduction in hospital admissions and a 40% reduction in emergency room visits among the group checking blood ketones, compared with the group checking urine ketones during a 6-month follow-up.[645] Among patients and families using blood ketone measurements, 70% reported they would check blood ketones more often than urine ketones.

It may be difficult to interpret a morning urine test showing ketones as you will not know at what time during the night the ketones were produced. However, if the level of ketones in the blood is raised above 0.5 mmol/l, you can interpret the results like this:

Ketones + high glucose level = lack of insulin.
Ketones + low glucose level = lack of food (carbohydrates)

If you, or your child with diabetes, feels nauseous or is being sick, you should test for ketones. This is because nausea and vomiting are common signs of insulin deficiency. Measuring ketones in the blood is more effective than urine tests for following progress and making sure that the level is decreasing when extra insulin is given. This is very important because if the level continues to rise, there is a risk of developing ketoacidosis. In such a case you should always contact your diabetes team.

After you have taken extra insulin, your body will stop producing ketones. Measuring blood ketones will give you accurate readings of a decreasing level. However, ketones will still continue to be passed into the urine for several hours and can sometimes be measured 1-2 days after ketoacidosis (see page 29).[280,410] The reason for this is that ketones are partly trans-formed into acetone which is stored in fat tissue. Acetone is slowly released to the blood and excreted via the urine and lungs, giving the breath a fruity smell. [280]

The advantage of measuring ketones in the blood is that an increased level can be detected earlier, for example when the level of insulin is insufficient because of an infection. Occa-sionally, only the level of beta-hydroxybutyric acid is increased when the body becomes insulin-deficient, and urine strips will then not give any reaction.[644] Ketones produced if a per-son is not eating enough ("starvation ketones") also show up on a blood test. Ketone levels of 0.1-0.2 mmol/l are common in adults with dia-betes if the test is taken before breakfast.[14] Among children with diabetes aged between 1 and 10, 12% had a morning blood ketone of 0.2 mmol/l or above.[928] People without diabetes who have not eaten overnight usually do not have levels above 0.5 mmol/l.[921] After pro-longed fasting of 24 hours or more, the ketone levels can rise to as high as 2-3 mmol/l in young children.[471]

Remember always to check ketones whenever you are ill or feeling sick and/or vomit. All children and adoles-cents, and especially those using pumps should be able to test blood ketones at home, if at all affordable. Adults using pumps will also benefit from being able to measure blood ketones. A ketone meter is a very good travelling companion and helps you to evaluate the situation if you become ill when you are far from home. Check blood glu-cose and ketones, and then try to call your diabetes team on the phone if you are not certain what to do.

Correcting high glucose levels

➡ The general recommendation is to give 0.1 U/kg as an extra dose when both glucose and ketones are high. A higher dose might carry a risk of hypoglycaemia a couple of hours later. It is then better to repeat the dose of 0.1 U/kg (0.5 U/10 lb) or according to the correction factor if the blood glucose is still high. The most important concern is that the level of ketones in the blood should have gone down within 2 hours, even if the blood glucose remains high, and the dose of 0.1 U/kg should be high enough for to ensure.

➡ However, if the family/person with diabetes has experienced a higher dose of insulin being necessary in a situation like this, it should be safe to recommend for example 0.15 U/kg to begin with. If you have a higher total daily dose (TDD = add meal boluses + basal insulin) than 1U/kg (2U/lb), you can try by giving 10% of the TDD in this situation.

➡ The correction factor gives too high numbers at very high blood glucose levels, for example 30 mmol/l (540 mg/dl) (and perhaps a small elevation in ketones) after a day's outing of physical exertion with a poor fluid intake. The calculated correction dose will then be far too high while 0.1U /kg is a more appropriate dose.

Mild infections associated with vomiting and diarrhoea in children without diabetes com-monly cause ketone levels to rise to above 1.0 mmol/l.[644] If the ketone level is 3 mmol/l or above, this indicates that there is a high risk of ketoacidosis.[465,1082] You should contact your di-abetes team or the hospital for further advice as soon as possible. In a study of 37 children and adolescents with ketoacidosis, only 3 had blood ketone levels below 3.0 mmol/l (1.8, 1.9 and 2.9 mmol/l).[437]

The measuring of ketones in the blood is partic-ularly helpful for people using an insulin pump, as the risk of insulin deficiency goes up when

Interpreting blood ketones (adapted from [645,928])

Blood ketones mmol/l	Blood glucose			
	< 10 mmol/l < 180 mg/dl	10-14 mmol/l 180-250 mg/dl	14-22 mmol/l 250-400 mg/dl	> 22 mmol/l > 400 mg/dl
< 0.6	No need to worry.		Measure again after 1-2 h.	
0.6-0.9	Measure again after 1-2 hours. Eat or drink something containing carbohydrates.	Take extra insulin according to correction factor, ½ dose before exercise.	Take 0.05 U/kg (0.25 U/10 lb).	Take 0.1 U/kg (0.5 U/10 lb). Repeat if needed after 2 hours.
1.0-1.4	"Starvation ketones" Eat or drink something rich in carbohydrates.	Eat or drink and take 0.05 U/kg (0.25 U/10 lb).	Take 0.1 U/kg (0.5 U/10 lb).	Take 0.1 U/kg (0.5 U/10 lb). Repeat if necessary.
1.5-2.9	"Starvation ketones". Eat or drink, then take insulin when blood glucose has risen.over 5-6 mmol/l (90-110 mg/dl) Risk of developing ketoacidosis. Contact your diabetes team!	Eat or drink and take 0.1 U/kg (0.5 U/10 lb).	Take extra insulin (0.1 U/kg, 0.5 U/10 lb). Repeat dose after 2 hours if ketones do not decrease.	
3.0 or above	There is an immediate risk for ketoacidosis if the ketone level is 3.0 mmol/l or above - treatment is needed urgently! Contact your diabetes team or emergency department.			

*Take extra insulin according to the correction factor (see page 146) if your blood glucose is > 8 mmol/l (145 mg/dl).

➠ Check for ketones when your blood glucose is repeatedly above 14 mmol/l (250 mg/dl) and during days when you are unwell. High blood glucose and elevated ketones indicate a lack of insulin. "Starvation ketones" are usually below 3.0 mmol/l.

➠ If you feel sick or vomit, you must try to drink sugar-containing fluids in small portions to keep your blood glucose up in order to give extra insulin. Always contact your diabetes team or the emergency department in this situation. When your ketone levels are raised, the number one priority is to give extra insulin. Never mind if your blood glucose doesn't decrease as much, the important thing is that the ketone level decreases after you have taken extra insulin. The ketone level may increase slightly within the first hour after taking extra insulin, but after that it should go down.

➠ If you use an insulin pump, you should remember to take extra insulin with a pen or syringe, *not* with the pump, and to replace the insulin/tubing/infusion set.

the continuous supply of insulin is interrupted. If your blood glucose is high (> 14-15 mmol/l, 250-270 mg/dl) for a few hours, and giving extra insulin via the pump does not decrease it, you should check for ketones. It is also advisable to check for blood ketones if the blood glucose is > 14-15 mmol/l, 250-270 mg/dl in the morning or at bedtime. An increased level indicates problems with the pump and you should take an extra dose of insulin with a pen or syringe (see page 200). It is common to have ketone levels of 1.0-1.5 mmol/l when there has been an interruption of the insulin supply for 5-7 hours (see page 202). Pregnant women should check for ketones each morning, and more often if they feel sick, vomit or have an infection with a raised temperature (see page 322).

The strips for one of the older meters (Optium Xtra, Precision Xtra, will give an error message (E-6) after the expiration date has passed. However, you can "fool" the meter by resetting the date on it. It is of course not the best thing to do, but if it is in the middle of the night and you cannot get hold of any newer strips, at least you will get an estimate of the ketone level.

The HbA$_{1c}$ test

HbA$_{1c}$ is the name for the test used to measure average glucose control over a longer period of time. It is named after a subgroup of adult haemoglobin, the red pigment in blood cells (in contrast to fetal haemoglobin, HbF), in which glucose molecules are hooked to the haemoglobin molecules in the red blood cells. Haemoglobin binds and transports oxygen in the red blood cells. The HbA$_{1c}$ test is based on red blood cells living approximately 120 days. They are produced in the bone marrow and are normally destroyed and recycled in the spleen. During the red blood cell's life span, glucose is bound to its haemoglobin depending on how high or low the blood glucose level is.[410]

HbA$_{1c}$ is a measure of the percentage of the haemoglobin in the red blood cells that has glucose bound to it. This reflects an average measurement of the blood glucose levels during the last 2-3 months.[31,677,1016] The blood glucose levels from the week prior to testing will not be included in the reading as this fraction of HbA$_{1c}$ is not stable. If HbA$_{1c}$ is monitored at regular intervals (at least every 3 months) at the diabetes clinic, the results will provide a good summary of how your glucose control has been throughout the year.

Haemoglobin in the red blood cells takes up oxygen in the lungs and transports it to the cells. Red cells take carbon dioxide from the cells back to the lungs. During their lifetime in the blood circulation, glucose also sticks to haemoglobin, which can be measured by HbA$_{1c}$.

It is important to remember that HbA$_{1c}$ reflects an average of your blood glucose levels. You can get an acceptable HbA$_{1c}$ reading with a combination of high and low blood glucose values. More often than not, you will feel better when your blood glucose level is relatively even. Although it is much discussed today, there is no scientific evidence that you will have more complications as a result of your diabetes if your blood glucose level is unstable than if your blood glucose readings are all the same, assuming that HbA$_{1c}$ is unchanged too.[607,732]

It is more difficult to obtain an acceptable HbA$_{1c}$ value during puberty, since the secretion of growth hormone will raise your blood glucose levels.[307] During puberty it is not uncommon to have an increase in HbA$_{1c}$ of up to 1% or 10 mmol/mol (for example from 7 to 8%, 63 to 73 mmol/mol),[762] if you do not follow-up closely and increase the insulin doses.

What level should my HbA$_{1c}$ be?

It is difficult to state an interval within which your HbA$_{1c}$ should be because different laboratories have different reference values. Many laboratories have the reference values of their

---

HbA$_{1c}$

- ⇒ Glucose is bound to haemoglobin in the red blood cells.

- ⇒ The level of HbA$_{1c}$ depends on the blood glucose levels during the life span of the red blood cells.

- ⇒ A red blood cell lives for about 120 days.

- ⇒ HbA$_{1c}$ reflects the average blood glucose during the previous 2-3 months.[1016]

DCCT units, %   **HbA$_{1c}$ and plasma glucose**   IFCC units, mmol/mol

Average plasma glucose   mmol/l

Your HbA$_{1c}$ value depends on the average blood glucose levels during the last 2-3 months. The graph and table show results from an international study including individuals with Type 1 and Type 2 diabetes and volunteers without diabetes from USA, Europe, Africa, and Asia.[777] A 1% increase in HbA$_{1c}$ (measured with a DCCT-equivalent method) means that you have had an average increase of approximately 1.6 mmol/l (29 mg/dl) in blood glucose levels compared with when your last test was taken.[899]

HbA$_{1c}$ DCCT units	Plasma glucose		HbA$_{1c}$ IFCC units
%	mmol/l	mg/dl	mmol/mol
5	5.4	97	31
6	7.0	126	42
7	8.6	154	53
8	10.2	183	64
9	11.8	212	75
10	13.4	240	86
11	14.9	269	97
12	16.5	298	108

This table from reference [777] shows the mean glucose values that a certain HbA$_{1c}$ value represents. However, these are average numbers, and the relationship between and glucose levels can quite different in some people, both in children [1111] and adults.[777] One should therefore be cautious about saying that the numbers above apply to all people with diabetes. It also seems as if the relationship between HbA$_{1c}$ and glucose levels is dependent upon the type of insulin regimen used (see page 368).[608] HbA$_{1c}$ results can be reported by clinical laboratories worldwide both in IFCC units (mmol/mol) and DCCT units (%).[458]

methods at the same level as the DCCT (Diabetes Control and Complications Trial) reference laboratory,[260] and this has been the recommended standard in the UK and US.[722] The American Diabetes Association recommends that the goal of therapy in adults and adolescents should be an HbA$_{1c}$ below 53 mmol/mol (7.0%) and that the treatment regimen should be re-evaluated in patients with repeated HbA$_{1c}$ above goals.[31] Both ISPAD [885] (International Society for Pediatric and Adolescent Diabetes) and NICE (National Institute for Health and Clinical Excellence)[785] recommend a target of < 58 mmol/mol (7.5%) in children of all age groups. See the fact frame on page 119.

To know what your HbA$_{1c}$ value really means, you should compare it with the results of one of the long-term studies (see "Lowering the risk of complications" on page 366). Many studies have shown that with an HbA$_{1c}$ value of less than 53 mmol/mol (7.0%) the risk of long-term blood vessel complications will be considerably less.[261,882]

The NGSP (National Glycohemoglobin Standardization Program) has developed a standardization allowing laboratories to relate their results to those of the DCCT, and most studies up until 2010-2011 have been published using only DCCT percentage numbers.

A true reference method for measuring HbA$_{1c}$ has been developed for calibration of laboratory instruments.[516,625] The IFCC (International Federation of Clinical Chemistry and Laboratory Medicine) HbA$_{1c}$ method gives percentage numbers that are approximately 2% below the DCCT standard.[517]

Everyone agrees that the new IFCC standard should be used for calibration of laboratory instruments worldwide, which means that HbA$_{1c}$ reports will be comparable all over the world. This is a substantial improvement from the previous situation when many countries had their national calibrations, and many even had several different calibrations within the same

HbA$_{1c}$ targets by age

	DCCT units %	IFCC units mmol/mol
Normal value, person without diabetes	4.1-6.1%	21-43
Toddlers and preschoolers (< 6 years) [885,785]	<7.5%*	<58
School-age (6-12 years) [885]	<7.5%*	<58
Adolescents and young adults (13-19 years) [299]	<7.5%*	<58
Adults [272]	<7.0%**	<53
Needs improving and re-evaluation of treatment [31]	8-9%	64-75
Not acceptable High risk of complications	>9%	>75
May have higher risk of severe hypoglycaemia (if not in honeymoon phase)	<6%	<42

The above numbers show the recommendations of ISPAD and the American Diabetes Association.[970] However, the Canadian Diabetes Association [169] recommends higher targets in children (< 8.0% for 6-12 years, < 8.5% below 6 years) because of an assumed risk of damage on the developing brain from severe hypoglycaemia. But clinicians and families often find that with intensive insulin therapy, one can actually achieve a HbA$_{1c}$ below 53 mmol/mol (7.0%) (and without severe hypoglycaemia) in younger children where parents are in full control.[459]

There may be individual differences in the HbA$_{1c}$ value it is realistic to achieve. It is important to take the child's age into consideration (see "Does severe hypoglycaemia damage the brain?" on page 50). Discuss with your diabetes team what value may be realistic for you.

* A lower target of 51-53 mmol/mol (6.8-7.0%) is recommended if it can be achieved without excessive hypoglycaemia.[786,970,975]

** The HbA$_{1c}$ goal for the individual patient is an HbA$_{1c}$ as close to normal (6%, 42 mmol/mol) as possible without significant hypoglycaemia.[272]

NICE = National Institute for Health and Clinical Excellence
ISPAD = International Society for Pediatric and Adolescent Diabetes

country. However, there has been a lively debate about which units to present to the individuals with diabetes, now that we have the IFCC system for calibration of laboratory machines. Changing the percentage numbers may affect the way people with diabetes relate to their HbA$_{1c}$ levels,[452] and therefore the new IFCC units are expressed in mmol/mol rather than per cent (see table on page 118).[795]

According to a consensus reached at a 2011 meeting between organizations that represent clinical chemists, diabetes doctors and people with diabetes, HbA$_{1c}$ should best be presented in both DCCT units and the new IFCC units, especially when research data is presented in scientific journals.[458] However, most countries in Europe have now standardized to reporting in IFCC units, while other countries, such as the US, Canada and Australia continue to use DCCT numbers.

The "blood glucose" numbers in this book refer to plasma glucose values unless otherwise stated, as this is what most new patient meters display. Plasma glucose is approximately 11% higher than whole blood glucose.[357] Although the table on page 118 shows which plasma glucose level that a certain HbA$_{1c}$ level represents, one must remember that there proved to be a large individual variation between these, both in children [1111] and adults.[777] It seems as if the relationship between HbA$_{1c}$ and blood glucose to some extent can depend on the type of insulin treatment.[608] There are also differences between races, as exemplified by young African Americans having higher HbA$_{1c}$ levels for the same mean blood glucose when compared to Caucasian young people.[585] As the risk of complications follows HbA$_{1c}$ levels independently of previous mean blood glucose levels,[731] some individuals need to have lower blood glucose levels than others if they are to avoid complications. This may explain why young African Americans (and young people in Africa) appear to be at an increased risk of diabetes complications.[184]

Most countries in Europe are introducing the IFCC HbA$_{1c}$ units which are expressed in mmol/mol, while the DCCT/NGSP units which are expressed in per cent will continue to be used in the US, Canada and many other countries. Previously, Japan and Sweden had their own levels of HbA$_{1c}$, with the Japanese being 0.4% and the Swedish 1% lower than DCCT. In times of increased international communication it is very important to check the level of the HbA$_{1c}$ method if you read about the results of studies from different countries, and want to compare with your own readings. See the table on page 118 for comparison between the IFCC and DCCT units. There is an Internet calculator available at www.hba1c.nu/eng for conversion between the two units.

Studies of adults have shown that those with a lower HbA$_{1c}$ experience better levels of psychological well-being. This includes less anxiety and depression, improved self-confidence and a better quality of life.[507] This has also been confirmed in children and adolescents (see page 405).[518]

The occurrence of severe hypoglycaemia will limit how low an HbA$_{1c}$ the individual person can achieve. An HbA$_{1c}$ within the range for individuals without diabetes usually means they are at high risk of severe hypoglycaemia and/or hypoglycaemia unawareness. In the DCCT study, patients with low HbA$_{1c}$ had a significantly higher risk for severe hypoglycaemia.[264] However, the risk decreased during the years of the study. At centres where intensive insulin treatment has been routinely implemented for a longer time, the relationship between the HbA$_{1c}$ value and severe hypoglycaemia is not as pronounced.[791,1068] An American adult study using pumps and continuous glucose monitoring, found that those with a baseline HbA$_{1c}$ of < 53 mmol/mol (7.0%) did not have any severe hypoglycaemia at all, and they lowered their mean HbA$_{1c}$ to 46 mmol/mol (6.4%).[556]

Is checking your HbA$_{1c}$ worthwhile? For whose benefit is the HbA$_{1c}$ test being done? Many patients feel as if they are visiting a "control station", and being examined by health professionals to see how well they have "behaved themselves". From the professional point of view, however, the HbA$_{1c}$ test is most valuable to individuals with diabetes themselves. When you see the reading, you will know if your way of life over the last 3 months has allowed you to achieve the average blood glucose level you want for the future. It may be difficult to manage this every time but we often see teenagers taking such a degree of responsibility for their own health that it seems natural for them to say: "Oh, now my HbA$_{1c}$ has increased again. I will have to do something about it." And without anything more being said at the clinic, the HbA$_{1c}$ value comes right down by the next visit.

When the HbA$_{1c}$ method was introduced, 240 adults with diabetes measured it every third month without otherwise changing their diabetes treatment.[653] After 1 year, the average HbA$_{1c}$ value was unchanged but it turned out that those with very low values had increased them and those with high values now had lower ones, showing the benefit of knowing your HbA$_{1c}$ level.

How often should you check your HbA$_{1c}$?

HbA$_{1c}$ should be checked regularly every third month in all people with insulin-dependent diabetes.[31] A high level, > 64-75 mmol/mol (8-9%), is not acceptable, considering the risk

Set up your own personal goal for your HbA$_{1c}$ in collaboration with your diabetes team. This goal will be different for different people and perhaps also different during different times of your life. It may be more difficult to achieve the same HbA$_{1c}$ level, for example at times when you are having problems at home or at work. By competing with yourself and setting a reasonable goal you will have a fair chance of winning your race.

A good way to do so is to keep track of your average glucose level over 7, 14 and 30 days. You will then quickly see if it begins to increase, and when you need to interact. Compare the glucose levels with those in the table on page 118 to see what the matching HbA$_{1c}$ is. You can either look on your meter or download it to a special computer program that is available with your meter.

of future complications. If your HbA$_{1c}$ is this high, it is a good idea to check it every month until it has gone back to an acceptable level. In children and adolescents, the HbA$_{1c}$ value is usually slightly higher, around 4 mmol/mol (0.4%), in the autumn and winter than in the spring or summer.[792]

After a visit to your diabetes healthcare team you may feel more motivated to "get your act together", and keep your blood glucose readings low. However, after a few weeks this determination can slip to the back of your mind, as daily life gets back in the way again. It is important to remember that it was not only insulin treatment that was intensive in the DCCT study. HbA$_{1c}$ was taken at every visit with monthly intervals, and telephone contact was made between the visits. So get into a routine of visiting your diabetes healthcare team every month to check HbA$_{1c}$ until it has come down

below 64 mmol/mol (8.0%), preferably to 58 mmol/mol (7.5%) or lower.

Some clinics send their HbA$_{1c}$ tests to the laboratory, so it may be some days before you get the result, while others ask you to send in a blood sample a week before the clinic. Others use a desktop method (such as DCA-Vantage®) that gives a result after a few minutes.

Even if your blood glucose control is improving and your tests are showing lower readings, it will still take some time for this to show in your HbA$_{1c}$. Half the change will show after about 1 month, and three-quarters of the change after 2 months.[1016] If you start with a very high HbA$_{1c}$, 108-119 mmol/mol (12-13%), and normalize your blood glucose levels completely (as often happens at diagnosis) it will go down by approximately 11 mmol/mol (1.0%) every tenth day.[1015]

Can I measure HbA1c at home?

At times you will be surprised that the HbA$_{1c}$ level has increased since your last visit. You can measure HbA$_{1c}$ at home with a point of care method, but they are often not so accurate. However, by checking the mean glucose level on your meter over 7, 14 and 30 days you will get a very good picture of how your HbA$_{1c}$ will be at the next visit. You can compare the mean

Send an HbA$_{1c}$ test by mail to your diabetes healthcare team if you are away from home for any length of time, or bring along a HbA$_{1c}$ home test kit.

value with the table on page 118. If you keep your mean blood glucose at 8 mmol/l (145 mg/dl) or below, you will probably have an HbA_{1c} matching around 52 mmol/mol (6.9%).

Can my HbA_{1c} be "too good"?

If you have a very low HbA_{1c} your average blood glucose is low and you may have a high risk of developing serious hypoglycaemia without any warning symptoms ("hypoglycaemic unawareness", see page 52), unless you are in the remission phase (see page 221). If you have a low HbA_{1c}, 42-53 mmol/mol (6-7%), and problems with severe hypoglycaemia or hypoglycaemia unawareness, it may be a good idea to aim for a slightly higher blood glucose level.

In very young children (under 2 years of age) the brain is still developing and repeated severe hypoglycaemic episodes and seizures can damage the brain (see page 50). In preschool children, avoiding severe hypoglycaemia should have the highest priority and it may be necessary to accept a slightly higher HbA_{1c}.

In clinical reality, children before puberty can achieve low HbA_{1c} values of 53-58 mmol/mol, 7.0-7.5% or even lower without risking severe

---

For how long do blood glucose levels affect HbA_{1c}?

Your recent blood glucose level affects HbA_{1c} much more than that from 2-3 months ago. However, your values during the last week will not show on most methods since this fraction of HbA_{1c} is very unstable. Of a given HbA_{1c} value, the contribution of the blood glucose is (counting backwards): [1016]

Day	1-6	very low
Day	7-30	50%
Day	31-60	25%
Day	61-90	15%
Day	91-120	10%

---

hypoglycaemia thanks to dedicated parents, frequent blood glucose testing (or continuous glucose monitoring, CGM) and daily adjustments of insulin doses. A Swedish study from 2013 did not find any severe hypoglycaemia with unconsciousness or seizures since the onset of diabetes in prepubertal children in spite of low mean HbA_{1c} of 54 mmol/mol (7.1%) in those younger than 6 years and 51 mmol/mol (6.8%) in the age group 7-11 years.[459] So as a parent you need not be worried even if your child has an HbA_{1c} within the range that is normal for people without diabetes (< 42 mmol/mol (6.0%), provided the child does not have severe or difficult hypoglycaemia. However, the child might have unrecognized night time hypoglycaemia. It is a good idea therefore, to check blood glucose during the night regularly (every week or second week) or use CGM.

HbA_{1c} when travelling

Sometimes you will want to know your HbA_{1c} but, for one reason or another, it may be difficult to visit a diabetes clinic. For example, you may want to test your HbA_{1c} at shorter intervals after a change in your insulin dose. A home test for monitoring HbA_{1c} may then be practical (like Metrika A1C Now). Another way is to put a few drops of blood on a filter paper and send it to the laboratory. This might be particularly useful if you are travelling, and cannot get hold of a doctor who knows enough about you or your diabetes. If you have well-controlled diabetes, sending an HbA_{1c} test every 3 months may be fine. You can call your diabetes team to discuss the result. A good way to keep track of your HbA_{1c} is to check your mean glucose every week. If you take 4-6 test per day, you will get a good understanding of what your HbA_{1c} would be at the clinic. See the table on page 118.

If your healthcare team uses "HbA_{1c} by mail" for routine testing, make sure you have taken the test long enough in advance to have the results ready in time for the visit.

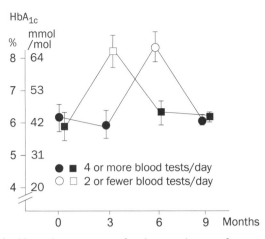

In this study, two groups of patients took two or four blood glucose tests per day during 3-month periods. The glucose control was significantly better in both groups when they were taking four tests a day.[946] The HbA$_{1c}$ values are recalculated from HbA$_1$, an older method of analysis.

Fructosamine

Monitoring fructosamine is a method of measuring the amount of glucose that is bound to proteins in the blood. The value reflects the blood glucose level during the last 2-3 weeks. Fructosamine can be good indicator during times of rapid changes in glucose control, for example when you start with a new method of treatment. However, if you only take a fructosamine test every third month you will not get a representative measurement of your glucose control over a longer period of time. This method, therefore, is not recommended for routine monitoring of long-term glucose control.[31]

Injection technique

The only way insulin can work on the cells is by binding to the receptors on the cell surface. Because of this, insulin will take effect only when it has entered the bloodstream and the bloodstream has supplied it to the cells. Today, the only practical methods of administration are by subcutaneous injection or infusion (in an insulin pump). However, a great deal of research is currently being carried out to explore alternative ways of administration (see page 384).

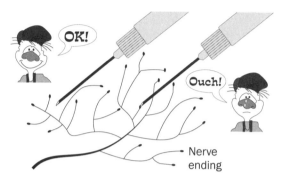

Nerve fibres look like thin branches of a tree. If you hit a nerve you will feel more pain than if you inject between the nerve fibres.

Getting used to injections

Having an injection is never going to be pleasurable. It is an annoyance at best, and at worst it can be painful, certainly at the beginning. But most people can adapt to most things, if they are allowed to take them at the right pace. Most school-age children learn quickly how to give themselves injections. The average age for learning this is 8 years.[1122] However, there are a few children and adolescents who find them close to unbearable even after many years of diabetes.[444] The use of indwelling catheters (Insuflon or i-port, see page 137) may help to decrease the injection pain for someone who is new to injections, especially if they use multiple injections from the start.[451]

Injections for parents

How do you teach yourself or your child to take or give insulin injections? It helps if the child can play with the pen or syringe and inject

teddy bears or dolls. The first step is usually to practise injecting oranges and then to inject a nurse or parent. After this, they may be ready to try an ordinary injection on their own. It is very important for adults to show the children in their care that giving themselves injections is not such a big deal. If mum and dad can overcome their fear of needles, the child will find it a lot easier to learn how to self-inject. Let small children try injections (giving saline, not insulin) and blood glucose monitoring on their parents (and perhaps also on a brave brother, sister or grandparent) as often as they want to, as this will demonstrate that injections are not dangerous. But remember that needles should not be shared! Use a new needle for each person. If you are the parent of a young child with diabetes, try to put yourself in the child's situation and think how it would appear if your parents appeared to be scared of having injections. "I am supposed to take several injections every day for the rest of my life and yet my mum doesn't want to have one. Nor does dad, but they are grown up and can do just about anything. Having an injection must be something terrible!"

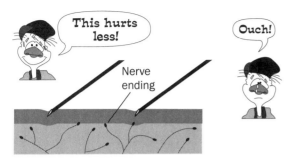

Try to find an injection site that hurts less when you press the needle against your skin!

Don't tell younger children too far ahead when it's time for an injection or blood glucose test. Many children will become anxious if they know something unpleasant will happen too far in advance. Other children want to know exactly and in plenty of time what will happen and when. Try to find out which approach suits your child best.

Taking the pain out of injections

Pain is generated by thin nerves and their endings. The nerves spread like the branches of a tree. If you hit a nerve directly, this will be painful. You can test out the position of nerves by pressing the needle carefully against your skin, and feeling where it hurts more and where it hurts less. Remember to hold the needle so that the sharp end of the needle will penetrate the skin (see picture on page 126). Certain areas on your abdomen and thighs will probably hurt less than others. However, the disadvantage of always using the same places for injections is that you will soon start to develop fatty lumps (lipohypertrophy, see page 217). Insulin will be absorbed more slowly from such lumps.[1128] If you insert the needle quickly with thrust, you will feel less pricking. However, some people prefer to push the needle slowly and carefully through the skin.

Where do I inject the insulin?

In the fat or in the muscle?

Insulin should be given by subcutaneous injection, i.e. into the fat beneath the skin, not into the muscle. The recommendations for how to avoid injecting insulin into the muscle have changed considerably over the years. With old (25 mm, 1 inch) needles it was natural to use a raised skin fold when injecting. When the 12-13 mm (0.5 inch) needles were introduced, it was thought that a perpendicular injection would deposit the insulin within the subcutaneous (fatty) tissue. However, as mentioned below, you risk injecting into muscle when using this technique, and people are now being advised again to inject at an angle into a raised skin fold.[1038]

**Research findings:
Injection technique**

♠ In a British study, the distance from the skin to the muscle was measured using ultrasound. The conclusion was that most boys and some girls who used the perpendicular injection technique risked injecting into muscle or even into the abdominal cavity.[982]

♠ In a French study, 31% of children who used a whole-hand skin fold with a perpendicular injection technique performed the injection intramuscularly. The figure was as high as 50% in young slim boys.[856]

♠ Even with an 8 mm needle there is a considerable risk of injecting into the muscle when using a perpendicular injection technique (despite lifting a skin pinch-up with a correct two-finger technique).[1047]

♠ The safest way to inject using the 5-6 mm needles is to lift a skin fold with two fingers and inject at a 45° angle.[520]

The right technique consists of lifting a skin fold with the thumb and index finger ("two-finger pinch-up") (see illustration on page 129).[371,1038] Lifting a skin fold is important, even if you are using an 8 mm (1/3 inch) needle. With 5-6 mm needles, injections can be given without lifting a skin fold if there is enough subcutaneous fat (at least 8 mm as skin layers may be compressed when injecting perpendicularly [97]). Lean boys, however, usually have less fat, especially on the thigh.[97,982]

Wiggle the needle slightly before injecting. If the tip feels "stuck" you have probably reached the muscle. If this is the case, withdraw the needle a little before injecting. You can also inject insulin into your buttocks where there is usually a layer of subcutaneous fat that is thick enough to insert the needle perpendicularly without lifting a skin fold. The speed of injection (varied between 3 and 30 seconds) does not affect how rapidly the insulin is absorbed according to a Danish study.[498]

Some research has found that injecting into the muscle is not necessarily more painful,[489,1121] but the insulin is absorbed more quickly. An

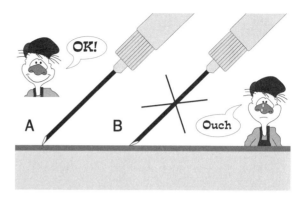

Look closely at the needle tip before pushing it through the skin. The tip of the needle is cut very sharp so that it will pierce the skin easily. If you prick the skin with the eye of the needle facing towards the skin (B) you will feel more pain than if you prick the skin with the sharp tip pointing towards the skin (A).

injection into the muscle can be experienced as uncomfortable, even if it is not particularly painful. The uptake of short-acting [371] and intermediate-acting [1059] insulin is increased by at least 50% from an intramuscular injection compared with a subcutaneous injection in the thigh. However, the insulin absorption is the same when comparing intramuscular and subcutaneous injections into the abdomen.[371]

The thicker the layer of subcutaneous fat, the smaller the blood flow. This results in a slower absorption of insulin. In one study, short-acting insulin (8 units were injected into the abdomen) was absorbed twice as fast from a subcutaneous fat layer of 10 mm (3/8 inch) compared with 20 mm (3/4 inch).[500] The same result was found in patients using insulin pumps. You can take advantage of this phenomenon by injecting where the subcutaneous fat is thinner, if you wish the insulin to take effect more quickly. Also, insulin that is injected above the navel will be absorbed slightly more quickly than insulin injected below or beside the navel.[374]

Some people find it more convenient to inject themselves through clothing. Although this can cause unpleasant skin reactions, these seem to be unusual.[356] However, it is more difficult to

---

Recommended injections sites

Rapid-acting insulin	Abdomen (tummy)
Short-acting insulin	Abdomen (tummy)
Intermediate-acting insulin	Thighs or buttocks
Long-acting (Ultratard, Humulin Zn)	Thighs or buttocks
Long-acting analogues (Lantus, Levemir)	Abdomen, Thighs or buttocks

The buttocks are the preferred injection site for intermediate- and long-acting insulin in children with thin subcutaneous fat on the thigh.[221] They may also be used for injecting short- and rapid-acting insulin to spread the injection sites and lessen the development of fatty lumps (lipohypertrophies). The buttocks may be a better injection site for pregnant women, especially once the abdomen has become large and tight.

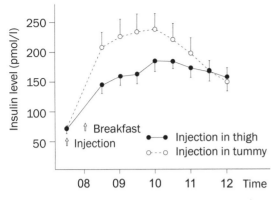

In an American study, adults took the same dose of short-acting insulin before breakfast in the tummy one day and in the thigh one day.[64] The injection in the tummy gave both a faster onset of insulin action and a higher peak level of insulin in the blood.

Blood glucose values from the same study as above. Because insulin enters the blood more quickly after an injection in the tummy, this will cause the glucose content from breakfast to enter the cells more effectively, resulting in a lower blood glucose level.

get hold of a proper skin fold through clothing, and this increases the risk of accidentally injecting into muscle. There is also a risk of blood staining your clothes.

In the tummy or the thigh?

In adults, insulin is absorbed more rapidly after a subcutaneous injection in the abdomen (tummy) compared with an injection in the

thigh, and the blood glucose-lowering effect is also increased [64,371] (see figures, page 127). The absorption from a subcutaneous injection in the tummy is comparable to that of an intramuscular injection in the thigh.[371] This is caused by an increased blood flow in the subcutaneous fat in the tummy compared with that in the thigh.[64] The insulin uptake from the buttocks is quicker than from the thigh but not as quick as from the tummy.[807] In some countries, the upper and outer area of the arm is used for subcutaneous injections as well, the uptake being similar to that in the thigh.[1027] This injection site is not recommended in other countries (like Sweden) since the subcutaneous layer is very thin and it is difficult to lift a skin fold at the same time as injecting at an angle of 45°.

The absorption of intermediate-acting insulin (NPH-insulin) is better balanced after an injection in the thigh and will give a lower insulin effect in the middle of the night and a higher insulin effect later in the night, compared with an abdominal injection.[490]

As insulin is absorbed faster from the tummy than from the thigh, we recommend giving the premeal doses of rapid-acting (or short-acting) insulin in the tummy and the bedtime injection of intermediate- or long-acting insulin in the thigh (or in the buttocks). Changing the site of injection between the thigh and the tummy from day to day is not recommended, as this will vary the effect of the insulin.[63] A young child has a smaller area on the abdomen or tummy that is suitable for injections, so it is advisable to use the buttocks for rapid- and short-acting insulin as well.

A small child using indwelling catheters for injecting short-acting insulin can try using this device for the bedtime insulin as well if it is NPH or Lantus insulin. However, if you encounter problems with night time hypoglycaemia or high blood glucose readings in the morning, it is better to give the bedtime insulin in the thigh as a separate injection (see also page 139).

The abdomen is usually used for injections of short-acting and rapid-acting insulin (NovoRapid, Humalog or Apidra). It will be absorbed slightly faster above the tummy button compared with other areas of the abdomen.[374] Always use the same area for a given type of insulin, e.g. the tummy (or buttocks for small children) for short-acting insulin and the thigh for bedtime insulin. It is important to rotate the injection sites within each area to avoid the development of fatty lumps (lipohypertrophies, see page 217).

You can also use your buttocks for injections. Inject a few centimetres below the edge of the hip bone. The buttocks can be used for injections in small children who have a thin subcutaneous fat layer on the abdomen or a tendency to develop fatty lumps (lipohypertrophies). The absorption of insulin is slightly slower from the buttocks than from the tummy. The illustrations are from reference [975].

Put one hand above the knee and one below your groin. The area between your hands is suitable for injections in the thigh. Remember that insulin will be absorbed more slowly from the thigh than from the tummy.

Don't give short-acting insulin in the thigh late in the day. The slower uptake may result in hypoglycaemia early in the night.[489]

Rapid-acting insulin

The difference in uptake between injection sites is not as pronounced when using rapid-acting insulin. If you are using NovoRapid [766] or Humalog [1027] the uptake is only slightly faster from the abdomen than the thigh. There was no difference in absorption between subcutaneous and intramuscular injections when using Humalog for thigh injections in a German study.[875]

Long-acting insulin

The long-acting analogue Lantus (glargine) gives the same effect when injected into the tummy, thigh or arm.[813] Exercise does not affect the action of a subcutaneous injection of Lantus.[835] However, if you inject Lantus in the muscle, the absorption is much quicker and you risk getting hypoglycaemia.[590]

The absorption of insulin is affected by many other factors as well (see page 90).

Subcutaneous injection technique 4-5-6 mm needle

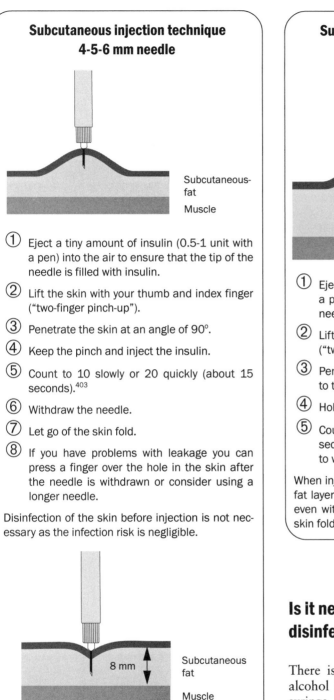

Subcutaneous-fat

Muscle

① Eject a tiny amount of insulin (0.5-1 unit with a pen) into the air to ensure that the tip of the needle is filled with insulin.

② Lift the skin with your thumb and index finger ("two-finger pinch-up").

③ Penetrate the skin at an angle of 90°.

④ Keep the pinch and inject the insulin.

⑤ Count to 10 slowly or 20 quickly (about 15 seconds).[403]

⑥ Withdraw the needle.

⑦ Let go of the skin fold.

⑧ If you have problems with leakage you can press a finger over the hole in the skin after the needle is withdrawn or consider using a longer needle.

Disinfection of the skin before injection is not necessary as the infection risk is negligible.

8 mm

Subcutaneous fat

Muscle

The 5-6 mm needle can be used for perpendicular injections if the subcutaneous tissue is at least 8 mm thick,[97] otherwise you need to pinch a skinfold.

Subcutaneous injection technique 8-13 mm needle

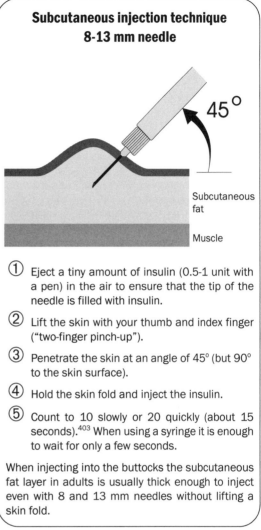

45°

Subcutaneous fat

Muscle

① Eject a tiny amount of insulin (0.5-1 unit with a pen) in the air to ensure that the tip of the needle is filled with insulin.

② Lift the skin with your thumb and index finger ("two-finger pinch-up").

③ Penetrate the skin at an angle of 45° (but 90° to the skin surface).

④ Hold the skin fold and inject the insulin.

⑤ Count to 10 slowly or 20 quickly (about 15 seconds).[403] When using a syringe it is enough to wait for only a few seconds.

When injecting into the buttocks the subcutaneous fat layer in adults is usually thick enough to inject even with 8 and 13 mm needles without lifting a skin fold.

Is it necessary to disinfect the skin?

There is no need to disinfect your skin with alcohol before injecting with an insulin pen or syringe. The risk of skin infection is negligible[734] and alcohol disinfection often causes a stinging pain when the needle is inserted. Good hygiene and careful hand washing are more important.

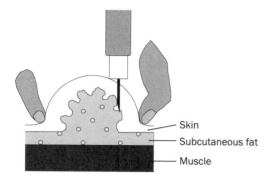

Skin
Subcutaneous fat
Muscle

The safest way to inject with the 5-6 mm needles is to lift a skin fold with two fingers and to inject at a 45° angle.[520] However, if you inject slightly to one side with a 5-6 mm needle, there is a risk of an injection into the superficial skin (intracutaneous injection, see figure) from which the insulin may be absorbed more slowly.[1000] With 5-6 mm needles, the injections can be given perpendicularly without lifting a skin fold to avoid intracutaneous injections [1000] if there is enough subcutaneous fat, which often is the case in girls (at least 8 mm as the skin layers often are compressed when injecting perpendicularly [97]). Lean boys, however, have a thinner subcutaneous fat layer, especially on the thigh.[97,982] When injecting into the buttocks, the subcutaneous fat layer is usually thick enough to inject without lifting a skin fold.

If you lift the skin with a whole-hand grip there is less risk of a superficial injection with a 5-6 mm needle. This technique, however, should not be used with the longer 8 and 13 mm needles since the muscle will be lifted as well, resulting in a risk of intramuscular injection.[856]

If you use an insulin pump or indwelling catheter (see page 137) you should wash the skin

Subcutaneous fat
Muscle

If you inject at a 90° angle with a 12-13 mm needle, there is a considerable risk of accidental intramuscular injection. This risk is substantial even with the shorter 8 mm needle if you inject in areas with a thin subcutaneous layer, such as the outside of the thigh, the upper arm or the sides of your body.[1047] Insulin from an intramuscular injection is absorbed more quickly into the bloodstream and this will give you a stronger but shorter effect from the insulin dose. However, you can take advantage of this type of injection in the thigh if you want your insulin to start working more quickly, or if you have problems with lipohypertrophies (see page 217).

If you inject with the needle held at right angles to the body with an 8 or 13 mm needle, into the abdomen or tummy, you run a considerable risk of injecting the insulin directly into your abdominal cavity.[373]

with an antiseptic solution or use chlorhexidine in alcohol or a similar disinfectant if you have problems with skin infections. Some skin disinfectants contain skin moisturisers which may cause the adhesive to loosen more easily.

Storage of insulin

Insulin withstands room temperature well. Most manufacturers recommend that insulin in use should be discarded after 4 weeks at room temperature (not above 25-30° C, 77-86° F).[413] Check the package leaflet for the type of insulin you are using and the expiry date on the bottle or cartridge. At room temperature, insulin will lose less than 1% of its potency every month.[413]

According to one study, regular, Lente and NPH insulin used for up to 110 days kept the insulin concentration at 100 U/ml.[872] Even after a year or more of being stored at room temperature, as long as it is kept in darkness, the insulin will lose only 10% of its effect.[810] Recommendations on expiration date are generally more based upon sterility issues than losing potency.[413]

A practical routine is to have your spare insulin supplies stored in the refrigerator (4-8° C, 39-46° F) and the bottle or cartridge that is currently in use, stored at room temperature. Storing it at room temperature makes the preservatives more effective in killing any bacteria that may have contaminated the vial during repeated use for injections.[872] Humalog that is diluted (with sterile NPH medium) to 50 U/ml (U-50) and 10 U/ml (U-10) is stable for one month when stored at 5° C and 30° C (41° F and 86° F).[997]

Don't put your insulin too close to the freezer compartment in the fridge as it cannot withstand temperatures below 2° C (36° F). Don't expose insulin to strong light or heat, such as the sunlight in a car or the heat of a sauna. Insulin loses its effect when it is stored at temperatures above 25-30° C (77-86° F). Above

Insulin is sensitive to heat and sunlight, so don't leave it in the sun or a hot car.

35° C (95° F) it will be inactivated four times as fast as it is at room temperature.[418] A practical way on holiday is to store insulin in a cooled thermos flask or wrapped in moist flannel to keep it cool.

In very hot climates where there is no refrigerator available, insulin vials and cartridges can be stored in a box that is floating in an earthenware pitcher (matka) filled half way with water without losing its effect. The pot should be kept in the shade. An Indian study showed that insulin stored in this way did not lose any of its effectiveness after 60 days with temperatures up to 40° C (104° F).[870]

You need not store human insulin in the dark as it keeps just as well in daylight (but not sunlight).[418] However, beef insulin degrades more rapidly in daylight.[418] Human insulin carried in a shirt pocket for 6 months did not deteriorate significantly more quickly than when it was stored at room temperature.[418] Never use insulin that has become cloudy if it usually is clear (applies to rapid- and short-acting, Lantus and Levemir). Intermediate- or long-acting insulin that contains clumps or that has a frosty coating on the inside of the vial should not be used either.[908]

If you mix Lente-type insulins (Monotard, Humulin I, Ultratard, Humulin Zn) with short-acting insulin in the same syringe immediately before injecting, the insulin will start acting more rapidly if you use insulin from refrigerated bottles [830] (see also page 86).

Different ways of administering insulin

♠	Syringes	1-3 injections per day.
♠	Insulin pen	4-6 injections per day.
♠	Insuflon	Indwelling Teflon catheter. Can be used if injection pain is a problem.
♠	Insulin pump	Delivers a basal rate over 24 hours and bolus doses at mealtimes.
♠	Jet injector	Injection without a needle. A thin jet stream of insulin is shot through the skin.

Syringes

Disposable syringes have been used since the 1960s and are still the standard injection device in many countries. They are graded in units for U-100 insulin, containing 30, 50 or 100 units. Syringes are used when mixing two types of insulin into the same injection or for types of insulin that are not available in pen cartridges. You will need to be careful when travelling, especially if you are visiting countries that use a different concentration of insulin. It is particularly important not to use U-40 insulin in a U-100 syringe or vice versa. In countries where pen injectors are less common, syringes are used for multiple injection therapy. In many countries with lower economic standards, non-disposable glass syringes with needles that require manual sharpening are still used. Needles for syringes cannot be made shorter than 8 mm to ensure that they can safely penetrate the rubber membrane on the insulin vials.

Mixing insulins in a syringe

➠ Start by injecting air into the bottle of intermediate-acting insulin (cloudy insulin).

➠ Take the syringe out of first bottle.

➠ Inject air into the bottle of the premeal rapid- or short-acting insulin (clear insulin).

➠ Draw up the short- or rapid-acting insulin (clear insulin).

➠ Take the syringe out of the second bottle.

➠ Carefully insert the needle into the bottle of intermediate-acting insulin (cloudy insulin).

➠ Draw up the correct dose (without injecting into the bottle).

➠ Take the syringe out of the first bottle.

➠ It is best to draw up the insulins in this order as it matters less if a drop of premeal insulin enters the bottle of intermediate-acting insulin than the other way around.

A small syringe can be experienced as a huge, frightening thing by someone who is afraid of injections. Daniel made this drawing of his insulin syringe on one of the first days in the hospital.

Injections with syringes

Cloudy insulin (intermediate insulins and the old long-acting lente type insulins) needs to be mixed before use. This is done by gently turning or rolling the bottle between the hands at least 20 times.[559] Do not shake the bottle as this will lead to problems with air bubbles in the syringe. Start the injection by drawing air into the syringe corresponding to the dose of insulin you will inject. Then inject the air into the insulin bottle, turn it upside down and then draw up the correct dose of insulin. Hold the syringe with the needle upwards, then tap on it a couple of times to get rid of the air bubbles.

Pen injectors

A pen injector (insulin pen) is a practical tool that is loaded with a cartridge of insulin for repeated injections. The standard cartridges contain 300 units (3 ml). Pen injectors will give a more accurate dosage compared with syringes, especially in the low doses.[324,539] Some pens can be adjusted to half units and are therefore well suited for children: NovoPen Echo® (fits with NovoRapid and Levemir), HumaPen Luxura HD® (Humalog) and Junior Star® (Apidra, Lantus). Many teenagers and even adults find that they also appreciate being able to adjust the doses in half-unit increments. The HumaPen Memoir® has an electronic memory for 16 injections and the NovoPen Echo® for one injection. This is very helpful, for example if you are not sure whether or not you took your injection, and your blood glucose is high when you measure it several hours later. However, compared with pumps that have a memory for all doses given over the course of several months, insulin pens still have a very limited memory.[456] When you use a pen injector, start by holding the pen with the needle upwards and eject 1-2 units into the air to ensure insulin flow (an "air shot", see also page 136).

Disposable pens are also available for most insulins. They are a practical alternative for carrying spare insulin, for example when you are travelling. Make sure that you have an extra disposable insulin pen at school, at work, with your grandparents or anywhere else you visit often. According to the ISO standard, insulin pens should have a dosing error of <10% at 10 U (±1 U) and <5% at 30 U (±1.5 U). In one study, all but one doses with Flexpen® were within this limit while 12% of the injections with Optipen® gave the wrong dose, most often not enough insulin.[778]

Why aren't all insulins available for pens?

Traditional intermediate- and long-acting insulins are cloudy and the bottle must be turned or rolled (not shaken!) at least 20 times before the insulin is injected to mix it up well.[559] The pen cartridge contains a small glass or steel marble that will help stir the insulin when the pen is turned. Lente (Monotard, Humulin L) and Ultralente-type insulins (Ultratard, Humulin Zn) are in crystal form and the crystals will break if a glass marble is present. Therefore, no pens are available for these insulins. They are not for sale in the UK or US.

Needles for insulin pens

Brand	Diameter of needle	Size of needle	Length
B-D Micro-Fine+	0.23 mm	32G	4 mm
Insupen	0.23 mm	32G	6 mm
Insupen	0.23 mm	32G	8 mm
B-D Micro-Fine+	0.25 mm	31G	5 mm
NovoFine, Insupen, Penfine, Unifine	0.25 mm	31G	6 mm
B-D Micro-Fine+, Penfine, Unifine Insupen	0.25 mm	31G	8 mm
NovoFine	0.30 mm	30G	8 mm
Omnican mini	0.30 mm	30G	8 mm
Penfine	0.33 mm	29G	10 mm
Penfine	0.33 mm	29G	12 mm
Omnican fine	0.33 mm	29G	12 mm
Unifine	0.33 mm	29G	12 mm
B-D Micro-Fine+	0.33 mm	29G	13 mm
NovoFine	0.36 mm	28G	12 mm
Optipen	0.36 mm	28G	12 mm

Even 4 mm needles have been shown to penetrate the skin well with decreased risk of intramuscular injections,[98] and adults preferred these over 5 and 8 mm needles in a study.[514]

Replacing pen needles

Sterile, disposable pen needles and syringes are designed for single use only. However, many patients reuse them for several injections. The risk of infected injection sites when reusing disposable needles seems to be negligible.[198,955] However, the injections may hurt more [186] since the needle becomes blunted due to tip damage after repeated use [685] and the silicon lubricant wears off. There is also some evidence that reusing needles with damaged tips causes repeated small injuries to the tissue when injecting. This can cause a release of certain growth factors that may lead to the development of fatty lumps

(lipohypertrophy) which may affect the amount of insulin required and its absorption.[999]

You should replace the needle of intermediate-acting insulin after every injection, because of the risk of leakage of fluid from the cartridge or air entry (see page 136) if the needle is left on.[539] The needle may also be blocked by insulin that has crystallized inside the barrel. Remove the needle directly after the injection and put the new one on immediately before the next injection. Eject a unit or two into the air with each new pen needle (the "air shot") to make sure that the tip of the needle is filled with insulin.

Insulin pens should not be shared, as there is a risk of blood-borne infections like hepatitis and HIV even if you change the needle.[175]

Different pens for day and night time insulin

It is easy to take the wrong pen injector by mistake if the pens for day time and night time insulin are similar.

To avoid taking the wrong type of insulin we recommend that you always use two completely

Needle choice guidelines [375]

Age	Needle recommended
Children	4-6 mm
Adults	4-8 mm

All injections should be given with a lifted skin fold ("two-finger pinch-up") at a 45° angle regardless of the needle used, except for injections in the buttocks where perpendicular injections without pinch-up can be used. Injections using 5-6 mm needles can be done without pinch-up if the subcutaneous fat layer is at least 8 mm.[97]

different pens for day time and bedtime insulin, so that you can feel the difference even if it is completely dark. If you have experienced taking the wrong type of insulin even once, having two completely different pens can start to look like a cheap form of life insurance.

Variations in insulin concentration

When the cartridge warms up with the needle attached (e.g. when you carry it in an inner pocket), the liquid in the cartridge will expand and a few drops will leak out through the needle. When the temperature falls again, air will be sucked in. In one study the surrounding temperature was lowered from 27° to 15° C (81° to 59° F). This caused air corresponding to 4 units of insulin to be sucked into the cartridge.[185]

A particular problem will occur with intermediate-acting insulin when the temperature is increased. As the insulin is in the cloudy sub-

If there is air inside the pen cartridge, you may see a drop of liquid coming out from the needle tip after your have withdrawn the needle from your skin.

stance that sinks to the bottom of the cartridge, only the inactive solution will leak out through the needle. The result will be that the remaining insulin will become more potent, up to a concentration of 120 or 140 U/ml. If the pen is stored upside down the problem will be reversed. The insulin crystals will then be closest to the needle and leak out when the temperature increases and the liquid expands. The remaining insulin will then be diluted.

Another possible cause of changes in the insulin concentration is not mixing the NPH insulin thoroughly every time before using it. In one study the insulin concentration in used vials and cartridges of NPH insulin that had not been mixed thoroughly varied between 5 and 200 U/ml.[559] The problem of altered concentration will not occur with clear insulins as the insulin is completely dissolved in the liquid. You will be less likely to have problems caused by changes in temperature if you remove the needle after each injection and store the pen with the top pointing upwards, for example in the pocket of your jacket.

Daniel made this drawing before he was discharged from the hospital. The giant syringe is now a small insulin pen and on his stomach he has placed a small indwelling catheter. The initial fear of needles has been substituted by a more realistic view of the modern injecting equipment that is now available. Compare with the drawing on page 132, which he made before his first injection.

Is it dangerous to inject air?

It is possible, on occasion, to accidentally inject a bubble of air from the syringe or cartridge

Elsa

B-D Safe-Clip® can be used to cut off the needle point from both syringes and pen needles.

Used needles and syringes

Discard used syringes, pen needles and finger-pricking lancets in an empty jar or milk bottle so that no one will be pricked by mistake. You can get a special cutter to remove needle points (B-D Safe-Clip®).

along with the insulin. Subcutaneously placed air is quite harmless to the body and will soon be absorbed by the tissue. The real problem is that you will have missed out on a certain amount of insulin (as much as was displaced by the air). You may need to take a unit or two extra to compensate for this. The same applies if you are using an insulin pump. Air injected through the tubing is completely harmless but you will have missed a certain amount of insulin at the same time which may cause problems.

Insulin on the pen needle

Sometimes a drop of insulin will leak from the tip of the needle after it has been withdrawn from the skin. The drop contains up to 1 unit of insulin and is caused by air in the cartridge which is compressed when you press the pen mechanism.[403] You can avoid this problem by waiting about 15 seconds for the air to expand before withdrawing the pen needle.[403] You can also remove the needle after each injection which will prevent air from being sucked into the cartridge. This problem will not occur when you are using a syringe because you inject all the insulin it contains. Remove the air in the pen cartridge according to the figure on page 136. Even if all air is removed, it is a good idea to hold the needle in for 10 seconds to prevent insulin dripping from the tip of the needle.[45]

How to get rid of the air in the insulin cartridge

When you replace the needle you can get rid of the air by following these steps:

① When the needle is removed, depress the pen mechanism a few times so that the pressure inside the cartridge will be increased. Tap on the cartridge to make the air bubble rise.

② Slowly push the needle through the membrane on the cartridge.

③ Air will leak out as soon as the needle penetrates the membrane. If you push the needle through the membrane too quickly an air pocket will remain in neck of the cartridge (see illustration).

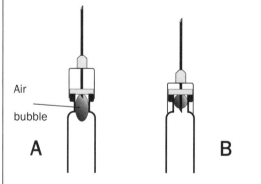

A   B

Push the needle slowly through the membrane when you replace it to allow air to leak out (A). When the needle is pushed quickly all the way in, a small pocket of air is formed in the neck of the cartridge (B).

Injection equipment

The development of thinner needles means that injections for adults are now less painful than they used to be.[703] However, in a double-blind study, children and adolescents did not appear to feel a difference in the amount of pain experienced from 0.30-0.40 mm needles.[448] "Placebo injections" (no needle was attached to some pen injectors, but the people in the study were not aware whether this was the case) caused significantly less pain. This contradicts the common belief that the needles of today are so thin that most of the experienced pain is psychological in origin.

Automatic injectors

An automatic injector will thrust the needle very quickly through the skin, and this keeps pain to a minimum. With one type (Injecto-matic®, Inject-Ease®) the syringe needle is pushed through the skin automatically, but you have to push the insulin in yourself. A similar device (PenMate™) is available for the pen injectors from Novo Nordisk. With another type (Autoject®) the syringe needle is pushed in and the insulin is injected automatically. The Diapen® both inserts the needle and injects the insulin automatically. The Autopen® is a pen injector that injects the insulin automatically after you have pricked the skin yourself with the needle.

The Inject-Ease will insert the syringe needle automatically when you press the spring.

Jet injectors

A jet injector uses very high pressure to form a thin jet stream (thinner than a needle) of insulin that penetrates the skin. The insulin is absorbed quickly and the glucose control can be as good as it is with an insulin pump.[195,539] Some find the device less painful while others experience the pain of a jet injector to be comparable to that of an ordinary injection needle. Bleeding, bruising and delayed pain after the injection have been described.[536] A jet injector might be a good alternative for patients with pronounced needle phobia if the person is not helped by using Insuflon. However, some children may find the device very noisy when the insulin mechanism is triggered.

Indwelling catheters

We like to make the introduction of injections at the onset of diabetes as painless as possible. Our present policy is to give all children below the age of 10 their injections by means of indwelling catheters or injection ports (such as Insuflon® or i-port®) when their diabetes is newly diagnosed. Older children and adolescents are also given the chance to try this

With a jet injector, the insulin is pressed through the skin by using a very high pressure. Once inside, it will spread more widely (left picture), compared with the depot from a regular injection with a pen or syringe (right picture).

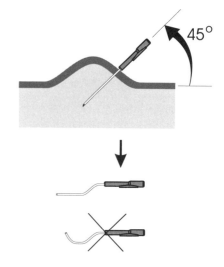

Use the shaded area of the abdomen for insertion of the indwelling catheter (or pump needle). Insert it in a horizontal position or up to 30° from a horizontal line. Otherwise there is a risk of kinking the catheter when you lean forwards. If you have problems with fatty lumps (lipohypertrophies) you can insert the indwelling catheter in the buttocks instead.

Aim at an angle of 45° to the skin when you are inserting Insuflon or a pump needle/catheter. After removal, you can check the catheter profile to see how it was inserted. A "fish-hook" appearance (lower picture) indicates that it was inserted too superficially.

method during their first week of subcutaneous injections after diagnosis. We take all the blood glucose tests by means of an intravenous cannula. These procedures ensure as little pain as possible in the early stages of what will be a life-long relationship with diabetes. After a week or so, the child has had time to adjust psychologically and learn the correct injection techniques. When this has been mastered, he or she can start to try regular injections. Children are given a choice of which injection method to use when they are discharged from hospital. Some 20-25% continue with indwelling catheters while the others choose to start giving themselves regular injections. Insuflon is even used

by many adults who find the injections painful or uncomfortable. In children and adolescents, the use of indwelling catheters from the onset of diabetes has decreased pre-injection anxiety, injection pain and other injection problems significantly.[451]

The use of indwelling catheters makes multiple injection treatment for small children much easier. It is also helpful for people who are not used to giving insulin by injection. Such people may include grandparents, babysitters or day care staff. In addition, an indwelling catheter also makes it easier to give extra injections if they

When using Insuflon you pierce a silicon membrane with the needle instead of the skin. The soft Teflon catheter is placed under the skin, and you inject the insulin through it. The catheter is replaced on average every 4-5 days. This can easily be done at home. If it is painful, you can use a topical anaesthetic cream before replacement.

are needed, as an additional injection will not involve the child in any extra pain. This can be particularly useful in situations such as, for example, choosing to give a child half an insulin dose before a meal even though you cannot be sure just how much that child will eat. This leaves you with the option of giving the child some extra insulin after the meal depending on how much he or she actually has eaten.

Children using indwelling catheters are probably at less risk of developing needle phobia through having been spared traumatic injections during their early experience of diabe-

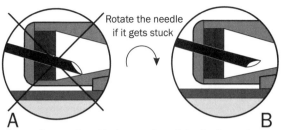

Insert the needle with the opening of the tip directed towards your skin and it will slide in more easily (picture B). Wiggle the needle sideways and rotate it if it still gets stuck.

tes.[451] One study showed that, in particular, the younger patients using indwelling catheters and multiple injection treatment would have found this method more difficult to accept if indwelling catheters had not been available.[444] An American study showed both decreased injection pain and a 10 mmol/mol (0.9%) lowering of HbA_{1c} 6 months after a group of children with elevated HbA_{1c} levels, 64 mmol/mol (8.0%), started using Insuflon.[160]

When should the catheter be replaced?

The average time between replacements is 4-5 days.[442] Some patients will be quite comfortable replacing their catheter once a week while others may need to replace it twice a week. If you disinfect the site with alcohol before inserting the catheter, you will cut the risk of infection. The i-port can be used with an automatic inserter.

Which insulin can be given in the catheter?

Small children usually use the same indwelling catheter both for rapid- or short-acting insulin at mealtimes and for bedtime insulin of NPH-type (Insulatard, Humulin I, Insuman Basal). Mixing Lantus and rapid-acting analogue insulin in a syringe before injection did not affect the 24-hour glucose values in one study,[588] nor HbA_{1c} after 3 months in another.[352] However, in studies looking more closely at the insulin effect, the action of the

---

**Tips for using
indwelling catheters**

⇒ Use topical anaesthetic cream (EMLA®, Ametop®) when inserting the catheter in small children and when new to the technique. Apply it for 1.5 -2 hours before insertion.

⇒ Lift a skin fold and insert Insuflon at a 45° angle (see figure on page 138). Lift the skin with three or four fingers if the subcutaneous tissue is thin, as is likely to be the case in small children.

⇒ Insert with a slight thrust and there will be less risk of "peel-back".

⇒ Apply the part of the adhesive that covers the insertion site first. Never try to remove an adhesive that is already stuck to the skin.

⇒ Insert the injection needle with the opening turned towards the skin and it will not get stuck on the plastic wall. Rotate the needle gently. (See figure on page 139.)

⇒ Use an adhesive of stoma-type (such as Compeed™) if you experience itching or eczema from the enclosed adhesive.

⇒ Use an 8-10 mm needle for both pens and syringes and there will be no risk of piercing the Teflon catheter by pushing the needle too far in. With newer designs of indwelling catheters, different needle lengths may be used. Check this with the inserted instructions.

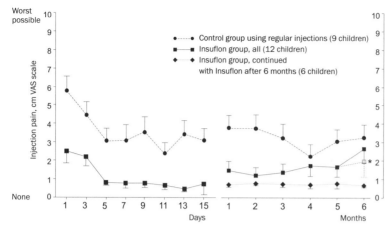

Injection pain in children younger than 8 years using indwelling catheters for introducing insulin injections at the onset of diabetes.[451] This study demonstrated a reduction in pre-injection anxiety, injection pain and other injection problems over a 6-month period. Those children who continued to use Insuflon throughout the whole study scored the pain even lower.

(*Data from two children were excluded; one skipped Insuflon for a week due to eczema problems, one had pneumonia).

rapid-acting insulin is blunted if it is mixed with Lantus.[178] Mixing NovoRapid with Levemir did not affect blood glucose levels negatively in one study,[784] but when studying the insulin effect more specifically the results were the same as for Lantus above.[179] You should therefore always discuss with your doctor before mixing long-acting and rapid-acting insulin. If long-acting insulin is to be given via Insuflon, this insulin should be given first.

Dead space

The dead space of the Insuflon catheter (the hollow inside that will be filled with insulin with the first injection) is approximately 0.5 U of insulin, measured in a clinical setting,[450] the same as for i-port. If the doses are very small, one can add an extra half-unit with the first injection after replacing an indwelling catheter.

When you give yourself your bedtime insulin, the catheter will already be filled with rapid- or short-acting insulin. This will partly be exchanged for intermediate-acting insulin dur-

ing the injection. Remaining in the Insuflon will be a mixture of approximately 0.3 units of bedtime insulin and 0.2 units of rapid- or short-acting insulin.[450] In practice, these tiny amounts of insulin are usually insignificant.

Infection and redness

A very small number of patients develop infections requiring antibiotic treatment (one out of 140 patient months or one out of 850 used catheters). If you develop an infection of the catheter canal in the subcutaneous tissue, it is likely to cause redness and/or pain around the insertion site. If you have problems with redness or infections at the insertion site, we recommend you to use chlorhexidine in alcohol (Hibiclens™ or similar disinfectant) for skin disinfection and hand-washing. Don't use products containing a skin moistener since this causes the adhesive to come loose more easily.

Hygiene is more important if you use an insulin pump or indwelling catheter. Always wash your hands before replacing the catheter. We recommend using chlorhexidine in alcohol for disinfection of the insertion site.

The catheter can peel backwards on the metal needle (called "peel-back") if you penetrate the skin too slowly. This is a typical beginner's problem.

Problems with indwelling catheters?

Problem	What to do about it
Adhesive comes off	Wash the anaesthetic cream (EMLA®, Ametop®) off carefully with water. Apply Skin- Prep™, Masti-sol™ or Tincture of Ben-zoin™ that leave a sticky film when drying. Warm the adhesive with your hand after application. Apply extra tape if necessary.
Itching, eczema from adhesive	Apply hydrocortisone cream. Use a stoma-type adhesive (e.g. Compeed®).
Sticky traces of adhesive	Wipe off with remover such as Detachol™ or Uni-Solve™.
Infection/irrita-tion at the injec-tion site	Wash hands and skin with chlorhexidine in alcohol (Hibiscrub™). Replace the catheter more frequently.
Leakage of insu-lin	An increased pressure when injecting indicates a bent catheter. Replace it! Use 8-10 mm needles.
Sore skin from plastic wings	Apply a piece of tape beneath the wings.
Scars in the skin from old cathe-ters	Caused by an infection of the injection site. Replace Insuflon more frequently. See infection advice above.

Research findings: Insulin absorption and Insuflon

♠ HbA$_{1c}$ test results, blood glucose levels and insulin were all unaltered when using Insuf-lon during a 2-month so called cross-over study.[443]

♠ Studies of insulin pump users have shown both an unchanged insulin absorption during 5 days' use [808] and an increased absorption after 3 days of using the same injection site.[679]

♠ Studies from Finland with indwelling cathe-ters show no change in insulin absorption during 5 days of use.[582]

♠ A Swedish study using radio-actively labelled insulin did not show any change in absorp-tion during 4 days of using indwelling cathe-ters.[445]

apply a skin film (for example Tegaderm®) first, and insert the Insuflon through it, putting the regular adhesive on top of the skin film. Itching can also be caused by perspiration in hot weather or during sports activities. The itching usually disappears when the individual stops sweating.

See page 194 for additional tips if you have problems with dry skin or eczema.

Redness and/or itching can be caused by an allergic reaction to the adhesive. Application of 1% hydrocortisone cream usually helps. If the problem continues, we have successfully used a stoma-type adhesive (such as Compeed® or Duoderm®). Cut a hole for the catheter hood before applying it. Another alternative is to

ROBERT 8 years

An 8-year-old boy made this drawing of himself using an indwelling catheter. Before he started using this, his father had to come home from work twice a day to help his mother hold him, so they could give him his insulin injections.

Adjusting insulin doses

Starting insulin treatment

When type 1 diabetes is first diagnosed, treatment with subcutaneous insulin is started without delay. The total dose may be as high as 1.5-2 U/kg per day (0.7-0.9 U/lb per day) in the period immediately after diagnosis, but it soon goes down. Smaller children are more sensitive to insulin and usually need fewer U/kg. However, insulin dosages are very individual and two children of the same age often need quite different amounts.

Two-dose treatment

In the UK and many other countries, most children are started on two injections per day. Many children will use combinations or mixtures of rapid- (Humalog, NovoRapid) or short-acting insulin (Actrapid, Humulin S, Insuman Rapid) and intermediate-acting insulins (Insulatard, Humulin I, Insuman Basal) before breakfast and before dinner/tea. These doses and mixtures are adapted to the size of meals and usual activity levels. With a two-dose treatment it is essential that the last meal of the day is taken immediately before going to bed (bedtime snack) to prevent night time hypoglycaemia.

Many things need to be balanced in your body to keep the blood glucose level steady. It isn't easy to make all the pieces fit, and it can often be difficult to work out exactly what went wrong. Sometimes, we just have to accept that there is no obvious explanation for why the blood glucose level was high or low at a given time. In this drawing, Robert uses a shark to illustrate how it feels when his body loses this balance.

Three-dose treatment

A three-dose insulin treatment usually consists of a combination of rapid- or short-acting and intermediate-acting insulin for breakfast, rapid- or short-acting insulin for the afternoon snack after returning from school or for dinner/at tea-time, and intermediate-acting insulin at bedtime. This may be a suitable regimen for a smaller child, especially if it is difficult to find someone who can give the lunchtime dose at school or in the day nursery. A combination of rapid- or short-acting and intermediate-acting insulin at breakfast may also be a good solution for the teenager who tends to forget lunchtime insulin doses when at school or out with their peer group. In situations like this, pre-mixed insulin that can be administered with a pen may be an alternative choice.

Multiple injection treatment

In Sweden, the US and many other countries, it is common to use a multiple injection treatment with premeal doses of rapid-acting insulin from the onset of diabetes, even for younger children and toddlers. In some places, young children are started on insulin pumps within a few weeks from the onset of diabetes but usually this form of therapy is started later. With multiple injections, premeal injections will be given for the main meals of breakfast, lunch, dinner/tea and evening snack. An extra bedtime snack will usually be given only if the blood glucose level is low with this type of insulin regimen.

Insulin is adjusted in relation to the carbohydrate content of the meal. Before breakfast, higher doses of insulin are needed in relation to

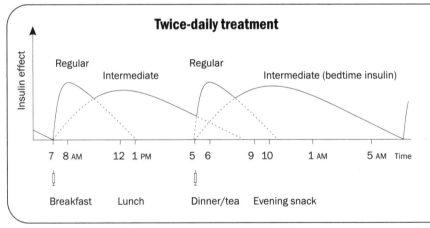

Twice-daily treatment

Before the introduction of the insulin pen in 1985, the usual regimen was twice-daily injections, mixing short-acting and intermediate-acting insulin. The advantage was fewer injections per day. But the disadvantage was difficulty in adjusting doses to take account of changes in food intake or physical activity, and problems with night time hypoglycaemia when the dinner/tea time dose was increased.

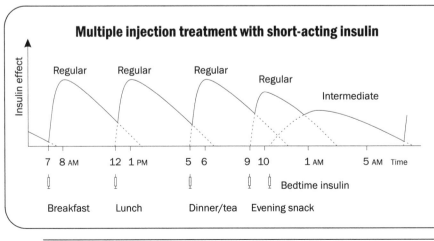

Multiple injection treatment with short-acting insulin

Five daily insulin doses (four doses of short-acting insulin and one dose of intermediate-acting) will better mimic the body's normal mealtime insulin secretion. The system is easy to understand as each insulin dose affects only one meal. Today, rapid-acting insulin is more often used for multiple injection therapy (see page 156).

the size of the meal. This is due partly to increased levels of growth hormone (the dawn phenomenon, see page 58) and partly to a reduction over time in the effect of the bedtime insulin dose. In addition, breakfast usually con- tains a greater proportion of carbohydrates than other meals (e.g. from juice, bread, cere- als). It is becoming more common, however, to start counting carbohydrates just as soon as diabetes is diagnosed.

Premeal rapid-acting insulin + bedtime insulin

If you use rapid-acting insulin (NovoRapid, Humalog or Apidra) for the premeal bolus doses you will have a better effect with that meal. However, you are likely to be short of insulin by the time of the next meal as rapid-acting insulin will not last for more than 3-4 hours at the most.

Rapid-acting + 2 doses of intermediate-acting insulin

You can take a dose of interme- diate-acting NPH insulin (Insula- tard, Humulin I, Insuman Basal) for breakfast to attain a better insulin effect before lunch and dinner/tea. However, it is difficult to get this dose to last until the evening snack without risking too strong an insulin effect at lunchtime, especially in children and adolescents. A third dose of intermediate-acting insulin at lunchtime may solve the prob- lem.

Rapid-acting + 2 doses of long-acting insulin

With long-acting insulin you will have a level of basal insulin in between meals. Previously, Ultra- tard and Humulin U were used this way, but today Lantus is the first choice. It gives a more even effect and is usually given only once daily, in the evening, morn- ing or for dinner. When using small doses you may need to give it twice daily. Compare this insulin curve with the curve of a person without diabetes on page 23.

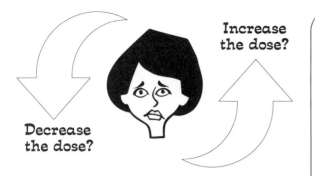

Increase the dose?

Decrease the dose?

The instructions for adjusting insulin doses in this chapter apply mainly to multiple injection treatment. However, many of the principles can be applied even if you are using a two- or three-dose treatment. If you are in the remission (honeymoon) phase and produce insulin of your own, you should reduce the recommended doses (see page 177).

Different types of insulin treatment

Multiple injection treatment with rapid-acting insulin
(Humalog, NovoRapid, see page 156)

Meal	Type of insulin	% of 24 h. dose
Breakfast	Rapid-acting	15-20
	Basal insulin	15-20
Lunch	Rapid-acting	10-15
Dinner/tea	Rapid-acting	10-15
Evening snack	Rapid-acting	10-15
Bedtime	Basal insulin	25-30

If the basal insulin is Lantus or Levemir, around 50% is given as one dose in the evening or morning but some may need two doses of this insulin, especially younger children (see page 174).

Multiple injection treatment with short-acting insulin
(Actrapid, Humulin S, Insuman Rapid)

Meal	Type of insulin	% of 24 h. dose
Breakfast	Short-acting	20-25
Lunch	"	15-20
Dinner/tea	"	15-20
Evening snack	"	10-15
Bedtime	Intermediate-acting	25-30 (-40)

Two-dose treatment

Meal	Type of insulin	% of 24 h. dose
Breakfast	Rapid-acting or short-acting	20-25
	Intermediate-acting	35-40
Dinner/tea	Rapid-acting or short-acting	10-15
	Intermediate-acting	25-30

The pre-dinner/tea intermediate-acting insulin can be given with the evening snack or before bedtime if a three-dose treatment is preferred.

Questions before taking insulin

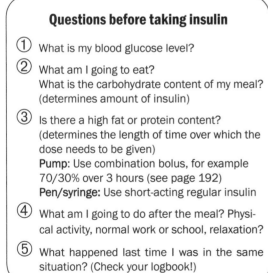

① What is my blood glucose level?

② What am I going to eat?
What is the carbohydrate content of my meal? (determines amount of insulin)

③ Is there a high fat or protein content? (determines the length of time over which the dose needs to be given)
Pump: Use combination bolus, for example 70/30% over 3 hours (see page 192)
Pen/syringe: Use short-acting regular insulin

④ What am I going to do after the meal? Physical activity, normal work or school, relaxation?

⑤ What happened last time I was in the same situation? (Check your logbook!)

How much does 1 unit lower blood glucose?

Units/24 hours	Rapid-acting	Short-acting Regular
20	5.0 mmol/l	4.2 mmol/l
30	3.3 mmol/l	2.8 mmol/l
40	2.5 mmol/l	2.1 mmol/l
50	2.0 mmol/l	1.7 mmol/l
60	1.7 mmol/l	1.4 mmol/l
70	1.4 mmol/l	1.2 mmol/l
80	1.3 mmol/l	1.0 mmol/l
90	1.1 mmol/l	0.9 mmol/l

The figures are from the "1800 Rule" for rapid-acting insulin [1086] (divide 1800 by total daily insulin dose for mg/dl, divide 100 for mmol/l) and "1500 Rule" for regular short-acting insulin [255,285] (divide 1500 by daily insulin dose for mg/dl, divide 83 for mmol/l). The glucose-lowering effect of one unit of insulin is called "correction factor" or "insulin sensitivity factor".[1092]

If a person takes 40 units per day and has a blood glucose of 14 mmol/l (250 mg/dl) before the meal, an extra dose of 2 units will lower the blood glucose level by an additional 5 mmol/l (90 mg/dl) with rapid-acting insulin, or 4.0 mmol/l (70 mg/dl) with short-acting insulin. Do not use the correction factor to subtract units from the premeal dose if the blood glucose level is low and you have taken glucose. The blood glucose level will rise to normal within 10-15 min., and you will then need a normal bolus dose for your meal (see page 66).

Units/24 hours	Rapid-acting	Short-acting Regular
20	90 mg/dl	75 mg/dl
30	60 mg/dl	50 mg/dl
40	45 mg/dl	38 mg/dl
50	36 mg/dl	30 mg/dl
60	30 mg/dl	25 mg/dl
70	26 mg/dl	21 mg/dl
80	23 mg/dl	19 mg/dl
90	20 mg/dl	17 mg/dl

The actual blood glucose-lowering effect of an extra unit is of course dependent upon many factors including food intake, insulin dose, exercise, variable absorption etc. For this reason, the tables must not be used to predict the exact lowering of blood sugar in any individual. They only show the estimated effect. These rules are determined for adults and can be used as starting points for children and adolescents as well.[332] However, do not give more than 0.1 U/kg at one time to begin with (see page 115). By experimenting, you can find out how well they work for you. During the night, a correction dose will usually have a higher effect so you can try by giving half the above-mentioned doses.

How much does insulin lower the blood glucose level?

The actual blood glucose-lowering effect of a given insulin dose depends on many factors: the meal size, the amount of insulin taken earlier in the day, the amount of exercise and even the level of stress. A dose of 0.1 U/kg (0.5 U/10 lb) body weight will give a substantial blood glucose-lowering effect and extra doses in the home should rarely exceed this amount as it will only increase the risk of hypoglycaemia after a couple of hours (although the newer rapid-acting insulins will be safer in this respect).

When does the insulin dose have the peak effect?

Time of injection	Effect when?
Rapid-acting: (NovoRapid, Humalog, Apidra)	
Before meal	For that meal
Short-acting: (Actrapid, Humulin S, Insuman Rapid)	
Before breakfast	Until lunch
Before lunch	Until dinner/tea
Before dinner/tea	Until the evening snack
Before evening snack	Until midnight
Intermediate-acting: (Insulatard, Humulin I, Insuman Basal)	
At bedtime 10 PM (multiple inj. treatment)	During the night until breakfast
Two-dose treatment: Morning	Lunch and afternoon
Dinner/tea	Evening and night
Long-acting: (Lantus, Levemir)	
At dinner/tea	During the night and the morning thereafter
Morning	Afternoon, evening and part of the night

One unit of insulin given between meals will lower your blood glucose by about 1 mmol/l (20 mg/dl) if you use 90-100 units of insulin per day and about 2 mmol/l (40 mg/dl) if you use 45-50 units. To use the "correction factor", divide 100 (83 for short-acting insulin) by your daily insulin dose in units and you will have the blood glucose-lowering effect of 1 unit in mmol/l (1800 for rapid-acting and 1500 for short-acting insulin to get the results in mg/dl).[285] See key fact box on page 146. Modern insulin pumps can use the correction factor to calculate how much extra insulin should be given if your blood glucose is high, and you enter your blood glucose level into the pump.

What to do if your blood glucose level is high

Don't go looking for high blood glucose readings. If you change your ordinary insulin doses or carbohydrate ratios on a daily basis in line with every individual blood glucose reading, you will soon find it impossible to identify which dose actually does what. The blood glucose can swing up and down like a roller coaster, resulting in frequent, and often difficult, hypoglycaemic episodes without your understanding why.[77] While you may often know the reason for a temporary high or low blood glucose reading, sometimes things go wrong with no obvious explanation. If you do not understand what has caused a weird glucose pattern one day, then try to give just the same doses (same carbohydrate ratios and cor-

rection factors) to see if the pattern repeats itself the next day.

A temporary high blood glucose level from time to time is impossible to avoid in everyday life. A person with diabetes, whether child or adult, will not necessarily feel at all unwell when this happens, nor will it affect long-term diabetes control. HbA_{1c} will mirror the value of all blood glucose values, and then a temporarily high glucose level will not make much of a difference. But if the blood glucose is high in the night when you measure it on single occasions, it may influence HbA_{1c} as the night is long and it will affect the mean blood glucose if repeated on many nights.

Important

Never decrease the amount of food to regulate your blood glucose level if you are ill. Drink sugar-containing drinks if your appetite is poor!

Don't adjust insulin doses in relation to food quantities "by eye" or carbohydrate counting when you are ill. See the chapter on illness, page 301.

High blood glucose and ketones

If your blood glucose level repeatedly tests high (15-20 mmol/l, 270-360 mg/dl) and particularly if you have ketones in your blood or urine (as a sign of insulin deficiency), you need extra insulin.

(1) Give 0.1 U/kg (0.5 U/10 lb) of insulin, preferably rapid-acting (NovoRapid or Humalog). See algorithm on page 149 if you are using a two-dose treatment. *If the child uses an insulin pump, this extra dose should be given with a pen or syringe!*

(2) Test your blood glucose and blood ketone levels again after 1-2 hours.

(3) Give another 0.1 U/kg (0.5 U/10 lb) if your blood glucose level has not gone down after 2 hours. If the blood ketones have not gone down considerably, you should suspect that something is wrong with the insulin and get a fresh cartridge from the refrigerator.

Do not give extra rapid-acting insulin more often than every second hour (every third hour with short-acting), or you will risk dose overlap resulting in hypoglycaemia after a couple of hours.

Contact your diabetes team or doctor if you vomit or are in the least unsure about what you should do. This is equally, if not more, important if you are looking after a child with diabetes.

What to do if your blood glucose level is high

① Your blood glucose is high but you are feeling perfectly well

➠ **A temporarily very high blood glucose level (> 25-30 mmol/l, 450-540 mg/dl)**
This can often be caused by not drinking enough, for example during a school outing. If the person is able to pass plenty of urine, the blood glucose level can go down to approximately 20 mmol/l (360 mg/dl) without extra insulin.[701] If you find your blood glucose reading is very high when you are feeling fine, therefore, it may be a good idea to drink plenty of extra water or sugar-free drinks. You should also check your blood or urine for ketones (see below).

➠ **Blood glucose > 8 mmol/l (145 mg/dl)**
This is the recommended level for correcting a high glucose. Rapid-acting insulin has its highest effect after 1-2 hours, so wait at least 2 hours after a given dose before giving a correction dose. Give extra insulin according to the correction factor in the table on page 146 when you correct in between meals. Note that you should not correct a high blood glucose if it is caused by a rebound effect (high blood glucose after being low) or if the high glucose level has been caused by stress. See key fact frame on page 155.

➠ **Your blood glucose often goes high after a certain meal**
Increase the dose (if adjusting by eye) or decreasing the carbohydrate factor (if you count carbohydrates, see page 246). If your blood glucose usually comes down again without extra insulin, you can wait until the next meal and then increase your insulin dose by 1-2 units (or use your correction factor, see below) if the blood glucose level still is high. Breakfast, in particular, can be difficult in that the blood glucose level often rises after you eat, but will go to low if you give extra insulin 2 hours after breakfast. You can then try taking the dose 15-30 minutes before breakfast (see also page 192 if you use a pump).

➠ **Your blood glucose is high (> 15 mmol/l, 270 mg/dl) on 2 occasions with a few hours in between**
Check for blood or urine ketones and give extra insulin according to the correction factor on page 146 even in between meals, but not more than 0.1 U/kg to begin with. If the ketones are increased, see table on page 115.

② Your blood glucose is high before a meal

See the table on page 146 if you are using the correction factor. Increase your premeal rapid- or short-acting dose by 1-2 units if you are eating a standard meal and use your "measurement of eye".

③ Your blood glucose is high at bedtime

➠ **The blood glucose level is high (> 8-10 mmol/l (145-180 mg/dl))**
Give an extra dose of rapid-acting insulin according to your correction factor (see table on page 146). See the algorithm on page 149 if you are using a two-dose therapy.

➠ An extra dose given in the night usually has a stronger effect, and you can therefore try half the dose according to the correction factor table on page 146 if you give the dose after 10 PM ("200-rule" for mmol/l or "3600-rule" for mg/dl). However, many younger children have an increased need of insulin during the hours before midnight,[205,787] and can therefore need the higher dose ("100-rule" for mmol/l or "1800-rule" for mg/dl) if you give the correction dose before midnight. Check your blood glucose at 2-3 am if you have taken extra insulin at bedtime or changed the dose.

④ You are feeling unwell (feeling very hungry, sick or vomiting)

Check for ketones in your blood or urine. **The presence of ketones is a sign of insulin deficiency!** Give an extra dose of insulin (0.1 U/kg, 0.5 U/10 lb) according to the table on page 115 to lower your blood glucose and block the production of ketones in the liver. Avoid giving extra doses more frequently than every second hour to avoid stacking of insulin.

⑤ Your blood glucose level is high at the same time of the day, several days in a row

Take a blood glucose test around 1½-2 hours after the meal several days in a row. If it rises more than 2-3, you need to adjust the dose. Adjust the carbohydrate ratio, so that you will get more insulin (lower ratio) or increase the dose by 1-2 units if you measure by eye. It is important that you wait a couple of days between each dose increase, otherwise it will be difficult to see which change led to what.

The blood glucose level in a non-diabetic person seldom goes above 8 mmol/l (145 mg/dl), and this is the recommended level for a correction dose. If your blood glucose often goes high after a certain meal, you will need more insulin to that meal.

This can be addressed in different ways. If you are using a correction factor based on your insulin sensitivity (see table on page 146), add the amount of insulin needed to lower your blood glucose to your target level. See the fact frame on page 148 for concrete advice on high blood glucose in different situations.

Instead of increasing the insulin dose you can decrease the carbohydrate content of the meal if you are using multiple injection therapy (see page 150). You are usually not as hungry when the blood glucose level is high (see "Hungry or full?" on page 244). Drink water instead of milk or juice with your meal. If your blood glucose is high (> 12-15 mmol/l, 215-270 mg/dl) at snack-time, you will probably not need the snack at all.

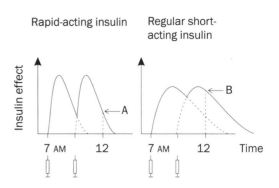

Rapid-acting insulin (NovoRapid, Humalog or Apidra) is preferable when the blood glucose level is high. You can give an extra dose at snack-time without risking dose overlapping and hypoglycaemia, since much of the effect is gone after 2-3 hours. Compare the insulin effect at noon (arrow A) with the right chart illustrating regular short-acting insulin (arrow B). When taking an small extra dose of rapid-acting insulin before going to bed in case of a high blood glucose, the effect of this dose will have waned before the effect of the bedtime dose starts.

If you are feeling unwell, sick or vomiting you should check for ketones in blood or urine and give extra insulin according to the table on page 115. It is better to give rapid-acting insulin (NovoRapid, Humalog or Apidra), as the effect of this will usually disappear before the bedtime insulin has begun to act. There is always a risk of night time hypoglycaemia when you take additional short-acting regular insulin before going to bed. Extra insulin should not be administered more often than every second (rapid-acting) or third (short-acting) hour in case the insulin effects accumulate and cause hypoglycaemia. Rapid-acting insulin (Novo-Rapid, Humalog or Apidra) is the best type to use in this situation. Its quick effect means there is less risk of the doses overlapping.

If you are caring for a child with diabetes, and he or she is hungry, some chewing gum may be a good idea as it will give them something to hold in their mouth until the insulin begins to work. Also, encourage the child to drink some water or diet squash, as high blood glucose causes people to pass a lot of urine.

Extra doses when using two-dose treatment

When you are using a two-dose treatment, this table can be used for extra doses of rapid-acting insulin (NovoRapid, Humalog) that can be given any time up to 10 or 11 PM depending on age.[1013]

Blood glucose

Age, years	15-17 270-305	17-20 305-360	> 20 >360	mmol/l mg/dl
0-6	0.5-1 U	1-2 U	2-3 U	
7-11	1-2 U	2-3 U	3-5 U	
12-15	2-3 U	3-4 U	4-8 U	
16+	3-4 U	4-6 U	6-12 U	

Different ways of adjusting insulin doses

There are many different ways of adjusting insulin doses. Check with your diabetes team which method they recommend for you.

Fixed insulin doses

With this system you eat your meals and snacks at the same time of the day each day. The meal plan emphasizes having the same amount of carbohydrates for a given meal each day. A two-dose treatment usually works along this line.

Varied insulin doses but not counting grams of carbohydrate

With this system you take premeal insulin for each meal and vary the size of the dose according to the carbohydrate content, but without counting the exact grams of carbohydrate in each meal. I call this "measurement by eye" in this book.

Counting grams of carbohydrate to determine insulin doses

With this system you need to determine the grams of carbohydrate in each meal and you use the insulin:carb ratio to determine your insulin dose (see page 246). A correction dose for high or low blood glucose is calculated using your insulin sensitivity factor (see table on page 146).

What about the food you eat?

It is easiest if you count carbohydrates, since the dose will automatically be correct when you adjust the amount of carbohydrate in the calculations. For a description of how to count carbohydrates in a more exact manner, see page 246. The alternative is to use the "measurement

by eye" method. Once you have learnt about the way the carbohydrate content of a meal relates to your individual insulin dose, it is often possible to determine the effect of your meal on blood glucose levels just by looking. If you eat a little more carbohydrate (for example, an extra potato or some more pasta) than usual, you can take (0.5-) 1-2 units of rapid- or short-acting insulin extra if you are on a multiple injection or pump therapy. However, if you eat some more meat, chicken or fish, you need not increase your insulin dose since this type of food does not contain carbohydrates. If you eat a little less, you can decrease the dose by (0.5-) 1-2 units. If you are counting carbs, correct the dose according to your insulin:carb ratio. Measure your glucose level after around 2 hours to determine whether the dose was correct. Make a note in your logbook for future reference in case you are confronted with a similar situation another time.

Changing the content of the meal to affect blood glucose

At times it may be an option to change the size of the meal depending on the actual blood glucose level. The feeling of fullness after a meal is often increased when the blood glucose level is high.[571] If the blood glucose before the meal is increased (8-14 mmol/l, 145-250 mg/dl) it may be a good idea to wait a while after taking the insulin to let the glucose level begin to decrease before eating. You can drink water instead of milk with the meal or decrease the carbohydrate content of the meal by eating less pasta, potato, rice or bread.

Reduction in food should be used very cautiously with growing children. Children themselves should be involved in discussions and any decisions about this. They should also be offered increased amounts of food later in the day to compensate. In general, witholding food in an effort to control blood glucose should be discouraged.[365] But it can be a practical solution on occasions when a child whose blood glucose

Temporary changes of the premeal insulin dose, e.g. during illness

1-2 U in the advice below implies changing the rapid- or short-acting dose by 1 unit for a premeal dose of < 10 U and 2 units for a premeal dose of > 10 U. If the dose is < 3 U, change by only 0.5 units. The table is modified from reference [507]. If you use the correction factor for extra doses, it will give you the amount of extra insulin.

Blood test before meal	Measure / Change in dose
< 3.5-4 mmol/l < 65-70 mg/dl	1) Take 10 g of glucose (three dextrose tablets) or half a glass of sweet juice (see table on page 66). 2) Wait 10-15 minutes before eating anything else to allow glucose to pass into the bloodstream. 3) Take ordinary dose of premeal insulin.
4-8 mmol/l 70-145 mg/dl	Take your ordinary dose.
8-11 mmol/l 145-200 mg/dl	1) Increase the dose by 1-2 U or drink water with the meal.* 2) Take the insulin just before you eat (at least 30 min. before with short-acting).
11-14 mmol/l 200-250 mg/dl	1) Increase the dose by 2-3 U or drink water with the meal.* 2) Take the insulin 10 min. before you eat (45 min. before with short-acting).
14-20 mmol/l 250-360 mg/dl	1) Increase the dose by 2-4 U and drink water with the meal.* 2) Take the insulin 20 min. before you eat (60 min. before with short-acting), or wait until the blood glucose level returns to normal before you eat.
> 20 mmol/l > 360 mg/dl	1) Increase the dose by 0.1 U/kg (0.5 U/10 lb) body weight. 2) Same as 14-20 mmol/l.
Consider for a moment...	Why the blood glucose might be high? Missed insulin dose? Other illness or fever? Have you eaten more than usual?
Ketones?	Contact your diabetes staff, clinic/ward or A&E department if you vomit or feel generally unwell.

* if you normally drink something containing carbohydrates with the meal.

What if your blood glucose level wasn't what you expected it to be?

➡ Have you eaten the usual amount of food?

➡ Was the timing between your meal and the injection correct?

➡ Have you been more active physically than usual?

➡ Were you feeling ill, with a cold or fever?

➡ Could you have had hypoglycaemia with rebound phenomenon?

➡ Was your injection technique different from usual? Did you change the injection site for your premeal injection (e.g. from abdomen to thigh)?

➡ Did you inject into muscle rather than fat?

➡ Did you inject into a fatty lump (lipohypertrophy)?

➡ The variability in effect of injected insulin doses is huge, even when two identical doses are given under the same conditions. This variation lies outside the "human factor" and may explain much of the frustration of trying to find correct doses.

is high does not feel hungry. The feeling of fullness can be the same if the amount of non-carbohydrate food is increased although the decreased amount of carbohydrate contributes to a lower glucose level after the meal.[365]

The stomach empties more slowly when the blood glucose level is high.[957] This makes it much more likely that food will still remain in your stomach from the previous meal if you have a high blood glucose level. Food will then continue to empty into the intestine (where glucose can be absorbed into the blood) even though you have not necessarily eaten recently.

Fluids are emptied from the stomach more quickly than solid food.[1062] Drink early in the course of the meal if your blood glucose is low.

If it is high, it is better to wait until the end of the meal before drinking as your stomach will be more slow to empty. See also "Emptying the stomach" on page 231.

You may feel hungry even if your blood glucose level is high. This is due to a lack of glucose inside the cells which signals hunger. If you eat as usual (without taking extra insulin) despite a high blood glucose level, your blood glucose will remain high. If this continues for some time it will result in increased insulin resistance, e.g. a given insulin dose will be less effective than usual (see page 223).

Feeling ill, especially with fever, is likely to depress your appetite. In spite of this, the blood glucose level will often be high, due to an increased need for insulin during illness. You should then increase the insulin doses and try to eat the usual amount of carbohydrate. Do not attempt to reduce the carbohydrate content in the meal to compensate for a high blood glucose level if you are ill! If your appetite is poor, it is important to drink plenty and eat food with a high carbohydrate content, e.g. bread, potatoes, rice, pasta or cereal. This will give the insulin "something to work with" (see page 301 for further advice on insulin treatment when ill).

Changing insulin doses

Check your blood glucose before and around 2 hours after meals and during the night. (See the key fact box on page 100.) Aim for blood glucose values not below 4.0 mmol/l (70 mg/dl) and not above 10 mmol/l (180 mg/dl) when adjusting insulin doses, and that it does not change by more than 2-3 mmol/l (35-55mg/dl) when the dose is accurate. See key fact box on page 153 for recommended levels before and after meals. If there are difficulties in finding a pattern in regular blood glucose monitoring, a continuous glucose measurement will give much more information (CGMS, see page 107).

Basic rules

① You cannot interpret a 24-hour glucose profile correctly if you have had hypoglycaemic episodes. A high blood glucose level could be the result of a rebound phenomenon following a hypoglycaemic episode. Begin by decreasing the doses to avoid hypoglycaemia before attempting long-term adjustments. If you have a hypoglycaemic reaction without an apparent reason (such as exercise or too little food) you should decrease the "responsible" insulin dose the following day (see table on page 66).

② Symptoms of hypoglycaemia should appear at a normal level, i.e. at 3.5-4.0 mmol/l (65-70 mg/dl). If they first appear when your blood glucose has fallen below 3.5 mmol/l (65 mg/dl), you should take great care to avoid all low blood glucose levels for the next 1-2 weeks. This will help improve the situation. If you have hypoglycaemic symptoms at levels above 4.0-4.5 mmol/l (70-80 mg/dl), you should resist the temptation to eat until the blood glucose has fallen to 3.5-4.0 mmol/l (65-70 mg/dl). After a couple of days, the symptoms will appear at a lower blood glucose level (see pages 44 and 63).

③ It is a good idea to try and keep the carbohydrate content of the meals and amount of physical activity as consistent as possible when you are adjusting insulin doses.[1092] The total carbohydrate content of meals and snacks is more important for the pre-meal insulin dosage than the type or source.[365]

④ Don't change more than one dose at a time. It is otherwise easy to end up in a vicious cycle where you don't know what has caused what.

⑤ Don't make large changes in your doses all at once. If you use carbohydrate counting, a change of the ratio by 1 g is usually sufficient if the ratio is below 10, 2 g if it is between 10 and 20 and 3-5 g if it is above 20 g. Change doses of less than 3 U by 0.5 U at a time, 3-10 U by 1 unit, and those more than 10 U by 2 units at a time if using measurement by eye.

⑥ Wait a couple of days between insulin changes so that you can see clearly what the outcome is. There is always a depot of insulin in your body and it will take a couple of days before this has reached equilibrium (see "Depot effect" on page 86). Intermediate-acting insulin (Insulatard, Humulin I, Insuman Basal) should not be changed more often than every 2 or 3 days. When using long-acting insulin (Lantus, Levemir) you should not change the dose more often than 2 or 3 times per week.

What is the best blood glucose level to have?

Ideally, your blood glucose readings during the day should be between 4.0 and 10.0 mmol/l (70-180 mg/dl).[39,206] If you have problems with hypoglycaemic unawareness you should be careful to avoid all readings below 3.5-4 mmol/l (65-70 mg/dl, see page 52).

Blood glucose	Before meal	2 h. after meal
Ideal	4-6 mmol/l 70-110 mg/dl	5-8 mmol/l 90-145 mg/dl
Acceptable	5-7 mmol/l 90-125 mg/dl	8-10 mmol/l 145-180 mg/dl
Hypoglycaemic unawareness*	5-9 mmol/l 90-160 mg/dl	8-11 mmol/l 145-200mg/dl

*When symptoms of hypoglycaemia have returned to a level of > 3.5 mmol/l (63 mg/dl), normal targets for blood glucose can be used. See "Hypoglycaemia unawareness" on page 52.

---

⑦ Review blood glucose readings and insulin doses once a day when you have time to sit down and make notes of your carbohydrate ratios and correction factors (when carbohydrate counting) or plan preliminary doses for the following day (when measuring by eye) in your logbook. If you do this, you will be much less likely to make rash decisions.

⑧ Be careful about extra insulin on days when you are making adjustments to the longer-acting insulins. You will otherwise distort all the information you have built up relating to the usual doses. If you feel that you need to give yourself extra insulin (if you are ill, for example) it is better to stop your blood glucose monitoring for the 24-hour profile. Start over again after a couple of days or a week when you are back to normal doses again.

For the same reason, you should not eat anything extra if you measure a low blood glucose level, between 3.5 and 4.5 mmol/l (65-80 mg/dl), but feel well when doing a 24-hour chart. This applies also to the 2-3 AM blood glucose test (but be sure to check again after 0.5-1 hour). You want to know the blood glucose values during a night with normal sleep, not when you have been eating. As you have no symptoms, you would have slept on without eating if you had not set the alarm to take the test. If you have hypoglycaemic symptoms, you may get a rebound effect which will make it difficult to interpret the following blood glucose levels and then it is better to restart the 24-hour testing another day.

⑨ If you don't understand why your blood glucose reading turned out the way it did, try keeping to the same doses for another day or two. You will often see the pattern better then.

Keeping good records

Register all blood glucose readings in your log-book, otherwise you can never make an adequate judgement. If you have difficulties remembering to write them down, an electronic logbook can be a good alternative. Most blood glucose meters have memories and can be connected to a computer to be read. In an American study, patients who recorded their blood glucose readings in a logbook had lower HbA_{1c} values (54 mmol/mol, 7.1%) compared with 63 mmol/mol (7.9%)] than those who did not record their tests.[109]

What is the best order for changing the doses?

(multiple injection treatment)

① Lower the doses to avoid hypoglycaemia. Then concentrate on one dose at a time for a couple of days.

② Start by adjusting the dose for the evening snack if you are on multiple injections so that you will have an appropriate blood glucose level when going to bed.

③ Adjust the bedtime insulin dose (dinner/tea dose if on two-dose therapy) to obtain good overnight and pre-breakfast blood glucose levels.

④ Adjust the breakfast insulin dose.

⑤ Adjust the doses for lunch and dinner/tea (if on multiple injections).

Just as all fingerprints are different all insulin doses are different and unfortunately they often seem to work differently every day. This is perfectly logical if you think about it — we are all very different as individuals and insulin must be adjusted to fit the individual lifestyle.

When should you take your pre-breakfast insulin?

Timing the breakfast dose will be easier if you are using rapid-acting analogue insulin. This may be difficult to accomplish as part of a stressed morning routine if you use regular short-acting insulin, since it is then more important to take the insulin some time before breakfast. Measure your blood glucose as soon as you wake up, then adjust the time of your breakfast accordingly. Use this as a baseline for experimenting with different times:

If you find that your blood glucose goes high very soon after the meal (for example if you are using a CGM, see page 107), you will probably do better if you take the dose of rapid-acting insulin up to 15-30 minutes before breakfast even at normal blood glucose levels.

Insulin at breakfast

Blood glucose level		Rapid-acting insulin	Ordinary short-acting insulin
mmol/l	mg/dl		
< 3	< 55	just before*	just before
3-5	55-90	just before	15 min. before
5-8	90-145	15 min. before	30 min. before
8-12	145-215	20 min. before	45 min. before
> 12	> 215	30 min. before	60 min. before

* After taking some glucose, wait 10-15 minutes before eating. Your glucose level will then be corrected and you can take a normal meal dose before you begin eating. Do not lower the dose, since this will only result in a high blood glucose and a rebound effect after the meal.

Premeal bolus doses

Insulin for breakfast

It is more difficult to obtain a good blood glucose level during the night than during the day. Ideally, you want to start the morning with a normal blood glucose level. If you have problems with your blood glucose early in the morning when using NPH as bedtime insulin, you may be better off with Lantus as your basal insulin. The premeal insulin dose for breakfast will usually need to be slightly higher in relation to the amount of carbohydrates (see "Starting insulin treatment" on page 142). So even if the breakfast does not contain more carbohydrates than other meals, the breakfast injection is likely to contain the largest premeal dose of the day. It may be difficult to give sufficient amounts of insulin for breakfast without getting low at lunchtime, especially if the breakfast contains more than 60 g of carbohydrates.[721] You can try by exchanging one slice of bread or some cereals for an egg to decrease the amount of carbohydrates. If you use a pump, a so called superbolus might be an alternative (see page 192).

Insulin for lunch and dinner/tea

Measure your blood glucose level before and 2 hours after the meal. The same strategy applies for lunch and dinner/tea doses as for breakfast. If lunch at school is very early, the dose can be divided into two, where one dose is taken with the early lunch and one with a larger snack in the afternoon.

It is very important to take the insulin dose before the meal. If you take it after the meal, the effect on the blood glucose will be too late and children should therefore be trained in estimating how much they will eat. Children aged 10-12 years should be able to handle this, and it is important for parents to follow this up during high school. Unfortunately, we see many teenagers who have learnt to take the dose after the meal doing so even after they have become adults.

Insulin for evening snack

When using multiple injections, premeal insulin is usually given with the evening snack. Aim to start the night with an appropriate blood glu-

cose level by monitoring it shortly before the evening snack and adjusting food and the dose of rapid- or short-acting insulin thereafter. This system works especially well for younger children and for those going to bed fairly early, as long as they do not have too much physical exercise after eating.

Two units of rapid- or short-acting insulin per open sandwich (15 g of carbohydrates) is usually an appropriate dose for a person taking around 50 units in total over 24 hours, if you

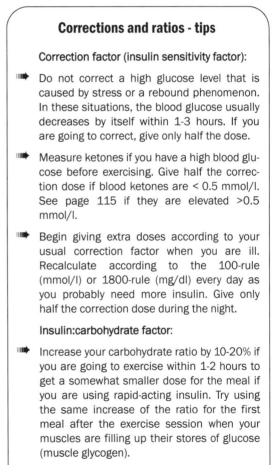

Corrections and ratios - tips

Correction factor (insulin sensitivity factor):

➠ Do not correct a high glucose level that is caused by stress or a rebound phenomenon. In these situations, the blood glucose usually decreases by itself within 1-3 hours. If you are going to correct, give only half the dose.

➠ Measure ketones if you have a high blood glucose before exercising. Give half the correction dose if blood ketones are < 0.5 mmol/l. See page 115 if they are elevated >0.5 mmol/l.

➠ Begin giving extra doses according to your usual correction factor when you are ill. Recalculate according to the 100-rule (mmol/l) or 1800-rule (mg/dl) every day as you probably need more insulin. Give only half the correction dose during the night.

Insulin:carbohydrate factor:

➠ Increase your carbohydrate ratio by 10-20% if you are going to exercise within 1-2 hours to get a somewhat smaller dose for the meal if you are using rapid-acting insulin. Try using the same increase of the ratio for the first meal after the exercise session when your muscles are filling up their stores of glucose (muscle glycogen).

➠ If you have an infection with fever, your ordinary doses are usually not sufficient. Lower the ratios by 10-20% to get more insulin and adjust according to blood glucose readings after the meals.

have a glass of milk (10 g of carbohydrates) along with the sandwiches for the evening snack (1 U per 10 g carbohydrates). For advice on carbohydrate counting and weighing your food, see page 246.

Pre-school children often have a greater need of insulin before midnight,[205,787] and it can then be a good solution to give a dose of short-acting regular insulin for the last meal of the day if you use rapid-acting insulin for meals and Lantus or Levemir as basal/night time insulin. See page 186 if the child uses an insulin pump.

When using a two-dose treatment, no insulin is given at bedtime. A bedtime snack is essential to avoid night time hypoglycaemia with this type of insulin regimen.

Holiday or weekday?

Your physical activity level can vary a great deal depending on whether you are at school, working or enjoying the weekend. It is normal, and relaxing, to have a lie in at the weekend, and the time-table for meals may be different. Having a lie in will be easier if you use the basal insulin analogues Lantus and Levemir as they have a longer-lasting insulin effect. Factors such as these may make it appropriate to have different insulin doses for weekdays and weekends. Make notes in your logbook and try to find a schedule that works well for you. Rapid-acting analogues are probably a better alternatives if you work shifts (see page 94).

Physical exercise or relaxation?

If you will be exercising within a few hours of a meal, you may need to eat a little extra or decrease your short- or rapid-acting premeal dose by 1-2 units (see also the chapter on physical exercise, page 278). If you will be resting more than usual, you may need to increase the doses by 1-2 units.

If you use rapid-acting insulin (NovoRapid, Humalog) you can try increasing the breakfast dose by 1-2 units in both examples above. If you are using regular short-acting insulin and your blood glucose readings look like the chart on the left, you can try increasing the breakfast dose by 1-2 units. If the blood glucose level decreases before lunch (as on the chart on the right) you will have problems with hypoglycaemia if you increase the pre-breakfast insulin dose of short-acting insulin. It is then better to take it earlier, i.e. 45 minutes before breakfast, if you usually have a 30-minute interval.

Using rapid-acting insulin analogues

The action of rapid-acting insulin will begin much more quickly than regular short-acting insulin when given as an abdominal injection, but not as quickly as the insulin that is produced in the beta cells of a healthy pancreas. This means you can administer it just before meals and still get a good insulin effect when your blood glucose level starts rising.[675]

The rapid-acting insulins NovoRapid, Humalog and Apidra have led to major improvements in the treatment of diabetes. These insulins more

How do you adjust insulin doses?

*indicates a change > 2-3 mmol/l (35-55mg/dl)	Dosing "by eye"			Carb. counting with insulin:carb ratio		
	Normal dose	BG rises* after 2 h.: Increase to	BG decreases* after 2 h.: Decrease to	Normal ratio	BG rises* after 2 h.: Decrease to	BG decreases* after 2 h.: Increase to
Breakfast	8 U	9 U	7 U	5 g	4 g	6 g
Lunch	6 U	7 U	5 U	8 g	7 g	9 g
Dinner	6 U	7 U	5 U	8 g	7 g	9 g
Evening meal	5 U	6 U	4 U	8 g	7 g	9 g

The thinking is similar when adjusting doses "by eye" or when using carbohydrate counting. You monitor your blood glucose before and 1½-2 hours after the meal. If the level increases more than 2-3 mmol/l (35-55mg/dl) the amount of insulin needs to be increased; in the example from 8 to 9 U for breakfast. When carbohydrate counting, you change the ratio, i.e. how many grams 1 unit of insulin covers. In the example, the ratio is changed from 5 to 4 grams per unit, i.e. a decreased ratio gives more insulin. **The difference in counting between the two methods is that an increased dose gives more insulin, while a decreased ratio gives more insulin.** It feels a bit backwards if you are not used to carb. counting, but you quickly get used to it.

closely resemble the insulin release of a healthy pancreas during the eating of a meal (see page 23). The rapid effect is caused by the splitting of the insulin into smaller parts directly after the injection, allowing it to be absorbed into the bloodstream very quickly (see page 75). The three rapid-acting insulins NovoRapid (aspart), Humalog (lispro) and Apidra (glulisine) have identical effects on blood glucose control, whether they are given as injections [847,852] or via an insulin pump.[116,530] Rapid-acting insulins can be taken just before meals, so there is no need to be punctual twice as with the older short-acting insulins that were recommended to be taken 30 minutes before meals.

At the present time, we in Sweden give all those children and adolescents with newly diagnosed diabetes an intensive insulin treatment with multiple premeal doses. This regimen consists of rapid-acting insulin before meals (3-4 doses) and basal insulin (long-acting once or twice daily).

Blood glucose before evening snack

When taking the rapid- or short-acting dose before the evening snack when using multiple injections, you should aim to have a blood glucose level of around 6-8 mmol/l (110-145 mg/dl) at bedtime. If you are using a correction factor, see table on page 146.

Test before evening snack	Measure
< 3.5-4 mmol/l < 65-70 mg/dl	Take glucose, wait 10-15 min. and then take a normal meal dose.
> 8 mmol/l (145 mg/dl)	Increase the dose by 1-2 units or according to the correction factor.
> 14-15 mmol/l (250-270 m/dl)	Think about what can have caused the high blood glucose. Increase the dose according to the correction factor, but do not give more than 0.1 U/kg extra.

By how much at a time should the dose be changed?

If you need to change the rapid- or short-acting insulin dose, for instance when you are running a temperature, while you are exercising, or when ill, we recommend the following changes to start out with:

Carbohydrate counting		Measurement "by eye"	
Carb. ratio	Increase or decrease by	Ordinary insulin dose	Increase or decrease by
> 20	3-5 g	1-3 U	0.5 U
10 - 20	2 g	4-9 U	1 U
< 10	1 g	> 10 U	2 U

A higher ratio gives less insulin and vice versa. The ratio is not to be changed if you eat less or more food, Instead recalculate the dose according to the ratio. However, you should adjust the ratio if your blood glucose 1½-2 hours after the meal is 2-3 mmol/l (35-55mg/dl) higher or lower compared to before the meal. See page 246 for details on how to change the carbohydrate ratio.

If you use measurement "by eye", you can use the above table for increments of dose changes. Avoid changing the dose too much since this will cause fluctuations in your blood glucose levels, and it will be more difficult too see any patterns.

Many parents find it difficult to estimate how much food their toddlers will eat at a meal. In this situation it would be an advantage to be able to give the injection after the meal when they know how much the child has actually eaten. Although several studies show that rapid-acting insulin is effective early enough even if it is taken after the meal,[75,152,248,912] clinical experience from continuous glucose monitoring shows that this is more likely to result in a high glucose peak after the meal. It is therefore best practice to give at least part of the dose before the meal, which easily can be done if the child is using a pump or an injection aid (Insuflon® or i-port®).

Rapid-acting insulin works well during the remission phase (honeymoon phase, see page

How to correct a high glucose level?

Use the 100-rule for mmol/l (1800-rule for mg/dl) to get the correction factor (how many mmol/l or mg/dl one unit of insulin will lower your blood glucose): Divide 100 for mmol/l (1800 for mg/dl) by TDD (Total Daily Dose = meal boluses + long-acting insulin counted in units). The insulin sensitivity is increased during the night, and you can the try using 200/TDD for mmol/l (3600/TDD for mg/dl).

Correct blood glucose levels above 8 mmol/l (145 mg/dl), and calculate a dose to bring you down to 6 mmol/l (110 mg/dl). When you get used to the method, you can try correcting to 5.5 or -5.0 mmol/l (100 or 110 mg/dl).

If you have used the 100/1800-rule to calculate the correction dose, and you find that it gives too much insulin or too little, you can try by using the increments below:

Correction factor (with mmol/l)	Increase or decrease factor by
> 20	3-5 mmol/l
10-20	2 mmol/l
3-10	1 mmol/l
< 3	0.5 mmol/l

Correction factor (with mg/dl)	Increase or decrease factor by
> 400	100 mg/dl
200-400	50 mg/dl
60-200	20 mg/dl
< 60	10 mg/dl

If you use measurement "by eye" to correct high glucose level, you can increasing changing the dose by the below increments. Double the extra dose if your blood glucose is above 12-15 mmol/l (220-270 m/dl).

Ordinary insulin dose	Increase dose by
1-3 U	0.5 U
4-9 U	1 U
> 10 U	2 U

Blood glucose 2 hours after breakfast

The pre-breakfast dose of rapid-acting insulin can be adjusted by referring to the results of tests taken 2 hours after breakfast. With regular short-acting insulin you can use readings taken before lunch. See the chart on page 156. If you are using a correction factor, see table on page 146.

Blood glucose	Measure
< 4 mmol/l < 70 mg/dl	Decrease the breakfast dose by 1-2 units or increase the carbohydrate ratio.
> 8 mmol/l > 145 mg/dl	Increase the breakfast dose by 1-2 units or decrease the carbohydrate ratio.
> 12-20 mmol/l > 215-360 mg/dl	Think! Is there any particular reason for your blood glucose level to be high just now? Did you miss your breakfast dose? Are you unwell?
Hypoglycaemia between breakfast and lunch?	Decrease the breakfast dose by 1-2 units or increase the carbohydrate ratio.

Switching from short- to rapid-acting insulin

Always talk to your diabetes team if you are interested in changing type of insulin. A rule of thumb is that the total number of units per day should be about the same with the new type of insulin. However, when using Lantus you may need a slight reduction. It is very important to take frequent tests, especially when you are new to a certain type of insulin.

① **Premeal doses**
A - You are on multiple injections:
Decrease the premeal doses by 1-2 units and add these units as an extra injection of basal insulin for breakfast. If you will be using NPH insulin (Insulatard, Humulin I, Insuman Basal) or Levemir, you can continue taking the same number of units of bedtime insulin as before. If you plan to use long-acting basal insulin (Lantus) you will probably need to decrease the premeal doses by 2-3 units.

B - You are on two doses per day:
You already take basal insulin twice daily as NPH or Lente insulin (alone or in a mix). Begin by distributing 50-60% of your total number of units per 24 hours as rapid-acting insulin on the number of main meals you eat (usually 3-4 depending if you eat an evening or bedtime snack). The breakfast dose usually needs to be slightly larger than the dose for other meals.

Divide the remaining number of units per day as shown below:

② **Distribution of basal insulin:**
See key fact box on page 169 for advice.

221) for premeal doses as you are likely to be producing insulin on your own to provide part of the basal requirement during the day. A study of adults in the remission phase found a fall in the numbers of low blood glucose readings some hours after the meal, when this type of insulin treatment was being used.[815]

Snacks become less necessary if you use rapid-acting insulin. This is because the insulin effect coincides better with the blood glucose-raising effect of a meal. As a result, insulin levels between meals are lowered. So if you do have a snack between meals, you will need an extra dose of insulin to be sure you avoid an increase in blood glucose.

Rapid-acting insulin may be a good alternative if you have irregular eating habits. Some people find they can even manage to skip a meal (and the dose of NovoRapid or Humalog), especially if they use a basal insulin regimen with Lantus or Levemir or take NPH twice daily. Check your blood glucose more frequently if you try this.

When can rapid-acting insulin be used for premeal injections?

Since the effect of rapid-acting insulin is too short to cover the periods between meals, you will need to take a basal insulin (i.e. another type of insulin that covers the basal need for insulin between meals) as well. You can try using rapid-acting insulin (NovoRapid or Humalog) in the following situations:

➡ If you take two injections of intermediate-acting NPH (Insulatard, Humulin I, Insuman Basal) or Levemir or one to two of long-acting Lantus as basal insulin (see page 144).

➡ If you use NPH as basal insulin only for bedtime, NovoRapid or Humalog may still be a good alternative if you eat frequent, regular meals (not more than 3-4 hours apart). However, you will need to be more strict with your mealtimes.

➡ If you are in the remission phase (honeymoon phase), your pancreas may produce enough insulin on its own to partially cover the basal needs between meals.

➡ NovoRapid and Humalog are very good alternatives if you use an insulin pump since the pump will supply the basal insulin (see page 214).

➡ If you have insulin antibodies (see page 218) you will produce your own long-acting insulin by binding insulin to the antibodies. One sign of having insulin antibodies is that you get redness in the skin after injections. If you are using regular short-acting insulin you can try replacing it with rapid-acting insulin. The chemical structure of this insulin is slightly different and it may give you fewer problems with antibodies and redness after insulin injections.

Adjusting the basal insulin

When using rapid-acting insulin for meals, you will also need another insulin to ensure that your need for basal insulin between meals is met. Without basal insulin, your blood glucose will begin to rise 3-4 hours after an injection of rapid-acting insulin.[540,675] If you are using Lantus, one dose per day may cover your need for basal insulin. Younger children using small doses often need to take Lantus twice daily to be sure it is effective round the clock. See page 174 for further advice on using Lantus.

When using NPH (Insulatard, Humulin I, Insuman Basal) as basal insulin you will probably need to take a second injection in the morning to avoid lack of insulin and a rise in blood glucose before the next meal. This is often also the case with Levemir as basal insulin, especially in children. If you take basal insulin in the morning, you will have more freedom to adjust your mealtimes, even if your meals are irregular with up to 6-7 hours between them.

Adults may try using only one dose of NPH basal insulin to start with. In a US study, only 20% of the adults needed to be switched to twice-daily basal insulin.[1133] In an Australian follow-up of 100 adults transferred to Humalog, 54% required an additional NPH dose in the morning.[201]

The basal insulin should give a steady level of insulin between meals during the day. Check the blood glucose before meals and, if necessary, change the dose of basal insulin (see the graph on page 161). See page 166 for advice on NPH insulin, page 173 for Levemir and page 174 for Lantus. It may be a bit difficult to decide how to adjust the doses of basal insulin. Ask your diabetes team for advice, especially when you are new to using rapid-acting insulin.

High blood glucose levels

The rapid-acting insulins are well suited as "emergency insulins" in a situation when you need to lower a high blood glucose level quickly (e.g. if you have nausea and ketones). Give according to the correction factor on page 146.

Achieving a better HbA$_{1c}$ with rapid-acting insulin

Rapid-acting insulins have a very quick but fairly short span of action. This may result in a lack of insulin in your body by the time of the next meal, especially if your meals are widely spaced. Many research studies do not show any significant improvement in HbA$_{1c}$ when switching to Humalog unless this change is combined with other measures. Below are some alternatives that have been tried with good results:

➠ Need for basal insulin between meals.
  1) Intermediate-acting (NPH) or long-acting insulin (Ultratard, Humulin Zn) also in the morning.[315,900]

  2) 10-40% intermediate-acting insulin (NPH) mixed with the rapid-acting insulin for all main meals.[283,315]

  3) Use Lantus [552] or Levemir [494] as basal insulin.

➠ Adjust your diet to the action profile of the rapid-acting insulin (smaller snacks [900] or no snacks at all [631] and larger main meals).

Many teenagers appreciate the possibilities of increased mealtime flexibility, which may be a reason for the change to rapid-acting insulin.[130] In a US study, teenagers using Humalog found coping with diabetes less difficult and reported less negative impact of diabetes on quality of life and fewer worries about diabetes.[419]

When adjusting your premeal doses of rapid-acting analogue insulin, it is a good idea to check your blood glucose before and 2 hours after the meal. If the blood glucose readings are like the graph on the left, you should try increasing your breakfast dose of rapid-acting insulin by 1-2 units or adjust your insulin:carb ratio to a smaller carb number if you are counting carbohydrates. The dose of basal insulin (intermediate- or long-acting) or basal rate (if you are using an insulin pump) seems to be correct since the glucose level doesn't change much more until lunchtime.

On the right graph, the blood glucose doesn't rise until 2 hours after breakfast. The breakfast dose is correct but the dose of basal NPH insulin in the morning needs to be increased by a unit or two. If you are taking one dose of Lantus in the evening, you can try increasing this dose. However, if increasing Lantus or Levemir in the evening results in morning hypoglycaemia, you may be better off dividing the dose and taking part of it in the morning.

However, you rarely need to take more than 0.1 U/kg (0.5 U/10 lb) body weight as an extra dose at one time. A higher dose will increase the risk of having hypoglycaemia a couple of hours later. Test your blood glucose level again after 2 hours. Give another 0.1 U/kg (0.5 U/10 lb) if the level has not gone down. Some people need to take more than 0.1 U/kg in this situation. Increase the dose slightly if you need to, as you work out what is appropriate for you.

You can take an extra injection of rapid-acting insulin at snack-time, and the effect of this injection will be almost over by the time you are ready for your next meal 2-3 hours later.[522] If you inject yourself with short-acting insulin at regular 2-hour intervals, you run the risk of the effects of these injections overlapping. This would make you more likely to experience hypoglycaemia later on (see figure on page 149).

If your blood glucose level is high at bedtime, you can take a small dose of rapid-acting insulin and have less risk of hypoglycaemia later in the night compared with short-acting insulin. The correction factor is most often adjusted so that you will get a lower extra dose after 10 PM (often not until midnight for younger children). The risk of having a too low blood glucose level in the middle of the night is small as the effect of the rapid-acting insulin will decrease before your night time insulin has really begun to take effect. To be on the safe side, always check your blood glucose level during the night to help you work out the best dose for you in this situation.

Examples of doses when switching to rapid-acting insulin

Beware! These doses are only suggestions for your first doses when switching to rapid-acting insulin. In the early days you must test your blood glucose before and after every meal as well as during the night.
You must not change insulin types on your own before discussing them with your doctor or diabetes nurse. See action profile graphs on page 144:

Example 1: 8-year-old weighing 32 kg (70 lb)

		Breakfast	Lunch	Dinner/tea	Evening	Bedtime	U/24 h.
Previous dose	Two-dose treatment	18 U Mix 30/70 (=5 Reg. + 13 NPH)	–	14 U Mix 30/70 (=4 Reg. + 10 NPH)	–		32
	Multiple injections with Reg.	6 U Reg.	5 U Reg.	5 U Reg.	4 U Reg.	12 U NPH	32
New dose	Rapid-acting and NPH or Levemir	6 U HL/NR 5 U NPH/LE	4 U HL/NR	5 U HL/NR	4 U HL/NR	8 U NPH/LE	32 (40% basal)
	Rapid-acting and Lantus	5 U HL/NR 6 U LA	5 U HL/NR	4 U HL/NR	3 U HL/NR 9 U LA	–	32 (42% basal)

Example 2: teenager (50-60 kg, 110-130 lb) or young adult (70-80 kg, 150-180 lb)

		Breakfast	Lunch	Dinner/tea	Evening	Bedtime	U/24 h.
Previous dose	Two-dose treatment	14 U Reg. 18 U NPH	–	10 U Reg. 26 U NPH	–		68
	Multiple injections with Reg.	14 U Reg.	12 U Reg.	10 U Reg.	8 U Reg.	24U NPH	68
New dose	Rapid-acting and NPH or Levemir	12 U HL/NR 10 U NPH or LE*	9 U HL/NR	8 U HL/NR	7 U HL/NR	22 U NPH or LE*	68 (47% basal)
	Rapid-acting and Lantus	12 U HL/NR	10 U HL/NR	7 U HL/NR	7 U HL/NR 32 U LA	–	68 (47% basal)

Reg. = regular short-acting insulin, NPH = NPH insulin, NR = NovoRapid, HL = Humalog, LA = Lantus, LE = Levemir. With smaller doses of Lantus, it is sometimes necessary to give it twice daily.
*With larger doses of Levemir, you can try giving it once daily.

Meal bolus doses are usually decreased when switching to rapid-acting insulin. The difference in premeal rapid-acting doses with Lantus or NPH as basal insulin is caused by different insulin profiles. NPH insulin gives a higher level of basal insulin at lunch compared to Lantus. The lunch dose of rapid-acting insulin is therefore usually not decreased when switching to Lantus. Levemir may give a greater insulin effect at lunch, so you can try the same lunch dose as with NPH insulin to begin with.

Hypoglycaemia

If you are using rapid-acting insulin, your premeal dose will be "responsible" for hypoglycaemia that occurs within 2-3 hours of the meal (see key fact box on page 66). Due to the very short time action of rapid-acting insulin, you will need to rely more upon carbohydrates with a high glucose content (glucose, honey, sugar) to treat hypoglycaemia. If hypoglycaemia occurs later, the basal insulin usually contributes more. Due to the rapid decline of the insulin effect after 2-3 hours, hypoglycaemia caused by NovoRapid and Humalog will resolve more quickly than those caused by regular short-acting insulin.

A meta-analysis (analysis of many studies) suggests that people who use rapid-acting insulin are at lower risk of hypoglycaemia than those who use short-acting insulins.[151] In a study where the participants were free to adjust their premeal doses, the number of hypoglycaemic episodes decreased by 11% among those people who injected Humalog immediately before the meal compared with those who took regular short-acting insulin 30-45 minutes before.[43] The risk of hypoglycaemia has also been shown to decrease among people using NovoRapid.[527] In a clinical follow-up of 100 adults switching to Humalog, 86% reduced their HbA_{1c} and 57% reduced the frequency of hypoglycaemia.[201] 47% managed to reduce both HbA_{1c} and the hypoglycaemia frequency.

In several studies, the frequency of hypoglycaemia decreases even during the night when using NovoRapid [528] or Humalog.[43,151,487,845] This may be because a dose of regular short-acting insulin for the last meal of the day gives a long enough effect to last into the night.

Exercise

If you take a dose of rapid-acting insulin within 1-2 hours before exercising, you may often need to lower the dose (see page 290).[1050] If you have exercised late in the evening you may need to

Tests when changing type of insulin

When you change the type of insulin you take, you will need to take more tests than usual. It is advisable to keep in touch with your diabetes nurse or doctor every day by telephone, fax or e-mail for the first few days or even a week.

Blood tests:

1) Before each meal
2) 1.5-2 hours after each meal
3) One test during the night depending on which bedtime insulin you use:
   2-3 AM: NPH insulin (Insulatard, Humulin I, Insuman Basal)
   3-5 AM: Long-acting insulin (Lantus, Levemir)

decrease your breakfast dose of rapid-acting insulin. Remember to decrease your bedtime insulin by 2-4 units after strenuous exercise. When using a pump, use the temporary basal function to lower 10-20% during the night.

Pre-mixed insulin

Pre-filled mixtures of rapid-acting and intermediate-acting insulin are available (NovoMix 30 Humalog Mix 25). If you have a long wait (4-5 hours or more) between lunch and dinner/tea, you may have problems with rising blood glucose before the next meal. This is caused by the waning of the breakfast intermediate-acting insulin. In such a situation, it may be a good idea to take a pre-mixed insulin (e.g. 50/50) at lunchtime or add some NPH insulin to the syringe. When you calculate the doses, try to think in terms of half-quantity NovoRapid or Humalog and half-quantity intermediate-acting insulin (Humulin I, Insulatard). A mixture of 70% rapid-acting and 30% NPH insulin has shown good results in adults, but is not yet commercially available.[1041] In children, it is generally preferable to mix insulins in a syringe rather than using pre-mixed insulin (see page 78).

Sometimes people can feel burdened by so many tests and changes in insulin doses. If this applies to you, take a break for a week or two, taking blood glucose tests only when necessary to avoid hypoglycaemia. Make sure that you concentrate instead on having as good a time as possible. (The same principle applies to parents monitoring their children.) You can then come back to monitoring again afterwards with renewed commitment and enthusiasm.

Short-acting regular insulin

Regular short-acting insulin, when used for premeal injections, covers both the carbohydrate content of the meal and the need for basal insulin until the next meal, but it needs to be taken 30 min. before the meal. If you are using rapid-acting insulin, you can inject yourself immediately before your meal, then you will not have to worry about the time interval before eating. In practice, many individuals using short-acting insulin end up taking their premeal doses shortly before eating. This will risk the blood glucose level rising sharply after the meal, only to be followed by a low blood glucose some hours later when the effectiveness of the short-acting insulin has reached its peak.

To avoid a lack of insulin between meals when using premeal doses of regular short-acting insulin, the gap between major meals preceded with insulin injections should not be more than 5 hours. If you switch to rapid-acting insulin,

you need not be so strict about timing if you have a sufficient supply of basal insulin.

Switching to rapid-acting analogues

Because rapid-acting insulin better matches the blood glucose profile after a meal, you will probably have to reduce your premeal doses by about 10% when starting with Humalog.[815] Otherwise there will be a risk of hypoglycaemia 2-3 hours after the meal,[631] especially if it contains pasta (giving a slow rise in blood glucose) or fewer carbohydrates and more fat, e.g. meat with a cream sauce.[161]

Adjust the premeal doses for rapid-acting insulin in the same way as for regular short-acting insulin, depending on the carbohydrate content of the meal and your actual blood glucose level. If you are using NPH insulin (Insulatard, Humulin I, Insuman Basal) for basal insulin, you should adjust the bedtime dose as you did before. Long-acting insulin (Ultratard, Humulin Zn) takes effect so slowly that you should probably take it around 5-7 PM to get the benefit during the night. However, long-acting Lantus can be given later in the evening.

In a Finnish study, patients were advised to transfer at least half of their snack carbohydrates to the previous main meals, when starting with Humalog.[900] This resulted in a 3 mmol/mol (0.25%) decrease of HbA$_{1c}$ (for those who followed the dietary advice) and less hypoglycaemia, even during the night.

With regular short-acting insulin, the dose for the last meal of the day will also contribute to the insulin levels during the early part of the night. Adults who switched to Humalog found that a 20% decrease of the evening snack dose combined with a 25% increase in the bedtime NPH dose resulted in better glucose levels after the meal and unchanged glucose levels overnight.[15] In our experience, younger children using rapid-acting insulin often experience a rise in blood glucose level shortly after falling asleep. One way of compensating for this is to

Do you need regular short-acting insulin while using rapid-acting insulin for meals?

Short-acting insulin (Actrapid, Humulin S, Insuman Rapid) will give you a longer effect (around 4-5 hours compared with 2-3 hours for rapid-acting insulin (Humalog, NovoRapid) and may be better in certain situations (sometimes we call it the "party-insulin"):

➠ A meal with 2-3 courses that takes longer than usual to eat.

➠ A birthday party where food will be served several times within a couple of hours.

➠ A meal rich in fat (such as pizza) or protein (such as a large steak).

➠ A meal with a low glycaemic index (GI, see page 240)

➠ Many young children need a higher level of basal insulin just after falling asleep (i.e. before midnight),[205,787] and this may be achieved by giving short-acting insulin for the last meal of the day.

Rapid-acting insulin can be mixed with short-acting insulin to give a slightly prolonged insulin effect for example:

➠ To cover a mid-morning snack.

➠ When the interval between meals is longer.

➠ When eating a meal with high fat content.

If you have a pump you can use an extended bolus dose to achieve a longer insulin effect for meals like this. The only way to find out what works best for you is to experiment while checking your blood glucose.

give short-acting insulin (Actrapid, Humulin S, Insuman Rapid) for the evening snack, and increase the dose until the right balance is achieved.

Do you need regular insulin when using analogues?

Cereals with milk for breakfast will work fine with rapid-acting insulin, but food that is absorbed slowly such as lasagne (pasta with a sauce rich in fat) or beans (with a low glycaemic index, see page 242), which had previously been covered well by regular short-acting insulin, may give you problems now. This also applies to meals rich in fat, since fat causes the stomach to empty more slowly. With rapid-acting insulin the result may be a lowering of the blood glucose level within ½-1 hour after the meal, before the glucose in the food has been absorbed into the blood. If your blood glucose is low (below 4.0 mmol/l, 70 mg/dl) before such a meal, it is a good idea to take your injection of rapid-acting insulin after the meal to stop your blood glucose from dropping even lower before the carbohydrates in the meal have time to enter your bloodstream.[546]

If you start the meal by drinking something containing sugar, such as a glass of juice, your blood glucose may be prevented from falling. You could take an injection of regular short-acting insulin with this type of meal while using rapid-acting insulin for the other meals.

Rapid-acting insulin has a quick effect that fits well with sugary sweets. However, for treats containing fat, such as ice cream, chocolate and crisps, the effect may be too quick. A dose of regular short-acting insulin may then be more appropriate. The alternative is to inject Novo-Rapid or Humalog after a treat of this type.

If you eat very slowly, or eat many small meals (rather than main meals) during the day, regular short-acting insulin may be a better alternative.[120] If you are having a dinner with a lot of courses, you can try to divide your meal dose of rapid-acting insulin and take part of it for the starter and part for the main course. An alternative is to take regular short-acting insulin for meals when you are sitting still for longer than usual, or a prolonged bolus when using a pump.

Basal insulin

When more than 2-3 hours have passed since the last meal, the liver will supply glucose to prevent the blood glucose level from falling too low. A low basal level of insulin is necessary to keep the blood glucose level stable, and allow the cells to use the glucose as fuel. If there is no insulin available at all, the counter-regulatory hormones (adrenaline and glucagon, see page 35) will raise the blood glucose level by increasing the output of glucose from the liver even more. Basal insulin (background insulin) should give a low and steady level of insulin in between meals and during the night. The night is long and high blood glucose levels during the night can have a substantial effect on your HbA_{1c}.

Many different factors contribute to a high blood glucose level in the morning. The most widely used bedtime NPH insulins (Insulatard, Humulin I, Insuman Basal) have their greatest effect in the middle of the night. At the same time, the body's insulin sensitivity is increased between midnight and 2 AM compared with 6-8 AM [129] (the night time secretion of growth hormone increases the blood glucose early in the morning, see "Dawn phenomenon" on page 58). When combined, these factors result in an increased risk of hypoglycaemia in the middle of the night. See page 174 if you are using Lantus as your long-acting insulin.

Night time insulin action

It is difficult to state the best blood glucose to go to bed on. Studies have shown that blood glucose levels of more than approximately 7 mmol/l (120-130 mg/dl) when going to bed,[83,947] or at midnight,[728] decrease the risk for night time hypoglycaemia. When using Lantus or Levemir as basal insulin, you can probably aim at a slightly lower blood glucose level when going to bed, 5-6 mmol/l (90-110 mg/dl). A higher dose will last longer, and thus have a bet-

ter effect on the morning blood glucose level (see page 78).

Later in the night, the effect of the bedtime insulin decreases at the same time as the insulin sensitivity also decreases due to the dawn phenomenon (see page 58). This causes a morning rise in the blood glucose level. Night time hypoglycaemia followed by rebound phenomenon (so called Somogyi phenomenon) can occur if the insulin levels are low during the later part of the night and can further contribute to a high

---

Tests to take when adjusting the night time dose

The tests will be more representative if your day has been routine, without heavy physical exercise or hypoglycaemia. The bedtime blood glucose level for children should be about 5-6 mmol/l (90-110 mg/dl) with Levemir and Lantus, and 7-8 mmol/l (125-145 mg/dl) when using NPH insulin, when you take the bedtime dose to ensure a "normal" night. It is advisable to take a test in the middle of the night every 1-2 weeks to make sure that you are not at risk of night time hypoglycaemia.

☞ Blood tests: Before evening snack
                   Evening at 10 PM
                   Night at 2-3 AM with NPH,
                   3-5 AM with Lantus and
                   Levemir

☞ Urine tests: Morning (if short in supply of
                   blood glucose strips)

Getting up in the middle of the night to take a test is not much fun. Try to take tests during "normal" nights when you will obtain most information.

morning glucose (see charts on page 60 and 167).

In adults on multiple injection treatment, the risk of night time hypoglycaemia seems to follow a different pattern, probably due to a lower degree of hormonal activity. In one study,[81] only 30% of the night time hypoglycaemia would have been detected by a 3 AM blood glucose

r-a = rapid-acting insulin, LE = Levemir

8 U r-a	6 U r-a	4 U r-a	6 U r-a	9 U	37 U/24 h.
4U LE				LE	

The blood glucose level rises early in the night and is still high in the morning after a night with high values. With a large dose of rapid-acting insulin for breakfast, the blood glucose level falls in the morning, and there is hypoglycaemia in the afternoon.

Start by decreasing the pre-meal bolus at lunchtime to avoid the afternoon hypoglycaemia. Then increase the pre-evening snack bolus dose (or perhaps eat slightly less). Alternatively lower your carbohydrate ratio, and increase the bedtime insulin (remember to check the blood glucose at 3-4 AM!). Then you can adjust the dose before breakfast when you have obtained a better blood glucose level during the night.

Blood glucose monitoring before bedtime insulin

Younger children will usually allow blood tests and injection of bedtime insulin to be done while they are asleep. On the other hand, giving food to a newly awakened child can be very tricky, especially when the blood glucose level is low. It is often more practical to test before eating the evening snack. You can then adjust the amount of food and insulin dose, in order to start the night with the best possible blood glucose level.

Test before bedtime insulin	Measure
5-6 mmol/l (90-110 mg/dl) (Lantus, Levemir) 7 mmol/l (125 mg/dl) NPH insulin	Give ½-1 glass of milk. A good alternative with a pump is to use the temporary basal rate to decrease by 30% over 2-3 hours, and you will not need to wake up the child
6-10 mmol/l (110-180 mg/dl)	Give the ordinary dose
10 mmol/l (180 mg/dl)	Give 1-2 units of short- or rapid-acting insulin or according to the correction factor

If you give a larger snack at bedtime, you may need to give some extra insulin as well. Giving an extra dose of insulin along with the bedtime insulin may increase the risk of a hypoglycaemia early in the night. It is best to use rapid-acting insulin (Novo-Rapid or Humalog) as the peak effect of this insulin will decline before the bedtime insulin of NPH type begins to act. With Lantus there will be less risk of night time hypoglycaemia in this situation, and you can also safely give short-acting insulin in this situation.

test. In another study,[1069] 29% of the patients had night time hypoglycaemia (< 3 mmol/l, 55 mg/dl) but none of these occurred between 1.30 and 3.30 AM. This suggests a longer time to peak action of the bedtime insulin (of NPH type) which was taken at 11 PM. The conclusion from this study was that after midnight (e.g. 1-2 AM) hypoglycaemia was always preceded by a bedtime glucose reading of < 7.5 mmol/l (135 mg/dl) and that early morning hypoglycaemia did not occur if the blood glucose level on waking was > 5.5 mmol/l (100 mg/dl).

If the blood glucose level in the middle of the night is higher (about 7 mmol/l, 125 mg/dl in this study) than it would be in an individual without diabetes, the blood glucose level as

| 5 U Reg. | 4 U Reg. | 4 U Reg. | 3 U Reg. | 5 U NPH | 21 U/24 h. |

Reg. = Regular short-acting insulin

This person used NPH insulin as bedtime insulin. The dawn phenomenon (see page 58) contributes to a rising blood glucose level during the later part of the night. If you increase the insulin dose for bedtime you will have a lower morning blood glucose level (dashed line) but you will also increase the risk of night time hypoglycaemia. You must therefore check the blood glucose at 2-3 AM when adjusting your bedtime insulin dose. Compare with the graphs on the top of page 174.

such will cause insulin sensitivity to decrease (increased insulin resistance). The result will be that increased insulin sensitivity, present at a normal blood glucose level, will not occur.[129] This is an important part of the explanation for why it is so difficult to adjust the bedtime insulin dose. You will have a sort of either/or situation when it will be practically impossible to find the "correct" insulin dose.

Either:

If the insulin dose is high enough to bring the blood glucose down to about 7.0 mmol/l (125 mg/dl) or less in the middle of night, the insulin sensitivity increases and there will be a risk of night time hypoglycaemia.

The difficult, often impossible, balance of night time insulin

Either...

You must increase the bedtime insulin dose to lower the blood glucose level in the morning...

Or...

... but if you increase it too much, the insulin sensitivity in the middle of the night will increase when the blood glucose is lowered and you will be at risk of hypoglycaemia. This will happen not only if you increase the bedtime dose too much, but also if you forget to decrease the bedtime insulin when needed, e.g. after a game of football. See the text for a strategy to address this "either/or" dilemma. The very variable absorption of injected insulin further adds to the frustration of finding a correct bedtime dose. If you recognize these problems you may be better off trying Levemir, as its effect varies less from night to night, or Lantus which has an effect that is longer and more even compared with NPH insulin.

Dosing of basal insulin

Begin with approximately 40-50% of your daily dose as basal insulin. You will probably end up with 40-60%, often slightly higher for teenagers (to compensate for missed meal doses) than for children or adults.

NPH: Begin with approximately 40% of your daily dose as basal insulin, one third in the morning and two-thirds at bedtime.

Lantus: Begin with 50% of your daily dose as a single dose at your evening snack or at bedtime. Young children may be better off taking Lantus in the morning to avoid low glucose levels in the night. When using small doses, it may be better to split the dose into two and to take around half the dose in the morning and half in the evening.

Levemir: Give approximately 50% of the daily dose as basal insulin, half in the morning and half in the evening. Children with newly onset diabetes and teenagers with large doses (that give effect over a longer time) can try giving the whole dose in the evening.

Or:

If the insulin dose is too small causing the blood glucose to increase above 7.0 mmol/l (125 mg/dl) after midnight, the insulin sensitivity will decrease. This will result in even higher blood glucose later in the night and in the morning.

In practice, the blood glucose level will vary a great deal from morning to morning due to this either/or effect. The dawn phenomenon on the other hand is mostly constant from night to night. The large and often frustrating variability in morning blood glucose, despite the same insulin dose, is caused by variations in the speed of absorption of the injected dose of bedtime NPH insulin, in combination with a waning insulin effect early in the morning.[129] Levemir may be a better alternative in this case, since it gives a more predictable effect with a considerably smaller "day to day" variation in absorp-

tion.[482] The long-acting insulin Lantus gives a more even insulin level during the night, resulting in both a decreased risk of night time hypoglycaemia and less rise in the early morning blood glucose level (see page 174).[873] Continuous glucose monitoring can often help you decide which basal insulin will give you the best overnight glucose profile.

What should you do next?

Increase the bedtime dose by 1-2 units at a time until the blood glucose level approaches 6-8 mmol/l (110-145 mg/dl). Check at 4-5 AM when using Lantus or Levemir, at 2-3 AM with NPH. The blood glucose level should be at least 5-6 mmol/l (90-110 mg/dl) when you take the 2-3 AM test to avoid night time hypoglycaemia. A level of 6 mmol/l (110 mg/dl) as such is not disturbingly low but you should have some leeway as the blood glucose level another night might very well be 1-2 mmol/l (20-40 mg/dl) lower, even if you take the same insulin doses. When the blood glucose level in the morning is fine, the basal effect of Lantus or Levemir should also last during the day if you take only on dose of the basal insulin. You can check this by looking at the glucose level before lunch and dinner. If the blood glucose level is normal 2 hours after the meals but there is a tendency for it to rise before the next meal (see graphs on page 161), you may be better off taking Lantus or Levemir twice daily.

High blood glucose in the evening?

If you are using rapid-acting insulin (Novo-Rapid, Humalog or Apidra) you can administer a small extra dose along with the bedtime insulin if your blood glucose level is high. This is because this insulin will have ceased to be effective before the intermediate-acting NPH insulin kicks in. However, we don't recommend giving extra short-acting insulin at bedtime to decrease a high blood glucose level, not even if you inject it in the abdomen. The effect of such a dose will overlap with the bedtime NPH injection,

High blood glucose levels in the morning: what can you do?

Night time hypoglycaemia with rebound phenomenon?

You can wake up with a high glucose reading after a night time hypoglycaemia followed by a rebound phenomenon. It is therefore very important to monitor your blood glucose in the middle of the night before increasing your basal insulin if you wake up with high blood glucose levels.

Long-acting insulin (Lantus, Levemir)

① Increase the dose by 1-2 U at a time until the morning glucose is OK, but check your blood glucose around 3-5 PM so it is not too low then.

② With long-acting insulin, you can probably go to sleep with a blood glucose of 5-6 mmol/l (90-110 mg/dl) without risking a night time hypoglycaemia if your dose is correctly adjusted.

③ If the dose is large (> 15-20 U), it may be better to split it into two: one dose before breakfast and one in the evening. You usually begin with the same size for both doses, and can then adjust the day and night dose separately. Many find that 2 doses work much better, even if it means an extra injection per day. See page 174 for more details on Levemir and Lantus.

Bedtime insulin of NPH type insulin (Insulatard, Humulin I, Insuman Basal):

This insulin may cause problems because its effectiveness can cease before the morning. In order to make it last longer, you will need to increase the dose (see page 78). However, if you are to do this without risking night time hypoglycaemia, you may need to start the night with a slightly higher blood glucose than usual, tentatively 10-12 mmol/l (180-215 mg/dl). Try following these steps:

① Lower your evening premeal dose by 1-2 units at a time, until your blood glucose level is 10-12 mmol/l (180-215 mg/dl) at the time you take your bedtime insulin.

② Increase your bedtime insulin dose slowly. However, your blood glucose should always be at least 5-6 mmol/l (90-110 mg/dl) at 2-3 AM.

③ If your blood glucose level still is high in the morning, it is better to change to Levemir or Lantus, which have a much longer duration than NPH, up to 24 hours.

putting you at risk of hypoglycaemia 4-5 hours later. With Lantus or Levemir as basal insulin, it is usually safe to give short-acting insulin in this situation.

Blood glucose levels at night

If you are taking tests from a child for a 24-hour profile, you should not give anything to eat if the blood glucose is low in the middle of the night (4-5 mmol/l, 70-90 mg/dl) and the child is not showing any symptoms of hypoglycaemia. After all, the child would not have woken up if you had not taken the test — and what you are interested in is what happens during an ordinary night. Instead of giving the child food, check the blood glucose once again

after 0.5-1 hour and don't forget to check the morning blood glucose as well. This will be a tiresome night but you will learn a lot about how your child's diabetes works. An adult with diabetes may find it more difficult to reset the clock and go back to sleep. It is therefore best to eat something in this situation. Don't forget to record all test results in your logbook.

Possible causes for high blood glucose in the morning

① Insufficient insulin effect late at night due to the dawn phenomenon (see page 58) or too low a dose of bedtime insulin?

Morning tests

Morning tests: Blood glucose   8 mmol/l (145 mg/dl)
                 Urine glucose   0.1%
                 Ketones   0

When the blood glucose level rises above the renal threshold, glucose passes into the urine. Since the blood glucose level is not so high in the morning you know that it has been higher some time earlier in the night. You will need to know what your renal threshold is if you are to interpret urine tests correctly (see page 101).

Morning tests: Blood glucose 12 mmol/l (215 mg/dl)
                 Urine glucose   0.5%
                 Ketones   0 (or +)

The blood glucose level has been adequate during most of the night since the urine glucose concentration is low. Only blood glucose monitoring during the night can determine how low the blood glucose level actually has been. What you do know from the urine test is that the blood glucose level only has been above the renal threshold for a short while, since the urine glucose concentration is low. If ketones are present when urine glucose during the night is low, this indicates that the blood glucose has been low as well ("starvation ketones"),

Morning tests: Blood glucose   14 mmol/l (250 mg/dl)
                 Urine glucose   5%
                 Ketones   ++

The blood glucose level has been high during most of the night due to a lack of insulin. This has caused a large amount of glucose to pass into the urine. The ketones in the urine are caused by a lack of glucose inside the cells.
.

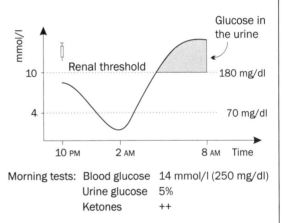

Morning tests: Blood glucose   14 mmol/l (250 mg/dl)
                 Urine glucose   5%
                 Ketones   ++

There has been a rebound phenomenon after hypogly-caemia in the night. Ketones were passed into the urine during hypoglycaemia (starvation ketones) and glucose was passed into the urine when the blood glucose level was high. The morning tests are exactly the same as in the example above. If you misread this, believing that the blood glucose has been high all night, you may very well increase the insulin dose instead. The blood glucose level would then fall even lower the following night, giving an even more pronounced rebound phenomenon. This type of reaction is called the Somogyi phenomenon (see page 59). The only way to distinguish it from the pattern in the upper right example is to check your blood glucose at 2-3 AM.

② Rebound phenomenon after night time hypoglycaemia?

③ Not enough insulin to cover the evening snack or bedtime snack?

④ Too high a blood glucose level in the evening?

⑤ Forgot to mix the bedtime insulin thoroughly when using cloudy insulin? (Levemir and Lantus don't need mixing.)

Night time hypoglycaemia

The first thing to do is to decrease the bedtime or basal insulin dose and/or make sure that a reasonable bedtime snack is eaten every night. See page 55 for further instructions. If you practise competitive sports or do hard physical training some days or evenings every week, you will probably need less insulin before your evening snack and at bedtime on these days (see "Physical exercise" on page 278).

The only way to know for sure what your blood glucose level is in the middle of the night is to take a test. The best time to take it is usually at 3-5 AM when using Lantus or Levemir, and at 2-3 AM if you use NPH insulin (Insulatard, Humulin I, Insuman Basal).

NPH basal insulin

Try giving the bedtime insulin of NPH type (Insulatard, Humulin I, Insuman Basal) as late as possible to ensure that it lasts until morning. Giving it at 10 PM usually works well for most people. You must of course consider your family routines, particularly if the family member with diabetes is a young child. It is not a good idea to sit up late in order to give the bedtime dose. For many children, it may be possible to administer a late (10 PM) bedtime insulin dose without them waking, or even stirring. If the child has an indwelling catheter (Insuflon or i-Port, see page 137), it will be easy to give the late-night dose while he or she is sleeping.

Night time glucose monitoring

Test your blood glucose levels at the time when you expect them to be at their lowest. This may differ from person to person. See page 100 for suggestions on times for monitoring.

① Monitoring for a 24-hour chart
If you have something to eat in the night, the entire night's blood glucose values will be affected and the chart will be difficult to interpret. Eat only if the blood glucose level is less than about 4-5 mmol/l (70-90 mg/dl) or you are feeling unwell. The same applies if you are caring for a child. If the level is above 4-5 mmol/l (70-90 mg/dl) it is better to take another test 0.5-1 hour later to see in which direction the level is heading.

② Monitoring because of actual risk of night time hypoglycaemia
If you (or your child) have not eaten well or have exercised more than usual during the afternoon/evening, you should take precautions to avoid hypoglycaemia during the night. Eat or drink something if your blood glucose level is < 6-7 mmol/l (110-125 mg/dl), and you will be able to sleep on safely.

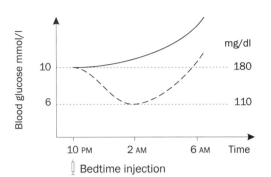

⚕ Bedtime injection

A small difference in insulin dose can cause a large difference in the blood glucose level due to an either/or effect (see page 168). The insulin sensitivity increases (decreased insulin resistance) in the middle of the night, causing the blood glucose to fall, but only if the blood glucose is within normal levels for people without diabetes, below about 6 mmol/l (110 mg/dl), dashed line. If the blood glucose increases after midnight, the insulin resistance will increase as well and the bedtime insulin dose will not be able to lower the blood glucose level sufficiently (solid line).

It is often difficult to ensure that bedtime insulin of intermediate NPH-type (also called isophane insulin) will last till morning. A smaller dose is not only less effective, it also lasts for a shorter period of time. If you still have a high morning blood glucose level (more than 10 mmol/l, 180 mg/dl), you might need to try another bedtime insulin with a slightly longer (Levemir) or much longer (Lantus) duration. See key fact box on page 170. Discuss this with your doctor or diabetes nurse.

Basal analogues: Levemir

The new basal insulin Levemir has a longer action than NPH insulin, but usually not long enough to be given only once daily. Most children need to take one dose in the morning and one at bedtime, i.e. approximately the same times as with NPH insulin. A larger dose has a longer duration (see page 78), so some teenagers and young adults may find that one dose at bedtime is sufficient. The doses can be adjusted in much the same way as for NPH insulin (see above), and it is important to check night time

Research findings: Levemir

♠ A study in children and adolescents showed lower and more predictable fasting glucose levels and lower risk of night time hypoglycaemia with Levemir compared with NPH insulin.[894]

♠ Approximately 70% of the participants were on a twice-daily Levemir dose both before and at the end of the study, but several shifts occurred during the study.

♠ Of those taking Levemir once daily, the dose was on average 42% of the total daily insulin dose, while those on two doses took 61% as basal insulin (half of the total Levemir dose in the morning and half in the evening).

♠ In another study, 82 children aged 2-5 used NPH or Levemir as their basal insulin during one year.[1031] There was no difference in HbA$_{1c}$, but less severe hypoglycaemia in the Levemir group (0 vs. 6 episodes in 3 children).

♠ Both these studies showed a weight reduction or less weight gain with Levemir.[894,1031]

♠ In a study from Israel, one dose of Levemir was initially given in the morning to young people aged 6-18 years as part of a multiple daily injection (MDI) regimen. After 4 months, half of them had gone over to twice-daily Levemir (2/3 of the dose in the morning and 1/3 in the evening) due to difficulties in having enough effect until the next morning without problems with hypoglycaemia between meals during the day. Those that needed to split the dose into two were mainly the younger children and those in mid-puberty (when the insulin resistance is most difficult, see page 226).[790]

♠ Children below age 12 that were using a 2-dose regimen and teenagers with MDI lowered their HbA$_{1c}$ with 8 mmol/mol (0.7%) and 4 mmol/mol (0.4%) respectively after 1 year with Levemir. The risk of severe hypoglycaemia also decreased.[144]

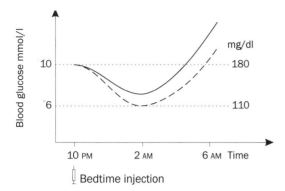

⊔ Bedtime injection

The blood glucose level during the night usually assumes a "hammock-like" curve when you use insulin of NPH type for bedtime injections (Insulatard, Humulin I, Insuman Basal) in a multiple injection therapy. This insulin will have its greatest effect 4-6 hours after the injection.[923] If you increase the dose, the morning blood glucose will be lower (dashed line) but the risk of night time hypoglycaemia will increase. The blood glucose level at 2-3 AM (approximately 4 hours after injection) can therefore be used as an indicator when adjusting the bedtime insulin dose.[129] Ideally, you should aim for a blood glucose of about 10 mmol/l (180 mg/dl) when you take the bedtime insulin and then let it fall about 4.0 mmol/l (70 mg/dl) to reach 6 mmol/l (110 mg/dl) at 2-3 AM (which usually is the lowest point during the night).

If your blood glucose level is below 7-8 mmol/l (125-145 mg/dl) at the time of taking the bedtime NPH insulin, you may need a bedtime snack to prevent night time hypoglycaemia.

blood glucose at 3-4 AM every second week or so and also after a change in dose.

Levemir has a much more predictable effect than NPH insulin.[911] It may therefore be a good option for a person who experiences widely differing effects from NPH insulin from day to day, for example resulting in problems with night time hypoglycaemia.

Clinical studies performed with Levemir have shown that this analogue is associated with lesser weight gain than NPH insulin.[651,894,911] The explanation for this effect is so far unclear. Thus, for the adolescent or young adult with a weight problem, switching to Levemir may be worth trying. Usually one can start with the

same doses of Levemir as the person had when using NPH insulin.

Basal analogues: Lantus

It usually takes about 3-6 hours after a Lantus injection to reach the plateau level of insulin effect.[664] In clinical practice, the effect of Lantus in doses given to adults often decreases after around 20-22 hours,[49,438] meaning that there will be less basal insulin effect just before you take the next Lantus injection. You can give the Lantus dose at lunch, dinner/tea or bedtime depending on the individual effect of the insulin.[49,438] A dinner injection can affect the blood glucose during the early night better, since it takes a couple of hours for the effect to set in.[49] If you find that you have a tendency towards lower glucose levels before lunch than when you wake up, you could also try taking Lantus at dinner/tea or at lunch. Where hypoglycaemia after midnight is a problem, a bedtime injection may work well.[49] If you have problems with hypoglycaemia during the later part of the night, Lantus can be given at breakfast time.[438]

Research findings: Levemir vs. Lantus

♠ A review of several studies comparing Levemir and Lantus in adults found the duration of action to be very much the same (21.5-23 hours for Levemir and 22-24 hours for Lantus) but Levemir gave a more stable insulin effect from day to day in the individual person.[483]

♠ A paediatric study also found less variation in effect for Levemir when comparing the 2 insulins.[251]

♠ Treatment with twice-daily insulin Levemir or once-daily insulin Lantus, each in combination with NovoRapid, resulted in similar HbA$_{1c}$ levels in an adult study.[849] The risks of both severe and nocturnal hypoglycaemia were significantly lower with Levemir and the fasting blood glucose was lower with Lantus.

Come down to earth gently! Don't change too much at any one time when you are adjusting your insulin doses, or you will have difficulty establishing what caused what afterwards.

One study even found Lantus to be more effective when given in the morning. HbA_{1c} decreased significantly, 15 mmol/mol (1.4%), in this group vs. only 3 mmol/mol (0.3%) in the group that took Lantus in the evening (mean age 13 years in both groups).[589]

Since the effect of Lantus lasts for up to 24 hours [813] it is best not to change the dose more often than two or three times in any week.[813] Use your morning blood glucose to adjust the dose but make sure that you also check some night time glucose levels (for example at 4-5 AM) especially when you just have started with Lantus. Aim for an ideal blood glucose of 4-6 mmol/l (70-110 mg/dl) on waking but 7-9 mmol/l (125-160 mg/dl) is also acceptable.[873,950] Lower the dose if your morning glucose level is low (< approximately 4.0 mmol/l, 70 mg/dl).

Younger children taking one dose of Lantus per day often benefit from taking it in the morning. A smaller dose of Lantus will last for a shorter time, meaning that many children will need two injections every day. In such cases, the basal insulin effect between meals has been too low in the afternoon, but increasing the evening dose has led to morning glucose levels that are too low. This may also be helpful for adolescents and adults who have problems with rising blood glucose levels during the hours before their Lantus injection.[49] When dividing the Lantus dose, between half and one third is injected in the morning and the rest at dinner/tea or with the evening meal.

If you eat an afternoon snack after school you are likely to need a premeal injection when using a single dose of Lantus as basal insulin. If the afternoon snack is small, it may work without a premeal dose if you split the Lantus dose and take part of it in the morning. Another solution is to add a small amount of NPH insu-

Research findings: Lantus

♠ Lantus given once daily in adult doses is equally effective if given at bedtime, for dinner or in the morning.[438]

♠ When compared with NPH insulin given once or twice daily, one dose of Lantus at bedtime results in a lower fasting blood glucose, and less hypoglycaemia but unchanged HbA_{1c}. This is the case for children from age 5, adolescents [282,950] and adults.[873]

♠ In most countries, Lantus is approved from the age of 2 years, and, there are reports of successful use of Lantus in children from under 1-5 years of age.[293] Night time severe hypoglycaemia decreased when bedtime NPH insulin was changed to Lantus (given in the buttocks) while HbA_{1c} was unchanged. Most children also injected NPH in the morning (with no lunch premeal injection) in this study.

♠ Overnight profiles when Lantus has been given at 8-10 PM have shown lower levels of insulin and a smaller drop in night time blood glucose compared with NPH.[752]

♠ When Lantus was given as a supervised injection at lunchtime in school to children with an HbA_{1c} of > 64 mmol/mol (8.0%), there was a drop in average HbA_{1c} from 87 mmol/mol (10.1%) to 74 mmol/mol (8.9%).[552]

♠ Exercise does not increase the absorption of glargine.[835]

♠ There is a risk of hypoglycaemia if injecting Lantus intramuscularly, particularly in young and lean individuals.[590]

♠ In rare cases, nausea and vomiting have been described as a side effect of Lantus therapy (without a deterioration of glucose control).[294]

lin to the lunchtime dose of rapid-acting insulin or to take an injection of NPH in the morning as additional basal insulin.[1019]

Although Lantus is a long-acting insulin, the action of this insulin may cease quite abruptly. If you forget your evening Lantus dose, you may not feel well at all when waking up. In fact, some people can experience high blood glucose, nausea and even vomiting in this situation, all symptoms of lack of insulin delivery caused by an increased amount of ketones in the blood. In this situation, you can take an extra dose of approximately 0.1 U/kg of rapid-acting insulin and delay breakfast for an hour or two until you feel better. Take approximately half your evening dose of Lantus in the morning and the next Lantus dose in the evening as usual.

After extra exercise in the afternoon you may need to reduce the Lantus dose in the evening by 2-4 units to avoid night time hypoglycaemia, although this may give you less basal insulin effect during the next day. You can also try reducing the evening Lantus before a daytime exercise session that will last more than 2-3

hours. Due to its prolonged action, Lantus has been used successfully in people who are being fed continuously by means of a stomach tube.[864]

When switching to the long-acting insulin analogue Lantus from intermediate-acting NPH insulin (Insulatard, Humulin I, Insuman Basal) you can begin with the same number of units if you take NPH at bedtime only.[873] If you take NPH twice a day, it is advisable to decrease the total NPH dose by around 20% and give it as one dose of Lantus.[950,1019] Be careful to monitor blood glucose during the night after the change. Severe hypoglycaemia with seizures has been described within the first week after initiating Lantus therapy.[950]

Puberty

During the teen years and puberty, when the body is developing quickly, the need for insulin is increased and young people are likely to find they must increase their doses considerably. Girls grow fastest the year before their first menstrual period, while boys have their growth spurt later on in the teen years. During puberty the levels of growth hormone (see page 40) in the body increase, especially during the night, increasing the blood glucose levels.[307] This leads to a decreased sensitivity for insulin (increased insulin resistance, page 223),[3] thus requiring large doses of bedtime insulin. Individuals without diabetes have increased levels of insulin in the blood from around 5 AM in the morning to manage this.[307]

If too little insulin is given during these "growth spurt" years, the young person's final height may be one or several centimetres less than predicted.[307] In earlier years, it was common for children with diabetes to be stunted in their growth, but today this is very rare (see also page 220).

Switching to Lantus

Example of doses:

Morning NPH	Bedtime NPH	Lantus
-	12 U	12 U
-	36 U	32 U
8 U	14 U	18 U
12 U	26 U	30 U

If you take Intermediate-acting NPH insulin once daily, you can begin by taking the same number of units of Lantus in the evening. With twice-daily NPH, it is best to decrease the combined doses by approximately 20% and give it as one dose of Lantus. If you are taking large doses of NPH, it is a good idea to lower the dose even more to reduce the risk of hypoglycaemia. You can then increase the Lantus dose, aiming at a wake-up blood glucose of 5-8 mmol/l (90-145 mg/dl).

Try to make diabetes part of your daily routine. For example, you could test your blood glucose when you get up in the morning and then inject insulin before taking a shower. You would then get a good effect on your breakfast rise in blood glucose.

If you are growing fast, you are likely to need to increase your bedtime insulin considerably. For example, teenagers often find they have to increase their NPH insulin (Insulatard, Humulin I, Insuman Basal) from 12 to 20 or 24 units within a short period. This may then need to be increased even further, up to 30 units, a couple of months later. One teenage girl using multiple injection treatment increased her bedtime dose of NPH insulin from 6 to 20 units within a year. A teenage boy increased his 24-hour dose from 1.2 U/kg to 1.7 U/kg (0.5 to 0.8 U/lb) during his growth spurt.

Increase your bedtime insulin by 2 units at a time until the blood glucose at 2-3 AM approaches 5 or 6 mmol/l (90-110 mg/dl, see page 174). Wait a few days before increasing the dose again to make certain that the effect is fully established. If your blood glucose level is still high in the morning, despite your 2-3 AM being 6 mmol/l (110 mg/dl), you may need to try another type of insulin for bedtime injections, for example Levemir. Long-acting-type insulins, such as Lantus (see page 174), may also be a better alternative. An insulin pump (see page 181) that will deliver sufficient amounts of insulin during the later part of the night could be even better.

No one can claim that remembering to take all your insulin injections is easy. But missed doses can contribute to a raised HbA$_{1c}$, especially during puberty. One study in children and adolescents using insulin pumps showed that two missed premeal bolus doses in a week raised HbA$_{1c}$ by as much as 6 mmol/mol (0.5%).[159] A Scottish study compared the amount of insulin that young people (under the age of 30) with diabetes collected from the pharmacy, against the amount that was actually prescribed for them by their doctor.[760] As many as 28% obtained less insulin than their prescribed dose. On average, these individuals left themselves short of insulin adding up to 115 days in the year. People obtaining less insulin had higher HbA$_{1c}$ levels, and were more likely to be admitted to hospital with ketoacidosis.

Try to find a way of reminding yourself or your child to take your insulin regularly without getting repetitive or boring yourself. Unfortunately, most pen injectors have no memory, so you are unable to see how long ago you took the last injection, and how many units it was. One pen (Memoir™) can show 16 doses, which may be very helpful, and another can show how long time ago the last dose was taken (NovoPen Echo®). If you are using an insulin pump, it will have a memory that records the premeal doses, along with the total amount of insulin given per day. It may be a good idea for parents and teenagers to read this memory together every now and again.

Insulin adjustments during the remission phase

A couple of weeks after the onset of your diabetes, your insulin doses will probably have been lowered considerably and they will go down even further in the weeks to come. There is no reason to worry if your blood glucose level is high on one occasion. Don't take extra insulin immediately. Rather, you should wait and check

It can be tough if your parents seem to be nagging you about your diabetes during your teen years. But at the same time you need their support. Try to look upon them as "diabetes coaches" instead of "diabetes parents". A successful team player always has a good coach in the background. Even David Beckham wouldn't score so many goals without a good coach.

the level again before your next meal. It is likely that it will have returned to normal by itself. If not, give extra insulin according to the correction factor (see page 146).

When the daily insulin dose is less than 0.5 U/kg of body weight and has an HbA_{1c} level close to that of individuals without diabetes, < 42 mmol/mol (6%), the individual has entered the remission phase (honeymoon phase, see page 221). The duration of this phase varies widely among individuals but will often last 3-6 months, sometimes even longer.

Rapid-acting insulin (NovoRapid and Humalog) can be used for premeal doses during the remission phase since the body's own insulin production will often be enough for the basal needs in between meals. The basal insulin injection in the morning can then be omitted for a longer or shorter period of time but you will usually need to take a small dose of NovoRapid and Humalog before each main meal. In a study of adults with diabetes, the frequency of hypoglycaemia after the meal decreased with this type of insulin treatment.[815]

Insulin requirements during the remission period may be very low, often only a few units to a meal. You may then need to temporarily withdraw the lunchtime and evening snack premeal insulin doses, if even one half or a single unit results in low blood glucose readings. This would leave only three doses per day (premeal insulin for breakfast and dinner/tea, and bedtime insulin). When the blood glucose level increases after lunch, or after the last meal of the day, this means it is time to reinstate these other doses. Another common policy is to give two-dose treatment during the remission phase, but it may then be more difficult to go back to multiple daily injections when the need of higher insulin doses appears again. Daily glucose monitoring is important during this phase, as it lets you know when to increase the insulin doses again. It is a good idea to check the average value of all blood glucose values taken every week. If the average is above 8 mmol/l (145 mg/dl), you need to increase the insulin doses. If the average does not go down under 8 mmol/l (145 mg/dl) by the next week, you need to contact your diabetes clinic.

During the remission phase it is important to increase the insulin doses if the blood glucose level is high on consecutive readings. This situation might occur if you have an infection, for example. Check your blood glucose levels before each meal and increase the dose according to the correction factor. The carbohydrate ratio needs to be lowered (gives less insulin) for the coming day. When making dose adjustments by eye, increase by one unit at a time (two if the dose is more than 10 units), if you find that the blood glucose is 8-10 mmol/l (145-180 mg/dl) or higher and your appetite is unaffected. You may have to get near to doubling the dose very quickly (more than 1 U/kg, 0.4 U/lb) during an illness accompanied by fever (see chapter on illness, page 301). Always telephone your diabetes healthcare team if you have a child with diabetes who is ill for the first time since being diagnosed.

During the remission phase, you need to take smaller doses of additional insulin if you eat something extra (for example, ice cream or pizza) compared with later in your diabetes life. This is because, during the remission phase, you will be producing some insulin of your own (see "How much extra insulin should you take?" on page 264).

There is some evidence that better blood glucose control and intensive insulin treatment early in diabetes makes the remission phase more likely to last longer.[817,962,269] High blood glucose levels seem to be harmful to the insulin-producing beta cells. The capacity to produce insulin is decreased, even at a blood glucose level of around 11 mmol/l (200 mg/dl), and at 28 mmol/l (500 mg/dl) one can see alterations inside the cells.[323] See also page 221. From this it follows that if your "aim" is better when adjusting the insulin treatment during the remission phase, the chances of a prolonged remission increase. It is important that you check your blood glucose regularly, even when you are feeling perfectly well, in order to be

"You must swim upstream if you want to find the spring"

Saying from Middle East

When you feel that you understand the basics of your diabetes, it is important to have the courage to explore new pathways.

able to see when the dose needs to be raised to deal with an increasing blood glucose level.

Hypoglycaemia

Problems with hypoglycaemia are less common during the remission phase. This is because the amount of insulin you produce yourself is regulated according to your blood glucose level. Therefore, it can be stopped completely if the blood glucose falls too low. For example, if you take 3 units of insulin for breakfast, your own pancreas can contribute by making another couple of units. These units will not be secreted at all if your blood glucose is decreasing to a low level, thereby preventing the hypoglycaemia. The ability of your pancreas to secrete the hormone glucagon that increases the blood glucose level is better during the remission phase.[817]

If you have symptoms of hypoglycaemia, with a blood glucose lower than 3.5 mmol/l (65 mg/dl), and you are not sure why (e.g. whether you are having too little to eat or more exercise than usual) you should lower the "responsible" dose of insulin (see page 152) by 1 U (0.5 if the dose is < 3 U, 2 U if > 10 U) the next day (see page 66).

Not everyone likes physical exercise. Some people feel more like having a lazy time fishing or sunbathing. You must find the approach that suits you best, and it is the job of your diabetes healthcare team to help you find a way of adjusting the insulin doses to your preferred life-style. However, you will undoubtedly be healthier in the long run if you can find some kind of exercise that you enjoy, and it will help you to have a more effective diabetes treatment by increasing the sensitivity for insulin in your body. We therefore encourage all forms of physical activity as part of your regular diabetes care. Both in Sweden [929] and Germany,[493] a higher frequency of regular physical activity has been associated with lower HbA$_{1c}$ without increasing the risk of severe hypoglycaemia.

Hypoglycaemia before a meal

Take glucose according to advice above, wait 10-15 minutes and then take a normal premeal dose. The next day you will need to lower the morning basal insulin if the low glucose levels were not caused by exercise. When using regular short-acting insulin, you may need to shorten the recommended interval between the injection and eating to 15-20 minutes.[815]

Low blood glucose readings

Reduce the insulin in the same way as above if your blood glucose is 4.0 mmol/l (70 mg/dl) or lower at the same time of the day for 2 days in a row (even if you have no symptoms of hypoglycaemia). Decrease the bedtime insulin if the blood glucose in the morning is below 4 mmol/l, 70 mg/dl. Remember that this is a normal level in the morning for a non-diabetic person so your pancreas will strive to achieve this level even if you have come down to very small doses of basal insulin. The morning blood glucose will not increase even if you lower the bedtime dose further. Instead you should adjust the bedtime basal insulin so that your blood glucose level is normal around 2-3 AM, i.e. 5-6 mmol/l (90-110 mg/dl).

Experiment!

We encourage young people to experiment with their injections in different situations. It is important to try and avoid terms like "permitted" or "forbidden". The point is to find out what is suitable just for you. Do remember to measure your blood glucose level and record the results in your logbook so that you know what you are doing. The worst situation you are likely to encounter (and it is not particularly serious anyway) is that you can find yourself hypoglycaemic after trying something new, or with a temporary high blood glucose level. Gradually, you will get to know yourself better, finding out which insulin doses your pancreas would have supplied if it had worked as usual. There is a saying that goes: "You can only learn by your own mistakes". Remember that most lessons in life are learned by trial and error!

Insulin pumps

An insulin pump delivers insulin to your body in a way that much more closely mimics that of a normal pancreas. If treatment by injections does not give acceptable glucose control, many children and teenagers will feel much better after changing to pump therapy. More than 40% of those in the intensive treatment group in the DCCT study (see page 367) chose an insulin pump. In 2008 there were approximately 400,000 people with diabetes on insulin pumps in the US.

Insulin pump therapy (also called CSII, continuous subcutaneous insulin infusion) is more expensive than conventional syringe or pen therapy. In countries where insulin pumps are not subsidized, they may be difficult to afford. If this applies to you, ask your diabetes team whether you might be eligible for any grants or other financial help from local organizations or national charities.

Only rapid-acting or short-acting insulin is used in the insulin pump. Today most pumps are started using rapid-acting insulin (Novo-Rap-

"How do I wear the pump at night?" is usually one of the first questions asked by someone interested in trying a pump. You will be surprised by how quickly you get used to this, and find a solution that fits in with your sleeping habits.

id,[112] Humalog [1132] and Apidra,[441,530] see page 214). A so called meta-analysis found a 3 mmol/mol (0.26%) lower HbA_{1c} among adult people using rapid-acting insulin compared with regular short-acting insulin.[202] A study comparing NovoRapid and Humalog found no difference between the two insulins in the effect on blood glucose levels and HbA_{1c} when used in pumps in children [1099] or adults.[116] There was also no difference in either study in the rate of hypoglycaemia or the number of blockages in pumps and infusion sets. Rapid-acting insulin can be diluted to U-50 or U-10 with sterile diluent and stored for 1 month for use in pumps for infants or very young children.[576,997] In the past, short-acting insulin with a special solvent was used to prevent the catheter becoming blocked (Velosulin BR Human, Insuman Infusat). The action time and effect of this insulin was similar to ordinary short-acting insulin (Actrapid, Humulin S, Insuman Rapid).

Disadvantages of using an insulin pump

⟱ A small store of insulin in your body means you will be sensitive to any interruption in insulin supply, which puts you at risk of rapidly developing ketoacidosis.

⟱ You need to do more regular monitoring tests if you are using an insulin pump.

⟱ The pump will be attached to you 24 hours a day (except when you disconnect it). Some people feel this makes them more tied to their diabetes.

⟱ The pump will be very obvious, for example if you go swimming in a public pool. So you will not be able to keep your diabetes secret. Other people may be curious about the pump, something people who are not yet entirely comfortable with their diabetes might find difficult to deal with.

⟱ The pump's alarm is likely to go off every now and then, and you might need to stop your activities to change the infusion set at an inconvenient time.

Advantages of using an insulin pump

⟱ The basal rate will give you sufficient amounts of insulin in the early morning to avoid a high blood glucose level when you wake up (dawn phenomenon).

⟱ Some people need more insulin than others between meals. An insulin pump can provide this.

⟱ The continuous supply of basal insulin makes it less essential to eat at regular intervals.

⟱ You will always have your insulin with you.

⟱ It is easier to take a bolus dose with the pump than to take an injection with a pen or syringe, especially if you don't feel like injecting when you are out.

⟱ Your premeal doses can be adjusted in 0.1 unit increments or even 0.05 units on some pumps.

⟱ You will be able to adjust the pump to take account of your differing needs for basal insulin during the day and night.

⟱ The pump uses only rapid- or short-acting insulin. These are likely to be more predictable in their effect than intermediate- or long-acting insulins.

⟱ The risk of severe hypoglycaemia is usually lessened by using an insulin pump.

⟱ The fact that the body's insulin store is small will mean that additional insulin is less likely to be released in an unpredictable fashion during physical exercise.

⟱ During and after exercise, a temporary basal rate can be used.

⟱ Pumps are easy to adjust if you are travelling across time zones.

The insulin pump will deliver a basal rate of insulin for 24 hours every day. Most modern pumps can be adjusted for different basal insulin rates during the day and night. Extra insulin is given with meals (a "bolus dose") by pushing a button on the pump. The insulin is pumped through a thin tubing (catheter) that is connected to a metal needle or indwelling cannula placed under the skin (subcutaneously). Another type of pump (like the Omnipod®) has the needle right under the pump patch, and uses no tubing.[1135] These types of pumps are called patch pumps.

A common problem with pen injectors and syringes is that the insulin will not always give quite the same effect even if the dose is exactly the same. With an insulin pump, the insulin will be deposited in the same site for several days and the absorption will be more even.[655] In a research study, insulin absorption after a pre-meal dose was constant for 4 days when the cannula was inserted in an area free of lipo-hypertrophy (fatty lumps).[808]

The total insulin requirement per 24 hours usually decreases by around 15-20% after starting

Reasons for starting with an insulin pump

➠ High HbA$_{1c}$.

➠ Incipient complications of diabetes.

➠ High blood glucose levels during the night or morning (dawn phenomenon).

➠ Wide fluctuations in blood glucose.

➠ HbA$_{1c}$ is OK with multiple injections but it takes too much work.

➠ Missed injections.

➠ Pain from insulin or injection needle.

➠ Recurrent severe hypoglycaemia.

➠ Hypoglycaemia unawareness.

➠ Possibility of having a lie in.

➠ Need for flexible meal sizes and schedules.

➠ Need to manage diabetes while exercising.

➠ Shift work/variable working patterns.

➠ Quality of life issues.

➠ Use of a pump from the time diabetes is diagnosed in preschool children [818]

At one time, we would only give people insulin pumps if there were definite medical reasons, but now more attention is being paid to quality of life issues and the use of pumps is becoming more widespread. We now have the routine of starting preschool children on pumps within a few weeks from the onset of diabetes, and the results are very good.[454] Preschool children often have an irregular lifestyle and the use of pumps for this age group can be very positive.[678,1046]

Changing insulin doses with a pump

① Meal boluses
Meal boluses are adjusted in the same way as when using multiple daily injections with a pen or syringes, i.e. changes by (0.5-) 1-2 units depending on how much you eat and your pre-meal blood glucose, or according to carbohydrate counting. There is a bolus guide in the pump that can suggest doses of insulin according to your intake of carbohydrates and current blood glucose level.

② Basal rate
It may be more difficult to relate to the basal rate, but it is important that you learn how to adjust this as well. If you need to change the basal rate in the pump, for example if you have an infection or if you have been exercising, you usually begin by setting a temporary basal rate i.e. increasing or decreasing the basal rate expressed as a percentage of the ordinary rate. You can try increasing the rate by 10-20 % if you have a fever or decrease by 10-20 % if you have a gastroenteritis (see page 304) or if you have been exercising.

average of 18%.[205] The amount of basal insulin given by the pump was reduced by around 40% compared with the basal dose (intermediate- or long-acting insulin) needed by young people on multiple injections. One study showed that the dose of basal insulin decreased by an average of 20% in children and adolescents after they started using an insulin pump.[787] The bolus doses decreased by approximately 25% in those who had a high HbA$_{1c}$ before starting with the pump and by approximately 15% in those who had other reasons for using a pump.

The glucose control often improves, resulting in a lower HbA$_{1c}$,[111,225,453] in young children as well.[678,1097] When used from the onset of diabetes, there was no difference in HbA$_{1c}$ compared with the control group using multiple injection treatment.[977] However, satisfaction with diabetes treatment was higher in the children and

with insulin pump treatment.[111,225,787,678] A US study of adults found an average decrease of 26%, with greater percentage reductions for patients on Humalog, and for those with higher daily dosages.[114] In a study of children with diabetes, those who had not reached puberty showed little change in insulin requirements, while those of the adolescents decreased by an teenagers who used a pump. Some patients (especially teenage girls) will gain weight when they start using an insulin pump if they don't decrease their food intake as their glucose control improves. The extra glucose that, beforehand, was lost in the urine now remains in the body and is transformed into fat instead.

The risk of severe hypoglycaemia usually decreases with pump treatment,[111,225] even when used in children under the age of 6-7 years.[678,1046,1097] The risk of ketoacidosis may increase according to some studies [225,455] but appears to decrease in others.[111,1046] The risk of ketoacidosis for young people using an insulin pump was approximately twice that of people taking multiple daily injections in a Swedish study.[455] Ketoacidotic episodes may occur soon after starting with a pump, before the person has got used to the new form of treatment.[453,739] Those teenagers who are prone to frequent episodes of ketoacidosis caused by interrupted insulin supply may find the frequency and severity of these to be drastically reduced by using an insulin pump that makes a continuous insulin supply possible.[101,992]

Starting the pump

We start new pumps on an outpatient basis, except for the very youngest children (under 3 or 4 years old) who are admitted to hospital for a night or two. Patients attend a 3-day pump school at the day care ward together with their parents (even older teenagers need to bring their parents to the sessions). No intermediate-acting insulin (Insulatard, Humulin I, Insuman Basal) is taken on the morning they start using the pump, and only half the dose the evening before for those using long-acting insulin once daily (Lantus, Levemir). Only the premeal bolus of short-acting or rapid-acting insulin is taken in the morning. The pump cannula is inserted after anaesthetizing the skin (with EMLA®, Ametop® or similar) and using a skin disinfectant. The first pump bolus is given at lunchtime. Today, we start almost all new pumps on rapid-acting insulin. For a few patients, the slightly larger

> ### Insulin pump treatment will be easier if you: (adapted from [1020])
>
> ⇒ Are comfortable with the pump cannula being constantly attached to your body and understand how it works.
>
> ⇒ Check your blood glucose regularly, at least four times a day (including morning and evening) and preferably before each meal.
>
> ⇒ Regularly monitor ketones (preferably blood ketones) when you are ill or feeling sick, or when your blood glucose is repeatedly above 14 mmol/l (250 mg/dl).
>
> ⇒ Recognize symptoms of low blood glucose. Always carry glucose tablets.
>
> ⇒ Recognize early symptoms of ketoacidosis. Always carry extra insulin and a pen or syringe to be able to treat this condition.
>
> ⇒ Make sure you keep in regular contact with your diabetes clinic.
>
> ⇒ If you live alone, you should make sure you can always contact a close friend or relative.
>
> MARRi

insulin depot when using short-acting insulin (Velosulin BR Human, Insuman Infusat) can help to avoid recurrent episodes of ketones/ ketoacidosis.

Even though the amount of insulin you are receiving goes down when you start using a pump, you will probably find your blood glucose levels will be in the lower range at first. If so, it is very important to lower your pump doses even further to avoid problems with hypoglycaemia. The reason you will need even lower doses is that when your blood glucose readings decrease, your insulin resistance will decrease as well (increased insulin sensitivity,

Daytime basal rate

These guidelines apply to pumps with programmable basal rates. When new to the pump, it is advisable to make changes in basal rates in collaboration with your doctor and diabetes nurse.

A good idea is to divide the hours of the day into different basal rate profiles where each contains a main meal. Measure the blood glucose level before the meal a couple of days in a row to evaluate the basal rate.[598] Change the basal rate profile *before* the meal:

Blood test before meal	Measure
< 5 mmol/l < 90 mg/dl	Decrease the basal rate by 0.05 U/h if the rate is < 0.3 U/h, 0.1 U/h if the rate is < 1 U/h, 0.2 U/h if the rate is > 1 U/h.
> 8-10 mmol/l > 145-180 mg/dl	Increase the basal rate by 0.05 U/h if the rate is < 0.3 U/h, 0.1 U/h if the rate is < 1 U/h, 0.2 U/h if the rate is > 1 U/h.

Another way of adjusting your daytime basal rate is to skip breakfast (and the pre-breakfast bolus) and adjust the basal rate to keep the blood glucose level constant until lunchtime.[110] Repeat the procedure with the other meals during the day. In children, this may be difficult to accomplish but parents can try serving food that contains only protein and fat (i.e. no carbohydrates).

One good opportunity for finding out the basal rate can be when you are having a lie in. If your parent or friend takes an early blood glucose followed by a few more tests until you wake up, you will get a good understanding of your basal rate. Many pumps have the ability to use different basal rate profiles, for example during weekdays and weekends, or during periods of intense physical activity.

see page 223). This implies that a certain insulin dose will be more effective at lowering your blood glucose level than the same dose was just a few days before.

The basal rate

The small amounts of insulin that the pump automatically delivers every hour is called the basal rate. An appropriate basal rate lets you keep your blood glucose levels stable when you are not eating, for example during the night or between meals. When starting a pump we usually set five basal rates: after midnight (12-3 AM), early morning (3-7 AM), morning (7 AM-12noon), afternoon (12-6 PM) and evening (6-12 PM). The charts on page 188 give more details. It is important to emphasize that starting doses are only estimates, and that it is essential to monitor your blood glucose very frequently (including at night) during the first few weeks in order to establish correct basal rates and bolus doses. If the basal rates are set correctly, the pump user will usually be able to delay or skip meals, and sleep longer in the morning when they want to.

Approximately 40-50% of the daily insulin requirement is given as the basal rate (often close to 1 unit per hour for an adult person).[507] The remainder is given as premeal bolus doses. Older children and teenagers may need to increase the basal rate up to 60% as basal rate with rapid-acting insulin (50% if using short-acting insulin in the pump),[598] most often because they miss out on taking bolus doses.[803] Younger children often need a lower percentage of their daily dose as basal insulin. In a US study, children before puberty had 41% of their daily dose as basal insulin and the pubertal group had 46%.[205] A lower percentage of basal insulin will give you more opportunities for continuous adjustments by giving small correction boluses, depending on the glucose level during the day.

After a change in the basal rate, it will take 2-3 hours before the blood glucose level is affected when using short-acting insulin,[499] and approximately 1-2 hours with rapid-acting insulin.[478] The basal insulin may be absorbed twice as rapidly if the person has a thin layer of subcutaneous fat (less than 10 mm in a lifted skin fold)

Night time basal rate

Check your blood glucose levels during a night after an ordinary day when you have been feeling well and have not had extra exercise. Adjust the premeal bolus dose before the evening snack to reach a blood glucose level of about 7-8 mmol/l (125-145 mg/dl) at 10-11 PM.[129]

Blood test at 3 AM and in the morning	Measure
< 6 mmol/l < 110 mg/dl	Decrease the basal rate after midnight and/or early in the morning by 0.05 U/h if the rate is < 0.3 U/h, 0.1 U/h if the rate is < 1 U/h, 0.2 U/h if the rate is > 1 U/h.
> 9-10 mmol/l > 160-180 mg/dl	Increase the basal rate after midnight and/or early in the morning by 0.05 U/h if the rate is < 0.3 U/h, 0.1 U/h if the rate is < 1 U/h, 0.2 U/h if the rate is > 1 U/h.

Teenagers often have a higher need of basal insulin early in the morning before they wake up (dawn phenomenon, see page 58), while pre-school children often have the highest basal rate during the hours before midnight (reversed dawn phenomenon).

If your pump cannot be adjusted for different basal rate profiles, you should adjust it to fit the night time need for basal insulin to reach a blood glucose level of 6-7 mmol/l (110-125 mg/dl) at 3 AM.[129]

Make the changes in basal rates in collaboration with your doctor and diabetes nurse to begin with. Then we would like you to make active changes as well!

with 5-7 AM.[129] If you have problems with night time hypoglycaemia, you can administer a lower basal rate from 11-12 PM to 3 AM to avoid this.[129] If you have problems with high glucose readings in the morning, you can try a slight increase in the basal rate (0.1-0.2 U per hour) between 3 and 7 AM.

Many children below the age of puberty need a higher basal rate late in the evening (9 PM to midnight) [125,205,787] and it is not uncommon for the basal rate to need to be higher in the middle of the night (midnight-3 AM) than later in the morning (3-7 AM).[1048] This may be caused by an early rise in the level of growth hormone shortly after the child falls asleep [205] or by the emptying of the child's stomach at this time.

Do not make too great a change in the basal rate at any one time. It is usually sufficient to change by 0.05 U per hour if the basal rate is < 0.3 U per hour, 0.1 U per hour if the basal rate is 0.3-1 U per hour and by 0.2 U per hour if the basal rate is > 1 U per hour. You should not change the basal rate more than twice in any week as, otherwise, it may be difficult to see which change leads to what. To avoid hypoglycaemia you should be prepared to decrease the basal rate (especially at night) when blood tests start to show lower readings.

Elsa

A modern insulin pump is small and easy to manage. You will soon master the different controls. Many teenagers with labile diabetes find life easier with an insulin pump. Even small children can benefit from using a pump. For example, one of our patients, a 3-year-old boy, had better morning blood glucose levels in addition to less night time hypoglycaemia after starting with an insulin pump.

compared with a thicker subcutaneous fat layer (more than 20 mm).[501]

The body's insulin requirement in adults is often about 20% lower between 1-3 AM compared

Temporary change of the basal rate

If you are using long-acting insulin, you are always faced with making an active decision about which dose to take and whether you need to change it. But since the basal rate in the pump is given automatically, you will not be prompted for a decision in the same way. One of the big advantages with a pump is that the basal rate can be changed throughout the day as the level of activity changes. With injections of basal insulin, it goes without saying that you cannot change the dose once it has been given,

⟹ Make use of the pump's potential to change the basal rate both during the day and night!

Temporary increase of the basal rate

⟹ Illness with an increased need of insulin: Increase by 20-30 %, often up to 50 %, during the remission phase (honeymoon phase). Sometimes even more, up to 100 %, as your own production of insulin will decrease rapidly if your blood glucose rises when you have a fever.

⟹ Decreased physical activity, for example if wet weather means a child is unable to play outside, or when travelling for long periods, or if a sports practice is cancelled.

Temporary lowering of the basal rate

⟹ Increased physical activity, for example a school outing, playing in the snow, jumping on the trampoline or skiing in the mountains.

⟹ If the activity takes place in the afternoon or evening, it is advisable to lower the basal rate during the night by 10-20 %. Your storage of glucose in the liver (glycogen stores) is used to fill up the muscle stores after a bout of physical activity, and this will cause your blood glucose to easily fall during the night.

⟹ If the blood glucose is in the low range when the child is going to sleep, it can be a good idea to lower the basal rate by 20% for a couple of hours. Check how much active insulin (see page 193) there is left that can affect the blood glucose level during the coming hours, and try out a suitable temporary basal rate.

⟹ You can preferably use a temporary basal rate if you discover a blood glucose in the lower range, < 5-6 mmol/l (90-110 mg/dl), during the night, and expect it to fall further. It is much easier than waking up the child and trying to get him or her to have something sweet.

⟹ If the blood glucose is below approximately < 4 mmol/l (70 mg/dl), you can try setting the basal rate to 0% for 1-2 hours instead of waking up the child.

The advice on basal rates in this chapter is written for a pump that can be adjusted for different basal rate levels throughout the day and night. Some pumps can be adjusted for different basal rates every hour, and others can be set for different profiles for a longer or shorter period of time. However, if you have a pump that can be programmed for only one basal rate, you should adjust it according to your night time blood glucose values. You will then have to adjust the premeal bolus doses to fit the fixed basal rate.

Temporary change of the basal rate

Most pumps allow you to make temporary changes of the basal rate for one or several hours. This is practical if, for example, you have problems with low blood glucose and repeated hypoglycaemia for sustained periods despite extra food intake. It will usually help to decrease the basal rate or stop the pump completely for an hour or two. If your blood glucose is high at bedtime you can temporarily increase the basal rate by 10-20% (around 0.1-0.2 U per hour) for a couple of hours. If your blood glucose is low during the early part of the night, you can temporarily decrease the basal

When should basal rates be changed?

(adapted from [110])

You should not change the profiles of the basal rate too often. When you are used to the pump it may be practical to change the basal rates once or twice in a month according to what your 24 hour blood glucose profiles show. Change the premeal bolus doses to adjust for temporary changes in diet or blood glucose readings or use the temporary basal rate. In the following situations it may be necessary to make changes to the basal rates:

⇒ Illness with fever and increased need for insulin.

⇒ Change in school or work activities with a new timetable or different physical activity.

⇒ Change in body weight of 5-10% or more.

⇒ Pregnancy.

⇒ Women may have different insulin needs during different phases of the menstrual cycle (see page 324).

⇒ Initiation of treatment with drugs that increase the need for insulin (such as cortisol or prednisolone).

⇒ Prolonged physical exercise (such as a hiking or cycling trip lasting 12-24 hours or more).

rate for a few hours by 10-20% (around 0.1-0.2 U per hour). The temporary basal rate is very useful for prolonged exercise. For example, during a 5-hour bike ride, try decreasing the basal rate by 50%. If you have exercised in the afternoon or evening, you should decrease the basal rate by 10-20% (around 0.1-0.2 U per hour) for the whole night.

If you work shifts, it may be a good idea to use the temporary basal rate during the nights you are working or use a separate profile programme if your pump has this feature. It is common to find you need to increase the basal dose during the latter part of the night to compensate for the stress effect of staying awake.

	4 U	3.5 U	3 U	3 U	26.9 U/24 h.
	0.6	0.6	0.6	0.4	0.5

Basal rate pump U per hour

Interpreting the 24 hour profile
(girl 30 kg, 66 lb)

See the previous profile for general interpretation.

Evening snack: No changes in premeal bolus. Young children often need to have their highest basal rates before midnight. The rise in blood glucose before midnight indicates that an increase in basal rate of 0.1 U per hour from 9 PM to midnight may be appropriate.

Night: The blood glucose does not change much between midnight and 3 AM. However, late at night it drops significantly, so reducing the basal rate from 3 AM to 0.4 U per hour is recommended. Young children often need less insulin during these hours and a further decrease to 0.3 U per hour may be appropriate.

Breakfast: The blood glucose rises quickly after breakfast and the dose should preferably be increased to 5 units. The basal rate is probably sufficient as the blood glucose is lowered at lunch again. However, when the breakfast bolus dose is increased to 5 units the basal rate might need to be decreased.

Lunch: The blood glucose 2 hours after the meal is only slightly increased indicating that the premeal bolus dose is correct. However, as the blood glucose rises prior to dinner/tea, the basal rate could be increased to 0.7 U per hour.

Dinner/tea: No changes.

mmol/l   Blood glucose   mg/dl

8 U	6 U	5 U	4 U	41.4 U/24 h.

0.9	0.7	0.9	0.5	0.7

Basal rate pump U per hour

Interpreting the 24 hour profile
(boy 40 kg, 88 lb)

It is best to take tests for a couple of days in a row to be sure that the results of any one day were not unusual. Start by looking at the evening snack since that affects the level your blood glucose will be on going to bed. The dotted line shows what the blood glucose values might have been with the suggested changes.

Evening snack: The blood glucose after the meal is a bit low. Decrease the dose by 1 unit. Adjust the dose so that you will have a blood glucose of about 6-8 mmol/l (110-145 mg/dl) when you go to bed.

Night: The basal rate needs to be increased slightly in the middle of the night to 0.6 U per hour as the blood glucose is rising until 3 AM. The blood glucose level from 3 AM to 7 AM is stable so this rate does not need to be changed.

Breakfast: The blood glucose rises very quickly after breakfast. If you use NovoRapid or Humalog you can try increasing the pre-breakfast dose to 9 U and lowering the basal rate to 0.8 U per hour. With short-acting insulin, the breakfast dose could have been given even earlier before breakfast to prevent the peak at 8 AM.

Lunch and dinner/tea: No changes.

Sit down when you have some time for yourself and consider all the doses for the next day. Don't change all doses at the same time as it can be difficult to see which change resulted in what. Let a few days go by between changes to make sure that the profiles look similar from day to day. Read the pump memory and write down in your logbook the total number of units your pump has delivered each day.

Premeal bolus doses

It is important to take a bolus dose every time you eat something, so you can try to imitate how a healthy pancreas would secrete insulin. In a European study of 1,041 children and adolescents, the pump memories were downloaded. Those taking more than five daily boluses had a lower HbA_{1c}.[252] Take the bolus dose just before the meal if you are using rapid-acting insulin (NovoRapid, Humalog, Apidra), and 30 minutes before the meal when you are using regular insulin. However, the timing will also depend on what your actual blood glucose level is (see pages 151 and 154). Adjust the bolus doses up or down in the same way as you would if you were on multiple injections. See graph on page 161 for adjusting rapid-acting insulin. The breakfast dose is usually slightly larger than the other premeal bolus doses. It will often have a better effect if you give it 15-20 min. before breakfast, especially if the glucose level is high. Since the basal need for insulin between meals is now supplied via the pump, your premeal bolus doses will be lower than when on multiple injections. You will probably need to decrease the size of additional insulin doses as well if you eat something extra. On most pumps the type of bolus dose can be varied from rapid delivery (standard bolus), administered over a period of time (square or extended bolus), or a combination of both (dual or combination bolus). See the figure on page 192.

You can calculate the amount of insulin needed for a given amount of carbohydrates by dividing the total amount of carbohydrate eaten during the day by the amount of insulin taken as premeal bolus doses.[255] One unit will usually cover 10-15 g of extra carbohydrate for a school-age child. If, for example, you eat ice cream containing 30 g of carbohydrate, 2-3 units of extra insulin will probably be enough. See page 243 for a list of carbohydrate contents in different foods. Modern "smart" pumps can calculate your bolus dose if you enter the amount of carbohydrate in a meal. They can

Changing the basal rate

Since it takes 1-2 hours with rapid-acting [478] (1 hour for basal rates < 0.5 U/h, 2 h. if it is 0.5-1.0 U/h. and 3 h. if it is > 1.0 U/h [615]) and 2-3 hours with regular insulin [499] before a change in the basal rate will take effect, you must plan ahead. The reason for this is that when you increase the basal rate, part of the insulin will stay in the subcutaneous tissue as an insulin depot. When you decrease the basal rate, the insulin from the depot will continue to be released and absorbed into the bloodstream for another 1-2 hours until the depot has decreased in size.

① Change the dose 1-2 hours before you want it to take effect, e.g. increase from 3 AM if you want an increased insulin effect from 5 AM on.

② If you want a rapid increase in the effect of the basal rate (e.g. if you are ill with fever) you should administer an extra dose of insulin (corresponding to 2 hours of the basal rate) before increasing the basal rate. This will result in a rapid increase of the insulin depot resulting in a quicker absorption of insulin into the blood.

③ If you want to decrease the effect of the basal rate fast (e.g. if you are going to exercise) you should stop the basal rate for 2 hours and then start it again at a lower level. The insulin depot will then rapidly decrease in size and the change in basal rate will take effect sooner.

④ In adults, the basal rate is often titrated by omitting meals.[1086] The basal rate should then keep the blood glucose level stable until the next meal. Some centres recommend to do this by omitting one meal per day; begin with dinner/supper one day, then lunch the next day and breakfast the last day.[615]

Repeat the schedule if glucose targets are not reached or confirmed, i.e. the blood glucose level increases or decreases when you do not eat and take no insulin. It does not work to eat food with little (< 10%) or no carbohydrates, as the blood glucose will rise anyway when the liver produces glucose from the contents of the carbohydrate free or carbohydrate low meal.

also correct for high or low blood glucose levels with the help of your correction factor (see page 146).[1138] See page 246 for advice on carbohydrate counting and insulin:carb ratio and the fact frame on page 193 for details on the bolus calculator (bolus guide). If you are using continuous glucose measuring, you can find the trend arrows useful for adjusting the bolus dose (see page 108).

When using a bolus calculator, there is less need for correction boluses for high blood glucose after the meal and less need for extra carbohydrates to correct hypoglycaemia after the meal.[423] When comparing adult pump users, those using a bolus calculator had lower blood glucose levels after the meal, but HbA_{1c} was not different.[622]

With an insulin pump, you will not be bound to maintain a regular interval between meals (and insulin doses) as when you were on multiple injection treatment with short-acting insulin. The basal rate will probably make it possible to increase the time period between meals to 6-7 hours, which might be an advantage if you keep irregular hours.

With a pump you can adjust the premeal bolus to match the carbohydrate content of your meal. Breakfast usually contains a high proportion of carbohydrates. You may find that 1 unit of insulin can take care of a slightly lower amount of carbohydrates for breakfast compared with other meals. See page 246 for further advice on counting carbohydrates.

Balancing the fine bolus line

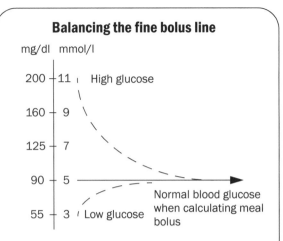

It is difficult for a child to get a reference for how much insulin a certain meal takes. While parents can use bolus guide or calculators to figure out the dose by entering the carbohydrate content and current blood glucose level, a child will often find these arithmetics confusing. One way of ensuring that the child will always judge the insulin dose according to a normal blood glucose level is to do this in two steps (assuming a target of 5 mmol/l (90 mg/dl)):

1) **Correct a high blood glucose:**
   Use the correction factor (also called ISF, insulin sensitivity factor, see page 193), and give this as a separate bolus dose first (without entering any carbs into the calculator). If you have time, and the child can wait without problems, delay the meal until the blood glucose has come down a bit. This is of course easier if you check the blood glucose 30 minutes before the meal. For example, a 30 kg child using 25 units/day as her total daily dose would have a correction factor of 1 U/4 mmol (70 mg/dl). If her blood glucose is 11 mmol/l (200 mg/dl), 1.5 U would be her correction dose in this example: 11-5=6 mmol/l (200-90=110 mg/dl), and 6/4=1.5 (110/70=1.5)

or:

   Correct hypoglycaemia:
   Do not use the bolus calculator, i.e. do not enter the low blood glucose value into the pump. Try instead to give just enough glucose to raise blood glucose into the normal range (i.e around 4-5 mmol/l (70-90 mg/dl). Three grams of glucose per 10 kg body weight will raise it by approximately 3-4 mmol/l (55-70 mg/dl) (see page 66). So a child weighing 30 kg would need 6 g of glucose to raise blood glucose around 2 mmol/l (from 3 to 5 mmol/l), 35 mg/dl (from 55 to 90 mg/dl.

2) If you do this, you will be able to calculate the bolus dose for the meal according to a normal blood glucose of around 5-6 mmol/l (90-110 mg/dl). This will help the child to learn what size bolus dose is appropriate for a particular meal.

Square or dual bolus doses: when can they be useful?

⇒ When you are eating pasta, as this gives a slower blood glucose rise.

⇒ When you eat a meal rich in fat or protein that is digested more slowly, for example a pizza.

⇒ When your meal is larger than usual.

⇒ When you eat a meal that takes a longer time than usual, for example a three course dinner.

⇒ When several small meals are eaten within a short period of time, for example at a birthday party.

⇒ When you eat slowly, for example popcorn or crisps while watching a movie.

⇒ Younger children often need a dual bolus for their last meal to prevent a rise in blood glucose after they have fallen asleep.

⇒ When parents are not sure if the child will finish eating. If you begin the dual dose before the meal and set it over 30-60 min., you can shut it off when the child stops eating.

⇒ If you have problems with delayed stomach emptying (see page 365).

Change of insertion site

The most common insertion site is the abdomen. With small children, it is preferable to use the buttocks as well to be able to spread the infusion sites, thereby decreasing the risk of fatty lumps (lipohypertrophies, see page 217). You can also use the thigh or the upper arm but both sites can result in an increased absorption

Different types of bolus doses

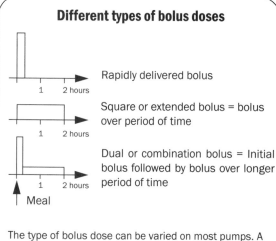

Rapidly delivered bolus

Square or extended bolus = bolus over period of time

Dual or combination bolus = Initial bolus followed by bolus over longer period of time

Meal

The type of bolus dose can be varied on most pumps. A square or dual bolus may be preferred for a large meal that is rich in fat or proteins, a meal with low glycaemic index (see page 240), or when you will be eating over a longer period, at a party for example. These bolus doses may also work well if you have problems with delayed emptying of the stomach (gastroparesis, see page 365). In a study of a meal high in carbohydrates, calories and fat, the square (whole dose over 2 hours) and dual (70% as an immediate bolus and 30% over 2 hours) bolus provided the lowest glucose levels over a 4-hour period.[190]

Superbolus for a high carb meal

Add to bolus dose 2.1U

Bolus dose 6 U

Basal rate 1.0 U/h

Meal

Temporary basal rate 30% for 3 hours

It may be difficult to give insulin for a meal that is very high in carbohydrates, for example breakfast. There is often a peak in blood glucose 1-2 hours after breakfast, and if you increase the dose, you will be low before lunch. One way is to try giving the dose 15-20 min. before the meal. Another way is the superbolus, a combination of temporary basal rate and an increased bolus without increasing your total insulin amount before lunch.[1086]

① Set a temporary basal for 3 hours to 30% If your basal is 1.0 U/h, you will get 0.7 x 3 = 2.1 U less.

② Use the bolus calculator in the pump to calculate the dose needed for your breakfast. Or estimate the dose "by eye", if you are used to that.

③ Add the decrease in basal rate to the bolus, and give it all as one dose. If your bolus for this breakfast is 6.5 U, then give 6.5+2.1=7.6 U

Simulator studies have shown that it is very difficult to find the right dose for insulin without decreasing the basal rate if the meal contains 60 g of carbohydrate or more.[133]

of insulin when exercising. There is also a greater risk of the cannula catching on the clothing and being pulled out.

Individual advice is needed on how often the cannula should be replaced. We usually start by recommending the use of a soft Teflon catheter, but some people prefer a short steel needle. You can usually let the catheter remain in place for 3 but not more than 4 days if your blood glucose readings do not become raised. Replacing the catheter twice a week on the same weekdays is often a good routine. However, some individuals, especially young children, will need to replace it every 2 days. The longer the catheter remains in one site, the greater the risk of developing fatty lumps (lipohypertrophies) and infections. A steel needle usually needs to be replaced every second day. If you have problems

with fatty lumps or redness of the skin you should replace the infusion set more frequently.

Disinfect the insertion site with Hibiclens™, IV Prep™ or similar product. Avoid your waistline, belt line and underwear line and a 5 cm (2 inch) circle around your belly button (see illus-

Smart pumps and the bolus guide: Settings when using the bolus calculator

Most pumps have several built-in functions that can make it easier to calculate correct insulin doses for meals and corrections of high blood glucose levels.

⟹ **Insulin:carbohydrate ratio (carb factor):**
This tells how many grams of carbohydrate one unit of rapid-acting insulin will cover. A simple way to get a rough estimate (the 500-rule) is to divide the number 500 by your total daily dose (called TDD) of insulin (adding all types of insulin, both premeal doses and basal insulin). See "Carbohydrate counting" on page 246 for further advice.

⟹ **Correction factor (ISF, insulin sensitivity factor):**
This tells you how many mmol/l or mg/dl one unit of insulin lowers your blood glucose during the next 4-5 hours. For mmol/l you divide 100 by your TDD (see above), for mg/dl you divide 1800 by your TDD. See the table on page 146. Remember that this only is an estimate to begin with. If you are exercising, your blood glucose will drop more, if you have an infection with fever, it will drop less.

⟹ **Duration of insulin action:**
This is the time that insulin is working in your body, i.e. the time when it still has some blood glucose lowering effect. This is usually best set to between 4 and 6 hours for rapid-acting insulin for adults,[1086] but children often need to lower it to 2-3 hours.[457]

⟹ **Active insulin**
Also called "Bolus on board" or "Insulin on board" since it means the amount of bolus insulin that you still have in your body that can lower your blood glucose (the basal insulin is not included). The pump calculates this from the duration of insulin action that you have set.

⟹ **Target blood glucose:**
This is the blood glucose level that you want to reach when using the correction factor. You can set this as a range, but most pumps will use the mean value for calculations (Medtronic uses the upper value). We often set this to 6 mmol/l (110 mg/dl) to begin with, and then lower to 5 (90)

The 100/1800 and 500 rules are originally set up for adults,[255] but can be used as starting points also in children and adolescents.[332] These settings are very individual and should be discussed with your doctor and diabetes team. See reference [1086] for more detailed advice.

When should you replace the accessories?

Teflon cannula	Start by replacing it 2-3 times a week. If there are no problems try using it 4-5 days before replacement. Some people, especially small children, may need to replace every second day.
Metal needle	Replace every second day, more often if signs of irritation are noted.
Tubing	Replace the tubing at least every other time you replace the cannula/needle and when you replace the reservoir.
Insulin reservoir	If your pump uses 3 ml reservoirs, you may find it more practical to refill from 3 ml pen cartridges than 10 ml vials. Do not reuse them as the silicon on the plunger wears off, resulting in an occlusion or blockage alarm.

tration on page 138). Straighten your back before you apply the adhesive to avoid tight skin. Insert the new infusion set at least 4-6 centimetres (2 inches) away from the old one to avoid developing fatty lumps.

The blood glucose level should always be checked 3 hours after changing the infusion set to ensure proper insulin delivery. It is not a good idea to change infusion sites just before going to bed. Since the basal rate runs very

Always use a topical anaesthetic cream such as (EMLA®, Ametop®) before replacing the infusion set when beginning with pump treatment in children. Apply the cream 1.5-2 hours ahead of time to get full effect. An alternative way of lessening the pain is to use an automatic inserter. Applying an ice cube is a quick way of lessening the pain of insertion in less difficult cases.

Replacement of infusion set

➠ If you replace the infusion set before taking a premeal bolus it will be flushed by the larger volume of fluid.

➠ Avoid replacing your infusion set before bedtime as you will need to be awake for a couple of hours to see that it functions properly.

➠ Start by washing your hands with soap and water.

➠ Choose an insertion site well away from your beltline.

➠ Disinfect a skin area that is a little larger than the adhesive you are going to apply. Use Hibiclens™, IV Prep™ or a similar product. Applying Skin-Prep™, Mastisol™ or Tincture of Benzoin™ will make the adhesive stick better. Use a disinfectant for hand-washing as well if you have problems with skin infections. See page 194 for advice if you have problems with a sensitive skin.

➠ Be careful not to touch the sterile needle. Do not breathe or blow directly onto the needle, as this may contaminate it.

➠ Pinch a two-finger skin fold and insert the needle at a 45° angle (see illustration on page 138) or according to the instructions for other types of needles.

➠ Remove the protective tape and apply the adhesive carefully. If it sticks unevenly don't try to move it. There is a considerable risk of removing the catheter at the same time if you try to move the adhesive.

➠ Fill the cannula with insulin after removing the insertion needle. Depending on the length of the cannula, it needs to be filled with 0.3-1 unit of insulin to fill up the dead space.

➠ Withdraw the old catheter **after** the insertion of the new one. Pull the adhesive from the side where the tip of the infusion set is located and it will come off more easily. If you remove the old catheter first, there is a high risk of contamination of your fingers as there are likely to be bacteria present at the old insertion site.

➠ If you have problems removing sticky traces of adhesive, try a remover such as Detachol™ or Uni-Solve™.

slowly during the night, it may take longer for the alarm to be triggered if something is wrong with the new insertion site. Many pump users find it more convenient to replace the infusion site straight after coming home from school or work. This leaves plenty of time to find out if something is wrong with the new infusion site. If you replace the cannula and tubing before taking a meal bolus dose, this will clear away any tissue from the cannula or needle.

Some sets of tubing and cannulas need to be filled with insulin before the needle is inserted. With others you need to give a small amount of extra insulin (around a half to a full unit) after insertion to fill up the air inside it (called dead space). Even if you have filled the tubing by pressing the reservoir plunger you need to build up the pressure in the tubing by giving a priming dose with the pump to make sure insulin appears at the tip of the tubing.

Problems with needle coming loose?

Skin-Prep™, Mastisol™ and Tincture of Benzoin™ leave a sticky film after drying to help the adhesive get a firm grip. Don't use products containing skin moisturizers, as these may cause the adhesive to loosen more easily. Reinforce by applying extra adhesive already at the time of inserting the needle. The extra adhesive needs to be replaced if it begins to come off.

Problems with dry skin or eczema?

If you are allergic to the adhesive, it can cause redness or itching. Try another type of adhesive or infusion set. Another solution is to apply a thin transparent adhesive (like Tegaderm™, IV 3000™ or Polyskin™) and then insert the cannula through it. In this way the cannula adhesive will not come into contact with the skin. A thicker stoma type adhesive (like Duoderm™ or Compeed™) will often help in especially difficult cases. A small hole needs to be cut for the catheter in these thicker types of adhesives. EMLA and other topical anaesthezisers may

For young children it may be a good idea to put the tubing in a sling and fix it with some adhesive to minimize the risk of pulling the cannula loose if the tubing is pulled or jerked, for example if you drop the pump.

How many tests should you take when using an insulin pump?

➠ Blood glucose at least four times daily (including morning and before going to bed), preferably before every meal, especially if you are using NovoRapid or Humalog in the pump.

➠ One or two 24-hour profiles every week or every other week with readings taken before and 1.5-2 hours after each meal and at night.

➠ Before and 1.5-2 hours after each meal if you are ill or feeling unwell for any reason at all.

➠ Check for ketones if you are nauseous, when you are ill, or when your blood glucose level is high (> 14 mmol/l, 250 mg/dl), and does not decrease after an extra bolus.

The adhesive should not cover a previous infusion site until it has healed completely. It is best to change sides on the abdomen (left/right) with each replacement. Apply an over-the-counter steroid cream if you have a tendency to develop eczema. For a stronger steroid effect, ask for a prescription. Apply a skin softener as a prophylactic measure to prepare your next insertion site, or use a cream that contains carbamide that binds water to the skin twice daily as a protective measure, especially during wintertime. A dry skin is sensitive, and will easily become irritated.

Problems with infected insertion site?

Insert the new infusion set before you remove the old one. If you do it the other way around, you will be at greater risk of contaminating your hands on the old site and therefore of transferring bacteria to the new site.

If the redness doesn't disappear soon after you have replaced the cannula, you can speed up the healing process by applying a dressing soaked in warm soapy water for 20 minutes four times daily. Topical antibiotic cream or hydrogen peroxide cream can be smeared on an infected infusion site, and may prevent spreading of an infection if applied early. If the redness increases or starts hurting, you might need antibiotic

irritate the skin. It may be better to try to numb the skin with a piece of ice just before insertion. Wash with water after wiping off the topical anaestiziser.

Don't use alcohol for disinfection as this will cause your skin to dry out for around 10 minutes. Instead use a mild soap, and let the skin dry thoroughly. A good tip is to replace the needle shortly after a shower, as both your hands and insertion sites will be properly cleaned. Don't tear off the adhesive from a used site, as the outermost layer of the skin then may come off. Cover the adhesive with baby oil and loosen it carefully once the adhesive has dissolved. If you use Remove™, wash carefully with soap and water afterwards.

Smart pumps: Things to think about

When you begin using the bolus calculator, you will probably know better than the calculator which doses are correct. It is then tempting to override the recommended dose. However, if you really want the pump to become smart, you need to learn it your way. It is then better to take exactly the dose it suggests, and then see in which direction it errors, i.e. if the blood glucose goes too high or too low. You can then adjust the settings in the pump yourself to achieve a better match.

Insulin:carb ratio:
Try experimenting with combination boluses (see page 191). If the carb content decides on the insulin dose for the meal, then let the glycaemic index (see page 243) guide you as to how long the duration of the combination dose should be. It needs to be longer for a meal containing a higher amount of carbohydrates. Fat slows down the emptying of your stomach, so a meal rich in fat also needs a longer dual dose. Adults needed 2 hours extension of the dose for a pizza meal in one study (given as 70/30%),[190] up to 8 hours in another (given as 50/50%).[573] A Big Mac needed a duration insulin of more than 3 hours when the dose was given intravenously.[1076]

Correction factor:
Use different setting for different parts of the day. To begin with, we usually set the factor twice as high during the night (which gives half the insulin dose), from 10 PM in older children and adolescents. However, younger children usually need to have their daytime correction factor until midnight. It is usually best to give a correction bolus at the earliest 2 hours after a meal.

Active insulin:
When your correction factor seems to be set correctly, next see if there is any difference depending on if there still is active insulin remaining. A common reply is: "Yes, the pump suggests a correct amount of insulin, but not when there is active insulin left!" Children often need a short time setting for active insulin, as their doses are small. Try decreasing the active insulin setting by 0.5-1 hour, and check the correction factor again. We find that 2-3 hours often works well.[457] Some pumps can even be set to 2.5 hours. One author suggests 3 hours if the average bolus is 2 U, 5 h. if the bolus is 10 U and 7 h. if it is 20 U.[614]

Some pumps (Medtronic, Animas, Roche) will dedicate insulin given for meals when you have entered carbs, and not make it available as active insulin when you take a meal or correction bolus later. This is correct as the insulin will be used to cover the carbohydrates that are absorbed from the intestines after the previous meal. Only insulin given as correction boluses will be counted as active insulin. However, all insulin doses will be counted as active insulin and will be subtracted from calculations if you do not enter carbs with your meals. It may then be better not to use the correction factor algorithm in the pump when there still is active insulin showing in the display.

Other pumps (Dana, Cozmo) count all types of boluses as active insulin, including those given with carbs entered in the pump. Some set the duration of insulin action down to 2 hours to avoid this interference.

Active insulin at bedtime:
Check active insulin before going to bed. If the blood glucose is below 6-7 mmol/l (110-125 mg/dl) there might be a risk of night time hypoglycaemia if there still is active insulin present. Instead of giving something to eat, you can use the temporary basal rate to set a lower basal rate for a couple of hours. You can even set it down to zero if there is a hypoglycaemia (and give some glucose), but do not do so for more than 2 hours, otherwise you will risk a high blood glucose level afterwards.

Low Glucose Suspend:
One pump (Medtronic Veo) can shut down the basal rate for 2 hours if there is a hypoglycaemia. You need to use a sensor and can define the glucose level where this will happen yourself. The pump will automatically restart, but will shut off again after another 4 hours if the glucose level still is low. In one study, severe hypoglycaemia with unconsciousness or seizures was completely avoided by using this feature.[702]

Use an App
There are several apps available that can help you to estimate the carb contents of your meal. Many have food lists and some even have picture of different sizes of meals (like Carbs & Cals). Some pumps also have food lists.

treatment. Contact your diabetes healthcare team or doctor. If you often have problems with infected insertion sites, it may be a good idea to carry antibiotics with you if abroad.

Problems with irritation or infection at the insertion site can be prevented by careful hand washing, disinfection and infusion set replacement every second or third day. Use chlorhexidine in alcohol (Hibiscrub™) or a similar agent for hand washing. If you have recurring problems with infected sites in spite of good hygiene routines, it might mean that the bacteria originate from your armpits or nostrils. If tests show you have bacteria (staphylococci) in your nasal cavity, you may need antibiotic treatment. Another approach is the application of local antibiotics to each nostril nightly, and chlorhexidine body washes on a daily basis.

More frequent home monitoring

Since there is a greater risk of insulin deficiency with a pump, you must be willing to test your blood glucose level more often. At the very least, you will need to be doing four tests a day including morning and late evening. Preferably you should test before each meal. You must also be careful to check for ketones if your blood glucose is high, or if you are feeling unwell, as ketones are a sign of insulin deficiency. It is a good idea to keep reagent strips for blood ketone monitoring at home, so that you can monitor the effect of extra insulin doses given in this situation (see page 113). A 24-hour blood glucose profile with tests before and 1.5-2 hours after each meal is needed every week or every second week to allow you to adjust your doses correctly. You should also take night time tests when compiling a 24-hour profile (at 2-3 AM and if necessary at 5 AM as well).

Record your test results in a logbook where you can document clearly the pump's basal rate. We find it best to use a logbook where every entry is written on a blood glucose chart. Doing this will help you to see patterns in your blood glu-

There is an increased risk of ketoacidosis in pump users if there is any interruption to insulin delivery as the insulin depot is so small. Ketoacidosis must be treated in the hospital with intravenous insulin and fluids. To avoid risking ketoacidosis, **always use a pen or syringe** when taking extra insulin if your blood glucose is high and you have ketones in your blood or urine.

cose readings (see charts on page 189). Make it part of your routine to check the pump daily for the total number of units delivered every 24 hours and record this in your logbook.

Insulin depot with a pump

The disadvantage of using an insulin pump is that the insulin depot will be very small, since no long-acting insulin is used. This will be important if the pump gets blocked, or if you intentionally turn it off when playing sport or swimming, for example. If the insulin supply is interrupted you will very soon develop symptoms of insulin deficiency such as high blood glucose, nausea and vomiting (see "Depot effect" on page 86).

If you are not feeling well, remember to test your blood or urine for ketones as a matter of course!

KETONE ALERT!

If you are using an insulin pump, you are at greater risk of ketoacidosis because you have a very small insulin depot. Ketones are a sign of lack of insulin delivery, indicating something may be wrong with your pump or tubing/needle.

ALWAYS check your blood glucose and ketones when you are not feeling well. Check for ketones in the following situations too:

⇒ If your blood glucose is more than 14 mmol/l (250 mg/dl) when you wake up or go to bed.

⇒ If your blood glucose has been higher than 14 mmol/l (250 mg/dl) for more than a couple of hours.

⇒ If you are ill and running a temperature (for example with a cold or flu).

⇒ If you have any symptoms of insulin deficiency (nausea, vomiting, abdominal pain, rapid breathing, or your breath smells "fruity" or of "pear drops").

If your ketone levels increase, this means that you are becoming more and more insulin-deficient. You will need to contact your doctor to discuss what to do next!

Be aware that insulin deficiency leading to increased ketone production shows in the urine within a couple of hours. With a blood ketone test, you will detect ketones even earlier. If you take extra insulin, the production of ketones will stop and the level of blood ketones will decrease within an hour or two (you may notice an increase in the first hour after extra insulin is given but the level should then drop considerably). The excretion of ketones in the urine will continue for many hours but you should notice the concentration stabilizing, then decreasing, as the hours pass.

If you are the least bit concerned, or cannot get hold of someone who is familiar with insulin pumps over the phone, you should take an injection of insulin by pen or syringe and then go to your nearest hospital accident and emergency department.

Always bring extra insulin to give with a pen or syringe wherever you go, even if you expect to be away from home for only a couple of hours or so. Disposable syringes containing 30 U are so small that they fit in the case of a blood glucose meter. If you always carry a couple, you can fill insulin from the pump reservoir if you have problems with high blood glucose and ketones.

Causes of ketoacidosis

⇒ Insulin delivery is interrupted, for example by a leak in the piece connecting the tubing to the reservoir or a cannula that has come out.

⇒ Increased insulin requirements caused by illness (e.g. a cold with fever) without the insulin dose being increased.

⇒ Inflammation or infection at the infusion site (indicated by redness or pus).

⇒ Decreased insulin absorption, for example caused by inserting the infusion set into a fat pad (lipohypertrophy).

⇒ Decreased insulin potency, for example after it has been frozen or exposed to heat or sunlight.

⇒ Alcohol intake may cause ketoacidosis to develop much more quickly.[952]

Thicker layers of subcutaneous fat will result in a larger insulin depot of the basal dose. In one study a basal rate of 1 U per hour of short-acting insulin was used. The insulin depot for those people with a subcutaneous fat layer of 40 mm (1.5 inch) was close to 6 U while those with less than 10 mm (0.3 inches) subcutaneous fat had only 1 U in their depot.[501] This suggests that thin people will be more sensitive to an interrupted basal rate since their insulin depot is smaller.

Ketoacidosis

A small insulin depot will result in early insulin deficiency symptoms if something goes wrong with the pump or the tubing. Your blood glucose will be high within 2-4 hours of interrupted insulin delivery (see chart on page 202). One night's interrupted insulin supply may be enough to cause incipient ketoacidosis in the morning with symptoms of insulin deficiency such as nausea and vomiting. Be extra careful to check both blood glucose and ketones whenever you are feeling at all unwell.

Tips and tricks with the pump

➠ Check how much "bolus on board" you have before going to bed. This will give you an indication if you need to eat something or lower the basal rate temporarily to avoid the risk of night time hypoglycaemia.

➠ If you are going to eat something that will raise your blood glucose very quickly (a very high GI meal, see page 240), the dose needed to avoid too high blood glucose will probably give you a risk of hypoglycaemia afterwards. You can try using a temporary basal rate of only 0-30% for 2-3 hours after the meal to avoid this. This has been called the "Superbolus" by John Walsh,[1086] and the function has been confirmed in a scientific simulation study.[133] See also page 192.

➠ Fill from 3 ml cartridges instead of 10 ml vials. The cost is only slightly higher, and you can use the same cartridges for your spare pen as for the pump. When the cartridge has been in the pen for 3 weeks, you can use it to fill the pump and put a new one in the pen. In this way, no insulin will be wasted.

➠ Another practical way to ensure you always have insulin for an injection when there is a pump failure is to carry some syringes for single use. They are small and you can put a few in the blood glucose cover, at school and in the glove compartment of the car and other places where they may come in handy. If you have problems with your pump, you can draw insulin from the pump reservoir and inject with the syringe.

➠ For younger children, it is a good idea to give a bolus by injection every now and then, so the child will be familiar with the procedure in case of a pump failure.

➠ Steel needles may seem tough to use, but many children and teenagers prefer them, once they have dared to try them. They can work very well especially for active children, since even if the needle is pulled slightly out of place during play or other physical activity, it will go back in without problem. A teflon catheter might easily kink in this situation.

➠ Skip setting the blood glucose in the bolus guide if < 2 hours have passed since your previous meal or correction bolus. There is still a lot of insulin active from your previous bolus, so the bolus calculator may give incorrect advice if you add your current blood glucose level when the insulin effect is at its greatest.

➠ If >10% of your total daily dose is made up of corrections, consider changing the basal rate or the carb. ratio and/or correction factor settings.

➠ Many young children need extra insulin with their last meal to cover the hours until midnight. This can be performed in several different ways:
1) Give a normal bolus of for example 3.5 U first, and then an extended bolus over 3-4 hours. This can be a fixed amount (e.g. 1.5U) or for example 40% of the meal bolus. Keep the normal ratio for the meal in this example.
2) Give a combined bolus with a fixed ratio, for example 5 U as 70/30% over 3 hours. The carb ratio then needs to be lowered so that the meal dose remains the same (multiply ratio by 0.7 (70%) in this example)
3) Give a combined bolus with a fixed amount as extended bolus. Dial in 5 U and then change the percentage of the extended part to match the amount you want to give. For example, you can lower the percentage until this equals 1.0 U if this is what you want to give over 3 hours. The carb. ratio needs to be lowered as in 2) above.

➠ If you have a late breakfast at a weekend, the pump might be set to a higher carb. ratio for lunch, which will give you less insulin. However, many pumps allow you to adjust the carb. ratio manually before giving the dose.

➠ Never plan to change infusion site after the last meal of the day. A meal bolus will flush the needle and alert an alarm if there is a blockage. The low basal rate might not trigger the alarm until next morning when the blood glucose has risen considerably and ketones are high. If you have to replace the needle set in the evening, you need to check the glucose level in the night to see that the new set is working correctly.

➠ Gravity may play a role in your pump treatment by a siphon effect. If the pump is placed higher than the insertion site, the basal rate may increase slightly. And if it is placed lower, it may decrease slightly.[1137] This can have a clinical effect if, for example, you sometimes use a bra, thigh or calf holder for your pump. It should make no difference if the pump always is located at the same level in relation to the insertion site of the needle.

High blood glucose and ketones?

If your blood glucose is higher than 14 mmol/l (250 mg/dl) and you have ketones in the blood (> 0.5 mmol/l) or urine (moderate or large), this indicates a blocked insulin supply or increased need for insulin, for example, because of an infection.

① Take 0.1 U/kg (0.5 U/10 lb) body weight of preferably rapid-acting NovoRapid, Apidra or Humalog (otherwise short-acting insulin) *with a pen or a syringe*. Don't use the pump as you cannot be sure whether or not it works properly.

② Measure blood glucose every hour. If it doesn't decrease, the insulin dose of 0.1 U/kg (0.5 U/10 lb) body weight can be repeated (every second hour with rapid-acting insulin, or every 2-3 hours with regular short-acting insulin). Measure blood ketones if you have such strips available (see page 113). Often there will be an increase in the first hour after insulin is given but after that you should find the level decreases.

③ Check the pump by disconnecting the tubing from the cannula/needle. Activate a prime dose. Insulin should immediately appear from the tubing. If not, replace the tubing.

④ Replace the cannula/needle if the tubing works well. Check for signs of redness in the skin and of moisture close to the infusion site as this would indicate insulin leakage.

⑤ Be sure to drink large amounts of sugar-free fluids. If your blood glucose is approximately 10-11 mmol/l (180-200 mg/dl) or below and you still have high ketone levels in the blood, you will need to drink fluids containing sugar and repeat the extra dose of rapid-acting insulin.

⮕ The general recommendation of an extra dose by pen or syringe in case of pump failure is 0.1 U/kg. However, if you find your child always needing more than this, for example 1.5 U/kg, you can give this as the first dose. See also page 115 regarding extra bolus doses.

Causes of a lack in insulin delivery

⮕ The connector between the tubing and the insulin reservoir can be cracked. Feel it with your fingers. It may smell of insulin even if you do not see a leak.

⮕ Hole in the tubing. (A cat bite in the tubing resulted in leakage which led to ketoacidosis for a teenage girl.)

⮕ Air in the tubing is not dangerous as such but will give you less insulin.

⮕ If the tubing is squeezed or bent, e.g. by a belt or tight jeans, it will take several hours before the pump's blockage alarm is triggered.

sea, vomiting, abdominal pain, rapid breathing, fruity smell on the breath). To avoid episodes of ketoacidosis, we sometimes admit the pump user to the day care ward a few weeks after pump start and the pump is stopped for 6-8 hours (except in the younger children).[459] See graph on page 202. Pump wearers (and family members) will learn to recognize the individual symptoms caused by lack of insulin, and can practise taking extra insulin with a pen or syringe under safe conditions. None of the patients who have undergone this form of test have had more than a mild degree of nausea with ketone levels of up to 2 mmol/l (with a normal pH). This reassures them that they can tolerate being without the pump for 6-8 hours ("a night's sleep") without risk of ketoacidosis. This procedure has also been recommended for adult pump users.[884]

If your blood glucose is above 14 mmol/l (250 mg/dl) and you have ketones in the urine or blood you should take an extra dose (0.1 U/kg or 0.5 U/10 lb. body weight) of insulin (preferably rapid-acting NovoRapid, Humalog or Apidra if available). The dose can be repeated after 2 hours if necessary (2-3 hours with short-acting insulin). Contact the hospital if you

It is very important to be able to recognize symptoms of insulin deficiency early on (nau-

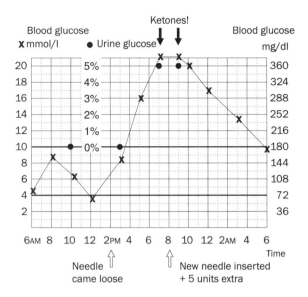

Blood glucose
x mmol/l   ● Urine glucose

Ketones!

Blood glucose
mg/dl

Needle
came loose

New needle inserted
+ 5 units extra

A few hours of interrupted insulin supply is sufficient to make the blood glucose rise quickly. The blood glucose will rise even if you don't eat because the liver will produce glucose when there is a lack of insulin (see page 34). When the blood glucose level was raised in the evening, this teenager was feeling nauseous. He checked for ketones and discovered that something was wrong. When he examined the needle, he found that it had come out so the insulin could not get into his body. He gave himself 5 extra units (0.1 U/kg, 0.5 U/10 lb.) with a pen injector, replaced the needle and started the pump. The blood glucose level returned to normal during the night.

If the blood glucose rises quickly you should remove the infusion set. Give a bolus dose and see if insulin comes out from the tip of the catheter. Kink the catheter and give another bolus dose. The pump should now give a blockage alarm. Check the tubing and connections for leaks. Replace the infusion set and check the blood glucose level frequently to make sure it goes down. Take an extra injection (with a pen or syringe) of 0.1 U/kg (0.5 U/ 10 lb) body weight if you have raised ketone levels, and check your blood glucose again after 1-2 hours. Repeat the dose if necessary.

vomit or feel sick and are unable to drink. If you often have episodes of raised ketones or ketoacidosis, it may be a good idea to replace part of the night time basal rate with an injection of long-acting insulin in the evening. This will make insulin deficiency less likely to occur.

We have found using a low dose of basal insulin (Levemir or Lantus, 0.1 U/kg) to be particularly effective in this situation (you may need to lower the basal rate in the pump slightly).

Disconnecting the pump

Sometimes you will want to disconnect the pump for one reason or another, for example when playing sports, doing aerobics, or swimming. Most infusion sets allow you to disconnect the tubing by using a silicon membrane as a one-way valve.

Taking a bath or shower

Most pumps can tolerate some water but we recommend disconnecting them when taking a bath or shower. You should also disconnect the pump if you have a sauna since insulin can't take the heat. The heat in a sauna will also

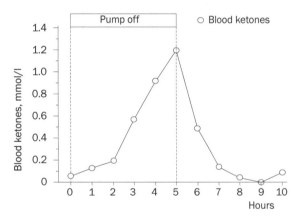

In this study of adults, the pump was stopped for 5 hours.[428] Blood ketone (beta-hydroxybutyric acid) levels increased rapidly to around 1.2 mmol/l. When the pump was started again, a bolus dose was given along with a meal and 1-4 U of extra insulin, resulting in a quick decline in ketone levels. Monitoring blood ketones is an effective method of monitoring the degree of insulin deficiency if you are having pump problems (see page 113). The ketone levels are comparable to those we have found in children and teenagers (see page 202).

Causes of high blood glucose

(adapted from [987])

① **The pump**
Basal rate too low
The pump has triggered an alarm and shut
itself off
Other problems with the pump

② **Insulin reservoir**
Wrong position in the pump
Empty reservoir or plunger is stuck
Leakage in the connection with the tubing

③ **Infusion set**
Forgetting to fill the tubing when replacing
Leakage in connections or hole in the tubing
(feel the tubing and smell your fingers)
Adhesive and/or cannula has come loose
Air in the tubing
Blood in the tubing
Infusion set has been in place for too long
The tubing was replaced in the evening
without checking blood glucose after
3 hours to ensure proper insulin delivery.
Bent or squeezed tubing
Blocked cannula/needle or tubing

④ **Infusion site**
Redness, irritation / infection
Fat pad at the infusion site
Placement close to belt or waistband

⑤ **Insulin**
Cloudy insulin
Expiry date passed
Exposed to heat / sunlight or extreme cold

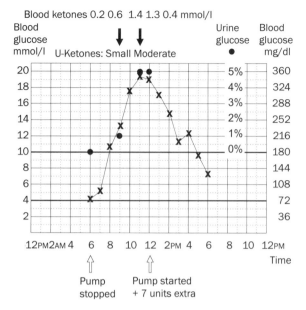

It is important to familiarize yourself with the symptoms of insulin deficiency (nausea, vomiting, abdominal pain, rapid breathing, fruity smell on the breath) and we therefore sometimes plan a "pump-stop" some weeks after pump initiation. This graph was recorded at our day care ward when a planned pump stop was performed (see page 200). This 15-year-old boy stopped his pump with Humalog at 6 AM. He was without insulin for 6 hours and felt slightly nauseous when his blood glucose increased and ketones were present. When he started the pump again at 12 AM he had his lunch and gave himself 7 units extra (0.1 U/kg) besides his normal premeal dose. Typically, blood ketones will rise to around 1.5-2.0 mmol/l (around 0.2 mmol/l rise per hour that the pump has been stopped) and blood glucose to around 20 mmol/l when performing a pump stop like this in children and adolescents.[454] Individuals still having some insulin production of their own will typically show a rise in blood ketones of ~0.1 mmol/l per hour. A few patients have been slightly nauseous, but the stop has not caused ketoacidosis in any of them (pH has not been affected).

If your blood glucose rises like this and you have raised ketone levels, you should take an extra dose of approximately 0.1 U/kg body weight (0.5 U/10 lb). **Always use a pen or syringe to be on the safe side!** Remove the cannula and take a bolus, watching whether insulin appears from the tip. Kink the cannula and take another bolus. The pump should now give an occlusion or blockage alarm. Check the tubing and connections for leakage (smell your fingers). Replace the cannula. Test your blood glucose again after 1-2 hours and repeat the bolus if necessary.

cause previously injected insulin to be absorbed much more quickly (see page 88).

Pump alarms

Insulin pumps seldom malfunction. If yours does, the pump will stop and give an alarm. There is no risk that the pump will pulse or surge, giving you too much insulin. The pump alarm will go off when something is wrong, for example if the tubing is blocked, the insulin container empty or the batteries flat. However, the pump cannot detect if the insulin is leaking somewhere, for example if the cannula has come out, the connections have come loose or there is a hole in the tubing (pets can bite through it). Check the operating instructions to see what the different alarms stand for and how to respond to them.

Most pumps have an alarm that is triggered if you have not pushed any of the buttons after a certain number of hours. It may wake you up early in the morning if you didn't take your evening snack insulin or forgot to push one of the buttons before going to bed. We usually recommend this alarm be set for 14-16 hours.

Occlusion or blockage alarm

The pump alarm will be triggered if there is an increased resistance when pumping insulin. But it cannot tell whereabouts in the system the problem may be. It may be that the insulin reservoir is empty, the plunger may be sluggish, or the tubing or cannula blocked. The tubing can be bent or squeezed, for example by a belt buckle. If the occlusion or blockage alarm is triggered, start by checking the tubing for kinks or pinches. Then give the remainder of the pre-meal bolus. If no alarm is triggered, all is well now and you have received the intended amount of insulin. If the alarm goes off again, the next step is to stretch out and try careful massaging of the infusion port and catheter under the skin (only for infusion sets that do not have perpendicular cannula). If the tubing hasn't been disconnected, there is no need to take any more than the remaining premeal dose of insulin if the pump now works without an alarm (unless the blood glucose level is still raised).

If the cannula or tubing is blocked it may take several hours before the pressure has increased enough to trigger the alarm. During this time you will not have received any insulin. Find out how much is needed to trigger the alarm in your

Disconnecting the pump

Time that the pump has been disconnected	Measure
< 0.5-1 hour	Usually no extra insulin needed.*
1-2 hours	Take an extra dose when you connect the pump corresponding to the basal rate you have missed.
2-4 hours	Take an extra dose before you disconnect the pump corresponding to the basal rate that you should have had during the missing 1-2 hours. Check your blood glucose when you connect the pump and take an extra bolus dose corresponding to 1-2 hours' basal rate if needed.
> 4 hours	Dose as above before disconnecting. Using a pen injector or syringe, take extra insulin every 3-4 hours corresponding to the missed basal rate. Take the pre-meal bolus dose with a pen or syringe.

If you disconnect the pump to exercise, you will probably need to lower the doses more than suggested above. Test this to find out what is right for you. Always leave the pump in "run" mode when disconnecting for a shorter time, as this prevents you from forgetting to turn it on again when you reconnect it.

Make sure there is no air in the tubing when reconnecting it. Prime it with some insulin if necessary. Do not put the pump lower than the insertion site when reconnecting (for example on the floor when in the gym). If you do, there is a risk that gravity will pull some air into the tubing.

*One adult study found that the blood glucose level continued to rise slowly (.1 mmol/l per 15 min. of disconnect, 1 mg/dl per min.) for around 1 hour after a 30 min. pump stop. The total rise before the blood glucose level was stabilized again after reconnecting was 1.7 mmol/l(30 mg/dl).[1136]

Problems with the pump?

Problem	Measure
Infection/irritation at the infusion site	Wash hands and skin with chlorhexidine in alcohol. Replace infusion set more frequently.
Blocked infusion set	It can be bent or blocked by coagulation or insulin crystals. Replace it.
Blocked tubing	Can be caused by precipitation of insulin. Disconnect the cannula from the tubing and give a prime dose. Replace if the alarm is triggered.
Blood in the tubing	Replace the infusion set.
Air in the tubing	No insulin delivered. See page 205.
White spots on the inner layer of the tubing	Most tubing is made from double plastic layers that can come apart, showing as white spots. This does not affect the function or the insulin.
Leakage of insulin at the insertion site	Has the needle/cannula come loose? Is there a bent cannula? Replace the infusion set.

Problems with the pump, cont.

Problem	Measure
Moisture under the adhesive	This indicates insulin leakage. Replace the infusion set.
Adhesive comes off	If EMLA® cream has been used, wash it off carefully with water. Disinfect the skin with Skin-Prep® that leaves a sticky film when drying. Warm the adhesive with your hand after application. Apply extra tape if needed.
Itching, eczema from adhesive	Apply hydrocortisone cream. Use a stoma-type adhesive.
Sticky traces of adhesive	Wipe off with special remover or medical benzine.
Sore skin from plastic on set	Apply a piece of tape beneath the hard plastic.
Scars in the skin from old catheters	Often more visible with dark skin. Replace cannula/needle more frequently. Try using a metal needle.
Redness of the skin over the cannula tip	Can be caused by insulin allergy. See page 218
Nothing works	Try running the pump with both insulin and tubing removed.

pump. It may also depend on what kind of tubing you have, and how long it is. Test it by pushing the steel needle into a rubber cork or pinch the end of the cannula. If you then give a bolus dose you will see how many units are pushed into the tubing before the alarm is triggered. For example, if your pump has given 4.3 units of the meal bolus dose when the alarm goes off and 2.6 units are needed to build up pressure to trigger the alarm, you will have only received 4.3 less 2.6 units, or 1.7 units of the bolus dose.

For smaller children we sometimes use insulin of 50 U/ml, for infants 10 U/ml. This means that fewer units are needed before the alarm goes off since the fluid volume is larger. If 2 units of 100 U/ml are needed to trigger the alarm, this will equal 1 unit of 50 U/ml.

Sometimes the pump will trigger the alarm for a block in the tubing even after you have replaced both the tubing and the cannula. If this happens, remove the insulin reservoir from the pump. Then start the pump again. If the alarm still goes off, the problem is an internal one,

The pump alarm will tell you if there is a blockage in the tubing or cannula/needle. The alarm is triggered by the increased pressure in the tubing. However, if the pressure goes down, for example because of a leaking connection, a cannula that has come out, or a hole in the tubing, the alarm will not go off. This type of delivery failure can only be detected by repeated monitoring of glucose and ketones. If you suspect a leak, feel along the tubing and smell your fingers; insulin has a very distinctive smell. **If the pump alarm goes off, and your blood glucose is high, you should first give yourself an extra injection with a pen or syringe and then check all possible reasons for the alarm.**

such as a motor problem. Don't reuse the pump reservoir. If doing so, the silicon on the plunger will wear off, and this may result in an occlusion or blockage alarm.

Leakage of insulin

The pump can't trigger the alarm if there is an insulin leak. It will only trigger if the motor runs against an increased resistance. Insulin can be deposited outside the infusion site if the cannula has been retracted. Often this can only be detected when you take a bolus dose. When the basal dose is running, the amounts of insulin are so small that it can be difficult to pick up leaks.

The tubing connector on the pump end can crack, causing leakage, especially if you apply too much force when connecting it. Feel the connector with your fingers, and then smell them. If it is leaking, you can often detect the smell of insulin. Sometimes a cat or dog may be able to warn you that there is a leak as they often like the smell of insulin.

Occlusion or blockage alarm

① Check the tubing for kinks and pinching. Try a careful massage of the infusion port and the catheter under the skin. If the alarm was triggered when taking a premeal bolus, take the remaining portion.

No alarm → OK, no problems
Alarm ↓

② Disconnect cannula/needle from tubing. Start a prime dose with the pump.

No alarm → Replace cannula/needle
Alarm ↓

③ Disconnect tubing from insulin reservoir. Start a prime dose with the pump.

No alarm → Replace tubing
Alarm ↓

④ Remove the insulin reservoir from the pump and start a prime dose.

No alarm → Replace reservoir
Alarm ↓

⑤ Something is wrong with the pump. Contact the pump dealer and deliver insulin with a pen or syringe.

Air in the tubing

When you connect the tubing to the pump there is always a risk of air coming in, especially if you fill it with cold insulin. Air will come out of the solution when the temperature rises. Always

When to call the hospital or your diabetes team

➠ The first time you become ill after you have started with the pump.

➠ If you have been feeling too sick to eat for more than 6-8 hours.

➠ If you have vomited more than once during a 4-6 hour period.

➠ If your blood glucose level has not come down, or the ketone level is still running high after the second extra dose of insulin.

➠ If your general well-being is deteriorating.

➠ If you are at all uncertain as to how to handle the situation.

make sure that the insulin is at room temperature before refilling the reservoir. Introducing air into the subcutaneous tissue is not dangerous in itself, but you will miss out on the corresponding amount of insulin. The alarm will not be triggered since the pump's microcomputer cannot tell the difference between air and insulin in the tubing.

If you see air in the tubing when you are about to take a premeal bolus dose you can compensate with a little extra insulin. Five to seven cm (2-3 inches) of air in the tubing usually corresponds to 1 unit of insulin. To find out the exact dimension of your pump tubing, give a bolus dose of 1 unit when you are priming the tubing. Make a mark on the tubing with a felt tip pen corresponding to the length that the insulin travels for that unit.

If the air in the tubing corresponds to more than 0.5-1 unit (or less for a small child) when the basal rate is running (e.g. between meals) it is best to disconnect the tubing from the cannula in the skin. Prime the tubing to purge the air and fill it with insulin once again.

Insulin pump and fever illness

➠ Continue with your ordinary meal bolus doses even if you eat less, and give extra insulin according to your correction factor if your blood glucose is high. Carbohydrate counting with your ordinary ratios will not give enough insulin in this situation. Try lowering them by 10-20% (see page 158) to get higher doses of insulin. If dosing "by eye", increase by 1 unit if necessary (2 units if your dose to start with is 10 units or more, 0.5 U if dose is < 3 U).

➠ Increase the basal rate if you have a raised temperature. Increase the rate by 10-20% (0.1-0.2 U per hour, 0.2-0.4 U per hour if the basal rate is > 1 U per hour) or more if your blood glucose continues to be high.

➠ Check your blood glucose every 2-4 hours. Check for ketones frequently. Keep good records in your logbook.

➠ Take extra insulin (1 U/10 kg or 0.5 U/10 lb body weight), preferably NovoRapid or Humalog, if your blood glucose is high and you have ketones. Give another 1 U/10 kg (0.5 U/10 lb) every second hour until the blood glucose is below 10 mmol/l (180 mg/dl) and the level of ketones is decreasing.

➠ Give all extra doses of insulin with a pen or syringe if your blood glucose has risen suddenly or your blood glucose does not decrease after you have given an extra dose with the pump. This is in case the high blood glucose has been caused by a problem with the pump.

➠ Try to drink large amounts of fluids as this will increase the excretion of ketones and lessen the risk of dehydration. As long as there is glucose in your urine, you will lose extra fluid. Drink glucose-free fluids when your blood glucose is above 10-12 mmol/l (180-215 mg/dl) and change to something containing glucose when the blood glucose is below this level. If you feel nauseous, try to drink small amounts (a couple of sips) at a time.

➠ Try to drink something sweet if hypoglycaemia is a problem. You may need to lower the basal rate but never discontinue it completely.

Sick days and fever

When you are ill, especially if you are running a temperature, your body will increase its insulin requirements, often by 25% for each degree Celsius (every 2 degrees Fahrenheit) of fever (see page 301). It is advisable to begin by increasing the basal rate. Start by a 10-20% increase when you notice that your blood glucose is rising. You will probably also need to increase the meal bolus doses in response to your blood glucose readings. It is important that you test your glucose level before each meal if you are ill, and preferably 1.5-2 hours after the meal as well. Usually, you will need to monitor your blood glucose levels during the night as well.

Many people with diabetes are successful in competitive sports. Others, like most children, just play for the fun of it. In either case, the pump helps keep the blood glucose at an appropriate level both during and after exercise.

Pump removal doses

It is very important always to carry extra insulin wherever you go in case your pump fails to work properly. Check to see that the insulin has not expired. You should have your pump removal doses written down and with you in case you need to use a pen or syringe as a temporary measure. The total number of units over 24 hours will probably need to be increased by 10-20% if you stop using the pump for a whole day or more.

Use the old doses

It is easiest to start with the same doses that you had when you used a pen injector or syringes, provided that you have written down the doses and not too much time has elapsed since then so that you still have more or less the same insulin requirements.

Adjusting doses by eye measure with rapid-acting insulin (NovoRapid, Humalog or Apidra) in the pump

You can continue taking the same premeal bolus doses with a pen or syringe. Replace the basal dose with intermediate-acting insulin. Divide the total basal dose during the day, taking one third in the morning as NPH insulin, and two-thirds at bedtime.

Adjusting doses by carbohydrate counting with rapid-acting insulin (NovoRapid, Humalog or Apidra) in the pump

If you count carbohydrates, long-acting insulin will be better (Lantus or Levemir). Take the total basal dose during 24 hours, and take the same dose of Lantus as one dose at dinner/tea or the evening snack.[117] Give half the dose in the morning, and half in the evening if you will be without the pump for a shorter time. Take the same amount and type of bolus insulin for meals as when on the pump. If you are going to use Levemir you can also begin with the same

Pump removal doses

Sometimes you must use an insulin pen or a syringe for a while, for example if something is wrong with the pump. The replacement with injections differs in calculation depending on which type of insulin you use in the pump.

Rapid-acting insulin in the pump:

➠ **Meal boluses:**
Continue with the same doses of rapid-acting insulin before meals as when on the pump,

➠ **Basal insulin:**
Every person using an insulin pump should have a basal insulin at home for use with a pen or syringe. Pump removal doses should be in writing. You can easily read the total number of units of basal insulin that the pump gives you, and which should be substituted. NPH-type of insulin works well for shorter pump stops. As your spare basal insulin must be discarded when it has expired, and since you seldom will have use for it, NPH insulin is often the best alternative since it is cheapest. But if you are carb. counting, the morning dose will give a slight peak effect at lunch time, in which case your insulin:carbohydrate ratio will not add up correctly.

➠ **Lantus or Levemir:**
Substitute the basal rate with the same number of units of Lantus or Levemir divided into 2 doses (morning and evening), With larger doses of Lantus, the whole dose can be taken once daily.[117]

➠ **NPH basal insulin**
Replace the basal dose with an intermediate-acting insulin (NPH) given twice daily. Take the basal rate in pump and divide it into two doses of intermediate-acting insulin. Give one third in the morning and two-thirds in the evening and adjust according to blood glucose monitoring.

Short-acting insulin in the pump:

With short-acting insulin, you can calculate which dose to use if you add the meal bolus dose in the pump with the basal rate during the hours until next meal (as short-acting insulin gives some basal effect as well during the day). You will probably need to increase the night dose since the pump is more effective, giving more insulin late at night and early in the morning than you would get from the intermediate-acting bedtime insulin. Check with your diabetes nurse if you are unsure what doses you used when you were on multiple injections.

An example of pump removal doses:

Time	6AM 8 10 12 2PM 4 6 8 10 12 2AM 4 6				

	6AM–12	12–2PM	2PM–8	8–12	12–6	
Premeal bolus dose (Pump)	7 U	5 U	5 U	4 U	42 U /24 h.	
Basal rate pump U/h.	0.9	0.8		1.0	0.7	0.9
Premeal bolus dose (Pen/syringe)	11 U Reg.	9 U Reg.	9 U Reg.	6 U Reg.	8 U NPH	43 U /24 h.
Calculation	7+ 0.9x5	5+ 0.8x5	5+ 0.8x2+ 1.0x2	4+ 1.0x2	1.0 x 2 0.7x3+ 0.9x4	

NPH = intermediate-acting bedtime insulin

DANIEL

dose as the total basal in the pump, but this insulin probably needs to be taken twice daily.

Regular short-acting insulin in the pump

Look at the pump doses. The breakfast dose with a pen will be the sum of the pump pre-breakfast bolus dose and the number of basal units the pump would have delivered between breakfast and lunch. If you have a high basal rate (> 1.5-2 U per hour), start by counting just 1-1.5 U per hour when calculating the dose when using a pen or syringe.

The bedtime dose of intermediate-acting insulin (Insulatard, Humulin I, Insuman Basal) is calculated by adding the basal rates between 10 PM and 8 AM (see example on page 208). You can also use short-acting insulin (*not* NovoRapid or Humalog) during the night, giving two doses, at 10 PM and 3 AM, corresponding to the sum of the basal rates during the night

Admission to hospital

If you are admitted to hospital in an acute situation, you may well find that none of the staff members on duty are familiar with your pump. So, if you have any problems using it, it would be best to begin injecting insulin with a pen or syringe until the daytime staff arrive. If you are being sick or have signs of ketoacidosis, the best treatment may be by intravenous insulin (see page 74).

Physical exercise

Try wearing the pump in a case on a strong elastic waistband during exercise. If you are involved in contact sports, you can disconnect the pump for 1-2 hours without taking any extra insulin. If you are exercising for longer than 2 hours, it will probably be better to keep the pump connected and temporarily decrease the basal rate. Try half the basal rate while exercising and for the following hour or two. You may need to lower the basal rate even more, but the only way to know for sure is to try it yourself. Another alternative is to connect the pump again for a short while when you are halfway through the exercise (for example at half-time in a game of sport), and take a small bolus dose.

If you have problems with hypoglycaemia early in your exercise session, you will need to dis-

connect the pump at least 2 hours before the session starts. [379] There was no difference in the rate of hypoglycaemia during 40-45 minutes of submaximal effort on an exercise bicycle (~60% of VO_2 max, maximal oxygen uptake) between having the pump off or reducing the basal rate by 50%.[10] However, late hypoglycaemia 2.5-12 hours after exercise was more common than hypoglycaemia during exercise, and occurred more often when the pump was not removed.

If your blood glucose is rising after exercise when the pump has been disconnected, you can try taking a small bolus (begin with 1-2 U) immediately after finishing, i.e. before taking a shower to counteract this (see also page 291). If you are practising carbohydrate counting, you may want to put in some carbs in the pump along with this dose (although you are not eating). Otherwise the pump will count this dose as active insulin (see page 193), and subtract it from your next meal bolus (unless the meal is after the active insulin has expired).

If you are using rapid-acting insulin, your blood glucose level may plummet if you exercise shortly after taking the premeal bolus dose (see graphs on page 290) without decreasing it. You can try taking half the meal bolus dose (see table on page 291), or even skipping it if the exercise is particularly strenuous. However, you will probably then need to keep the pump connected to get the basal rate during the entire period of exercise.[1083]

When you go to a diabetes or sports camp you will be very active for several days in a row. Try lowering the basal rate 10-20% (0.1-0.2 U per hour) when you arrive at the camp, and then adjust it according to your blood glucose levels.

Don't forget to refill your glucose stores after exercise (see page 284). After strenuous exercise (e.g. a ball game or skiing) you must decrease the basal rate by 10-20% (0.1-0.2 U per hour) or even more during the night to avoid hypoglycaemia. Try this out yourself and note the blood glucose test results in the logbook for future ref-

In the winter when it's cold, you must keep the pump close to your body. The tubing is very thin and no part of it must be outside the clothing, or it will easily freeze. It may be a bit awkward finding the pump to take the bolus dose but since the insulin can't be allowed to freeze, you must protect it from low temperatures.

erence should you be faced with the same situation again.

Another way of decreasing the basal insulin effect if you are having a full day of exercise (like a soccer cup) is to disconnect the pump in the morning after breakfast and take an injection of intermediate-acting NPH or long-acting Levemir or Lantus insulin. Try taking approximately one third of your daily basal rate by injection to begin with. When you eat, connect the pump to take bolus doses. Reconnect the pump when you are finished exercising.

If you are exercising regularly and need to disconnect your pump often, you can also replace part of the basal dose with long-acting insulin (Lantus or Levemir). This can be a good alternative if you swim a lot, for example. Try with 30% of the total basal rate as one dose in the morning to begin with and adjust according to blood glucose levels.[19] The effect should be correct for days with exercise so that the pump can be disconnected for many hours without your blood glucose rising. Connect the pump temporarily when eating and then after finishing exercise for the day. The basal rate during the evening and night can probably be quite low, as the long-acting insulin taken in the morning will still have some basal effect.

During the day (when the pump is disconnected) it can be set to 0.1U/hour to prevent clogging and make it easy to connect again. On days (and weeks) when you are not exercising (but continuing with the long-acting insulin)

An insulin pump needs to be looked after, and tubing and batteries need to be replaced. When the alarm goes off, you must know how to respond. You will be the "first-line pump mechanic" and will probably find that you soon learn how to take care of the practical details.

you will need to increase the basal rate slightly to match your need of basal insulin without exercise; begin by approximately 0.1-0.2 U/kg body weight during 24 hours. Alternatively, stop the long-acting insulin and set a full basal rate on the pump during this period without exercise.

Using the pump at night only

Some people feel that the pump has obvious advantages during the night but that multiple injections are better during the day. This may be the situation for a child who is not yet ready to manage the pump alone without adult supervision. Using a pump at night time may be a good alternative for children who are using intermediate-acting insulin (Insulatard, Humulin I, Insuman Basal) at bedtime and experience problems with night time hypoglycaemia or high blood glucose levels in the early morning.[599] It is perfectly acceptable to connect the pump in the evening, let it stay in place overnight, and disconnect it the next morning. During the day you can use a pen injector or syringe for premeal bolus doses. Talk to your diabetes doctor if this sounds like the right approach for you.

In a group of children aged 7-10 years, the pump was used for the dinner and evening snack bolus doses and for the basal rate during the night.[599] Intermediate-acting NPH was given in the morning and premeal boluses during the day were given as injections of rapid-acting insulin. The children's blood glucose readings were lower with the night time pump than when using bedtime NPH insulin. In one study of night time pumps in adults, the morning blood glucose levels were more even and the patients also experienced fewer episodes of hypoglycaemia in the daytime.[586]

A night time pump may be a good alternative if you are on a seaside holiday, for example swimming and surfing. Disconnect the pump in the morning and take your meal bolus doses with a pen or syringe; then connect the pump again when you come back to the hotel in the afternoon or evening. Since you will probably be exercising more than usual, your need for basal insulin is lowered, but you will probably still need an injection of basal insulin in the morning (some pump needles can be used also for giving injections). You can try giving approximately half or two thirds of the basal dose the pump should have given while disconnected as intermediate-acting NPH insulin or long-acting Levemir or Lantus.

Is the pump a nuisance?

You must keep your insulin pump next to you 24 hours a day. Many people ask us, "How do you sleep with it?", but they are then surprised by how quickly they get used to wearing the pump at night. Some people who lie quite still put the pump beside or under the pillow and wake up in the morning with it still there. Others, who are more restless, find it better to have the pump on a waistband, leg band, or in a pyjama pocket.

When should I disconnect the pump?

⇒ In the bath tub

⇒ In a public bath or swimming pool

⇒ In a sauna or jacuzzi

⇒ During an X-ray, CT (CAT) scan or MRI scan

Most pumps are waterproof when they leave the factory, but water can easily get inside if there is a small crack in the casing or display. You will then get a new pump on the warranty, but we feel the simplest advice is to disconnect the pump just before entering the water as long as you are not planning to stay for a longer period of time in a wet environment (if you are windsurfing, for example). If you go abroad for a beach holiday it can be difficult to have a new pump sent to you, so be on the safe side and disconnect the pump when swimming.

On rare occasions, some people have taken bolus doses while sleeping. It may well be that they have dreamt of eating and are so used to the pump that they have taken a bolus dose without waking up. If you have hypoglycaemia unexpectedly in the morning, it is a good idea to check the pump memory to find out if you have taken a dose in your sleep. If this is the case, you should wear the pump in a case at night to prevent you from pressing the buttons. in error. Another solution is to lock the pump at night, or to use a remote control for bolusing and place this far away from your bed at night.

An 18-year-old girl said that the first question friends asked her was, "What do you do with the pump when having sex?" Fortunately, it is

> ### Research findings:
> ### Rapid-acting insulin and pumps
>
> ♠ Long-term studies show that individuals can achieve a 6 mmol/mol (0.5%) lower HbA$_{1c}$ when using Humalog in the pump without increasing the risk of severe hypoglycaemia or ketoacidosis.[948,740]
>
> ♠ In a Canadian pump study, regular short-acting insulin and rapid-acting insulin were used in insulin pumps during a 3-month double-blind cross-over study.[1132] All bolus doses were given immediately before the meals. HbA$_{1c}$ was significantly lower, 61 mmol/mol (7.7%) compared with 64 mmol/mol (8.0%), when using rapid-acting insulin but there was no difference in the frequency of hypoglycaemia.
>
> ♠ In a French pump study, blood glucose levels were more stable and the number of readings below 2.0 mmol/l (36 mg/dl) decreased when using Humalog.[740]
>
> ♠ In a German study of adults, the pump was stopped from 10 PM in the evening until 7 AM in the morning. With Humalog, the changes in blood glucose and ketones developed 1.5-2 hours earlier than with regular short-acting insulin.[884] Blood glucose increased with about 11 mmol/l (200 mg/dl) in 6 hours using Humalog compared with about 6 mmol/l (110 mg/dl) with short-acting insulin. One patient stopped the test after 7 hours due to headache and nausea but no one developed ketoacidosis.
>
> ♠ In an Italian study of adults, the pump was stopped for 5 hours in the morning without eating breakfast. During these hours, glucose levels increased by 5.6 mmol/l (100 mg/dl) on average when using short-acting insulin (Velosulin) compared with 9.2 mmol/l (165 mg/dl) with Humalog.[428] Blood ketone levels rose to about 1.2 mmol/l when using Humalog compared with 0.9 mmol/l with Velosulin.
>
> ♠ In an American study, the differences between regular short-acting insulin and Humalog were not as pronounced when the pumps were stopped for 6 hours.[51]

easy to disconnect the pump for a short while to stop it getting in the way. Making love also involves physical exercise, so be aware that you might need a little less insulin for a while. Just don't forget to reconnect the pump afterwards.

Does using a pump cause weight gain?

If you have an increased HbA$_{1c}$, there is a risk of gaining weight when your blood glucose improves since less glucose will be lost via the urine. If you have frequent hypoglycaemic episodes you will be likely to gain weight since you will find yourself needing frequent snacks. If you start treating yourself to sweets and crisps you are bound to put on weight. Talk to your dietitian about how to find a way around these problems. It might be easier to lose weight without an increase in HbA$_{1c}$ if you have an insulin pump because you can then decrease both your food intake and meal bolus doses but be able to ensure you meet your basal insulin requirements.

Having a lie in

With an insulin pump it is easier to sleep longer in the morning as your basal need for insulin is covered automatically. To find a suitable basal rate, skip breakfast (don't take the breakfast bolus dose either) and test your blood glucose several times until lunch. If the level hasn't changed you know it will work well when you sleep late. Before you know how your body reacts, it is a good idea to have a parent or relative help check your blood glucose at 7-8 AM and adjust the basal rate accordingly. If it is below 3.5-4.0 mmol/l (65-70 mg/dl) it may be easier for them to shut off the pump for a while than to wake you up in order to eat something.

Travel tips

Always take extra insulin and an insulin pen or syringes wherever you go. Don't forget to adjust the pump's clock if you travel across time zones. Change the clock to the new time when you arrive at your destination. Since you will be sitting still on the plane, it may be a good idea to increase the basal rate slightly on a long trip. Measure your blood glucose before each meal and make necessary adjustments to the bolus dose. You may need a certificate for customs declaring that you need to wear an insulin pump. The pump does not usually trigger the metal detector at airports. Some companies will lend you a spare pump that you can take along on the trip in case something goes wrong with your own pump. Due to the change in pressure at flight cruising level, existing air bubbles at ground level will expand. New bubbles may also emerge in the insulin reservoir. This could cause some insulin to be pushed through the tubing, resulting in a lowering of your blood glucose level (see also page 349).[613]

If you travel in a very hot climate, the insulin may lose its potency. You may need to change insulin cartridges every 1-2 days. If you fill your reservoirs yourself, do not fill with more insulin than you will use in this time. Keep your insulin supply in a refrigerator, if possible. See page 343 for further travel tips.

Using an insulin pump works well for all age groups; no child is too young to try one. Even babies only a few weeks old have used insulin pumps successfully. If your child has unpredictable eating habits, it is very practical to be able to give small bolus doses every time he or she eats something. The best insertion site for the infusion set in toddlers is the buttocks.

Toddlers using pumps

No child is too young to use a pump. They have been used successfully even in babies only a few weeks old. In a US study of toddlers aged 2-5 years, HbA_{1c} decreased from 80 mmol/mol (9.5%) to 63 mmol/mol (7.9%) and the number of instances of severe hypoglycaemia decreased from approximately one episode every 2 months to approximately one episode every 10 months.[678] For young children with basal rates < 0.3 units per hour U-50 can be used, for babies often U-10. Small children may need a lower percentage of the total daily dose as the basal rate (down to 30-40%). Young children often need the highest basal rate in the late evening from 9 PM-12 AM.[205,787]

Especially picky and unpredictable eaters will benefit from repeated small bolus doses in accordance with their eating habits. Dual/combined or square/extended bolus can be very effective if there is any doubt about just how much a child will eat, as the bolus can be cancelled when the child has had enough to eat. The pump can be kept out of reach of the toddler by being worn in a harness between the shoulders. Children from the age of 4-5 years can often wear the pump in the same way as older children. In our experience, they very quickly learn not to interfere with the pump. If in doubt, lock the buttons on the pump.

The buttocks are often used for infusion sites for the very youngest, since the cannula is then out of sight. If the child wears nappies, position the insertion site so that it won't be soiled by the nappy contents.

Pregnancy

Using an insulin pump is an excellent way to obtain blood glucose values close to those of an individual without diabetes.[577] With a close to normal blood glucose, the risk of complications during pregnancy decreases to the same levels as for women without diabetes (see page 319). In pregnancy, basal needs are usually only 40% of

Remember to bring extra batteries and other accessories when you are away from home for more than a couple of hours. Most airlines don't allow you to pack spare lithium batteries in your checked baggage. Instead, carry any spare batteries with you in your carry-on baggage. Also bring a pen or syringe and rapid-acting insulin so you can take extra insulin if your pump stops working properly.

Many people come to look upon their pump as a reliable friend that they will use for many years. Little Linda has even given her pump a name; "Bloue Pumpis".

the total daily dose.[305] The insulin requirements will gradually increase during pregnancy, but will often plummet after delivery (see page 322). During the later part of pregnancy it might be difficult to have the pump cannula on the distended abdomen. Instead, it would be a good idea to use the buttocks, the upper part of the thighs or the upper arm.

There is an increased risk of ketoacidosis during pregnancy. You should check your blood glucose more often and also change tubing and cannulas more often (every day with metal needles and every other day with Teflon catheters). Contact the hospital immediately if your blood glucose level is high and you have raised levels of ketones in your blood or urine. Adding a bedtime dose of intermediate-acting insulin (0.2 U/kg) to cover part of the normal basal dose delivered by the pump has decreased the risk of ketoacidosis considerably.[717]

Rapid-acting insulin in the pump

As rapid-acting insulin (NovoRapid and Humalog) acts more quickly and more closely mimics the insulin response in a person without diabetes, it is the logical choice for use in insulin pumps.

One problem when using insulin with an even shorter duration is that your body's insulin depot will go down considerably as well (see

page 197). This implies that symptoms of insulin deficiency will arise fast if the pump fails. The production of ketones will start after approximately 4 hours when a pump with Humalog is stopped.[1041] One can compare a pump-free period of about 4 hours with rapid-acting insulin to about 6 hours with regular short-acting insulin. However, this can vary considerably from one individual to another.

NovoRapid and Humalog are now both approved for pump use in most countries and their use is increasing fast. The experiences to date are positive. In our department, we start all new pumps with rapid-acting insulin. However, if you develop symptoms very quickly after an interruption of the insulin supply, you may be better off using regular short-acting insulin.

When switching from short-acting to rapid-acting insulin in the pump, you may need to lower the bolus doses slightly (by approximately 1-2 units) since the bolus doses of regular short-acting insulin supplied part of the basal insulin, overlapping with the next meal as well. To compensate for this you may need instead to increase the basal rate slightly, when you are using either NovoRapid [115] or Humalog.[199]

The onset of action with a premeal bolus dose of NovoRapid or Humalog may be too rapid in certain situations, such as eating a meal that is digested slowly because it is rich in fat and carbohydrates (e.g. pasta or pizza), or a long drawn-out dinner with many courses. You can then try taking the bolus dose after the meal. If you have a pump that can deliver the dose more slowly (square or extended bolus, see illustration on page 192) this is an ideal solution in these situations. You can use this type of bolus dose even if you have problems with gastroparesis (slower emptying of the stomach due to diabetic neuropathy, see page 363). See the chapters on insulin adjustments on page 156 and diet on page 234 for further advice on the use of NovoRapid and Humalog.

If you use regular short-acting insulin in the pump and want to sleep half an hour longer in the morning, you can take the pre-breakfast dose with rapid-acting insulin in a pen or syringe immediately before eating instead of 30 minutes earlier. NovoRapid or Humalog is also a good alternative if your blood glucose is high before you eat.

Which type of treatment do the health professionals prefer?

In an American study, professional members of AADE (American Academy of Diabetes Educa-

tors) and ADA (American Diabetes Association), mainly nurses, doctors and dietitians, were asked how they treated their own diabetes.[412] The results showed that as many as 60% of the AADE members with diabetes and 52% of the ADA members with diabetes used insulin pumps (only 10% of the patients used pumps at the time of the study). Only 3-4% used 1-2 injections per day. The rest used multiple injections with 3-4 doses per day. The average HbA_{1c} for pump users was 50 mmol/mol (6.7%), for multiple injections 55 mmol/mol (7.2%). One interesting observation was that diabetes (type 1) was 13 times more common among the AADE and ADA members than in the general population. The explanation may be that since diabetes generally develops at a younger age (average age at onset in the US is 16 years), the disease may influence a person towards choosing a career involving diabetes care.

For further reading on insulin pumps, try any of the following: *Pumping Insulin* by John Walsh and Ruth Roberts, Torrey Pines Press, San Diego, USA; *Think like a Pancreas* by Gary Scheiner, Marlowe, New York, USA; and *Insulin Pump Therapy Demystified* by Gabrielle Kaplan-Mayer, Marlowe, New York, USA.

An insulin pump will enable you to "fine tune" your insulin doses and will give you more "horsepower under the bonnet" for taking care of your diabetes. However, greater knowledge and attention will be needed if it is to work well, just like a stronger and faster car. Used correctly, an insulin pump is a very good tool that can give you wonderful support on your long diabetes journey.

Side effects of insulin treatment

Pain

If an injection is particularly painful you have probably hit a nerve (see illustration on page 125). If you can stand the pain you can readily inject the insulin, otherwise you must pierce the skin once again. If your injections are often painful, see the chapter on injection equipment, page 137.

Insulin leakage

It is not uncommon for a drop of insulin to come out on the skin after the needle is withdrawn. Two to three drops from a pen needle contain approximately 1 unit of insulin (100 U/ml). In one study on children and adolescents with diabetes, 68% encountered leakage of insulin after injections during 1 week.[996] And 23% of these injections were followed by leakage of up to 18% of the injected dose (2 units out of an intended dose of 11 units).

It may be difficult to avoid insulin leaking, but the risk will be reduced if you lift a skin fold and inject at a 45° angle (see illustration on page 129). Try to inject more slowly. You can also try to withdraw the needle half way and then wait 20 seconds before withdrawing it completely. Some people find it helpful to press a finger on the injection site or to stretch the skin immediately after removing the needle. At one time, the standard advice was to stretch the skin sideways before injecting to avoid insulin leakage, but this is not a good idea because you risk giving yourself an intramuscular injection by mistake.

If you penetrate a superficial blood vessel with the needle it may bleed a little. Bleeding under the skin will feel like a small bubble, which is often bluish in colour.

Blocked needles

Sometimes the needle will be blocked when you inject long- or intermediate-acting insulin. This can be caused by the crystals in the insulin that build up. It seems to depend on how quickly you inject the insulin. The problem is more likely to occur if you perform the injection slowly (over a period of more than 5 seconds). Try to inject the insulin quickly (within 5 seconds) of penetrating the skin. The risk increases when you reuse needles as any remaining insulin may crystallize inside the needle barrel.

Bruises after injections

If you penetrate a superficial blood vessel in the subcutaneous fat layer, there may be a small amount of bleeding. However, the blood vessels in the subcutaneous fat are so small that there is no risk of insulin being injected directly into one of them. The bleed will feel like a small bubble under the skin and may be bluish in colour. Bleeding like this is quite harmless and is absorbed completely after a while. If you are worried about it, pressing over the injection site for 2 minutes may decrease problems with bruising.

Fatty lumps

Skin-related complications of insulin therapy are fairly common, and a review can be found in reference [886]. Fatty lumps (lipohypertrophies) are caused by insulin's effect of stimulating growth of fat tissue.[901,382] This is a common problem when you don't rotate your injection sites often enough. Fatty lumps contain both fibrous and fat tissue.[1039] Up to 30% of adult patients have problems with fatty lumps,[821,901] and as many as 50% of children and adolescents (18% had massive lumps).[632] In the paediatric study, those with lipohypertrophy had higher HbA_{1c}, more daily injections and longer duration of diabetes, but there was no association with needle length.[632] Sometimes these soft lumps can contain harder nodules of scar tissue.[1084]

A child usually wants to prick the skin where it hurts the least, resulting in injections too close together. It is important to explain carefully why this is not a good idea, and help to find a system for rotating the injections sites effectively. Younger children (aged under 10-12 years) should have a parent helping them with 1 or 2 of their injections each day. The parent can then inject into areas that the child might have difficulty in reaching, such as the buttocks (see "Where do I inject the insulin?" on page 125).

Insulin causes the subcutaneous tissue to grow if you inject frequently into the same spot. You will get a "fatty lump" (lipohypertrophy) in the skin that feels and looks like a bump.

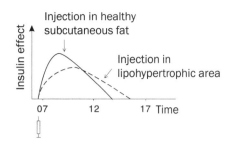

Insulin will usually be absorbed more slowly and probably more erratically if you inject in an area with fatty lumps (lipohypertrophy).

Re-using needles causes blunting which means that repeated injections are not only more painful, but they also cause more damage to the skin and may even contribute to an increase in the formation of fatty lumps.[999]

Injections in fatty lumps will usually result in a slower (and probably more erratic) absorption of insulin,[642,1128] because of a decreased number of blood vessels in the lump.[886] When using rapid-acting insulin, the maximum concentration was 25% lower after an injection in an area with lipohypertrophy.[567] An area with lipohypertrophy should be left alone for at least a couple of weeks. One way to accomplish this can be to use an indwelling catheter (Insuflon, see page 137) with which the injection sites can be actively rotated. Another way is to use a guide with a rotation scheme, designed with holes or sections for different days of the week.[367] In extreme cases it take up to a year before the fatty lumps disappear,[469] and fat suction has even been used to remove them.[886]

In one report, the problems with lipohypertrophies decreased among individuals using rapid-acting insulin (Humalog).[901] The explanation may be that, as this type of insulin enters the bloodstream much faster, the time for which the fat cells are exposed to the insulin will decrease.

Remember that insulin will start to act sooner if you inject it in an area free from lipohypertrophy. You may have to lower the dose to avoid hypoglycaemia when you switch your injections into a "fresh" site without lipohypertrophy.

Redness after injections

Redness, sometimes with itching, that occurs immediately after or within hours of an insulin injection can be due to an allergy towards the insulin or a preservative. This type of reaction will usually subside after some years as you continue with insulin treatment.[827] Inform your doctor if you have problems with redness after injections. There is a special skin test available to find out whether you are allergic to the insulin or the preservative. There is often an increased level of insulin antibodies in the blood as well (see later). If problems with redness continue, antihistamine tablets can be helpful. Adding a small amount of corticosteroids to the insulin may also help.[682] Switching to rapid-acting insulin (NovoRapid [17] or Humalog [640]) has decreased the problem with redness after injections in some cases. It may also be helpful to try switching to another brand of insulin as they contain very small amounts of residues from the manufacturing process (parts from yeast cells in Novo Nordisk insulins and parts from E. coli bacteria in Eli Lilly insulins).[594] The slow infusion rate of an insulin pump was helpful for building up tolerance to insulin (so called "desensitization") in a girl who had problems with burning local reactions to insulin.[310] We have the impression that the problem of redness after injections has decreased considerably since we began giving all patients rapid-acting insulin as part of a multiple daily insulin regimen right from the onset of diabetes. However, it has been described also when using Levemir [107] and Lantus.[711]

It is important to make sure your insulin has not passed its use-by date and that it is stored correctly (see page 130). Inappropriate storage conditions can result in the insulin breaking down and give rise to harmful substances that can cause local allergic reactions.[418] A generalized allergic reaction after insulin injection is very rare.[196,640]

Allergy to the nickel in pen and syringe needles can cause redness after injections. The needles are covered with a layer of silicone lubricant. If you are allergic to nickel you should not use the needles more than once as the silicone layer wears off and the nickel will come in closer contact with the skin. Needles on syringes have a thicker silicone layer since they need to penetrate the membrane of the bottle when drawing up insulin. For this reason, they will be more appropriate if you are allergic to nickel. You can have a skin test to see whether this is the case. If you are allergic to nickel, you will usually react to it in other items as well, for example earrings, belt buckles or wrist watches.

EMLA®cream (a topical anaesthetic used for taking blood samples or when replacing indwelling catheters) can cause an allergic redness that looks very much like an allergy to the adhesive.

Insulin antibodies

Your body will produce antibodies to "defend" itself against foreign substances. Insulin antibodies with pork and beef insulin were common. With the use of human insulin it is not common to have high enough levels of antibodies to cause problems. Higher levels of insulin antibodies are more common when using multiple injections or insulin pumps compared with conventional treatment with two doses a day.[226]

Insulin antibodies work by binding insulin when there is a high level of free insulin, for example after a meal bolus injection.[1064] When there is a low level of free insulin, for example during the night, they release insulin.[127] The effects have been studied both with short-acting [127,1064] and intermediate-acting insulin,[836] but since it is the free fraction of insulin in the blood that is bound to antibodies, they can affect any type of insulin. In this way the insulin concentration in your blood will be levelled off in a way that does you no good at all. When you want a high level of insulin after a meal, it will be lowered (resulting in high blood glucose); and when you want a low level in the blood many hours after a meal or during the night you will instead have too much insulin (resulting in hypoglycaemia that can be prolonged).[1064] It could be said that if you have high levels of insulin antibodies you will produce long-acting insulin on your own. In fact, one of the new long-acting insulin analogues (Levemir) is using the same principle: after entering the bloodstream, the insulin is bound to a protein (albumin) and then released very slowly.[477]

One possible method of reducing the impact of this reaction is to give yourself a fairly large dose of insulin in the morning to "saturate" the insulin antibodies. During the day, you can take smaller and smaller doses just before meals. At bedtime give only a very little dose of insulin to lessen the risk of night time hypoglycaemia. As the injected insulin will have a prolonged action, it may help to keep in mind that rapid-acting insulin (NovoRapid or Humalog) will work like short-acting insulin (Actrapid, Humulin S, Insuman Rapid) for a person with a high level of insulin antibodies; short-acting insulin will work like something in between short- and intermediate-acting (Insulatard, Humulin I, Insuman Basal) while intermediate-acting insulin will work as long-acting (Lantus) normally does.

Switching to rapid-acting insulin (Humalog) substantially decreased the level of antibodies and problems with early morning hypoglycaemia in one case report [647] and solved the problem of redness at the injection site and generalized insulin allergy in another.[640] Apparently, the structural differences between regular short-acting and rapid-acting insulin molecules prevented Humalog from binding to the human insulin antibodies. NovoRapid has also been used successfully in patients who are allergic to insulin.[17]

A blood test is available to measure how much of the total amount of insulin is bound to antibodies. Normally this level is below approximately 6%. Problems with antibody effects on insulin action as described above can be seen with levels > 10%.[836,1064] We have seen antibody levels above 90% in cases where the person has had particular difficulty both with redness after injections and with prolonged insulin activity. Insulin antibodies can be very troublesome but usually the negative effects will slowly subside after several years, even if you still have measurable levels of antibodies.

Lipoatrophy

Lipoatrophy appears as a cavity in the subcutaneous tissue. The reason for its development is not clear. It does not usually appear in areas that have been used too often as injection sites. Rather, it is believed to be an immunological reaction towards insulin which causes the breaking down of subcutaneous tissue.[827,886] Patients with lipoatrophy often have high levels of insulin antibodies. Lipoatrophy was more common when using older types of insulin, but has also been described in a person using Humalog in an insulin pump.[420] You can try treating the cavities by injecting insulin along the edges. This will cause the formation of new fatty lumps and eventually the cavities will disappear. Mixing a small amount of steroids in the insulin or topical sodium cromolyn has been effective in some cases.[905]

Insulin oedema

Sometimes, local or generalized oedema can follow a rapid improvement in blood glucose control (for example, shortly after diabetes has been diagnosed or when beginning with regular insulin doses again after having skipped a lot of them). This is caused by a temporary build-up of fluid in the body and usually subsides spontaneously over a period of days to weeks if the blood glucose control continues to be good.[968] In severe cases, ephedrine has been an effective treatment.[531] The diuretic furosemide may also help in severe cases.

Insulin requirements

How much insulin does your body need?

An adult without diabetes produces approximately 0.5 U of insulin/kg (0.23 U/lb) body weight every day.[8] After the remission phase (usually within 1-3 years after the onset of diabetes) the insulin requirement for a growing child stabilizes, generally somewhere between 0.7 and 1.0 U/kg per day (0.3-0.45 U/lb per day),[691,968] and usually close to the 1 U/kg per day (0.45 U/lb) mark (approximately 20% less when using an insulin pump). Sometimes only a few units less per day can result in quite a difference in HbA_{1c}. If the young person becomes unwell, it will usually be necessary to increase insulin doses, especially if the illness is accompanied by fever (see page 301).

During the growth spurt of puberty, insulin doses often need to be increased considerably.

Puberty and growth

During puberty, the young person starts to grow rapidly, so larger doses of insulin are needed. Boys usually have their growth spurt at around the age of 14, and girls at around 12 years (a year before they start menstruating) but this does vary considerably. Boys usually require much higher doses during puberty, often as much as 1.4-1.6 U/kg per day (0.6-0.7 U/lb per day),[689] sometimes even more. Girls may also need to increase their doses to exceed 1 U/kg per day during their growth spurt.[1056] After they start menstruating, their growth slows down, and they have usually reached their full adult height within a further 2 years. At this time it is very important to lower the insulin dose, and regulate food intake, to avoid "gaining width" instead.

Within a few years after puberty, insulin requirements decrease to an adult level, usually

0.7-0.8 U/kg per day (0.3-0.35 U/lb per day). It is a good idea to try and get used to counting insulin requirements in units per day in different situations as well as considering the number of units in each injection.

Height and weight should be monitored regularly. Children and adolescents with diabetes are often slightly taller than their healthy peers when they develop diabetes, but their final height falls within the normal range.[924,1129] Poor diabetes control, especially during early puberty, can slow down growth.[307,1112] Puberty may be delayed and girls' menstrual periods missed or their onset delayed.[307] Generally, the HbA_{1c} will be high, but it may not be if a lack of insulin is combined with poor nutrition. Because of this, it is very important to consider both insulin and nutritional requirements in relation to growth patterns. Treatment with an insulin pump can considerably improve growth rate in poorly controlled diabetes by establishing a reliable supply of basal insulin.[992]

Remission (honeymoon) phase

You are likely to need particularly large doses of insulin when your diabetes has just been diagnosed. This is because your body will not be as sensitive to insulin as it should be, on account of your high blood glucose levels during the weeks immediately before diagnosis (around the time you may have been feeling unbelievably thirsty). Once you start treatment, your body is likely to regain its sensitivity to insulin very fast so that, within a week or so, the amount of insulin you need will have come right down.

When your blood glucose level has been normal for some time, the beta cells usually start to produce some insulin again, and this makes it possible to decrease your insulin doses further. Often this natural insulin production will continue to rise. If the insulin doses can be lowered to 0.5 U/kg body weight or less, and the HbA_{1c} level is close to that of individuals without diabetes, < 53 mmol/mol (7.0%), you can be described as having entered the remission phase (also called honeymoon phase). The advantage of insulin coming from your own pancreas is that it is secreted in relation to the blood glucose level, which makes it easier to manage your diabetes.

Even if the beta cells produce only a small amount of insulin, this can be enough to counteract the production of ketones. Insulin inhibits the breakdown of fat into fatty acids, which then can be transformed to ketones in the liver. Because of this, patients who produce their own insulin over a period of several years have a certain "protection" against ketoacidosis.[570] But if they are faced with a stressful situation or an infection, their need for insulin will increase considerably. This is because the increased levels of cortisol and adrenaline result in more fat being broken down into fatty acids and causing more ketones to be produced.

The remission phase usually lasts 3-6 months, sometimes a year or longer. Insulin require-

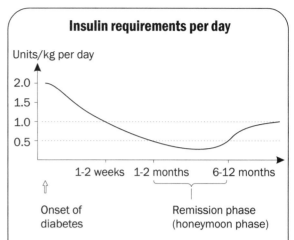

Insulin requirements per day

Units/kg per day

Large doses of insulin are usually needed during the first 1-2 weeks after diagnosis as blood glucose levels will have been high for a sustained period of time, resulting in considerable insulin resistance in your body. The amount of insulin needed usually goes right down during the first few weeks and months.

A growing child is likely to need an insulin dose of around 1 U/kg body weight per day. When children need less than this, their pancreas is probably producing some insulin of its own. This is common during the first 6-12 months after the onset of diabetes. A child who needs less than 0.5 U/kg per day (0.23 U/lb per day) has entered the remission phase (honeymoon phase).

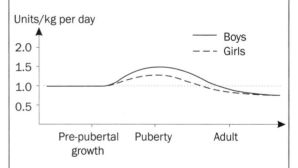

Units/kg per day

During puberty, teenagers grow fast, and larger doses of insulin will be necessary. It is important to be sure to take enough insulin at this time. Growth hormone is secreted mainly during the night and the bedtime insulin dose may need to be raised by a considerable amount. Young people who don't get enough insulin during puberty may lose a few centimetres (0.5-1 inch) from their final height. Once the final height has been reached, insulin doses will need to come down again.

ments are usually at their lowest between 1 and 4 months after the onset of diabetes.[691] However, this varies from person to person. Some will not have a remission phase at all; for others it can last for more than a year. After 2-4 years of insulin treatment in young people, it is very unusual to be producing any insulin at all. If you had symptoms (thirst, needing to pass a lot of urine, weight loss) for only a week or two before starting insulin treatment, your chance of having a remission phase is higher. Younger children usually have a shorter remission phase. Children who were below the age of 5, or who had ketoacidosis at the onset of diabetes, are unlikely to have a remission phase according to one Italian study.[134] Intensive insulin treatment and better blood glucose control from early on in the diabetes is thought to give the beta cells an opportunity to rest, increasing the chances of enough insulin subsequently being produced to allow a longer remission phase.[247,269]

Insulin doses can sometimes be brought right down during the remission phase, to the extent that the person requires only a few units of insulin a day. It almost feels as if the diabetes will disappear, but unfortunately this doesn't happen. If you have it, you will need to take insulin for the rest of your life or until a cure for diabetes has been found. The remaining insulin produced by the beta cells reduces gradually, then usually disappears completely.

An infection will often trigger an increased need for insulin, and cause your blood glucose levels to rise. Insulin doses must be adjusted accordingly. If you are prompt in modifying your doses in response to your blood glucose readings, there will be less stress for your pancreas and you will have better chances that your total insulin requirement per day will go down again, once the illness is over.

The term "remission phase" might more accurately be described as "partial remission". Complete remission would mean needing no insulin at all for a shorter or longer period of time. All the insulin is usually not withdrawn,

---

Insulin requirements (after the remission phase)

☞ Pre-pubertal growth	0.7-1.0 U/kg/day, usually closer to 1 U/kg/day (approximately 20% less with an insulin pump).
☞ Puberty	Boys: 1.1-1.4 U/kg/day, sometimes even more.[689] Girls: 1.0-1.2 U/kg.[1056]
☞ After puberty	Girls: < 1 U/kg/day from a couple of years after the first menstrual period. Boys: around 1 U/kg/day at 18-19 years of age, less after a couple of years. (1 kg = 2.2 lb)

You can estimate your own insulin production during the remission phase by comparing the total insulin dose given per 24 hours with the numbers for different ages in the above table.

---

although the insulin requirement may be very low.[74] An exception to this rule is when a person with diabetes finds themselves experiencing hypoglycaemia as a result of tiny doses such as 0.5-1 unit. The reason for not withdrawing insulin completely is that even small doses help to keep the beta cells working, which in turn makes a longer remission phase more likely.

How much insulin does the pancreas produce?

It is not possible to measure the insulin produced in the pancreas in a direct way as it is chemically identical to the insulin you inject. However, internal insulin production can be indirectly assessed by measuring C-peptide, a protein produced in equal measure to insulin in the healthy pancreas but not present in the insulin you inject (see page 373). A person with type 2 diabetes produces more insulin in his or her own pancreas, so measuring C-peptide can be used as a method of distinguishing between type 1 and type 2 diabetes.

Insulin sensitivity and resistance

The body's insulin sensitivity is essential for determining how much the blood glucose level will be lowered by a given dose of insulin. You might think that the same dose of insulin would have the same effect on the blood glucose in any single individual, but this is not the case. Certain factors increase insulin sensitivity while others decrease it (see key fact box on page 224).

Insulin resistance implies that a higher insulin concentration in the blood is needed to obtain

Think of your blood glucose level as similar to your body temperature, the blood glucose meter as a thermometer and the regulation of the blood glucose as a thermostat (the same type that radiators have to maintain an even temperature). If you are faced with insulin resistance, i.e. decreased sensitivity for insulin, it is as if the "glucostat" has been turned up. Your blood glucose will be higher and more insulin than usual will be needed to lower it again. This is similar to having a fever which raises your body's thermostat and causes your temperature to increase.

When you have recovered, your body will reset the thermostat so your body temperature returns to normal. In the same way the "glucostat" resets to a normal insulin sensitivity when the blood glucose level has been back to normal for a day or two.

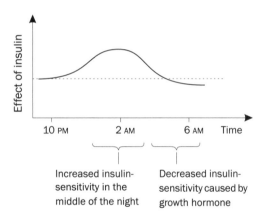

In the middle of the night (midnight-3 AM), when we don't eat, the body's sensitivity to insulin is increased. The secretion of growth hormone increases in the middle of the night but the blood glucose-raising effect does not appear for 3-5 hours.[129] Growing children have higher levels of growth hormone than adults do. Levels of growth hormone are even higher during puberty, which explains why the dawn phenomenon is more pronounced in adolescents. Young children who fall asleep early have their growth hormone peaks before midnight and it is common to see an increased need for insulin from 9 PM-12 AM.[125,205] Individuals whose glucose control is poor have increased levels of growth hormone which make increased blood glucose levels in the morning more likely, as well as retarding growth (see page 40).[129]

the same blood glucose-lowering effect. You could also say that the insulin sensitivity is decreased. The decreased effect of insulin is caused by a restrained transport of glucose through the cellular wall when the blood glucose level is high.[646,1125] The decreased uptake of glucose into the cells can also be caused by a constriction of the blood vessels, resulting in a decreased blood flow.[388] Insulin resistance will, in this sense, be a defence for the insulin-sensitive cells that are prevented from taking up too much glucose.[1126] These cells will not be exposed to glucose toxicity and will therefore not be affected by the long-term complications of diabetes. The cells that are not dependent on insulin for their glucose uptake (e.g. the eyes, the kidneys and the nerves) will, on the other hand, have a high uptake of glucose. This will expose them to glucose toxicity leading to long-term complications. See illustration on page 356.

If your blood glucose level has been high for a short period only (just 1 day, for example) such as during an infection, your body will require higher insulin doses to achieve the same blood glucose-lowering effect. A meal of a given size and composition will accordingly need a higher dose of insulin than usual. This increased insu-

Increased insulin resistance

Short-term factors

① High blood glucose level for 12-24 hours.[7,343,1124]

② Rebound phenomenon (see page 54).

③ Later part of night (dawn phenomenon).

④ Infection with fever.

⑤ Stress.[751]

⑥ Surgery.

⑦ Inactivity, bed rest.[1083]

⑧ Ketoacidosis.

Long-term factors

① Puberty.

② Pregnancy (the later part of).

③ Weight gain, being overweight.[44]

④ Smoking.[53,325,768]

⑤ High blood pressure.

⑥ Drugs, e.g. cortisol, contraceptive pills.

⑦ Other diseases like toxic goitre, chronic urinary tract infection, dental abscess.

Decreased insulin resistance

① Low blood glucose levels (improved glucose control).

② Weight loss.

③ After physical exercise.[1093]

④ Early hours of the night (midnight-3 AM).

Research findings: Insulin resistance

♠ In one study, the blood glucose level was held at 17 mmol/l (305 mg/dl) during part of the day and night, 15 hours in total.[343] The following day the subjects had a decreased sensitivity for insulin.

♠ Another study showed that if the blood glucose level had been sustained between 13 and 20 mmol/l (220 and 360 mg/dl) during a 24 hour period, the effect of a given insulin dose was decreased by as much as 15-20%.[1124] After 44 hours with a blood glucose level of 15 mmol/l (270 mg/dl) the insulin effect decreased by 32%.[361]

♠ In the same study it was found that admission to the hospital in itself resulted in a decreased insulin effect by 21%, probably caused by associated illness, bed rest and temporary changes in lifestyle. The effect seems to be due to an increased blood glucose level as such, since the levels of the blood glucose increasing hormones (adrenaline, cortisol and growth hormone) were not increased.

♠ In a healthy beta cell, the production of insulin will be decreased if it is being exposed to high glucose levels even for as short a period as 2 days.[660]

lin need may continue for a week or so after the infection has subsided if your blood glucose level has been high for a longer period of time. Some people have noted higher blood glucose levels during periods when the pollen count is high if they have hay fever. This may be because they are less active while suffering from pollen allergy.

After some time with high insulin doses (and normal blood glucose levels) you will start experiencing hypoglycaemia, even though you have not changed either your insulin doses or the amount of food you eat. The body's sensitivity to insulin will change when the blood glucose level is low, and the same insulin concentration in the blood will now lower the blood glucose more effectively,[216] resulting in a lower dose of insulin for the same meal. As you experience this you will learn to decrease your insulin doses slightly as a preventive measure when your blood glucose levels have been normal for a day or two (or up to a week depending on

A vicious cycle can easily develop, in which a high blood glucose level can give an increased insulin resistance within 24 hours.[1124] This will make your insulin less effective, you will find it more difficult to get your blood glucose levels down to normal, and your blood glucose levels will rise after some time, as will your HbA_{1c}. The graph above shows that a high HbA_{1c} implies that twice the amount of insulin is needed to obtain the same blood glucose-lowering effect.[1125]

To start with, you must increase the insulin doses if you are to break this vicious cycle. However, in the long run the key issue is to become more "accurate in aiming" your insulin doses, not letting the blood glucose increase too much or too often again. After just 1-2 weeks with lower blood glucose levels, you will be able to decrease the insulin doses again. If you have been using pump treatment for 3-6 months, it may be possible to lower insulin doses by 10-30% as the insulin resistance decreases after a period with lower blood glucose levels.[1125]

It is common to seek the "ideal insulin dosage". Just imagine, finding this would ensure "smooth sailing" for a long time to come. Unfortunately this is never as easy as it sounds. Sometimes you will find it very frustrating searching for the right insulin dose. It seems that no matter how you approach the problem you cannot make any sense of the relationship between your blood glucose measurements and the amount of insulin you take. This is made all the more frustrating by the fact that the speed at which injected insulin is absorbed varies enormously (see page 88). Often, your insulin doses are unlikely to be suitable for more than a couple of weeks at a time. After that, something in your daily life changes, the insulin sensitivity is affected and suddenly your doses are not appropriate any more. Of course, this can be very difficult to understand and to live with. But it is important not to have unrealistic expectations. Just as daily life differs slightly from week to week and month to month, so your insulin requirements will also change.

If you are unable to find a schedule that works, it can be helpful to keep to exactly the same doses for a week. You will then be better equipped to see a pattern in your glucose readings and insulin doses. Contact your diabetes healthcare team to discuss what to do next.

individual differences), thus preventing hypoglycaemia.

Compare your blood glucose level with a thermostat that regulates the central heating in a house. If the thermostat is adjusted to 20° C (68° F) more energy will be needed to maintain this temperature if the outside temperature is colder than usual. In the same way, more insulin will be needed to keep the blood glucose at the same level when insulin resistance is high. If the blood glucose level has been high for a while, the "glucostat" will adjust and you will start having hypoglycaemia at a higher blood glucose level than before. If you have had very low blood glucose levels for some time, the glucostat

will readjust in the opposite direction and you will not experience hypoglycaemia until your blood glucose level is very low (see also pages 44 and 62).

Weight gain increases insulin resistance while weight loss decreases it. This is one of the reasons why it is difficult to maintain a normal blood glucose level if you are overweight. Male pattern obesity ("apple fatness") is particularly likely to increase insulin resistance.[684] Other factors can also contribute to the level of insulin resistance (see key fact box on page 224).

Increased levels of stress hormones (adrenaline, noradrenaline) will induce an insulin resistance that develops within 5-10 minutes.[684] Stress also causes release of cortisol, which increases insulin resistance within hours.

During puberty, an increase in the secretion of growth hormone raises the blood glucose level. This causes a resistance to insulin that contributes to the need for increased insulin doses during puberty. Smoking leads to increased insulin resistance because nicotine decreases the uptake of glucose to the tissues of the body.[53]

Regular exercise (at least every other day) leads to a decrease in insulin resistance that lasts between exercise sessions, while inactivity (for instance caused by being bedridden) gives an increased resistance within days.[1083] Active athletes, for example, need to lower all their insulin doses considerably. When the training season is over, doses are likely to need considerable adjustment upwards if higher blood glucose levels are to be avoided. Sometimes 30-50% more

insulin will be needed during periods of reduced activity.

Ideal insulin doses?

Of course we all want to search for the ideal insulin doses, but unfortunately this is not a realistic goal since insulin requirements vary according to activity, other illnesses, insulin resistance (see page 223) and other factors. A good parallel can be seen with body temperature. Your body strives to maintain a temperature around 37° C (99° F) but this would be difficult if you always wore the same amount of clothing regardless of what the weather was like. Just as an outfit that is perfect one week can be much too warm the next, so a particular dose of insulin is likely to be ideal for a week or two only, before you need to readjust it. As with your clothing, you will need to make daily adjustments in your insulin doses if you are to remain comfortable.

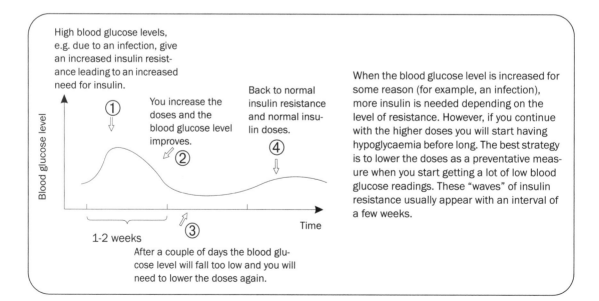

High blood glucose levels, e.g. due to an infection, give an increased insulin resistance leading to an increased need for insulin.

① You increase the doses and the blood glucose level improves. ②

Back to normal insulin resistance and normal insulin doses. ④

1-2 weeks ③ After a couple of days the blood glucose level will fall too low and you will need to lower the doses again.

When the blood glucose level is increased for some reason (for example, an infection), more insulin is needed depending on the level of resistance. However, if you continue with the higher doses you will start having hypoglycaemia before long. The best strategy is to lower the doses as a preventative measure when you start getting a lot of low blood glucose readings. These "waves" of insulin resistance usually appear with an interval of a few weeks.

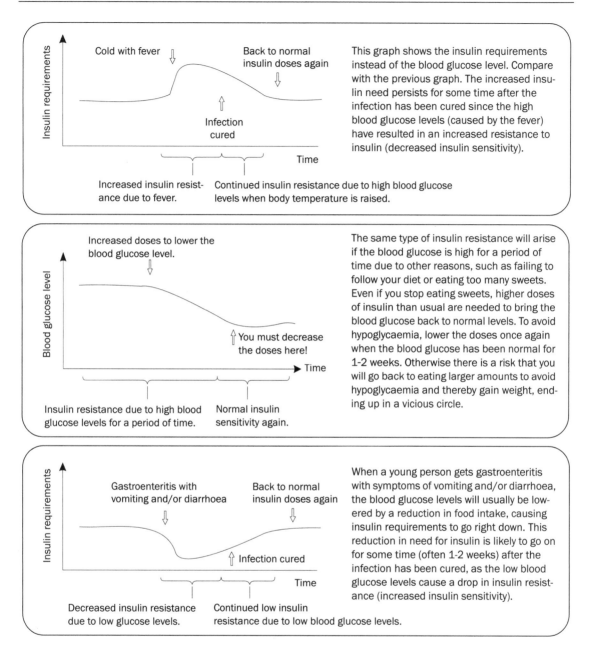

Cold with fever ⇓   Back to normal insulin doses again ⇓

This graph shows the insulin requirements instead of the blood glucose level. Compare with the previous graph. The increased insulin need persists for some time after the infection has been cured since the high blood glucose levels (caused by the fever) have resulted in an increased resistance to insulin (decreased insulin sensitivity).

⇑ Infection cured

Insulin requirements

Time

Increased insulin resistance due to fever.

Continued insulin resistance due to high blood glucose levels when body temperature is raised.

Increased doses to lower the blood glucose level. ⇓

The same type of insulin resistance will arise if the blood glucose is high for a period of time due to other reasons, such as failing to follow your diet or eating too many sweets. Even if you stop eating sweets, higher doses of insulin than usual are needed to bring the blood glucose back to normal levels. To avoid hypoglycaemia, lower the doses once again when the blood glucose has been normal for 1-2 weeks. Otherwise there is a risk that you will go back to eating larger amounts to avoid hypoglycaemia and thereby gain weight, ending up in a vicious circle.

Blood glucose level

⇑ You must decrease the doses here!

Time

Insulin resistance due to high blood glucose levels for a period of time.

Normal insulin sensitivity again.

Gastroenteritis with vomiting and/or diarrhoea ⇓   Back to normal insulin doses again ⇓

When a young person gets gastroenteritis with symptoms of vomiting and/or diarrhoea, the blood glucose levels will usually be lowered by a reduction in food intake, causing insulin requirements to go right down. This reduction in need for insulin is likely to go on for some time (often 1-2 weeks) after the infection has been cured, as the low blood glucose levels cause a drop in insulin resistance (increased insulin sensitivity).

⇑ Infection cured

Insulin requirements

Time

Decreased insulin resistance due to low glucose levels.

Continued low insulin resistance due to low blood glucose levels.

Nutrition

From a historical perspective, dietary advice for people with diabetes has been very restrictive when it comes to carbohydrate intake. Foods containing sugar were excluded from the diet. This created feelings of guilt in people with diabetes when the "rules were broken". To do as most other people do, i.e. to vary one's food intake and indulge in the occasional sweet "treat" was discouraged and by some looked upon almost as "sinning". But this is an outmoded and inappropriate approach. The inclusion of foods containing moderate amounts of sugar has not been found to worsen blood glucose control.

Sticking to a rigid pattern of mealtimes and selected food is unlikely to be necessary because of diabetes alone, especially if you are taking premeal insulin in a multiple injection or pump regimen, although regular eating habits and a knowledge of carbohydrate quantities is important. Many people with diabetes live full and varied lives, enjoy their food, and still manage to control their blood glucose levels effectively.

A kitchen scale can be useful for weighing food and extras to calculate the carbohydrate content when learning carbohydrate counting. Many centres recommend estimating helpings and nutritional contents by eye,[1079] after an initial learning period when diabetes is first diagnosed. Other centres teach carbohydrate counting as a more exact method of calculating premeal insulin doses when using multiple injections or a pump (see page 246).

The more knowledge you have about carbohydrate foods and their effects on your blood glucose, the more control you will have over your diabetes. This chapter will give you many details about blood glucose and different foods, but you will learn the general aspects of healthy eating from your dietitian.

It is important to be careful about what you eat, even if you don't have diabetes. But remember that food should not be looked upon as medicine. Food should look and taste good. Meals are meant to be pleasurable; we should enjoy food and feel satisfied afterwards. If you concentrate upon food being "good for you" to the exclusion of everything else, you will find no pleasure in it. It will be much more rewarding if you are able to discuss what you can eat with a dietitian who will help you draw up a meal plan based on the mealtimes, routines and preferences that are important to your family. "You should never eat what you don't like", says UK dietitian Sherry Waldron.

"What can I eat?", "What should I avoid?" Such questions are commonly asked by people newly diagnosed with diabetes. Usually, the comment after the first consultation with a dietitian will be: "I am glad to discover I can eat most of the things as I used to before getting diabetes". Dietary advice should be directed towards the whole family from the very beginning. In a Finnish study of young children with type 1 diabetes, all family members increased their consumption of skimmed milk, low-fat cheese and low-fat cold meats. They also ate more fruit and vegetables.[1075]

Nutritional recommendations will be based on requirements for all healthy children and adolescents.[365] Children need to double their energy intake between the ages of 6 and 12 years if they are to grow as much as they should.[1080] At this time, they need to eat more food rich in energy and protein. However, if they do not reduce their energy intake once the growth spurt stops, they are at risk of becoming overweight.[1080] At the present time, there is no good scientific evidence for recommending vitamin or mineral supplements.[1080]

It is very important to get back to the normal parent-child rules and roles in the family as quickly as possible. When talking about this with the family, we should always try to separate what works from a blood glucose point of view and what the child can or cannot do according to family rules. It should still be the family that decides if the child can have sweets, and the rules for this should be as close as possible to those of friends and other children in the family. To be able to handle this, you need to learn how different types of sweets affect the blood glucose level. Younger children need to actively hear that "you would not have been allowed this even whether or not you had diabetes", otherwise the child will believe that it is the diabetes condition that sets the limits and will in time begin to hate this illness that stops all fun in life.

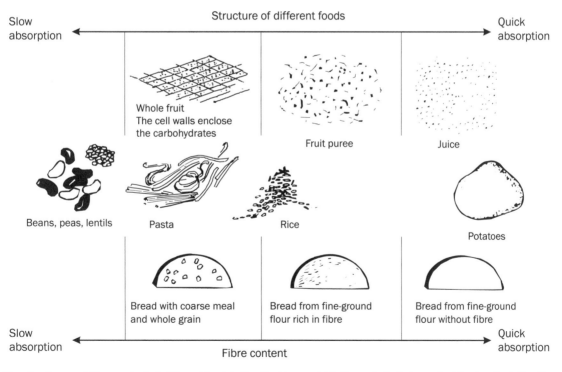

The structure and fibre content of different foodstuffs affect how quickly the carbohydrate content is absorbed. The illustration is from the book "Food and diabetes" by the Swedish Diabetes Association, printed with permission.

Absorption of carbohydrates

Glucose from food can only be absorbed into the bloodstream after it has passed into the intestines. It cannot be absorbed through the lining of the mouth, as used to be believed.[430,981] To reach the intestines, the food must first pass through the lower opening of the stomach (pylorus, see illustration on page 22) where a special muscle, the pyloric sphincter, acts as a "gateway" to the intestine below. The sphincter will only allow very small pieces to pass through.

Complex carbohydrates must first be broken down to simple sugars before they can be absorbed into the bloodstream. The length of the carbohydrate chain does not seem to affect absorption as much as was once believed since "cleavage" (breaking) is a fairly rapid process. Simple carbohydrates are cleaved by enzymes in the intestinal lining while more complex carbohydrates and starch are first prepared by amylase, an enzyme found in the saliva and pancreas. Starch fibre cannot be cleaved into carbohydrates in the intestine.

At one time, carbohydrates were divided into quick-acting and slow-acting, mainly depending on the size of the molecule. It is more accurate to speak of quick-acting and long-acting foods and to evaluate the composition, fibre content and preparation in order to determine the effect on the blood glucose level, rather than simply its content of pure sugar.[591,1079] The term "glycaemic index" (GI) is used to describe how the blood glucose level is affected by different food (see page 242).

Dietary fibre content and particle size seem to be particularly important according to recent studies.[44] The starch in vegetables is broken down more slowly than the starch in bread.[1034] The starch in potatoes is quick to break down to glucose. The starch from pasta products is broken down much more slowly, even though it

> ## Factors that increase the blood glucose level more *quickly* (*increased glycaemic index*)
>
> ① Cooking:
>
>   Boiling and other types of cooking will break down the starch in food.
>
> ② Preparing food:
>
>   Prepared food, e.g. polished rice will give a quicker rise in blood glucose than unpolished, mashed potatoes quicker than whole potatoes and grated carrots quicker than sliced.[1034] Wheat flour gives a higher blood glucose response when baked in bread than when used for pasta.[591]
>
> ③ Fluids with food:
>
>   Drinking fluids with a meal causes the stomach to empty more quickly.[1042]
>
> ④ Glucose content:
>
>   Extra sugar as part of a meal can cause the blood glucose level to rise, but not by as much as was once believed. Particle size and cell structure in different food compounds give them different blood glucose responses in spite of their containing the same amount of carbohydrates.[44]
>
> ⑤ Salt content:
>
>   Salt in the food increases the absorption of glucose into the bloodstream.[1035]

is made from white flour, which is low in fibre.[591]

How much you chew the food and the size of the food particles swallowed also influences the blood glucose response.[878] Industrially manufactured mashed potatoes contain a fine powder that is mixed with fluid. The glucose in mashed potatoes is absorbed just as quickly as a glucose solution.[1070] Pasta and rice are swallowed in larger bites and must be digested before they can be absorbed. Likewise, a whole apple will give a slower rise in blood glucose than apple

Factors that increase the blood glucose level more *slowly* (decreased *glycaemic index*)

① Starch structure:

Boiled and mashed potatoes give a quicker blood glucose response (as fast as ordinary sugar) while rice and pasta give a slower blood glucose response.[1070]

② Gel-forming dietary fibre:

A high fibre content (as in rye bread) gives a slower rise in blood glucose by slowing down the emptying rate of the stomach and binding glucose in the intestine.

③ Fat content:

Fat in the food will delay the emptying of the stomach.[1101]

④ Cell structure:

Beans, peas and lentils retain their cell structure even after cooking. Whole fruits affect the blood glucose level more slowly than peeled fruits and juice.[1070]

⑤ Size of bites: [878]

Larger pieces of food take longer to digest in the stomach and intestine. Larger pieces also cause the stomach to empty more slowly.

juice which contains smaller particles and is in a liquid form.

Heating decomposes starch, making sugar more accessible and faster to digest. Industrial food processing usually involves higher temperatures which gives food a quicker blood glucose-raising effect compared with home-cooked meals.[1034] Industrial baby food and semi-manufactured food (sometimes used in schools) can raise the blood glucose more than comparable home-cooked meals.

Indigestible carbohydrates (dietary fibre) cannot be broken down in the intestines and will therefore not give a blood glucose response. The amount of carbohydrate listed on a food label can be misleading as no distinction is made between digestible and indigestible carbohydrates. Your dietitian can discuss this with you further.

Emptying the stomach

Everything that causes the stomach to release food more slowly into the intestines will also result in a slower increase of the blood glucose level [44] (see illustration on page 70). From this, it follows that the composition of the meal will be important, and not only the amount of carbohydrates it contains. Fat [1101] and fibre [800] cause the stomach to empty more slowly while a drink with the meal will make it empty more quickly.[1062] A meal containing solid food (such as pancakes) is emptied more slowly than liquid food like soup.[1062] Swallowing without chewing also causes a slower rise in blood glucose.[878] Extremely cold (4° C, 39° F) or hot (50° C, 122° F) food will also slow down stomach emptying.[1005]

The emptying of the stomach is also affected by the blood glucose level. The stomach empties more quickly if the blood glucose is low and more slowly if it is high. Both solid and liquid food are emptied from the stomach twice as fast when the blood glucose drops from a normal level 4-7 mmol/l (70-125 mg/dl) to a hypoglycaemic level (1.6-2.2 mmol/l, 29-40 mg/dl).[956] If your blood glucose level has been lowered by a large dose of insulin, you want your stomach to empty as quickly as possible so that the glucose can be absorbed into the blood. In this situation you should take something with a high glucose content, such as glucose tablets, glucose gel or a sports drink.

A high insulin level in the blood (as if you have taken a too large dose) does not affect the emptying of the stomach in itself, it is the high blood glucose level that will cause a slower emptying.[630] Even small changes in blood glucose levels, well within the normal ranges for

Carbohydrates

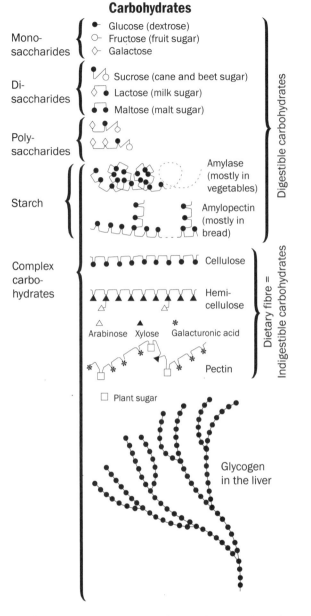

Carbohydrates are important for metabolism in the body. Only mono-saccharides can be absorbed from the intestine. Di-saccharides and starch must first be broken down by digestive enzymes. Dietary fibre cannot be broken down to saccharides in the intestines. The glycogen store in the liver is composed of very long chains of glucose.

The illustration is modified from reference [44].

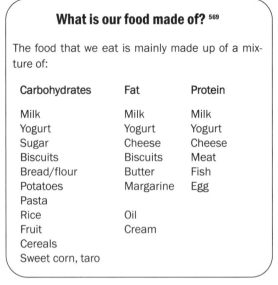

What is our food made of? [569]

The food that we eat is mainly made up of a mixture of:

Carbohydrates	Fat	Protein
Milk	Milk	Milk
Yogurt	Yogurt	Yogurt
Sugar	Cheese	Cheese
Biscuits	Biscuits	Meat
Bread/flour	Butter	Fish
Potatoes	Margarine	Egg
Pasta		
Rice	Oil	
Fruit	Cream	
Cereals		
Sweet corn, taro		

individuals without diabetes, seem to affect the rate of stomach emptying. One study of people without diabetes, showed a 20% decrease in the emptying rate when the blood glucose level was increased from 4 to 8 mmol/l (70 to 145 mg/dl).[957]

Non-strenuous exercise (like walking) will lead to unchanged or more rapid emptying of the stomach, while strenuous exercise or physical exertion stops the stomach from emptying for 20-40 minutes after muscular activity finishes.[149] A possible explanation for this delayed stomach emptying after physical exertion is an increased secretion of adrenaline and morphine-like hormones (endorphins).

Stomach emptying can also be delayed if you have gastroenteritis.[65] This may contribute to the problem of prolonged low blood glucose levels that are often associated with vomiting and diarrhoea.

There is a complication of diabetes known as gastroparesis in which the autonomic nervous system is damaged. This damage involves the nerves that coordinate the movements of the stomach and intestine, resulting in the emptying of the stomach being mildly or even severely delayed. See also the section on other complications on page 365.

Sugar content in our food

From a nutritional point of view, we do not actually need pure sugar at all. The liver is quite capable of producing the 250-300 g of glucose that a healthy adult normally needs per day. However, your body will produce a lot of ketones if you do not eat carbohydrates, see page 251.

Small amounts of glucose along with a meal do not cause an increased rise in blood glucose according to several studies in which a small amount of starch has been exchanged for glucose at a meal.[44,365] This means that you can add 5 g (1/5 ounce) of sugar to a meal without risk, for example in the form of ketchup.[1010] Where sugar is an integral part of the meal, it should be balanced by a comparable reduction in carbohydrate, or an appropriate increase in insulin.[365] Dietary sugar does not increase blood glucose more than an equivalent amount of starch.[365] This is great news for people with diabetes as it makes following the food plans much easier.

You can have a modest amount of ketchup with your food without any problems. However, if you use a large amount of ketchup, you will end up eating a lot of additional sugar.

However, sugar eaten between meals affects the blood glucose level much more. Your blood glucose level will rise just as quickly if you eat sweets or white bread (without butter or something on it) in between meals.[380] The important factor is whether the snack contains fibre or fat (like chocolate-covered biscuits) which delay stomach emptying. Far too many people in the UK, Australia, US, Canada and other countries

How is the emptying of the stomach affected?

More quickly	More slowly
Small bites	Large bites
Liquid food	Solid food
Hypoglycaemia	High blood glucose
Light exercise	Heavy exercise
Drink with food	Drink after food
	Fatty food
	Food rich in fibre
	Extremely hot or cold food
	Smoking
	Gastroenteritis

are now becoming overweight, often seriously so. Therefore, you should be very careful to avoid high fat snacks if you have a weight problem.

The recommendation to decrease the sugar content in food is based on more general factors:

① Sugar gives "empty calories", i.e. sugar gives only energy and contains no other nutrients. This energy will cause you to gain weight, while reducing your appetite for more healthy foods.

② Sugar is bad for your teeth.

In an American study where children took insulin twice daily, there was no difference in their blood glucose levels when they had a diet with 2% of the carbohydrates as pure glucose (in fruit and bread) compared with 10% (in fruit and bread, cereal and toast with jam for breakfast, chocolate chip cookies with lunch, chocolate for an afternoon snack and chilled milk with dinner).[683] This may be surprising, but can be explained by the fact that all the meals contained both fat and protein. The total carbohydrate content was the same for both types of meal.

It used to be common practice to decrease the carbohydrate content in a diabetes meal plan at all costs. The problem with this approach is that the fat content usually increases instead, and this results in the diet becoming inferior to the diet of many children without diabetes.[1012,1079] It is much more important to eat regularly and to adjust the insulin dose according to appetite and the content of carbohydrates in the meal.

Taking fluids with food

You can affect your blood glucose level considerably, depending on what you have to drink with your meals. Sweet drinks like fruit juice can be used to raise your blood glucose if it is in the low range. But if your blood glucose level is high, it is better to have water. It is a good idea to drink plenty of calorie-free drinks between meals if your blood glucose is high as this will help to bring it down (part of the excess glucose will be excreted into the urine). If you want ice cream for dessert, you can drink water instead of milk with your meal if you want to keep the amount of carbohydrate unchanged, or add insulin according to carbohydrate counting to take care of the ice cream (see page 264).

Dietary fats

The reason that individuals with diabetes should be careful with fat intake is that they have an increased risk of arteriosclerosis and heart disease (see page 356). A key goal for people with diabetes is to decrease the intake of total fat (including saturated fat and trans fatty acids) and cholesterol.[365] You need to be particularly careful with saturated fat and so called "trans fats".[365] Foods that contain large amounts of saturated fats include dairy products and red meats. They are also found in many snack foods such as chocolate, cakes and pastries and sometimes in crisps. Trans fats are often listed as "partially hydrogenated vegetable oil" or "vegetable shortening" on the food label.[1092] Try to use monounsaturated and polyunsaturated fats where possible instead. Ordinary margarine and butter contain only 3% polyunsaturated fat. An increased intake of monounsaturated fats may even improve your HbA_{1c}.[297] The softer the fat the better. Liquid margarine and oil do not contain any trans fats at all and also have a low content of saturated fatty acids. Be alert for palm and coconut oil as both are high in saturated fat and used widely in different products.

Today, dietitians promote monounsaturated fats (MUFA) which have a protective effect against heart disease.[850] Choose a margarine that contains monounsaturated fat. Light margarine is not recommended for very young children, however, as they have an increased need for fat in their diet. Olive oil and rapeseed oil contain large amounts of monounsaturated fat and are useful for frying. However, if the frying pan is very hot, the unsaturated fat can be broken down. Some types of light margarine cannot be used for frying. Sunflower oil is another example of oil which is good for frying as it is not broken down as readily as olive oil.

> ### Food rules of thumb
>
> ⇒ Regular eating habits are encouraged in all children and adolescents, with or without diabetes.
>
> ⇒ Plan mealtimes and contents with other daily activities in mind, e.g. will you be taking physical exercise or sitting at a desk?
>
> ⇒ Take extra insulin when necessary, e.g. at parties, or when eating lots of sweet things.
>
> ⇒ Eat fresh fruit as a snack rather than drinking fruit juice.
>
> ⇒ Cut down on snacks and what you eat at every meal if you have weight problems.
>
> ⇒ Aim for a high fibre content in your food.

Up to the age of 5 years, it is expected that the proportion of energy derived from dietary fats will fall from about 50% (as it is in breast milk and infant formula) to levels recommended for adults, but this moderation should not occur below the age of 2 years.[1080] Below this age the energy density of foods is important, and also low fat foods in toddlers may be associated with rapid gastric emptying and diarrhoea.[1080]

Although the total fat intake of children in the UK has gone down over the last decade, chil-

It isn't easy to balance food and insulin at all times. Many people seem to think that "It can't be that difficult, since a diabetes diet is what we all should eat". You may find well-meaning friends or relatives acting as "sugar-police", telling you shouldn't be doing this every time you eat something sweet, even if you have hypoglycaemia. Try to explain that at times it can be both healthy and necessary to eat sweet foods, and you may avoid some of the glances and remarks.

If the meal contains fat, the emptying of the stomach will be delayed, causing the blood glucose to rise more slowly. In this study, two helpings of mashed potatoes (50 g of carbohydrate) were given with or without corn oil (approximately 30 ml, 2 tablespoonfuls). The study was done in adults without diabetes, who can increase the amount of insulin in their blood very fast.[1101] Notice that the blood glucose level increased quickly despite this, with a significant change appearing in 30 minutes, in the group of people whose mashed potatoes did not contain oil. However, if you have weight problems you need to be careful about adding fat to your food.

dren with diabetes still seem to find it difficult to keep their intake within the recommended levels, and total fat intake remains above what is generally advised.[1080] The food habits of people in the UK and the unhealthy snack choices made by children may be responsible for this.[1080]

Many people believe that fat increases the blood glucose level since people with diabetes are usually advised to cut down on fat in their diet. However, fatty food has no direct effect on the blood glucose level. Fat affects the blood glucose level indirectly by slowing the rate at which the stomach empties.[535,681,1101] Studies on monkeys have found that their stomachs empty portions of food through the lower sphincter with the same amount of energy every minute.[737] As fat yields more energy than carbohydrate, the stomach is emptied more slowly when the fat content is high. A meal with a high fat content, therefore, will cause the blood glucose level to rise more slowly.

The fat in food must pass into the intestine before it can affect the emptying rate of the stomach.[1101] This means that if you start a meal with something rich in fat, the signal that slows down the emptying rate will reach the stomach more quickly.

If you eat a meal very rich in fat, you may still have food remaining in your stomach when you are about to have your next meal. If you are using multiple injections, you will need to decrease the amount of food you plan to eat (without changing the insulin dose), if you are to avoid an increase in blood glucose. If you are using rapid-acting insulin (NovoRapid or Humalog) you may be at risk of hypoglycaemia shortly after a meal rich in fat. If this happens to you, try giving yourself the injection after the meal instead of before.

It is the total amount of fat over time that is important in the long run. You can cut down on fat during the week and then have a festive meal at the weekend, complete with a delicious cream sauce, or a takeaway meal. Most fat substitutes, for example maltodextrin (modified food starch), are made of carbohydrate, which may affect your blood glucose.

Dietary fibre

The fibre content of food is healthy for many reasons. There are two kinds of fibre, soluble (gel-forming) and insoluble. Both help to prevent constipation but only the soluble fibres (found in fruit, vegetables, legumes and oats) affect the glucose control. You will feel full for longer after eating coarse rye or wholemeal bread with a high soluble fibre content, than you would after eating the same amount of white bread without fibre. A high soluble fibre content will also decrease the cholesterol level in your blood.[800] Adding fibre (such as oats and barley) to a meal will increase the viscosity, causing the contents of the stomach and intestines to empty more slowly.[800,1119] The fibre forms a thin film on the intestinal surface causing the glucose to be absorbed more slowly.[800]

When a glucose solution is mixed with large amounts of water-soluble, gel-forming fibre (i.e. guar, beta-glucan) the expected rise in glucose concentration will be reduced.[800] Soluble dietary fibre probably has the greatest impact on food intake with a high glucose content (such as many snacks) since it has been difficult to show in long-term studies that the addition of dietary fibre has resulted in a better HbA_{1c}.[800] These studies have mainly been done on individuals with type 2 diabetes. An Italian study of adults with type 1 diabetes compared a low-fibre diet with a high-fibre diet rich in fruit, legumes and vegetables.[396] Both diets contained exclusively natural foodstuffs. The high-fibre diet resulted in lower blood glucose levels, 0.5% lower HbA_{1c}, and decreased frequency of hypoglycaemia. In a European study on 2,065 adults with type 1 diabetes, the HbA_{1c} in people whose fibre intake was high was found to be approximately 3 mmol/mol (0.3%) lower than for the group with low fibre intake.[163]

Fruit and vegetables are good sources of fibre, but children in the UK eat on average fewer than half of the minimum of five portions recommended per day.[1080] A piece of fresh fruit and multi-grain bread can be a good basis if the rest of the meal is made up mainly of "quick-acting" carbohydrates. Parents can make use of the "fibre effect" by offering a slice of coarse wholemeal bread with some fat (for example margarine or cheese) to their child before other concentrated sugary foods or snacks. The combination of fibre and fat in the meal will help to slow down any rise in the blood glucose level.

Milk

Many children drink milk with their meals. Different types of milk have different fat contents. However, all types have the same amount of milk sugar (lactose, 5 g/100 ml) and usually the same amount of vitamins and minerals, including calcium. Small children (up to 2-3 years of age) need more fat in their diet and should drink whole milk. In practice, this means that the change from whole-fat milks to semi-skimmed or even skimmed milk should only be instituted after the age of 2 years.[1080] Which type of milk is most suitable also depends on how much the child drinks per day. Half a litre or 1 pint a day is recommended for its calcium content.

Milk contains 5 g and natural yoghurt around 4 g of carbohydrate/100 ml, while sweetened yoghurt contains the double amount or even more. The rise in blood glucose may perhaps not be greater with sweetened products if you practice carbohydrate counting. You may however gain in weight in the long run. However, it is very common to have a rise in blood glucose after breakfast, and it is difficult to increase the insulin dose without running low before lunch. It is therefore often a good idea to decrease the amounts of carbohydrate that you eat for breakfast.

The starch in vegetables is broken down more slowly than other types of starch. Vegetables also contain soluble fibre which is good for the digestion and prevents constipation.

Vegetables

You can eat freely from this food group (except sweet corn) as the carbohydrate content is very low (see table on page 238). Vegetables are also high in dietary fibre. Put the vegetables on the table before the children come to eat and they will probably help themselves to them while waiting for the food to be served.

Potatoes

Potatoes, sweet potatoes, taro and yam belong to this type of food stuff. The carbohydrate content of raw potatoes is absorbed slowly, but boiling causes the cell walls to burst. This allows the carbohydrates to be absorbed more quickly from the intestines. The carbohydrate content of mashed potatoes is absorbed as quickly as pure glucose [1114] (see graph on page 236). This can give a quick rise in blood glucose after the meal but may also result in hypoglycaemia 2-3 hours later, since all the carbohydrates in the mashed potatoes will have been absorbed during a fairly short time after the meal. If you change the surface of a potato (for example, by frying, deep frying, or storing it in the refrigerator after cooking) the glucose will be absorbed more slowly than if you eat it freshly boiled.[242] The manufacturing process and the high fat content of potato crisps cause the glucose contained in these to be absorbed very slowly (see graph on page 270).[177]

In one study of adults, chocolate cake was substituted for a baked potato without an increase in blood glucose levels.[837] If the chocolate cake was added to the baked potato, the glucose level increased. However, remember that chocolate cake and baked potato are very different in nutritional and energy value!

Bread

At one time, people with diabetes were strongly advised to eat unsweetened bread. Today, we know that white bread raises the blood glucose level every bit as rapidly as ordinary sugar. However, margarine and something with a high fat content (e.g. cheese) on the bread will slow

Vegetables

	Quantity	Carb.	% fibre
Bamboo shoots, canned	100 ml	4 g	50%
Broccoli, frozen	100 ml	5 g	60%
Carrots, raw	100 ml	5 g	27%
Corn, canned	100 ml	20 g	30%
Corn on cob, cooked, 1 medium size	19 g		10%
Cucumber	250 ml	3 g	< 1 g
Lettuce	250 ml	1 g	< 1 g
Onions, cooked	100 ml	11 g	18%
Peas, green, cooked	100 ml	13 g	31%
Peppers, green, raw	100 ml	3 g	33%
Radishes	100 ml	2 g	50%
Tomatoes, raw	100 ml	4 g	25%

Data from reference [525]

the rise in blood glucose by delaying emptying of the stomach. Bread (such as whole grain) that is high in fibre will also slow down any rise in blood glucose levels.

If you bake your own bread, it is perfectly acceptable to use an ordinary recipe. It should not be necessary to leave out sugar or experiment with alternative sweetening agents. Three to 6 tablespoons (45-90 ml) of sugar or syrup for a dough made from 0.5 litre (1 pint) of liquid can be used as only a small amount will remain in the bread after baking. If you buy bread, the carbohydrate content will be on the food label. When baking, a rough estimate is that 50% of the weight is from carbohydrates. It is more important to choose bread that is rich in fibre rather than omitting small amounts of sugar. Gluten-free bread gives a quicker rise in blood glucose compared with the same amount of bread containing gluten.[742]

Nutritious meals do not always need to be hot.[569] A sandwich or roll with tuna, egg, lean meat, chicken or cheese and salad, along with yogurt, fromage frais or fruit can be very enjoyable.

Unsweetened breakfast corn cereal (corn flakes) contains 90% starch, most of which rapidly becomes available as glucose. Sweetened (sugar-frosted) flaked corn cereal, on the other hand, contains around 50% starch and 50% sugar. Initially, both give the same blood glucose rise but sweetened corn flakes give slightly lower blood glucose levels after 3 hours.[1102] This may surprise you, but corn starch raises the blood glucose faster than ordinary sugar. The volume of sweetened corn cereal is around 25% less for the same carbohydrate content, so a small amount of pre-sweetened corn cereals can be used in a meal plan without increasing the blood glucose if the total amount of carbohydrate is taken into consideration when estimating the insulin dose. However, increasing the number of calories you consume will cause you to put on weight in time. It is healthier to eat muesli containing more of nuts, and you will be less likely to have a problem with raised blood glucose after breakfast.

Pasta

Pasta gives a slow rise in blood glucose since it is prepared from crushed or cracked wheat, not wheat flour, which causes the starch to be enclosed within a structure of protein (gluten).[523,743] This makes pasta a suitable food for people with diabetes. It has the additional advantage of being popular with children. If you are using rapid-acting insulin (Humalog), however, the rise may even be too slow, resulting in hypoglycaemia within 30-60 minutes.[545] If this applies to you, you should take your NovoRapid or Humalog after your meal, or use regular short-acting insulin when eating pasta (or beans as in chilli con carne). If you have a pump, you can use a prolonged bolus dose (see page 189).

Thinner pasta, such as macaroni, gives a quicker blood glucose response than spaghetti.[523] Cooking time does not affect the rate of blood glucose rise caused by spaghetti except in extreme cases of overcooking. Tinned spaghetti increases the blood glucose just as quickly as white bread.[523] As the gluten content of pasta contributes to the slow rise in blood glucose,[1119] gluten-free pasta allows blood glucose levels to rise faster.[814]

Meat and fish

Meat and fish have a high protein content. Sometimes the fat content is high as well. They do not contain any carbohydrates that will increase your blood glucose levels directly. Dietary protein does not slow the absorption of carbohydrate, and the adding of protein to a carbohydrate snack does not prevent late-onset or night time hypoglycaemia.[365]

Intake of protein does not increase blood glucose in people who do not have diabetes.[365] However, proteins stimulate the release of glucagon, and this in turn helps to convert protein into glucose (a process called gluconeogenesis, see page 34).[415] If there is not enough insulin, the blood glucose may be increased as a result. This increase comes rather late (after 3-5 hours)[838] so counteracting it with a premeal dose of rapid-acting insulin may not be the best approach. For a meal very rich in protein (like a big steak) it may be better to use regular short-acting insulin or, if you use an insulin pump, to use an extended dual type of bolus (see page 189). If you have diabetic kidney disease, you may need to reduce the amount of protein in your diet. Consult your doctor and dietitian about this.

If you are preparing food with a very low fat content (e.g. white fish such as cod or haddock, or very lean meat) it is a good idea to add a little extra fat. This can be in the form of oil or margarine when frying or baking, or with a sauce containing butter or cream. If your meal is entirely fat-free, your stomach will empty very quickly, leaving you at risk of hypoglycaemia after a couple of hours. As the energy content of boiled fish is fairly low, you may find having a larger helping is necessary to avoid getting hungry soon again. However, be careful about adding extra fat if you have weight problems, and check first with your dietitian.

Pizza

Pizza contains bread, cheese, meat or fish, and possibly vegetables. In other words, it is a balanced meal. One problem if you have diabetes is that a pizza meal will usually contain more bread than a traditional meal. The bread is baked hard which causes the carbohydrates to be absorbed more slowly. Cheese has a high fat content, which causes the stomach to empty more slowly. Try taking 1-2 extra units of insulin (or according to the actual carbohydrate content if you have calculated this) with the pizza or avoid eating the crust. If you use rapid-acting insulin (NovoRapid, Humalog, Apidra), it may be better to take this after the meal or substitute a dose of short-acting insulin (Actrapid, Humulin S, Insuman Rapid) instead. If you have a pump you can try a combined bolus with the extended part given over 3-4 hours (see page 192).

Salt

Salt intake is generally far too high. In Western countries, it is difficult to decrease this as salt is added to many processed foods (only 20% of total intake is added at the table and in cooking).[1080] Extra salt in the form of sodium chloride (table-salt) will increase the blood pressure and can be a risk factor especially as diabetes itself increases the risk of heart and vascular diseases (see page 356). Eating salty food can cause glucose to be absorbed more effectively from the intestine.[1035] Salt is also available as potassium chloride but this is more expensive than common table-salt and tastes rather different. Sea-salt and herb-salt usually contain the same amount of sodium as table-salt. In many countries iodine is added to table salt. If this is available, it is a good choice since iodine is important for the function of your thyroid gland (see page 351).

Herbs and spices

Herbs will not affect your blood glucose at all. However, it is important to be aware that some herbal "seasoning" preparations also contain a lot of salt. If the flavouring is strong enough to make you drink more, your stomach may empty more rapidly, resulting in a quicker rise in your blood glucose level.

Fruit and berries

Fruits and berries have a high carbohydrate content (see table on page 255). The higher the fibre content, the less the effect they will have on the blood glucose level.

Glycaemic index

The glycaemic index (GI) is an attempt to describe the blood glucose-raising effect of different foods. The glycaemic index of a mixed meal can be predicted from the GI of single foods.[193] It may be difficult to estimate the GI

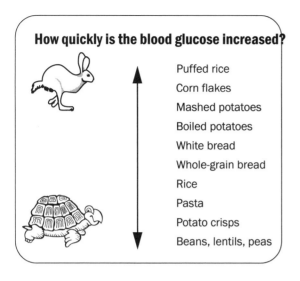

How quickly is the blood glucose increased?

Puffed rice
Corn flakes
Mashed potatoes
Boiled potatoes
White bread
Whole-grain bread
Rice
Pasta
Potato crisps
Beans, lentils, peas

for some combined meals from the GI of the single ingredients since the fat content also affects the speed with which carbohydrates are absorbed. A foodstuff with a low but easily accessible sugar content (for example carrots) has a high glycaemic index but you must eat a great deal if your blood glucose is going to be increased. Although the use of low-GI food may reduce blood glucose levels after meals, more research is required before GI can be used as a general tool in diabetes care. The Diabetes and Nutrition Study Group of the European Association for the Study of Diabetes recommends the substitution of high-GI by low-GI foods to improve glycaemic control.[312] A summary of many studies (called meta-analysis) found that a low-GI diet reduced HbA_{1c} by 5 mmol/mol (0.43%) compared with conventional or high-GI diets.[143] In Australia, the GI concept is much more accepted and widely used than, for example, in the US and UK.

Potatoes (GI 74) give a faster blood glucose response than pasta (GI 46-52). Adding a small amount of oil or polyunsaturated or monounsaturated margarine to mashed potatoes (GI 85) will slow down the glucose peak. If you replace one item in a meal with another (for example potatoes with pasta) the GI of the individual foods will help you determine the likely effect

on the blood glucose. For example, it may be a good idea to have something with a low-GI for supper as this could lower the risk of night time hypoglycaemia.

GI is very useful when you are looking at eating between meals (often single items of food such as yogurt, an apple, a bun, ice cream, crisps etc.). Professionals and parents alike have the difficult task of explaining to children how they should handle items such as these.

If you know that an ice cream made from dairy products has a GI of 37-61, you can recommend this as a good diabetes snack to be eaten in moderate amounts together with siblings or friends. When treating hypoglycaemia we want to use something with a high-GI to obtain a quick glycaemic response. Milk (GI 21) and chocolate bars (GI 43) are widely used for treating hypoglycaemia but the rise in blood glucose is actually very slow.[148,177] However, white bread (without margarine, GI 70) with some sugar soda (GI 68) will cause the blood glucose to rise much faster. Glucose tablets have a GI of 100 and are appropriate when symptoms are more pronounced or the blood glucose level is lower (< 3.5 mmol/l, 65 mg/dl).

It may be difficult to figure out the GI of a composite meal like lunch or dinner. GI may then be more useful when discussing eating between the main meals, as snacks often consist of only one item, like yogurt, an apple, ice cream or crisps.

Mealtimes

Each family has its own routines for mealtimes, and they are likely to be the ones that particularly suit them. A dietitian should use the family's own eating habits and routines as a starting point when drawing up dietary advice for a person with diabetes. If you are using rapid-acting insulin (NovoRapid or Humalog) it is less important to have strict mealtimes since the basal insulin covers the time between meals. An insulin pump will also give you freer mealtimes. However, if you use multiple injection treatment with regular short-acting insulin, you should usually not leave more than 5 hours between the meals accompanied by insulin.

Snacks

People who don't have diabetes have low insulin levels in between meals. If you are using rapid-acting insulin (NovoRapid or Humalog) with multiple injections or an insulin pump, you will be less dependent on snacks in between meals. This is because its action is closer to the way blood glucose rises after a meal. This results in a lower insulin level between meals. Most children can have a piece of fruit (10 g of carbohydrate) as a snack in the morning without extra insulin when they are active at school, but if it is larger they will need a small dose of insulin along with it.

Some younger children (up to 9-10 years of age) need a larger afternoon snack when they come home from school. When on multiple injections, many families find it easier to give insulin with this afternoon snack and have dinner/tea a little later. The evening snack is then omitted. Try giving the same amount of insulin with the afternoon snack eaten earlier, as you would have done with the evening snack (or according to the carbohydrate gram count).

When regular short-acting insulin is injected, its effect lasts for 4-5 hours, and that of intermediate-acting insulin even longer if taken in twice-daily injections. This results in having a higher insulin concentration between meals, than would be found in individuals without diabetes. This is why snacks are important with this type of insulin regimen. Since the morning injection is usually larger than the lunchtime one, it is even more essential to eat a snack in the morning. A child in school will usually require a sandwich (or something equally substantial) as the mid-morning snack. However, if the school lunch is served early, a piece of fruit might do. In the afternoon a piece of fruit will usually be an adequate snack.

> ### Glycaemic index
>
> The glycaemic index is an attempt to describe the blood glucose-raising effect of different foods. A certain amount of carbohydrate of the food is given (usually 50 g) and the area under the blood glucose curve is measured for 2 hours. Glucose is used to give a baseline glycaemic index of 100. The glycaemic index can be misleading if you want to know how the blood glucose level is affected during a shorter period of time (e.g. 30-60 minutes) or if the food has a low, but easily accessible, sugar content.
>
> The list on page 243 is based on reference [360].
> Use it like this:
> GI tells you how quick the carbohydrates are. For a low GI, you will probably do better with an extended or combined bolus if you are using an insulin pump. If you are on injections, you can try short-acting insulin which has a slightly longer duration than rapid-acting insulin (see page 165).
>
> "Carbs in 100 g" tells you what the carbohydrate content of the food is. Boiled potatoes contain 18 g per 100 g, i.e. 18% carbohydrates. If the potatoes you are going to eat weigh 145 g, 145x18/100=23 g are carbs. You will get the same result with the equation 145x0.18 = 23, i.e. 18% carbs means that you can multiply the weight by 0.16 to find the total amount of carbs. It is useful to have an accurate digital scale at home.

The school snack mid morning is often the most difficult of the day because it has to be taken from home or bought, be carried in the school bag and be acceptable to the school and peer group.[1080] This often allows for few alternatives

A piece of fruit is a good and healthy snack.

Glycaemic index and carb. content [360]

Type of food	GI	Carbs in 100 g	Type of food	GI	Carbs in 100 g
Beverages and juice			**Milk products**		
Apple juice	40	12 g	Ice cream	37-61	18-26 g
Gatorade	78	6 g	Milk, 3% fat	21	5 g
Grapefruit juice	48	9 g	Yogurt	36	5 g
Cola, sweet drink	58	10 g	**Pasta, rice and potatoes**		
Fanta	68	14 g	Bulgur	48	17 g
Lucozade	95	17 g	Couscous	65	10 g
Orange juice	50	10 g	French fries	75	19 g
Solo, lemon squash	58	12 g	Noodles, instant	47	22 g
Tomato juice	38	4 g	Pasta	46-52	26 g
Bread and flour products			Pasta, gluten-free	56 [814]	23 g
Apple muffin (with sugar)	44	42 g	Potato, baked	85	20 g
Apple muffin (without sugar)	48	28 g	Potato, boiled	74	16 g
Baguette	95	50 g	Potato, mashed	74	13 g
Pancakes, mix	67	73 g	Potatoes, instant mashed	85	13 g
Pancakes, gluten-free mix	102	29 g	Rice, Basmati	58	25 g
Pita bread	57	57 g	Rice, Jasmin	89	28 g
Rye bread (whole-grain)	46	37 g	Rice, long grain	56	28 g
Rye bread (wholemeal)	58	45 g	Rice, parboiled	46	24 g
Scones, mix	92	36 g	Rice, puffed	74	28 g
Waffles	76	37 g	Rice, white	64	24 g
White bread	70	45 g	Spaghetti	44	27 g
White bread (gluten-free)	76	50 g	Spaghetti, whole meal	43	24 g
Cereals and porridge			Sweet potato	61	19 g
All Bran	30	50 g	**Sweets, sugars and snacks**		
Corn flakes	81	83 g	Chocolate pudding	47	16 g
Muesli	40-66	53-80 g	Corn chips	63	52 g
Special K	69	23 g	Fructose (fruit sugar)	19	100 g
Oatmeal porridge (from flakes)	74	11 g	Glucose	100	100 g
Rice Krispies	82	87 g	Honey	55	71 g
Weetabix	75	71 g			
Fruit			Jelly sweets	78	77 g
Apple	38	13 g	Lactose (milk sugar)	46	100 g
Banana, all yellow	51	22 g	Milk chocolate	43	56 g
Banana, yellow and green	42	21 g	Peanuts	14	12 g
Banana with peel		13 g	Popcorn	72	56 g
Cherries	22	10 g	Potato crisps	54	42 g
Grapefruit	25	9 g	Sucrose (sugar)	68	100 g
Grapes	46	15 g	**Vegetables and legumes**		
Kiwi	53	10 g	Carrots, raw	16	10 g
Orange without peel	42	9 g	Chick peas	28	20 g
Pear	33	11 g	Corn, sweet	54	23 g
Peach, canned in juice	38	9 g	Green peas	48	9 g
Pineapple	59	11 g	Kidney beans	28	17 g
Strawberries	40	8 g	Lentils, green	30	11 g
Water melon	72	5 g	Soya beans (dried)	18	4 g

Contents may vary in different countries and with time, even with the same brand. Check the food label. The weight is for prepared food, unless otherwise stated. See also reference [742] for an extensive list of more foods.

Common meal planning

Time	Meal	Example of doses for a child weighing 33 kg (73 lb)
7.30 AM	Breakfast	9 U Premeal dose
12 Noon	Lunch	6 U "
5.30 PM	Dinner/tea	6 U "
8.30 PM	Evening snack	4 U "

Alternative meal planning

Time	Meal	Example of doses for a child weighing 33 kg (73 lb)
7.30 AM	Breakfast	9 U Premeal dose
11.30 AM	Lunch	6 U "
3.00 PM	Afternoon snack	4 U "
7.00 PM	Dinner/tea	6 U "

With a multiple injection therapy or an insulin pump, you can be more flexible. For example, you can eat dinner later (or earlier) at weekends. It is easy to adjust the dose when switching meals during the day if you use carbohydrate counting.

when children do not want to eat either fruit or other healthy items in front of their friends. The fat content of snacks such as fruit or a bag of crisps can range from nothing to 12 g of fat per portion with similar carbohydrate values. The lower- or average-fat products, such as corn chips, potato sticks etc. should be encouraged, if this type meal is eaten.[1080] Fortunately, the recent trends towards awareness of diet within schools, and the "Healthy Schools" initiatives (which engage pupils too), are likely to make this less of a problem. The National School Fruit Scheme in the UK is an example of implementing healthier eating habits for all children.

If your blood glucose level is high, you won't need a snack. Try having half the snack if your blood glucose level is close to 10 mmol/l (180 mg/dl) and skip it completely if it is above 13-15 mmol/l (230-270 mg/dl). If this happens more than occasionally, you will need to adjust your insulin doses.

Can mealtimes be changed?

If you eat your meal up to 1 hour earlier or later than usual, you are unlikely to have problems as long as you don't change the time gap between taking your insulin and eating. If you use rapid-acting insulin (NovoRapid or Humalog) and twice-daily basal insulin (or once-daily Lantus), you will probably not have to be so strict about the hours between meals. If you check your blood glucose, you could try shifting mealtimes by up to 2 hours. Just remember not to exceed 5 hours between the doses if you are using ordinary short-acting insulin. A child will usually be hungry and need something to eat every 3-4 hours anyway.

Hungry or full?

A person whose diabetes is well controlled can often rely on feeling hungry or satisfied at the appropriate time. In one adult study, where fullness after a meal was measured, individuals with higher blood glucose levels experienced more fullness.[571] It is particularly important, if you are caring for a child with diabetes, to trust the child to respond sensibly to the promptings of appetite. Continuing to tell children that they must eat more or less regardless of how hungry they feel, will cause them to cease recognizing these feelings after a while. Children often experience lowered appetite if their blood glucose level is high. It is important, therefore, to give children time to reflect and build up their own opinion about what size meals should be. On the other hand, it is important for parents to be vigilant about how much children drink with any meal, especially if the drink contains carbohydrate (e.g. milk) or sugar.

Dry weight or cooked food? Peeled or unpeeled fruit?

If not listed otherwise, the amount of carbohydrates in food is mentioned as per eatable substance, i.e. cooked food and peeled fruit. Many packages list the carbohydrate content of the uncooked substance, for example rice and pasta. It can make quite a difference if you use the wrong number when calculating, for example weigh cooked pasta but use the percentage carbohydrates in dry pasta.

	Carbs/100 g	
	Dry weight	Cooked food
Pasta	70 g	25 g
Rice	75 g	25 g
Rolled oats	55 g	porridge 23 g
Potato	raw 16 g	cooked 18 g
	Unpeeled*	Peeled
Orange (28% peel)	7 g	10 g
Banana (33% peel)	15 g	22 g
Grapefruit (35% peel)	5 g	7 g
Cherries (9% stone)	13 g	15 g
Peach (13% stone)	8 g	9 g
Pear (12% pip)	10 g	11 g
Apple (13% pip)	10 g	12 g

*data from www.fineli.fi

➠ Example with rice:
240 g boiled rice = 240 x 0.25 = 60 g carbohydrate. But if you count with dry weight you get 240 x 0.75 = 180 g carbs, i.e. the dose of insulin will be 3 times higher!

➠ Example with banana:
100 g banana = 100 x 0.22 = 22 g carbs. But if you weigh an unpeeled banana, it contains only 0.15 x 100 = 15 g carbs, i.e. the dose of insulin will be 1½ times too high if you use the weight of the unpeeled banana!

The insulin dose will always give a better effect if it is taken before the meal. For this to work well, the child (and many adults) need to practise estimating how much they are going to eat to feel omega full. The person who has prob-

Counting the carbohydrates in your food will help you determine the size of your premeal bolus doses. Main sources of carbohydrates in your food are bread, pasta, rice, potatoes, chapattis, tacos and tortillas. Meat and fat contain no carbohydrates at all.

lems with overweight need to practice understanding the difference between being full and not hungry. A good trick is to wait 10 minutes before taking a second helping; you will feel more full in the meanwhile.

Beware! If you are lacking insulin and your diabetes is badly regulated, you may feel hungry even when your blood glucose level is high (see page 47).

Infant feeding

The glucose content of infant formula is absorbed fairly quickly. With a multiple injection regimen, the child will need short- or rapid-acting insulin for every bottle of formula milk (5-6 insulin doses per day). You may need to adjust in half units or even lower increments to find the right dose. If the child drinks formula milk at night, a small dose of short- or rapid-acting insulin can be given with this. If the child has problems with night time hypoglycaemia, a corn flour mix or commercial products made with uncooked corn starch may help (see page 58).

Toddlers' food (adapted from [569])

Food fads, picky eating and food refusal are common in this age group. In fact, such behaviour can be considered almost "normal" for toddlers, even though it is frequently worrying and frustrating for parents. Not surprisingly, such problems will cause even more anxiety to the parents of a child with diabetes. The following tips may be useful:

♠ Most children grow and thrive without being "told" how much to eat. Don't worry. Even if you feel your child is not eating enough, it is likely he or she is. Talk to your dietitian and diabetes team if you feel concerned and check your child's growth chart with your paediatrician.

♠ Rigid meals and snacks don't work well. Try to think what sort of food you would have provided, and when, if your child did not have diabetes and try to adjust the insulin accordingly.

♠ Plan mealtimes and menus taking into account the child's other activities, e.g. has the child been running around or sitting still?

♠ Children never respond to being force-fed. Even though it can be difficult, try to play down the emphasis on food. Usually a falling blood sugar will make the child hungry and more inclined to eat.

♠ Avoid using sweet foods or sugary drinks to "make up" for a low carbohydrate intake. Children soon learn to refuse food if the "reward" is a sweet drink or chocolate biscuit.

♠ Fresh fruit, eaten as a snack, is better than fruit juice to drink.

♠ Give the child extra insulin when necessary, for example at birthday parties or when they are given sweets.

♠ Breakfast time can be difficult, as it is quite common for children not to feel hungry early in the morning. Try a glass (or half a glass) of juice or milk to start with. After half an hour or so, when the blood glucose has risen a little, the appetite often improves.

♠ Glucose gel (for example Hypostop®) and juice can be very useful in this age group as children need not chew the glucose tablets when they are hypoglycaemic.

♠ Toddlers are growing and may often change their food habits. Talk to your dietitian for further advice.

Foods that contain carbohydrate

⇒ Bread, cereals, grains.

⇒ Pasta, rice, potatoes.

⇒ Starchy vegetables, such as corn and peas.

⇒ Fruit and fruit juices.

⇒ Dairy products, such as milk and yoghurt (cheese usually contains no carbohydrate).

⇒ Chocolate, biscuits, sugar and sweets.

If the child is breast-fed and takes full meals, you can give insulin in the same way as described above for formula. However, if the child feeds more frequently, taking a little at a time, an insulin pump which is the best type of treatment in this age group will probably work better. Lantus or Levemir may also be good alternatives, but discuss this with your doctor (neither insulin is officially approved for use by children aged under 2 years).

Carbohydrate counting

Insulin is needed mainly to balance the carbohydrates eaten. The amount of insulin needed for a meal is in direct proportion to the carbohydrate content of the meal.[435] The practice of carbohydrate counting differs between centres and countries. In many countries, carbohydrate counting is part of routine diabetes care (see page 246) and detailed tables are available for this.[525] Another method is to "measure by eye" for the size of the helpings (mainly the carbohydrate content, for example potatoes) and adjust the insulin dose accordingly.

Check with your dietitian what the local traditions are. Young children can be unpredictable eaters, so carbohydrate counting can be valuable for calculating the appropriate insulin dose for this age group.

The total carbohydrate content of meals and snacks is more important for the premeal insulin dosage than the type or where they come from.[365] However, some carbohydrates that are listed on food labels do not have any effect on the blood glucose level (dietary fibre, resistant starch).[1115] If a food contains 5 g dietary fibre or more, the grams of fibre should be subtracted from the total grams of carbohydrate for that food.[402,1092] When counting carbohydrates, only half the amount of sugar alcohols (polyols) should be included.[1092] The glycaemic index and fibre content of foods do not affect the premeal insulin requirements,[365] but they can influence how the insulin should be taken, for example using a prolonged or combined bolus dose with a pump. In the DCCT study (see page 367), individuals who adjusted their premeal insulin dosages based on the carbohydrate content had 6 mmol/mol (0.5%) lower HbA_{1c} than those who did not adjust their premeal insulin.[284]

Different methods of carbohydrate assessment

Many methods of counting or estimating carbohydrate intake are used in clinical practice. There is no consensus in favour of one particular method and some methods are better suited to particular individuals, children and families. What is becoming clearer is that if we are aiming at really tight glucose control to improve diabetes outcomes, there seems to be a need for some form of carbohydrate estimation to counterbalance insulin doses.[1080] Three levels of carbohydrate counting have been identified by the American Dietetic Association and can be considered as a step by step approach:[402,1080]

Basic level

For counting carbohydrates, there are printed food tables in which you can find the carbohydrate content of different foods. Or you can use exchange lists where servings of (for example) starch, fruit and milk contain between 8 and 15 g of carbohydrate each. Your dietitian can help you compile lists giving the carbohydrate contents of different products in special categories such as treats, ice cream or Christmas fare.

In the simplest form of carbohydrate counting, your dietitian teaches you how to calculate the amount of carbohydrate you need for different meals and snacks during the day. You also learn to read food labels, and how to use food lists to count carbohydrates. With fixed insulin doses, it is important to eat about the same amount of carbohydrate for meals and snacks at the same time every day to keep your blood glucose levels within the target range.

Intermediate level

At this level you learn to recognize patterns of blood glucose response to carbohydrate intake and how it is modified by insulin and exercise. You make your own adjustments to insulin doses, or alter carbohydrate intake or timing of exercise to achieve blood glucose goals. Alterations of insulin should be made in response to a pattern of blood glucose results over a few days, not based on a single high or low blood glucose reading. A more flexible method is to correct the premeal dose for changes in size of the carbohydrate content of a meal (without counting the exact carbohydrate content). See page 151 for advice on how much to adjust the insulin dose. Simple insulin adjustments are used to manage the intake of extra carbohydrate (see page 264).

In an Australian study, children tested both a flexible meal plan (servings based on appetite) and a fixed carbohydrate exchange model (servings based on carbohydrate content).[399] The exchange model included recommending artificially sweetened alternatives whenever available. In the flexible model, by contrast, sugar-sweetened products were preferred except for diet drinks. The children on the flexible meal plan appreciated their food much more than those on the exchange model. They also had, on average, a 3 mmol/mol (0.3%) lower

How to find your insulin:carb ratio ("backwards counting")

① Calculate the carb. content of your usual breakfast:

2 slices of bread	30 g
1 glass of milk (~200ml)	10 g
Total	40 g

② What is your usual dose for this breakfast? (when your blood glucose is 5-6 mmol/l) For example: 8U

③ Find the breakfast ratio: 40/8=5
1 unit of insulin covers 5 g of carbohydrate

④ Calculate the carbohydrate content of a weekend breakfast:

1 cup of milk (~250 ml)	12 g
30 g of cereals (Special K)	21 g
1 glass of juice	20 g
Total	53 g

⑤ Apply your insulin:carb ratio: 53/5=11U. Use the bolus calculator in you pump for calculations. For injection therapy, you can use a hand-held calculator or an app for a smartphone.

⑥ If the ratio is correct, your blood glucose after 2 hours should ideally have risen no more than 2-3 mmol/l (35-55mg/dl). It should be back to within 1-2 mmol/l of your premeal glucose level after another 2-3 hours if your basal rate is set correctly.

⑦ Calculate the carbohydrate content for supper or evening meal (for simplicity suppose 40 g of carbohydrates again).

⑧ What would be your usual dose for this meal? (when your blood glucose is 5-6 mmol/l) For example: 5U

⑨ Find the insulin:carb ratio: 40/5=8
1 unit of insulin covers 8 g of carbohydrate

⑩ You can then use this ratio for all other meals during the day (except breakfast), and adjust as needed. It is quite common to need a higher insulin dose in the morning for a given amount of carbohydrates compared to the rest of the day. This is due to insulin resistance (decreased insulin sensitivity) in the morning (see page 223).

➠ If your blood glucose rises more than 2-3 mmol/l (35-55mg/dl) after the meal, you can use the correction factor (insulin sensitivity factor). An example with a correction factor of 6 mmol/l per unit of insulin. Your blood glucose rises from 4.5 to 10.5 after the meal. The rise amounts to 10.5-4.5=6 mmol/l. One more unit would then have made up a suitable insulin dose. Use 6U instead of 5U in the calculations above.

HbA$_{1c}$. In addition, children from this group experienced less family conflict. With multiple injection therapy or an insulin pump, you can enjoy flexible food habits together with the opportunity of adjusting your insulin doses in line with the carbohydrate contents of your meals.

Advanced level

Individuals taking rapid- or short-acting insulin before meals (via either injections or a pump) can vary the amount of insulin depending on the carbohydrate content of the meal. Use food labels and/or a food table to calculate how many grams of carbohydrate there are in the meal. In the advanced form of carbohydrate counting, you need to determine the amount of insulin to take for the amount of carbohydrate you wish to eat. This is called the insulin-to-carbohydrate (insulin:carb) ratio (or carbohydrate factor) and gives you the number of grams of carbohydrate covered by 1 unit of insulin. This method gives a more flexible meal schedule and, once you have learned it, you can apply it both at home and when eating out. Basically, you count the grams of carbohydrates in a meal and divide by the number of units of insulin required to keep the blood glucose at a similar level 2-3 hours later.

How many carbohydrates will 1 unit of insulin cover?[255]

Example:	Carbs (g)	Units	Insulin:carb ratio
Breakfast	60	6	1:10
Lunch	50	4	1:12
Dinner/tea	55	5	1:11
Evening snack	35	3	1:12
Whole day	200	18	1:11

The above example considers a 12-year-old boy (weighing 38 kg, 6 stone). One unit of insulin will take care of 10 g of carbohydrate for breakfast without changing the blood glucose level, and around 12 g of carbohydrate for the other meals.

Increase the ratio if blood glucose 2 hours after the meal decreases by more than 2-3 mmol/l (35-55mg/dl) (a higher ratio gives less insulin), and decrease the ratio if blood glucose rises 2-3 mmol/l (35-55mg/dl) or more. A change of the ratio by 1 g is usually sufficient if the ratio is below 10, 2 g if it is between 10 and 20 and 3-5 g if it is above 20 g.

It is very important to always follow the advice on dosing that you get when carbohydrate counting, whether you get the results from a pocket calculator, or a bolus guide in your smart phone or pump. You will then see if you blood glucose goes too high or too low after meals, and can adjust the insulin:carb ratio accordingly. Use a combined bolus dose for meals with a low GI (see page 243).

Taken a too high insulin dose? Use carbohydrate counting!

An 8-year-old boy weighing 25 kg, whose total daily dose is 19 U, accidentally took 8.5 U instead of 3.5 U for dinner with pasta. His mother counted the carbs based on the dry weight on the food label instead of cooked pasta. How can you manage this?

⮕ 8.5-3.5=5 U too much insulin

⮕ His carbohydrate ratio was 22 g (one unit of insulin will cover 22 g of carbohydrates)

⮕ 22 g/U = 22 x 5 = 110 g carbohydrates

⮕ Pasta contains slow carbohydrates

⮕ Therefore begin with fast carbs. He drank 2 glasses of apple juice (18 g carbs/glass)

⮕ And then??

⮕ Time for sweets!! He managed to eat 80 g containing approximately 70 g of carbs

⮕ Blood glucose readings: 5.3 mmol/l (95 mg/dl) before the meal, then 6.4, 6.1, 5.9 and 4.2 mmol/l (118, 110, 106 and 76 mg/dl)

What if you do not have a carbohydrate ratio? Well, then you can use the 500-rule:

⮕ Divide 500 by your total daily insulin dose (including basal insulin and mealtime insulin).

⮕ 500/19 = 26, i.e. one unit of insulin takes care of 26 g of carbohydrates.

⮕ Calculate according to above, but with 26 g as the carbohydrate ratio. It will not be as exact, but is still accurate enough to find the approximate amount of extra carbohydrates that the child needs to eat.

Test your insulin:carb ratio only when you have not had hypoglycaemia in the last 4 hours before the meal. Another method of calculating the insulin:carb ratio is to divide the total number of grams of carbohydrate consumed for all meals in a day by the total bolus (mealtime) insulin taken during the day (see key fact box on "How many carbohydrates will 1 unit of insulin cover?[255]" on page 249).[255] Do not include intermediate- or long-acting insulin (or pump basal rate) doses in this calculation.

A third method of calculating the insulin:carb ratio is the "500 Rule".[1086,1092] Divide the number 500 by your total daily dose of insulin (adding all types of insulin, both premeal doses and basal insulin). The answer is the number of grams of carbohydrate covered by 1 unit of rapid-acting insulin (NovoRapid, Humalog,

Should protein and fat be accounted for in the calculation of a meal bolus dose?

There is some discussion about whether fat and protein should be included in the calculations of a meal bolus. In Poland it is common to apply an equation with FPU (fat protein units):

➠ 100 kcal of fat or protein (one FPU) require the same amount of insulin as 10 g of carbohydrates. T

➠ The FPU part of the dose should be given as the extended part of as a combined bolus dose (see page 192) with a pump (3 hours for 1 FPU, 4 h. for 2 FPU, 5 h. for 3 FPU, and 6 h. for 4 or more FPU).

➠ In reality, this will give a higher basal rate for some hours after the meal.

A German study found reduced glucose levels after meals when including FPU, using an extended pre-meal dose for a pizza. This increased the total meal dose, and there was a higher rate of postprandial hypoglycaemic episodes (<3.9 mmol/l [70 mg/dL], 35.7% vs. 9.5% in the control group).[633] The basal rate was not changed in this study, and it is possible that a lowered basal rate would have decreased hypoglycaemia problems after the meals.

We do not generally include fat and protein in the calculations in Sweden, but if you eat a meal mostly consisting of protein and/or fat you may want to try the FPU method to find a feasible insulin meal dose.

Apidra). The number 450 can be used for short-acting insulin (Actrapid, Humulin S, Insuman Rapid).[1092] A more exact method of finding your carbohydrate ratio is described on page 248, so called "backwards counting".

Check the appropriate ratio by calculating the insulin dose from the carbohydrate content of the meal. When you take this dose, your blood glucose should ideally have risen no more than be within approximately 2-3 mmol/l (35-55mg/dl) from the initial blood glucose after 2-3

hours if you use rapid-acting insulin, or after 4-5 hours if you use regular short-acting insulin, if the ratios are correct. Checking your blood glucose after the meal is the only way to find out how well your bolus dose has worked.

One unit of insulin will usually cover 10-15 g of carbohydrate in a meal for an adult. For a school child who is more insulin-sensitive, 1 unit may cover up to 20 g of carbohydrate, perhaps even 30-40 g if they are in the remission (honeymoon) phase. A teenager or an overweight person who is extremely insulin-resistant may require one unit of insulin for every 5 g of carbohydrate.[255]

You may find that 1 unit of insulin covers a slightly lower amount of carbohydrate in the morning and you can try a 330 Rule for breakfast (1200 Rule for mg/dl), giving 50% more insulin compared to the 500-rule. This may be explained by temporary insulin resistance due to the dawn phenomenon (see page 58) and less physical activity at this time of the day.[255] In a Canadian study of adults, an average of 1.5 units was needed for every 10 g of carbohydrate for breakfast, 1.0 units for lunch and 1.1-1.2 units for dinner (carb ratio around 7 for breakfast, 10 for lunch and 8-9 for dinner).[866] In this study, the glycaemic index, fibre, fat and caloric content of the meals did not affect the premeal insulin requirements.

People who are physically active need to lower their insulin doses, changing the insulin:carb ratio. So, if you take part in seasonal sports you will probably need to adjust your insulin:carb ratio. If, for example, it is 1:15 (i.e. 1 unit per 15 g of carbohydrate) in the active season, you may need to change to 1:10 when the season is over.

All modern pumps can use the insulin:carb ratio to calculate which bolus dose is needed for a particular amount of carbohydrate in a meal. The pumps use the correction factor (see page 146) to calculate how much the bolus dose should be increased, depending on your premeal blood glucose level. In a Swedish study, the number of blood glucose results after meals within target (4-8 mmol/l, 70-145 mg/dl) was 53% in the group that used the "bolus wizard" in the pump, compared to 30% for those who used their pump without carbohydrate counting.[332] There are now apps available for smartphones that can help you in counting the carb content of different foods (for example the Carbs & Cals app).

When focusing on the carbohydrate content of a meal, food and insulin can be matched more precisely as you will eat different amounts of carbohydrates depending on your appetite or regime. However, if you concentrate only on the carbohydrate content, you may forget that some foods contain a lot of fat as well, and this is not healthy in the long run.

In the DAFNE (Dose Adjustment For Normal Eating) Study of adults in the UK, participants took part in a 5-day course that provided the skills to enable individuals to replace insulin by matching it to desired carbohydrate intake on a meal by meal basis.[222] One year later, the number of daily injections had increased from 3.6 to 5.3, HbA1c was improved by 6 mmol/mol (0.5%) without increasing severe hypoglycaemia, and psychological well-being had improved significantly.

General advice on balancing carbohydrate intake against the insulin action profile [1080]
⮕ Extra carbohydrate is required before, during and after increased exercise and sport to balance increased energy needs and prevent hypoglycaemia.
⮕ **2-dose conventional regimen:** Regular and frequent carbohydrate intake including snacks is advisable to prevent hypoglycaemia during inevitable periods of high insulin levels when the insulin regimen is twice-daily mixtures of quick and slower acting insulins.
⮕ Carbohydrate intake is required before bedtime to prevent night time hypoglycaemia with a two-dose treatment.
⮕ **Intensive insulin regimen:** A flexible carbohydrate intake is possible when mealtime doses of insulin are given with multiple injection regimens or during insulin pump treatment.
⮕ A "grazing" or "little and often" style of eating, often seen in younger children, will probably be easier to manage with a long-acting basal insulin analogue and small doses of regular insulin at mealtimes or an insulin pump.

How many (or how few) carbs should we eat?

Your body and especially your brain needs carbohydrates to function well. An adult brain needs approximately 120 g of glucose per day, which is about 60% of the total glucose requirements. If you eat less than 120 g, the remaining glucose needs to be produced in your body. This is done in the liver, which can produce glucose from fat and muscles.

ISPAD recommends that 50-55% of the energy should come from carbohydrates. The Nordic Food Recommendations from 2012 have become more flexible about the amount of car-

bohydrates and now recommends 45-60 energy per cent to be derived from carbs. It may be difficult to get a good enough insulin effect if you eat more than 60 g of carbs for a meal.[133,721] If you increase the dose to get a good effect on the blood glucose peak after the meal, you risk going low before the next meal. With a pump you can give a combination bolus, i.e. a larger part immediately before the meal, and a smaller part extended over 3-4 hours. Another alternative is the superbolus (see page 192).

You should always discuss the amount of carbohydrates you eat with your doctor or dietitian. It is not dangerous to make a moderate reduction of around 40 % if you like this type

Energy and carb requirements

The Nordic Food Recommendations from 2012 have become more flexible in that the limits of the energy distribution have been widened. The role of monosaturated fat has increased slightly, for example in the form of olive and rape oil and nuts. Due to this, the recommendation for the total fat intake has been adjusted to 25-40% (formerly 25-35 %), while the recommendation for carbohydrate intake has changed to 45-60% of the total energy intake (formerly 50-60 %).

	Boys/men			Girls/women		
E% = % energy	kcal/24 h.	Carbohydrates/day (g)		kcal/24 h.	Carbohydrates/day (g)	
		55 E%	40 E%		55 E%	40 E%
Child 6-11 months	765	98		765	98	
Child 13 - 23 months	980	128		980	128	
2 years	990	136	99	1080	149	108
3 years	1190	164	119	1260	173	126
4 years	1330	183	133	1420	195	142
5 years	1400	193	140	1500	206	150
6 years	1470	202	147	1560	215	156
7 years	1550	213	155	1680	231	168
8 years	1630	224	163	1740	239	174
9 years	1710	235	171	1840	253	184
10 years	1990	274	199	2150	296	215
11 years	2010	276	201	2140	294	214
12 years	2100	289	210	2260	311	226
13 years	2200	303	220	2340	322	234
14 years	2280	314	228	2580	355	258
15 years	2350	323	235	2770	381	277
16 years	2380	327	238	2930	403	293
17 years	2400	330	240	3040	418	304
18 - 30 y.inactive*	2940	398	294	2247	304	225
18 - 30 y.active**	3298	446	330	2557	346	256

Discuss with your dietitian or doctor if you want to reduce your intake of carbohydrates. However, a person with diabetes is not recommended to go below 40 % of their energy intake from carbohydrates.

Breakfast usually comes with a high carbohydrate load, and it is difficult to give enough insulin without risking a low before lunch. This is caused by a so called insulin resistance that is present at the time of your first meal during the day (see page 223). In clinical practice, it is often difficult to give a correct dose if the meal contains more than 60 g of carbs.[721] If you find that your blood glucose goes high 2 hours after breakfast, it is a good idea to exchange a sandwich or toast for an egg.

*Inactive implies sedentary work and limited physical activity during your leisure time.

**Active implies participating in sport or other physical activity 4-5 times per week for at least 30 minutes.

of diet. However, it may be dangerous to practise a LCHF (low carb high fat) diet with less than 50 g/day. If you decrease the carbs to 40 % of your energy intake, you should not have more than 20 % from protein. This implies that approximately 40 % of the energy

Carbohydrate counting at McDonalds?

Fast food is not good if you eat it often, but once in a while it can be a treat. The amount of carbohydrates is usually well presented. Note that the gluten-free bread usually contains considerably more carbs. It may be difficult to get a good insulin effect for meals that contain more than 60 g. With a pen, you can try regular insulin when the amount of carbs exceeds 60 g. See below for suggestions on how to dose with an insulin pump:

	carbs	Total	Type of dose
Hamburger	29 g		
French fries			
small	29 g	58 g	normal
medium	41 g	70 g	70/30%* over 2 h.
large	54 g	83 g	70/30%* over 4 h.
Hamburger with gluten-free bread	51 g		
French fries			
small	29 g	80 g	normal
medium	41 g	92 g	70/30%* over 2h.
large	54 g	105 g	70/30%* over 4 h.

*You can also try 50/50%

Nutrition behaviours associated with lower HbA$_{1c}$

⟹ Adherence to the prescribed meal plan.

⟹ Adjusting food and/or insulin in response to high blood glucose levels.

⟹ Adjusting the insulin dose for carbohydrate content.

⟹ Consistent consumption of agreed snacks within the meal plan.

⟹ Appropriate treatment of hypoglycaemia (not over-treating).

The average HbA$_{1c}$ among intensively managed patients in the DCCT study who reported that they followed specific diet-related behaviours was 3-11 mmol/mol (0.25-1.0%) lower than among subjects who did not follow these behaviours, who had a higher HbA$_{1c}$.[284]

⟹ Over-treating hypoglycaemia.

⟹ Consuming extra snacks outside the meal plan.

is derived from fat. It is then very important that you eat fat of good quality, i.e. mostly vegetable fat (for example different oils, nuts and seeds) and fat from fish (mackerel. salmon, herring). See also page 234.

At times, we get questions about the LCHF diet, which implies eating fewer carbohydrates and more of fat and protein. Usually the person wants to lose weight, but also people with diabetes ask whether they can reduce insulin doses if cutting down on carbs. My standard reply is that some adults find that they do better if cutting down on the amount of carbs, but not to such extreme levels. At the same time it is important to stress that if you don't eat enough carbs, your body has to produce carbohydrates (glucose) from fat and protein. This means

therefore that you need to take insulin even for a meal without any carbohydrates at all (see fact frame on page 250).

A young woman of 18 years with type 1 diabetes tried LCHF-diet on her own without consulting her doctor or dietitian. She ate only 20-30 g of carbohydrates/day, i.e. what would be called a ketogenic diet. Her ketone levels went up to 4.2 mmol/l with blood glucose levels below 10 mmol/l (180 mg/dl), but she said she was feeling well. The ketones disappeared quickly when she had some yoghurt, and she very quickly resumed eating a larger amount of carbohydrates. Another young woman ate a "normal LCHF-diet" with 20-30 g of carbohydrates/day and had an HbA$_{1c}$ of 51-55 mmol/mol (7.2%). She contacted her diabetes team a couple of times with ketones up to 3.3 mmol/l that were remedied by extra insulin after intake of carbohydrates. She was then admitted to hospital with ketoacidosis. This was caused by the very thin margin between her everyday increased ketone levels and ketoacidosis, so the balance could easily tip over in the wrong direction. After she increased the amount of carbohydrates to 50 g/day, she had no further problems of increased ketone levels. A 13-year-old boy who tried LCHF for half a year lowered his insulin doses considerably, and his HbA$_{1c}$ decreased. However, his height did not increase at all during this time due to lack of insulin which is the most important hormone for building your body (an anabolic hormone).

A teenager who has reached his or her full adult height who may want to try can cut down A LITTLE on the amounts of carbohydrates, but my recommendation would be to keep the ketones below 1.0 mmol/l, and I emphasize that there is no research showing that LCHF works better than a normal diet for adolescents with diabetes.

Breakfast is often a difficult meal for most people with diabetes as it usually contains a large amount of carbohydrates. Children often go low before lunch if they increase the amount of insulin for breakfast to prevent an increase in blood glucose. In such cases it often works better when replacing one piece of bread for an egg or some cottage or curd cheese. See also the section on superbolus on page 192 if you use a pump.

School

These days, it is unlikely that there will be any problem over a child with diabetes receiving appropriate types of food and snacks at school.

It may be difficult to get school staff to understand that a child with diabetes will not always eat the same amounts of food. When using multiple injection therapy or an insulin pump, the insulin dose can be adjusted according to the appetite and size of portion. Sometimes children may need additional snacks to avoid hypoglycaemia if there is a long interval between

School menu

It may be a good idea to note the relevant insulin doses on the school menu.
Children usually know what they like, and are put out if it doesn't taste as it should.

Units	Food
5U	Spaghetti and meat sauce
4U	Fish with rice
6U	Mashed potatoes and sausage
4U	Lasagne

If you use carbohydrate counting, you will find it helpful to write down the carbohydrate content of the different meals.

breaks. The dietitian can speak to the staff if necessary.

With a fixed meal plan, school lunches are best eaten at the same time every day, not too early since the time until the next insulin dose may be a long way off for a young person on multiple injection treatment. See the suggestions for meal schedules on page 244. Schools should be given the necessary information about appropriate mealtimes in order to be able to make the appropriate timetabling adjustments.

School and day care staff often find it easier when using carbohydrate counting, as they then have some rules to follow that can easily be adjusted to irregular eating habits.

When school friends buy sweets, children with diabetes may find it difficult to resist joining in. There is always a risk that, instead of being sensible, they will "show off" by eating even more sweets than the others. A compromise could be to buy a small amount of sweets to have after lunch, when the stomach already contains some food. At that time and under those conditions, the blood glucose level will not be affected to

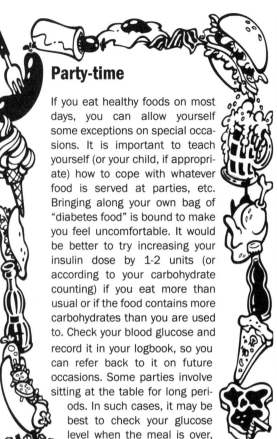

Party-time

If you eat healthy foods on most days, you can allow yourself some exceptions on special occasions. It is important to teach yourself (or your child, if appropriate) how to cope with whatever food is served at parties, etc. Bringing along your own bag of "diabetes food" is bound to make you feel uncomfortable. It would be better to try increasing your insulin dose by 1-2 units (or according to your carbohydrate counting) if you eat more than usual or if the food contains more carbohydrates than you are used to. Check your blood glucose and record it in your logbook, so you can refer back to it on future occasions. Some parties involve sitting at the table for long periods. In such cases, it may be best to check your glucose level when the meal is over, and take an extra dose of insulin if necessary.

Fruits

	Quantity	Carb.	Fibre	% fibre
Grapes	100 g	17 g	1.6 g	9%
Blackcurrants	100 g	16 g	4.9 g	32%
Blackberries	100 g	16 g	7.2 g	46%
Pineapple, canned	100 g	16 g	1.0 g	6%
Redcurrants	100 g	13 g	3.4 g	27%
Pineapple, fresh	100 g	12 g	1.2 g	9%
Cherries, sweet	100 g	12 g	1.7 g	13%
Strawberries	100 g	10 g	2.4 g	24%
Watermelon	100 g	9 g	0.6 g	7%
Raspberries	100 g	8 g	3.7 g	46%
Honeydew melon	100 g	8 g	0.9 g	11%
Banana	1 fruit	21 g	1.5 g	7%
Pear	1 fruit	16 g	3.0 g	19%
Apple	1 fruit	14 g	1.9 g	13%
Kiwi fruits	2 fruits	14 g	3.8 g	27%
Orange	1 fruit	13 g	2.0 g	16%
Plums	2 fruits	9 g	1.2 g	13%
Grapefruit	1 fruit	9 g	2.0 g	22%
Raisins	1 tbs	8 g	1.0 g	12%

A higher percentage of fibre will cause the glucose to be absorbed more slowly. Bananas contain very little dietary fibre and will raise the blood glucose level more quickly than other fruits. They are therefore suitable fruits to take if your blood glucose is low, or during exercise. When counting grams of carbohydrate, the fibre content should be subtracted if it is 5 g or more.[402,1092] Note that the weight of fruits can vary. See table on page 243 for carb. content per 100 g.

Carb. = carbohydrates

such an extent, especially if the lunchtime dose is adjusted to cover the sweets. Skipping lunch and buying sweets instead, as some teenagers do, can be harmful for those with diabetes. Children who do buy sweets would be better advised to buy chocolates than sweets made from pure sugar (see page 267) unless they have a weight problem.

Daycare

Using carbohydrate counting at daycare centres can work well, and the staff often find that it makes mealtimes easier if they have a relatively exact way of dosing insulin even if it can be a bit difficult to begin with.

Special "diabetic" food?

So called "diabetic" food (often found in health food stores) is not recommended for children with diabetes [968,1079] and is not suitable for adults either.[312] It is often both more expensive and higher in energy content than similar "normal" food. Besides, many find the taste unappetizing. Children may feel singled out as "different" if they are not allowed to eat the same food their friends eat. Diabetes food often contains sorbitol as a sweetener, which may produce side effects such as abdominal pain and diarrhoea. It is much better to learn how to handle ordinary food if you have diabetes.

"Fast food"

Many children, teenagers and adults like fast food, and it has become a fixture of modern life. As fast food often contains a lot of fat, it is not a good idea to make a habit of eating it. However, occasionally eating fast food shouldn't cause problems, and after a couple of times you will have found out what insulin doses are appropriate for your favourite items. However, you can easily find yourself with a meal that has a high carbohydrate content. See suggestions for insulin dosing on page 253.

Food at educational camps

Children who attend diabetes education camps are likely to be very active physically while they are there, and usually very hungry at mealtimes. It may be difficult for the staff to judge how much individual children are used to eating. The basic rule must be that they are allowed to eat enough to feel satisfied to compensate for the increased energy expenditure. Sometimes you see a child eating very large helpings, and it may then be a good idea to cautiously limit their food intake and then check with the parents how they handle such situations at home. This may present a good occasion for a discussion on how the carbohydrate amounts eaten, and what drinks are consumed with a meal, will

If you are a vegetarian you will need to talk to your dietitian about your meal plan so that you will get enough of all kinds of essential nutrients. This is especially important for young people.

affect the blood glucose levels. The increased activity will often require lowered insulin doses, especially at bedtime. A later evening snack (8.30-9 PM) will help young people withstand the night better. The total daily insulin dose was lowered by around one third, on average, in children aged 7-12 years attending a physically active (mainly water sports) camp in New Zealand.[142]

Vegetarian and vegan diets

A pure vegetarian or vegan diet may result in a disturbed balance between the amount of protein and carbohydrate in the diet. This is because vegetarian nutrients contain much less protein than animal nutrients. A lactovegetarian diet includes milk and milk products resulting in a higher protein content. A vegan diet including a high proportion of fruits and berries may even have a higher content of sugar than a mixed diet.[50]

However, if reasonable attention is paid to achieving a balanced diet, many vegetarians do very well and avoid vitamin and mineral deficiencies despite having diabetes. As many of these young people are in their mid teens or older, problems with growth are likely to be avoided too.

A strict vegetarian or vegan diet is not recommended for children, as it will put them at risk

People with diabetes are generally exempted from fasting during Ramadan. If you still want to take part in the fast, it is very important that you seek advice from your doctor before doing so.

of a deficiency of protein, vitamins and minerals. Not eating meat, fish or eggs is not necessarily synonymous with being a vegetarian. In vegan or lactovegetarian diets, the animal products are mostly replaced by products from leguminous plants. The intake of vitamin B_{12} will be cut in half if the vitamins in animal products are not replaced. This will lead to a considerable risk of anaemia which can show as tiredness. You should always talk to your dietitian or doctor before changing your diet.

Different cultures

Families from different cultures and different religions often have quite different eating habits. The number of meals can be fewer and sometimes certain foods are excluded due to religious reasons. According to tradition, Muslims and Jews do not eat pork, and Hindus are most often vegetarians. South Asian families often use Ghee (clarified butter) for cooking, which is very high in saturated fat and must be reduced or omitted where possible. The way of cooking is usually different. Lactose intolerance is more common among children from some countries.

In every case, it is of course important to take the family's customary food habits into consideration when discussing nutrition with a person who has diabetes. With a multiple injection treatment and premeal injections there are usually no difficulties for a person with diabetes in dovetailing healthy meal planning into the wider family routine.

Religious fasting days

Special religious fasting days, such as Yom Kippur for Jews, can easily be accommodated by appropriate attention to monitoring and adjustment (downwards) of insulin doses. Consult your diabetes healthcare team for advice if you are at all unsure about how to handle the situation, and keep records in your logbook for the next time!

Ramadan: the fasting month

During Ramadan, the ninth month of the Islamic year, Muslims fast from dawn until sunset. Sick people, and women who are pregnant, breast-feeding or menstruating, are exempt, as are young children. Fasting is not recommended for individuals with type 1 diabetes according to some health professionals [16] but even so, many devout Muslims with diabetes prefer to fast during Ramadan.

If you are going to fast during Ramadan, it is important that you find a way of accommodating both your body's need for a low basal insulin level during fasting hours, and the need for an increased insulin level for the meals you take just before sunrise and at sunset. This means frequent monitoring of your blood glucose and adjusting your insulin doses, so that you can avoid low levels during the day as well as high levels after ceasing your fast in the evening.

Fasting accelerates the breakdown of fat and ketone production, by increasing glucagon levels. So, if you cut down your insulin doses too much during the period of fasting, you will put yourself at risk of ketoacidosis. One patient, a 15-year-old boy, was admitted to hospital in ketoacidosis after fasting and omitting his lunchtime dose of insulin in combination with dehydration during Ramadan.[376]

In addition to the problem of fasting, there is risk of over-eating high-calorie sweets in the evenings during Ramadan.[16] Two doses per day of rapid-acting (Humalog) and NPH insulin gave better blood glucose levels and less hypoglycaemia than regular short-acting insulin and NPH in one study.[583] The two doses were taken before the morning and evening meals. Ask your diabetes team for practical advice if you plan to fast during Ramadan.

Research findings: Ramadan and diabetes

♠ Lantus once daily or Levemir twice daily have been recommended as good alternatives for basal insulin when participating in Ramadan, and they can be decreased by 10-20% to avoid hypoglycaemia according to one study where people took their basal insulin at the usual time of 9-10 PM.[20]

♠ These authors also recommended people with diabetes to take extra rapid-acting insulin if the blood glucose goes above 15 mmol/l (270 mg/dl) and to break the fast temporarily if it goes below 4 mmol/l (70 mg/dl) or if they develop ketones. Skipping the pre-dawn meal should be avoided, and carbohydrate counting is recommended to match the premeal dose, as the sunset meal often consists of extra sweet and savoury foods.

♠ For those on a 2-dose regimen the recommendation is to take the usual morning dose before the sunset meal and to take only short-acting insulin at the time of the dawn meal.

♠ In an investigation including 1,070 Muslims with type 1 diabetes from 13 countries, 43% fasted for at least 15 days during Ramadan, varying from 9% in Morocco to 72% in Saudi Arabia.[925] However, only 35% changed their previous insulin doses to match the difference in food intake.

♠ In the whole study population, episodes of severe hypoglycaemia leading to hospitalization were more common during Ramadan (0.14 vs. 0.03 episodes/month), and also episodes of very high blood sugar and ketoacidosis (0.16 vs. 0.05 episodes/month).

♠ The statistics were similar when a subgroup of people fasting for at least 15 days was considered. This suggested that the change in food habits made by other family members during Ramadan will also influence the way that the person with diabetes eats, even if they are not actually fasting themselves.

Sweeteners

Sugar-free?

When manufacturers state that a product has "no sugar added", this does not always mean it is completely devoid of sugar. It usually implies that no sugar is added, whereas the natural sugar from berries or fruits is still present. No added sugar chocolate or ice cream can contain more calories than ordinary alternatives. Sweet foods like this often contain sorbitol, which eventually will be transformed into glucose in the liver. Check the food label carefully.

Since prehistoric times, humans have craved sugar. This is believed to be because sweet natural products are seldom poisonous while many bitter ones can be so.

Non-nutritive sweeteners

Aspartame

Aspartame (E951) is 200 times sweeter than sugar and is used in such small amounts that

the energy content is negligible. It can lose its sweetness through cooking and baking.

Aspartame is made up of two amino acids called aspartic acid and the methyl ester of phenylalanine. Amino acids and methyl esters are found naturally in foods like milk, meats, fruits and vegetables. When digested, the body handles the amino acids in aspartame in the same way as those in foods we eat daily.[579] Although aspartame can be used by the whole family, individuals with a rare genetic disease called phenylketonuria (PKU) need to be aware that aspartame is a source of the protein component, phenylalanine. Those who have PKU cannot properly metabolize phenylalanine and must monitor their intake of phenylalanine from all foods, including foods containing aspartame. In many countries, including the UK, every infant is screened for PKU at birth.

Unfortunately, many myths about aspartame are circulating, scaring people with diabetes and others who use "diet" drinks. The fact is that aspartame has been studied extensively in humans. The safety of aspartame has been well established and it has been shown that eating or drinking products sweetened with aspartame is

Free from sugar?	
⇒ Unsweetened	No compound with sweet taste has been added to the product. However, it can contain natural sugar (fruit sugar, milk sugar).
⇒ Without added sugar No added sugar No sugar added	No sugars have been added. However it may contain sugar naturally, e.g. pure fruit juice.
⇒ Sugar-free	No more than 0.2 g sugar per 100 g or 100 ml.
⇒ Reduced sugar	At least 25% reduction on the original product.

not associated with adverse health effects.[579] A 240 ml (8-ounce) glass of milk has six times more phenylalanine and 13 times more aspartic acid than an equivalent amount of soda sweetened with NutraSweet. An 8 ounce glass of fruit juice or tomato juice contains 3-5 times more methanol than an equivalent amount of soda sweetened with NutraSweet.[579]

The UK's Committee on Toxicity, Consumer Products and the Environment (COT, a committee of independent experts who advise the Government on the safety of food chemicals) recently concluded that there is no evidence to suggest a need to revise their earlier statement that confirmed that aspartame is safe for use, or to revise the previously established Acceptable Daily Intake (ADI) of 40 mg/kg body weight per day. An adult would have to consume 14 cans of a sugar-free drink every day before reaching the ADI, assuming the sweetener was used in the drink at the maximum permitted level. In practice, most drinks use aspartame in combination with other sweeteners so that the level is considerably lower. Aspartame intakes have been shown to be considerably below the recommended maximum level, even among children and people with diabetes who consume large quantities of sugar-free drinks.

Saccharin

Saccharin (E954) is a synthetic product. It is 300-500 times sweeter than sugar and contains no energy. It gives a slight metallic taste when heated above 70° C (158° F) and should therefore be added only after cooking.

Acesulphame K

This sweetener (E950) is 130-200 times sweeter than sugar. It withstands heating well and can be used for baking. It is mixed with milk sugar (lactose) but in amounts too small to give any significant amount of energy.

Sucralose

Sucralose (E955) is 600 times sweeter than ordinary sugar. It is made from sugar but does not affect blood glucose. Sucralose tastes like sugar and is heat stable. It can be used both for baking and for cooking.

Cyclamate

Cyclamate (E952) is 30-50 times sweeter than sugar and contains no energy. It is stable in high temperatures and therefore suitable for cooking and baking. It is often used in soft drinks, dairy products and chocolate. The UK Food Standards Agency is advising parents to give young children no more than three beakers (about 180 ml each) a day of dilutable soft drinks, or squashes, containing the sweetener cyclamate. Drinking more than this amount could lead to children aged 1.5 to 4.5 years taking in more

Hot and cold drinks				
	Quantity	Carb.	Fat	Kcal
Low-fat milk	200 ml	10 g	1 g	75
1.5%-fat milk	200 ml	10 g	3 g	96
3%-fat milk	200 ml	10 g	6 g	120
Chocolate milk	200 ml	~20 g	*add milk	
Orange juice	200 ml	~25 g	-	100
Squash	200 ml	~15 g		60
Soft drinks	200 ml	~20 g		100
Lemonade	330 ml	~30 g	-	120
Diet Fanta	330 ml	0 g	-	1
Diet Cola	330 ml	0 g	-	1
Coffee	200 ml	0.3 g		2
Tea	200 ml	0 g		2
Herb tea	Can have a high sugar-content!			

Carb. = carbohydrates, kcal = kilocalories

* The fat and energy content of chocolate milk depends on how much fat there is in the milk used.

than the acceptable daily intake (ADI) of cyclamate. The Agency is also recommending that when preparing dilutable soft drinks containing cyclamate for young children, parents should dilute them more than they would for an adult.

Nutritive sweeteners

These all contain energy, which should be considered if weight is a problem.

Fructose

Fructose is almost twice as sweet as sugar. Even if fructose does not affect your blood glucose level directly, it is transformed into glucose in the liver, and the calorie content can cause weight gain. Because of this, fructose is not considered as a suitable sweetener for people with diabetes in some countries. In other countries (such as Finland and Germany) many "diabetes products" containing fructose are sold (see also page 70).

Sugar alcohols

Sugar alcohols (also called polyols) are used by food manufacturers to lower carbohydrate and/or fat content and are often used in chewing gum, "sugar-free" sweets, ice cream and pastry. Sugar alcohols provide approximately half the energy (2.5 kcal/g) compared with other carbohydrates (4 kcal/g). Chemically, they are neither sugars nor alcohols but eventually they will be converted into fructose and glucose by the liver. The names of sugar alcohols usually end in "-ol", for example sorbitol, xylitol, mannitol, maltitol, and lactitol. Hydrogenated starch hydrolysates and isomalt are also sugar alcohols. The sweetness of sorbitol is about half

Sweeteners without energy		
Substance	Trade name	Common in
Acesul-phame K	Sunett Hermesetas Gold (aspartame + acesulphame K)	Beverages, jams, baked goods,
Aspartame	NutraSweet Equal	Chewing gum Sweets Soft drinks Tabletop sweetener
Cyclamate	Sucaryl, Sugar Twin	Tabletop sweetener
Saccharin	Sweet'n Low Hermesetas Original	Tabletop sweetener
Sucralose	Splenda	Tabletop sweetener, drinks, baked goods, frozen and canned fruit

that of sugar. When counting carbohydrates, it is currently suggested that only half the amount of sugar alcohols should be included.[1092]

Sorbitol (E420) is a natural component of plums, cherries and other fruits and berries. Sorbitol and other sugar alcohols absorb water from the intestines and provide nourishment for intestinal bacteria. Large amounts of sorbitol can cause abdominal pains and diarrhoea, which may put an automatic limit on the amounts eaten.

Diet drinks and "light" foods

Diet drinks are usually sweetened with aspartame and do not contain any sugar. Most of these drinks are "unrestricted" for people with diabetes in the sense that they do not raise the blood glucose. However, cola drinks often contain caffeine so it is not healthy to drink large amounts of them.

It is best to get used to avoiding sugary drinks, for example Cola, as soon as you are diagnosed as having diabetes. There are many good alternatives without sugar. If you are hesitant, ask your parent to do a blind test, i.e. by pouring out different kinds of Cola (with sugar and without) in glasses without you knowing which is which. Try them and see for yourself which one you prefer. You might be surprised how difficult it is to taste the difference.

When a foodstuff is labelled "light", the situation is more complex. Such products are not necessarily sugar-free. In some countries a foodstuff may be described as "light" if the sugar content is decreased. Products containing fat

can be labelled "light" if the fat content has been decreased. Most countries have regulations to ensure that terms such as "light" or "low fat" are explained on food labelling. As the rules for labelling may vary from country to country, you should check with your dietitian about what is applicable where you live.

Light (low-fat) ice cream contains around one third of the fat content found in regular ice cream. "Fat free" means the product contains no fat, while "no sugar added" may mean sugar alcohols are added instead.

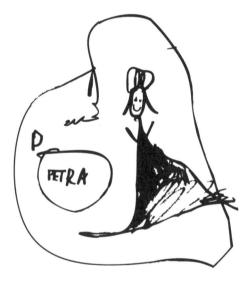

Sweets, treats and ice cream

Sooner or later all young people with diabetes will be tempted by their friends and peer group to indulge in treats like ice cream or sweets. At home, families often try to regulate this by allowing ice cream on special occasions and sweets only on certain days. This is something all parents may find difficult to enforce, regardless of whether or not a child has diabetes. The obvious problem for a young person with diabetes is that all these delicious things will also increase the blood glucose (if they don't take extra insulin or exchange for other sources of carbohydrates). This is often the reason parents feel they have to say, "No, you can't have that. It is bad for your diabetes".

In saying this, it is easy to forget that the answer is likely to have been "No" even if the child did not have diabetes: "No, you will damage your teeth", "No, we can't afford it", or "No, in our family we have sweets only on Saturdays". The practical effect will be the same (no sweets) but, for the child, the difference is important. If you always refer to the child having diabetes when saying "No!", the child will soon start hating the illness which appears to lie behind the limitations. He or she will start to believe that it is the diabetes alone that makes this and everything else impossible.

We don't want to ban sweets from children (or adults) with diabetes, but neither do we in any way want to say that they are unrestricted. The message is that **of course you can have some**

What is in "unhealthy" food?

	Quantity/Weight		Carb.	Fat	Kcal
Peanuts	¾ cup	100 g	15 g	53 g	630
Cheese Twisties		28 g	15 g	9 g	150
Potato crisps		28 g	15 g	8 g	130
Popcorn	0.5 litre	23 g	15 g	3 g	110
Milk chocolate	1 bar	28 g	15 g	9 g	150
Milk chocolate, no sugar added	6 squares		15 g	11g	170
Kit Kat ®	0.5 bar	20 g	14 g	6 g	103
Cream biscuit	1 piece		10 g	5 g	105
Plain biscuits	2 pieces		15 g	2 g	90
Jelly beans	5 pieces	19 g	15 g	-	65
Toffee	4 pieces	17 g	15 g	3 g	77
Boiled sweets	5 pieces		15 g	-	60
Glucose tablets	1 piece	3 g		-	12
Lifesavers	1 piece	2 g	2 g	-	8
Chewing gum	1 stick		2 g	-	8
Sponge cake with chocolate icing	1 slice	80 g	45 g	12 g	300

Carb. = carbohydrates, 1 kcal = 4.6 kJ

Read the list carefully! Fifteen grams of carbohydrate corresponds to one slice of bread. Which would you prefer? Four sweets or 0.5 litre of popcorn (25 g of unpopped popcorn)?

We can tell you how to handle insulin with different types of food, being "blood glucose technicians". But it is very important that these treats are "extras". It is not healthy for anyone to eat cakes every day and you must take this responsibility yourself.

sweets or ice cream — but you need to think about how and when to eat them so your blood glucose will not be affected too much. Most adults allow themselves a treat every now and again. So children, too, should be given opportunities to manage their insulin and food in a way that enables them to enjoy something sweet on occasion, without their blood glucose rising too high. Going to parties is far more fun if you can eat the same food as everyone else. However, just as adults won't feel well if they go out partying all the time, we emphasize to children that this is something they can do only on special occasions, not every day. Too many sweets are not good for people without diabetes either. They provide empty calories which increase the risk of weight gain and cause damage to your teeth.

It is all about freedom with responsibility and to master this you need to practise and experiment. It is important to monitor your blood glucose before and after you have tried something new. It will often not be perfect at your first attempt but after a few times you will learn better how your body works. The logbook is important so that, later, you will remember what you did and how it turned out.

How much extra insulin should you take?

Use your insulin:carb ratio if you have calculated this (see page 248). Otherwise, one additional unit of insulin for every 10-15 g of extra carbohydrate (i.e. sugar) is usually enough.[255] With fixed insulin doses, only the carbohydrate content which is in excess of that of your ordinary snack should be counted if sweets or ice cream are eaten instead of the usual snack. Of course, the effect on your blood glucose level will not be ideal, so this is not something we recommend you do on a regular basis. But it can be a good method for special occasions. Remember that exceptions must be exceptions — if you do it every day it will become a habit and such a habit is not compatible with your diabetes. How and when to eat sweets and ice cream is something that you and your family will need to discuss together. Your diabetes team can only tell you how the sugar in these treats works in your body and how to adjust your insulin.

The amount of extra insulin needed will depend on your total insulin requirement. If you are in puberty and your total insulin dose is high (more than 1 U/kg per 24 hours, 0.5 U/lb per 24 hours), you may need more than 1 unit of insulin for every 10 g of carbohydrate. If you are in the honeymoon phase (low insulin requirements during the first 6-12 months after the onset of diabetes, see page 221) you should only take a quarter to half a unit extra per 10 g of extra carbohydrate. Your own insulin production will supply the rest. Measure your blood glucose level 0.5-1 hour after you have eaten your

When should you test your blood glucose level?	
Sweets, ice lollies	After 0.5 hour
Ice cream, chocolate bar	After 1-1.5 hour
Potato crisps	After 2-3 hours

Ice cream cones

Ice cream cones usually contain:

Soft ice cream	20-30 g of carbohydrate
Ice cream (3 scoops)	20-25 g of carbohydrate

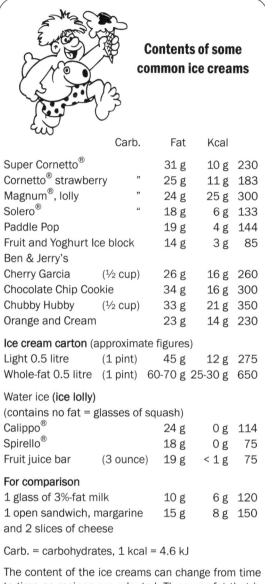

Contents of some common ice creams

		Carb.	Fat	Kcal
Super Cornetto®		31 g	10 g	230
Cornetto® strawberry	"	25 g	11 g	183
Magnum®, lolly	"	24 g	25 g	300
Solero®	"	18 g	6 g	133
Paddle Pop		19 g	4 g	144
Fruit and Yoghurt Ice block		14 g	3 g	85
Ben & Jerry's				
Cherry Garcia	(½ cup)	26 g	16 g	260
Chocolate Chip Cookie		34 g	16 g	300
Chubby Hubby	(½ cup)	33 g	21 g	350
Orange and Cream		23 g	14 g	230

Ice cream carton (approximate figures)				
Light 0.5 litre	(1 pint)	45 g	12 g	275
Whole-fat 0.5 litre	(1 pint)	60-70 g	25-30 g	650

Water ice (ice lolly)				
(contains no fat = glasses of squash)				
Calippo®		24 g	0 g	114
Spirello®		18 g	0 g	75
Fruit juice bar	(3 ounce)	19 g	< 1 g	75

For comparison				
1 glass of 3%-fat milk		10 g	6 g	120
1 open sandwich, margarine		15 g	8 g	150
and 2 slices of cheese				

Carb. = carbohydrates, 1 kcal = 4.6 kJ

The content of the ice creams can change from time to time as recipes are adapted. The more fat that is added, the slower the blood glucose rise will be but the more calories it will contain.

sweets and experiment to find out what works well for you. See "Carbohydrate counting" on page 246 for a more exact method of finding your individual need for insulin for a given amount of carbohydrates.

Rapid-acting insulins (NovoRapid or Humalog) are effective if you are eating sweets containing pure sugar, but may be too quick for treats containing fat, such as ice cream and chocolate bars. If you use a pump, you can set it to deliver a prolonged bolus dose if needed (see illustration on page 192). If you have short-acting regular insulin, you can take extra insulin at the same time as you have chocolate or a regular ice cream. But you should take it 30 minutes before having sweets containing only sugar as this will affect your blood glucose more quickly. Water ices and ice lollies (those that are not special "no added sugar" ones) contain a lot of sugar that can affect your blood sugar considerably. They may come in handy, however, if your blood sugar dips while you are on the beach, for example.

It is good idea to have your sweets or ice cream as dessert after a regular meal. The sugar content will then be mixed in your stomach with the rest of the food, so it will not affect your blood sugar too quickly. You can take your ordinary insulin dose if, for example, you replace a glass of milk (approximately 200 ml or 8 ounces) with 10 g of carbohydrates in sweets or ice cream. Substituting sweets for other carbohydrates in your meal plan is probably the best way to deal with this if you have a

It is easy to develop a "sweets-mania" if you have diabetes. Some children with diabetes eat more sweets than their friends although they know this is not healthy for them. Try not to make sweets too big a thing in your life. Aim at managing to eat only small amounts on appropriate occasions. Even if you can't manage this just at the moment, you can make a decision to do it when you are a little older. The question will then not be **if** you will succeed, it will be **when** you will succeed...

"sweet tooth". You can, for example, have smaller servings of bread, potatoes or fruit. If you add a dessert you will have eaten more carbohydrates than usual, in which case you will need to increase your insulin dose as described above or by carbohydrate counting. Like everyone else, eating extra often will put you at risk of gaining weight.

Ice cream

A summer without ice cream is no summer at all in the eyes of many children. Of course you can eat ice cream even if you have diabetes. The usual advice applies: think ahead and experiment to find out what is best for you. There are mainly two types of frozen treats: water ice (ice lolly, ice block) and ice cream made from dairy products. Water ices are like frozen fruit juice (often with added sugar or sweetener) and affect the blood glucose level in the same way as juice except that it takes longer to lick an ice lolly than to drink a glass of fruit juice. Ice lollies can be perfectly suitable if you have hypoglycaemia, for example while you are at the beach. You will need to be sure, however, that what you are eating is an ordinary ice lolly, and not a "light" or low-sugar variety, as the latter would have little or no effect on your blood glucose level.

Ice cream made from dairy products contains fat that causes your stomach to empty more slowly. Thus the increase in blood glucose level will not be seen until 45-90 minutes after eating ice cream.[773] From this it follows that dairy-based ice cream is not suitable for reversing hypoglycaemia. However, it can be a good alternative if you are playing football, for example, as an activity such as this requires extra sugar over a longer period of time.

During our educational holidays for young people with diabetes, we do some experimenting with ice cream and caramels. The dietitian tells the children about the contents of different ice creams. We then have an "ice cream test" at snack-time. The children measure their blood glucose levels beforehand and then discuss with their leaders what they should do next in order to have their favourite ice cream. If it is neces-

Ice cream gives a slower blood glucose rise than you might expect. The reason for this is that the high fat content causes the stomach to empty more slowly. The graph is from an American study of adults with diabetes who ate 100 g (3/4 cup) of vanilla ice cream (24% carbohydrate and 11% fat content). When they injected regular short-acting insulin (3-5 units) 30 minutes before the ice cream, the rise in blood glucose was reduced considerably.[773]

"Ice cream test"

① Measure your blood glucose level at snack-time.

② Calculate the carbohydrate content of your snack in grams (one open sandwich = 15 g, one glass of milk = 10 g, for fruit see table on page 255).

③ Decide which ice cream you want (not water ices — they only contain frozen sugar-water).

④ Calculate the carbohydrate content of the ice cream.

⑤ Take 1 unit of extra insulin for every 10 g of excess carbohydrate in the ice cream (or according to your insulin:carb ratio).

⑥ Decrease the dose by 1-2 units if your blood glucose level before the ice cream is less than 4-5 mmol/l (70-90 mg/dl) or if you are about to exercise. Increase by 1-2 units if the blood glucose level is above 10 mmol/l (180 mg/dl). You can also use the correction factors on page 146 if you are used to this system. If you are in the remission phase (honeymoon phase, see page 221) you should only take a quarter or half the above-mentioned extra doses of insulin.

⑦ Measure your blood glucose level 1-1.5 hour after you have finished the ice cream to see if things worked out the way you expected.

⑧ Record what you did in your logbook and you will be better placed to know what to do the next time you want to eat ice cream.

Remember that, whether or not they have diabetes, children do not eat ice cream every day. It is their parents who decide when they eat it, and the same rules should apply to children both with and without diabetes.

sary, they will take an extra dose of insulin along with the ice cream. It may not be the most sensible thing to have a large ice cream if your blood glucose level is 15 mmol/l (270 mg/dl) — but life is full of such situations and it is a good idea to know how to handle them. The children can have their choice of ice cream, but only if they take extra insulin. When the children measure their blood glucose level 1.5-2 hours after the ice cream, their average level is lower than it was before eating the ice cream.

Chocolate

Chocolate contains fat which will slow down the absorption of glucose by emptying the stomach more slowly. For example, you may eat a small chocolate bar (24 g, 1 ounce = 14 g carbohydrate) for a snack instead of an open sandwich, and take insulin with it if you are using rapid-acting insulin for meals. With regular insulin, snacks are usually needed without taking extra insulin. This may be fine occasionally, but (in common with anyone who does not have diabetes) you should not snack like this every day. However, when you are physically active you will probably be able to take a small chocolate bar in addition to your usual snack without problems.

Sweets

During our educational camps, we exchange the apple of the afternoon snack (on the "treasure hunt") for a box of sweets that contain jelly, making them tougher to chew, and causing the sugar to be absorbed more slowly. Other sweets which have a taste of sugar and easily break into small pieces during chewing contain mostly pure sugar. Sugar-free sweets usually contain sorbitol which is better for your teeth and raises the blood glucose level more slowly. We tell children these facts at the same time as they taste sweets of various types, in order to help them recognize the difference.

One box of jelly-type sweets sweetened with sorbitol (about 15 g) has the same blood glucose-raising effect as an apple or a pear. However, the contents of a box of sugar-type fruit pastilles gives the same effect as six lumps of dextrose (18 g). If a child chooses to eat one

Use the opportunity to eat your regular portion of sweets while you are doing some physical exercise. One girl had her "Friday sweets" every week while horse-riding and it did not affect her blood glucose level at all.

small sweet of this type at some stage in the course of an afternoon, it will not affect the blood glucose level at all. By saying this we don't mean that children should have sweets every day. Keeping sweet intake low is a good rule for all children whether or not they have diabetes. This situation should be the same for families without diabetes, in that it is the parents who decide which rules apply. The important thing is that children with diabetes feel that, as far as possible, they receive the same treatment as their friends without diabetes and siblings when it comes to sweets.

These principles for managing eating both ice cream and sweets combine freedom and responsibility. In order to learn how to manage different situations well, you will need to practise and experiment. It is important to measure your blood glucose level both before and after trying something new. It is likely that your blood glucose level will not be quite as it should be the first time around, but after a couple of times you will get to know your body better. The logbook is important — afterwards you can go back and determine what worked well and what did not.

Weekend sweets

In some families it is common to restrict sweets for children to the weekends. The best approach then is probably to give the sweets as part of a regular snack or meal, substituting the carbohydrates. If you want to have sweets for a snack, start by having a sandwich (preferably bread with a high fibre content). The combination of fat and dietary fibre contained in this snack will slow down the emptying of the stomach, thereby lessening any effect on the blood glucose level. Rapid-acting insulin (NovoRapid or Humalog) is effective much more quickly, so you may not need the slow absorption effect of the sandwich. Check your blood glucose before and after you eat sweets to find out what works best for you.

How much in the way of treats and sweet things can a young person have? You must try this out individually, but estimate that 70-80% of the candy weight is made up of carbohydrates. Eating too many sweets will cause you to gain weight, in exactly the same way as it would if you didn't have diabetes. A rule of the thumb is that one half to three quarters of the weight of any sweet is pure sugar. The carbohydrate content of an open sandwich corresponds to approximately 20-30 g (1 ounce) of sweets. Sweets containing fat give a slower blood glucose rise but contain more energy. This applies to treats such as milk chocolate or chocolate type sweets. Caramels, toffees and other sweets containing almost pure sugar will increase your blood glucose level much more quickly. The sugar content of liquorice sweets is about the same as of other types of sweets.

Weekend sweets

A child's typical afternoon snack:

1 sandwich	= 30 g carbohydrate
(2 slices of bread)	

Saturday snack:

½ sandwich	= 15 g carb.
20 g sweets	≈ 15 g carb.
	30 g carb.
15 g sweets extra	≈ 10 g carb. ➟ 1 U extra
30 g sweets extra	≈ 20 g carb. ➟ 2 U extra

If the sweets contain fat (e.g. chocolate, which contains around 50-60% carbohydrate), this produces a slower emptying of the stomach and thereby a slower rise in the blood glucose level. If you have access to both regular short-acting insulin (Actrapid, Humulin S, Insuman Rapid) and rapid-acting insulin (NovoRapid, Humalog, Apidra) you may find that short-acting insulin works better with sweets like these.

What does the labelling on sweet packets mean?

Types of sugar	Fructose
	Lactose
	Xylose
	Dextrose
Sugar alcohols	Xylitol
	Mannitol
	Sorbitol
	Isomalt
	Maltitol
	Lactitol
Other carbohydrate terms	Hydrogenated starch
	Hydrolysate (HSH)
	Maltodextrins
	Corn syrup
	High-maltose syrup
	High-fructose corn syrup (HFCS)
	Corn starch
	Unmodified starches

Tip: Ask your dietitian to help you learn more about food ingredients, sweeteners and types of carbohydrates and their impact on blood glucose.

Even when counting carbohydrates carefully, it is often difficult for the child with diabetes to find the right dose of insulin for 100 g of sweets (approximately 80 g of carbs. It is then better to maximize the amount of sweets to 50 g, and eat this much on two separate days if the child feels that 50 g is not enough for "Saturday sweets".

A good way to enjoy sweets is to eat them while you are engaged in some sort of active outdoor pursuit — for example, during an afternoon walk, playing football, or when you are out riding or running around on the beach. The additional activity will use up the extra calories gained from the sweets.

Taking a break from eating sweets

It is not easy to manage diabetes if you are eating large amounts of sweet things as everyone who has tried can testify. Even so, many individuals with diabetes do this. This is a bit like smoking for some people — just cutting down doesn't work. Try then to avoid eating sweets completely, at least for a while. If it is difficult to say "no" to yourself, do not keep them in the house. Unfortunately, excessive sweet eating must remain exceptional behaviour for any person with diabetes. And if you do something every day, it ceases to be exceptional.

Many families practise a system of taking a break from eating sweets, whether or not they have diabetes in the family. Children may then receive money instead or some other kind of bonus if they can manage without sweets for 6 months or a whole year. This system works well for children who benefit from not having sweets for other reasons as well, such as those who are overweight. Adults can try giving themselves

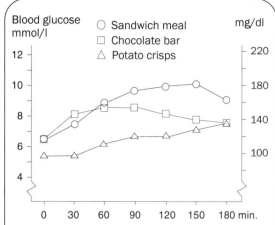

In a Swedish study, teenagers replaced two out of three open cheese sandwiches with jelly drops at snack time.[176] The blood glucose rise is slightly more rapid with jelly drops and the sandwich, but considerably less rapid than if they had eaten jelly drops alone. White bread contains almost no fibre but gives a larger volume compared with jelly sweets alone, causing the stomach to empty more slowly. The fat in margarine and cheese also leads to a slower emptying of the stomach.

A sandwich made of bread rich in fibre, along with the jelly drops, would probably have made the blood glucose response even less pronounced. From this it follows that a good way to eat your sweets is to eat it after a meal and your blood glucose level will be less affected.

In another study, different types of snacks with the same calorie content were compared: 2½ slices of dark rye bread with cheese and an apple, a bar of milk chocolate (67 g, 2.3 ounces) and potato crisps (70 g, 2.5 ounces).[177] The ordinary snack containing slightly more carbohydrates gave the highest blood glucose rise while potato crisps gave the slowest rise. The bar of milk chocolate gave a slow rise, making it unsuitable for anyone with hypoglycaemia.

The fat in chocolate and potato crisps causes the stomach to empty more slowly and the increase in blood glucose level will therefore be slower. The food processing used in the manufacturing of crisps causes the sugar to be less accessible to digesting enzymes, thereby being absorbed more slowly.

The message from the dietitian Gunilla Cedermark, who carried out these studies, is not that we should have chocolate and crisps for snacks every day. Most children don't, even if they would very much like to... The difference is that saying "No!" to crisps and bars of chocolate should be done on the same terms as it is for children without diabetes. It is very important to avoid referring to diabetes more often than necessary when saying "No!"

A bar of chocolate is a good snack for children with diabetes who are going on a hiking or skiing trip, in the same way as it is for friends and siblings without diabetes. One day a week you can replace a snack or parts of the evening snack with potato crisps. The whole family can enjoy these together with an easy conscience.

some kind of bonus, such as a new dress or a holiday, if they manage without sweets for a longer period of time.

If you have weight problems you will find it difficult balancing sweet eating with diabetes. If you eat sweets containing fat, this will have less of an effect on your blood glucose, but it will cause you to put on weight. If you eat sweets containing less fat, it will have a greater effect on your blood glucose level. A total break from eating sweets may be your only chance in this situation if you want to manage both your weight and your HbA_{1c}.

Different types of sweets

	Quantity	Carb.	Fat	Kcal
Gelatinous sweets	100 g	79 g	0 g	355
Caramels/ pastilles	100 g	97 g	0 g	400
Wine gums	100 g	75 g	0 g	300
Jelly beans	100 g	100 g	0 g	400
Marshmallows	100 g	80 g	0 g	360
Milk chocolate	100 g	54 g	33 g	570
Dark chocolate	100 g	60 g	32 g	560
Toffee	100 g	69 g	18 g	470

Carb. = carbohydrates

The contents are approximate as they vary from brand to brand. Chocolate with a high fat content increases your blood glucose level more slowly. Gelatinous sweets raise the blood glucose level slightly slower than sweets that are easy to chew. If you have access to both rapid-acting insulin (Novo-Rapid, Humalog, Apidra) and short-acting insulin (Actrapid, Humulin S, Insuman Rapid) you may find that short-acting insulin works better with chocolate sweets.

The best time to eat sweets is when you are physically active, when you have a low blood glucose level or immediately after a meal.

Popcorn makes a good "diabetes treat". Half a litre (1 pint) of popcorn contains about the same amount of carbohydrate as one open sandwich (one slice of bread). Microwave popcorn contains the same amount of carbohydrate as ordinary popcorn.

the palm of an adult hand) have approximately the same content of both fat (8 g) and carbohydrate (15 g) as an open cheese sandwich. It may be a good idea to eat crisps as an extra bedtime snack after a game of football to avoid night time hypoglycaemia. But remember that moderation is all and make sure you get crisps with unsaturated fat (vegetable oil). If you eat a whole 200 g (8 ounces) bag, your blood glucose will certainly rise.

Potato crisps

Potato crisps are not a healthy snack option since they contain a lot of fat and calories which can easily create a weight problem. In the UK it is common to have crisps at lunch time but lower-fat snacks (e.g. Quavers) would be a healthier alternative on an everyday basis. They can be OK to eat twice a week if you do not have them for lunch.

Potato crisps will raise the blood glucose very slowly over a period of at least 3-4 hours (see graph on page 270).[177] Twenty-five grams of potato crisps (the amount that can be held in

Chewing gum

Chewing gum contains such small amounts of sugar (about 2 g per stick) that chewing one piece at a time over a couple of hours will not cause you a problem. If you chew in this way, you will find little disadvantage, from the point of view of your diabetes, in using ordinary chewing gum, as opposed to the "sugar-free" variety. Your dentist will almost certainly recommend the latter of course. If you prefer chewing half a packet at a time, it is better to choose a brand with an artificial sweetener, like NutraSweet®.

Weight control

Many young people, particularly teenage girls, find they have problems with keeping their weight at a desirable level, whether or not they have diabetes. There are plenty of girls without diabetes who put on quite a lot of weight during the years following their first menstrual period (menarche), especially if they decrease the amount of regular exercise they do. This is caused by continuing to eat the same amount of food even though they have stopped growing in height. Most girls only grow another 6-8 cm (2-3 inches) after the menarche. The problem is made more complicated for girls with diabetes, as they find it particularly difficult to lose weight. It is very important, therefore, that teenage girls with diabetes reduce both their food intake and the insulin doses when their growth rate is slowing down and especially when they have reached their final height.

Body mass index (BMI) is an index for assessing body weight in relation to height. BMI can be calculated by dividing a person's weight by the square of their height in metres (kg/m^2). Overweight is defined as a BMI above 25.0, obese is above 30.0 and severely obese is above 35.0 kg/m^2. Overweight is a result of consuming more energy than is expended. Even moderate activity of just 30 minutes per day has been shown to improve insulin sensitivity, and this is what really helps weight loss.

A British study found females with diabetes to be overweight as adolescents, and both sexes to be overweight as young adults. Approximately 30% of the young women (but none of the young men) had given themselves less insulin than prescribed, in the hope this would help them control their weight.[153] A Swedish study found girls with diabetes to be on average 6.5 kg (14.3 lb) heavier than their peers without diabetes. Between the age of 18 and 22 their weight was unchanged but HbA_{1c} improved

and the daily insulin dose was significantly reduced.[295]

Satisfied or "feeling full"?

We believe children should always eat enough to satisfy them, but we should differentiate between being comfortably satisfied and "feeling full". Eating until you feel satisfied is not the same as eating as much as you want. Even children in their very early years at school should understand this distinction, and can be aware that over-eating will lead to weight gain.

Many children prefer to eat large helpings at every meal and this can easily become a habit. So, stop eating just as soon as you begin to feel satisfied and wait for 10-15 minutes. By this time, your feelings of hunger are likely to have disappeared without your having eaten any more. Vegetables will satisfy your hunger without providing significant amounts of carbohydrates or calories, and are a good alternative if you still want more to eat.

When a child or teenager has weight problems, some parents make a deliberate decision to avoid cooking more food than is needed for a normal helping for every family member. Once all the food prepared has been eaten, there will

be less room for discussion about second helpings and how much more it is appropriate to
eat. Parents can also make sure there are no
sweets, biscuits or cakes available at home to
tempt children to eat food when it is better they
don't.

Many parents are quite strict about their children finishing what is on their plate. But if you
are trying to lose weight, you might find it difficult to judge by eye how much you are going to
eat. If you have weight problems, therefore, you
should ask permission to leave food on the plate
if you find that you have taken too much and
feel satisfied before you have finished. If your
blood glucose level is high, you won't need to
eat as much as usual, and you are likely to find
you feel unusually full.[571]

Reducing weight

Talk to your dietitian about adjusting food
intake and insulin doses. Losing weight can easily lead to a vicious circle if you have diabetes.
Taking insulin forces you to eat even if you are
not hungry at the time. Try to decrease your
food intake and, at the same time, decrease the

It seems unfair that some individuals can eat as much as
they want, while others gain weight by just "looking at"
food. The reason for this is that our bodies work differently when it comes to using energy and storing it. During
the Stone Age it was useful for survival to be able to store
energy as fat when food was not available on a daily
basis. But in today's world, for those with an unlimited
supply of food, this ability has become a disadvantage.

amount of insulin you give yourself. It can be
difficult to find the appropriate balance
between insulin and food.

You may find it hard to know what foods you
can cut down on. Write down everything you
eat in the course of a 3-day period, recording
the exact quantities. Include everything, food,
drink, sweets, ice cream and so on. Ask your
dietitian to calculate the energy amounts and
advise you on reducing the amount of fat and
calories you consume.

If you decrease the amount of food you eat, you
run the risk of becoming hypoglycaemic — and
if this happens you will need to eat to reverse
the situation. But the next day you can think
about reducing both food and insulin to lose
weight sensibly. Remember to check that you
really have low blood glucose (less than 3.5-4.0
mmol/l (65-70 mg/dl) before eating something
extra. Be careful not to eat too much if your
blood glucose level is too low. Ten to fifteen
grams of glucose is usually enough (see page
66). Then wait 10-15 minutes before eating
anything else, even if you are still hungry, as this
will give your blood glucose level time to rise.

You should avoid losing weight too quickly. A
slow and steady loss resulting from a change in
habits is better than a quick loss caused by
reducing your food intake to a minimum. A sufficient rate is usually 1-3 kg (2-6 lb) per month.
It may not sound like much, but will result in
many kilograms in one year. Complete fasting
can be dangerous for a person with diabetes
and it is something that is positively discouraged. However, see page 257 regarding Ramadan. See also "Anorexia" on page 276).

There is a lot of debate about what to eat if you
want to lose weight, and you will constantly see
different examples in the news where a particular diet is claimed to be superior to others. In a
US study, 811 non-diabetic adults with a BMI
between 25 and 40 were assigned by lot to 4
different diets with the same energy content (a
daily deduction of 750 kcal from their usual
diet).[922] The study ran for 2 years, and they had

How do you count calories?

All food is made up of from different ingredients. Check the table of contents to calculate how many calories you will get.

Fat	9 kcal/g
Sugar	4 kcal/g
Protein	4 kcal/g
Alcohol	7 kcal/g
Sugar alcohol (e.g. sorbitol in sweets)	~2.5 kcal/g

Calorie table

The following will give you 100 kcal		Activities which will spend 100 kcal	
Whipped cream	200 ml	Walking	
Sugar	2 tbs (25 g)	slow	40 min.
Oil	2 teasp.	quick	15 min.
Mayonnaise	1 tbs		
Bun	1	Cycling	
Danish pastry	½	normal	35 min.
Crisps	20 crisps	quick	10 min.
Peanuts	15 g	Running	10 min.
Sweets	8-10 pieces		
Chocolate	20 g	Skating	25 min.
Snowball	1	Dancing	25 min.
Light beer	330 ml	Chopping logs	15 min.
Beer	250 ml		
White wine, dry	200 ml	Swimming	10 min.
Spirits	45 ml		
Liqueur	30 ml		

28 g ≈ 1 ounce, 100 ml ≈ 0.2 pints

counselling by a dietitian every 2 weeks. After 6 months, the average weight reduction was 6 kg, but thereafter the weight increased again, so after 2 years only 3 kg of weight loss remained. There was no difference between the different diets that were high or low in fat, protein or carbohydrates. From this study the conclusion is that it is the energy content as such, not the composition of the diet, that predicts the success of a weight-losing diet. Also, only those that did participate in the counselling sessions lost weight (on average 0.2 kg for every visit!). So the bottom line is to cut down on food and energy intake, and to use whatever support you can get to keep being motivated. See page 251 for a discussion on LCHF (low carb high fat) diet in people with diabetes.

The little extras

A little extra food, such as sweets, crisps or biscuits every day, will amount to quite a lot before the year is over. About 7,000 kcal are needed to build up 1 kg (2.2 lb) of fat in the body. An extra bun or some biscuits each day (100 kcal) will cause you to put on 5 kg (11 lb) of weight in one year! A small bag of peanuts (175 g, 6 ounces) extra *every week* will result in almost 8 kg (17 lb) weight increase in one year!

Never skip a meal. If you eat regularly, your blood glucose levels will be more steady and prevent you from getting too hungry. A missed meal is often followed by binge eating on something less healthy, such as crisps, which contain a lot of empty calories.

High HbA$_{1c}$ and weight loss

Having a high blood glucose level will result in the loss of large amounts of glucose in the urine. You might say that you "eat for two" since you eat not only to cover your daily energy requirements but also for the glucose lost in the urine. When your HbA$_{1c}$ is between 75 and 85 mmol/mol (9 and 10%), it is not unusual to lose glucose in the urine in amounts of up to 100-200 g of glucose in a day.

Having a high HbA$_{1c}$ can be an effective but dangerous way to lose weight.[245] Many teenagers will deliberately skip insulin injections to avoid gaining weight. In an American study, 15% of teenage girls with diabetes (but no boys) had used this method to diet.[842] You may get rid of a few pounds or kilograms temporarily, but the high blood glucose level that follows will increase your risk of long-term complications. If you feel tempted to use this method, try speaking instead to your diabetes team. They will make every effort to help you find a safe means of controlling your weight. The parents of young people with diabetes should be alerted if their teenager loses weight, or fails to show a normal weight increase at the appropriate time.

Increasing insulin doses will cause your body to take up the glucose that was being lost in the urine, and this will cause you to put on weight. Unfortunately, you have to increase the insulin doses initially because the high blood glucose level itself has induced increased insulin resistance (see page 224). What you must do is to increase the insulin doses for a short while (one or two weeks) to overcome the insulin resistance, and then lower them again as quickly as possible. This is because your blood glucose level goes down when the insulin resistance is back to normal. If you also reduce your food intake you will have a good chance of success.

Remember that if your blood glucose level has been high for some time you will have early symptoms of hypoglycaemia even at a low normal blood glucose level of 4-5 mmol/l (70-90 mg/dl).[140,508,574] Because of this, you should always take a blood glucose test when you feel hypoglycaemic. Eat only if your glucose level is less than 3.0-3.5 mmol/l (55-65 mg/dl). If your blood glucose level is higher, try to avoid eating despite symptoms. Your body may be giving

---

Exchange list

It is more important than one might imagine to choose an alternative with fewer calories. The table shows the difference (Diff.) between foodstuffs in calories and weight gain.

If you replace	with	Diff. in kcal	Diff. in Weight
0.5 litre of standard milk	0.5 litre of low fat milk	120 kcal/day	6 kg/year
3 open sandwiches with margarine and full fat cheese	3 open sandwiches with low-fat cheese but without margarine	205 kcal/day	10 kg /year
1 fried egg	1 boiled egg	40 kcal /day	2 kg /year
2 tbs mayonnaise	3 tbs sour cream	155 kcal	1 kg/ 45 times
1 bar of chocolate	1 apple	235 kcal	1 kg/ 30 times
1 helping of french fries	1 helping of boiled potatoes	145 kcal	1 kg/ 50 times
1 bottle of beer	1 bottle of light beer	45 kcal	1 kg/155 bottles
1 bag of peanuts (175 g)	0.5 litre of popcorn	1000 kcal	1.5 kg/ 10 bags
1 kg = 2.2 lb			

You might sometimes find it necessary to put a guard on the refrigerator in case you find yourself craving something tasty... One extra sandwich per day turns into 16 kg of extra fat in one year!

you warning symptoms, but remember that it believes you want a higher blood glucose level as this has been the case for some time. (See "Blood glucose levels and symptoms of hypoglycaemia" on page 44.) You must be prepared for a difficult time during the first 1-2 weeks, but after this you should start to experience warning symptoms at a lower blood glucose level. It is a good idea to have a friend or parent present while you are getting accustomed to this. You will need support and understanding from someone close to you, if you are to make it work.

Eating disorders

Both anorexia and bulimia (binge eating) are symptoms of weight-phobia, in that the person concerned finds it impossible to eat without worrying about putting on weight. A person with an eating disorder always has a distorted picture of their own body, but it is the emotional disturbance which is the most important. Eating disorders are much more common among girls, but can occur in boys as well. Anorexia usually starts between the ages of 13 and 16 years, bulimia somewhat later.[335] A person with an eating disorder is unlikely to appreciate the seriousness of the problem and may not feel it at all necessary to seek medical help. Physical or sexual abuse or any form of trauma can be the root cause of eating disorders such as anorexia and bulimia.[1085]

Anorexia

In anorexia there is a weight loss of at least 15% of the estimated normal weight for age or not being able to reach this weight at all. There is also an extreme fear of gaining weight and a very distorted idea of what the body looks like. Typically, someone with anorexia will see themselves as fat when looking into the mirror — even though, to others, they appear very slim. Food fixation is common, i.e. being interested in cooking for others while avoiding eating anything themselves. A person with anorexia is usually quite active physically, often running many miles a day in an attempt to keep their weight down.

The starvation that a person with anorexia is going through can result in physical symptoms such as headaches, lowered body temperature, increased body hair and irregular or disrupted menstrual periods. Psychological symptoms may include depression, feelings of inadequacy, sleeping difficulties and obsessions.

Having an eating disorder is difficult. It is common for young people with anorexia or bulimia to try and manipulate their insulin doses, and individuals often have problems with low or high blood glucose levels. Anyone with anorexia or bulimia will definitely need help. If this applies to you, tell your diabetes nurse or doctor, or another adult whom you trust. You will probably need to be referred to a specialist in these problems. It is also very difficult to calculate the insulin doses to match your irregular food intake if you have an eating disorder, so you will need help from your diabetes team with this.

Bulimia

People with bulimia engage in bingeing large amounts of food, much more than a person without the disorder would eat at one sitting. There is sense of loss of control and an inability to stop eating unless, for example, another person comes into the room. Self-inflicted vomiting or laxatives, excessive exercise or fasting may be used to control the weight. These individuals are often very impulsive and, if they also have diabetes, may find the regular routines necessary to manage it effectively, really very difficult.[897]

Diabetes and eating disorders

The combination of diabetes and eating disorders has been called "diabulemia".[146] A UK study found that 9% of 11-18-year-olds met the criteria for eating disorders, and that the proportion was the same among girls with or without diabetes.[842] However, a Swedish study found that teenage girls with diabetes were at greater risk of eating disorders (binge eating and self-induced vomiting) than their peers without diabetes.[335]

With the increased use of intensive diabetes therapy including carbohydrate counting and striving for lower HbA_{1c} targets, there has been concern that the risk of disordered eating behaviour will be increased. A German study compared adolescents aged 11-17 years with a long diabetes duration (10-16 years) and an HbA_{1c} of 67 mmol/mol, 8.3% using intensive insulin therapy (92% used multiple daily injections or pumps) with non-diabetic peers. They found the same frequency of disordered eating behaviour in both groups (around 30% in girls and 13% in boys).[60] However, 21% of the girls and 19% of the boys reported skipping their insulin or intentionally taking lower than needed at least 3 times per week.

Having diabetes and an eating disorder usually implies problems with blood glucose control and a tendency to manipulate insulin doses to control weight.[842,897,898] Not eating enough causes low blood glucose levels, and reducing insulin doses results in high blood glucose peaks.

Individuals with diabetes cannot starve themselves the same way as people without diabetes are able to, because insulin levels will not adapt to the situation of hunger as it does in people without diabetes. If you have diabetes, it is much more dangerous for you to make yourself vomit or take laxatives than it would be if you did not have diabetes. Your body will be easily thrown off balance, especially if you change insulin doses up and down as well. Your condition can deteriorate to a dangerous level and hospitalization may be necessary. A BMI below 14-15 (see page 272) usually indicates that you need medical attention. The risk of dying a diabetes-related death is considerably higher if you have anorexia too.[788] A high HbA_{1c} will increase your risk of developing late complications of diabetes in the future.

Anorexia and bulimia in someone with diabetes demand expert psychological and psychiatric care in addition to diabetes care. Anyone suffering from such a combination may also require a long hospital stay because of the risks of death and diabetic ketoacidosis if insulin is omitted. Family involvement should be an integral part of the treatment of eating disorders in young people.[245] Most people with these disorders can recover if they receive proper treatment.

Physical exercise

Everyone should do some form of physical exercise if they are to keep healthy. A body in good general condition can withstand hardships better. However, exercise must be enjoyable and should not be something one is forced into. Younger children usually run around a lot while they are playing, but older children are very different. Some like sports while others prefer to sit quietly with books, the television or a computer. We must adjust the insulin treatment to the individual, not the other way around, but as

Walking to and from school or riding your bicycle will give you some exercise every day. It is easier to find an appropriate dose of insulin when you are exercising daily than if you sit still one day and do a lot of exercise the next.

The effect of exercise on the blood glucose level

⟶ Exercise increases absorption of insulin from the injection site that you use during exercise, for example the thigh when running or playing football.

⟶ It also increases the consumption of glucose without increasing the need for insulin.

⟶ BUT — insulin must be available or the muscle cells will not be able to take up glucose!

⟶ **Beware!** Be careful with exercise when there is not enough insulin available in your body (blood glucose above 15-16 mmol/l, 270-290 mg/dl and elevated levels of ketones). You might need an extra insulin injection of approximately 0.05 U/kg (0.25 U/10 lb) and abstain from exercise for 2-3 hours until the blood glucose level has gone down.

⟶ You will be at risk of hypoglycaemia many hours afterwards (in the evening or night) because you have used the liver's store of glycogen after a lot of exercise.

⟶ If you exercise regularly you will know how much the blood glucose is affected but if you exercise only occasionally, your blood glucose may drop much more than you expect during and after exercise.

physical exercise increases the sensitivity for insulin in your body, we emphasize the importance of including exercise as part of your diabetes treatment right from the time that it is diagnosed. Schoolchildren and teenagers with diabetes actually tend to be more physically active than their friends without diabetes.[724,868] In a Spanish study, young people with diabetes aged 8-16 years had the same level of physical activity and fitness as their siblings. Moderate to vigorous physical activity was associated with better metabolic control and accounted for 30-37% of the difference in HbA_{1c}.[219] The selection of sporting activities is the same for both boys and girls with diabetes, compared with friends without diabetes.[868]

Everyone should be encouraged to take part in some form of regular physical activity, even if it is only riding a bicycle to and from work or school, and people with diabetes are no exception to this. Regular physical exercise lowers cardiovascular risk factors (overweight, hypertension, high blood lipids) in adults [662] and adolescents [55] with type 1 diabetes. In contrast, the pronounced lack of exercise and muscular activity in some teenagers seems to contribute

Exercise and insulin action

Insulin   Glucose (sugar)

Insulin

+ Oxygen

Energy
Carbon
dioxide
Water

Blood vessel   Muscle cell

Sitting still

Insulin "opens the door" to the cell for glucose to enter. The size of your insulin dose decides how quickly your blood glucose level will fall. Your regular insulin doses during school or work days are adjusted in line with your usual level of physical activity.

Insulin

+ Oxygen

Energy
Carbon
dioxide
Water

Physical exercise

If you play football or take part in some other type of intensive physical activity you will need to lower your insulin dose. Exercise will cause the same amount of insulin to keep the door open for a little longer, i.e. more glucose will be transported into the cell, and the blood glucose level can easily fall too low. Decrease the insulin dose slightly.

The effect of strenuous exercise may last for at least 8-10 hours which means that you should decrease your bedtime insulin as well (by 1-2, up to 4 units) and have a substantial bedtime snack to avoid night time hypoglycaemia.

to an increased insulin resistance, a tendency to be overweight and a deterioration in blood glucose control.[691]

When your muscles are working, the store of glucose in the muscles (muscle glycogen, approximately 400 g in an adult person) is used first. After this, glucose from the liver and fatty acids (breakdown products from fat) are used as fuel. Exercise lowers the blood glucose level by increasing glucose uptake into the muscle cells without increasing the amount of insulin needed. This is because more glucose is consumed by your muscles during exercise. After exercise, the muscles will have increased insulin sensitivity for 1-2 days [136,1083] (see also "Insulin

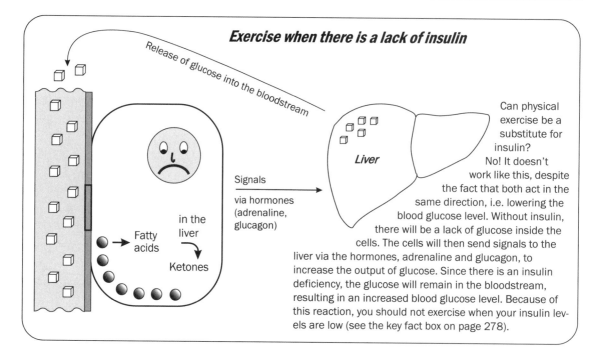

Exercise when there is a lack of insulin

Release of glucose into the bloodstream

Liver

Signals via hormones (adrenaline, glucagon)

Fatty acids

in the liver

Ketones

Can physical exercise be a substitute for insulin? No! It doesn't work like this, despite the fact that both act in the same direction, i.e. lowering the blood glucose level. Without insulin, there will be a lack of glucose inside the cells. The cells will then send signals to the liver via the hormones, adrenaline and glucagon, to increase the output of glucose. Since there is an insulin deficiency, the glucose will remain in the bloodstream, resulting in an increased blood glucose level. Because of this reaction, you should not exercise when your insulin levels are low (see the key fact box on page 278).

sensitivity and resistance" on page 223), leading to an increased risk of hypoglycaemia up to 24 hours after exercise.[706,891] This means that exercise 3-4 times a week will result in increased insulin sensitivity even between the training sessions, and the total insulin dose can probably be lowered. Sometimes the increased insulin sensitivity does not begin until 4-6 hours after the exercise [1083] and may occur during the night if you exercise in the evening.

Exercise and hypoglycaemia

Exercise can be classified into two forms: anaerobic and aerobic.[891] Anaerobic activities are characterized by higher intensities of muscular work (for example sprinting, power lifting, hockey). Aerobic activities involve lower intensities of muscular work (for example running, cycling, rowing, swimming and other endurance sports). Many aerobic activities include short bursts of anaerobic activity (like soccer and baseball). Anaerobic efforts last only a short time (sometimes only seconds) but may increase the blood glucose level dramatically

due to the release of the hormones adrenaline and glucagon.[891] This rise in blood glucose is usually transient, lasting typically 30-60 minutes, and can be followed by hypoglycaemia in the hours after finishing the exercise. Aerobic activities tend to lower blood glucose both during (usually within 20-60 minutes after the onset) and after the exercise.[891]

It is advisable to achieve a blood glucose level that is at least 6.5 mmol/l (120 mg/dl), if not higher, before the start of exercise to avoid hypoglycaemia.[1021] You may need repeated blood glucose tests, spaced about 30 minutes apart, to determine if your blood glucose is falling or rising prior to beginning your exercise. If the blood glucose is < 5 mmol/l (90 mg/dl), not rising, and the activity is primarily aerobic, there is a high risk of hypoglycaemia during the exercise.[891] If you have had an episode of hypoglycaemia prior to exercising (even during the previous night) you may have an increased risk of hypoglycaemia during your physical activity.[223] Due to this, it is a good idea to avoid exercising the day after an episode of severe hypoglycaemia.

If you exercise within 2 hours after a meal, you usually need to lower the bolus dose by 30-50%.[891,1050] For prolonged exercise (90 minutes or more), a greater reduction may be needed. The timing of exercise and risk of hypoglycaemia depends on what type of insulin you are using (see page 290). In one study, cross-country skiers with type 1 diabetes were able to carry on for several hours when reducing the premeal dose by 80%, compared with only 90 minutes if the dose was reduced by 50%.[933] Some people find that lowering their premeal insulin dose may cause an initial rise in their blood glucose which impairs their performance.[891] In such a case, it is probably better to rely on extra carbohydrate intake rather than dose reduction for best performance. If you take basal insulin only in the evening (Levemir or Lantus) and are going to exercise in the morning or take part in an all-day cup, the best way to decrease the basal insulin effect may be to switch to an injection of NPH insulin the evening before to get a shorter insulin action (try taking half your usual dose).

If you have been exercising your leg muscles, insulin injected into the thigh will be absorbed rather more quickly from the subcutaneous tissue (more so with short-acting than with rapid-acting insulin).[371] If you inject insulin deep enough to enter the muscle it will be absorbed much more quickly and you will risk having hypoglycaemia (see page 87). *It is important to remember that exercise alone will not lower the blood glucose level at all. Insulin has to be present to enable this to happen.* Glucose from the bloodstream needs insulin in order to enter the muscle cells.

The rate of glucose uptake into the muscles of an adult is approximately 8-12 g per hour when exercising at an ordinary rate, and is more than

doubled with heavy exercise.[1093] The levels of the hormones, adrenaline, glucagon and cortisol in the bloodstream increase during physical exercise. Glucose is released from the liver depot (liver glycogen, see page 34) and new glucose is produced in the liver from proteins. If the liver were unable to increase its glucose production, the blood glucose level would drop by about 0.1 mmol/l (2 mg/dl) per minute during exercise, soon resulting in hypoglycaemia.[1093] A high level of insulin in the blood counteracts the production of glucose in the liver which, in turn, increases the risk of hypoglycaemia. In people without diabetes, the level of insulin in the blood drops during exercise.[1093]

Your blood glucose level will rise if you exercise when the insulin level in your body is low. This is due to the lack of sugar inside your muscle cells causing different hormones to increase your blood glucose level. Your body still "thinks" as if it does not have diabetes, so it cannot adapt to the fact that you already have too much sugar in your blood. If your blood glucose level is high (above 14 mmol/l, 250 mg/dl) and you also have elevated ketone levels, you should take some extra insulin and wait a while for it to start working before exercising. The graph is from reference.[1078]

You can never replace insulin with exercise!
When exercising, you will need less insulin. But if you exercise without enough insulin in your body, your blood glucose level will rise.

How does the intensity of exercise affect my blood glucose?

Most team and field sports and also spontaneous play in children are characterized by repeated bouts of intensive activity interrupting longer periods of low to moderate intensity activity or rest. Contrary to what one may think, 30 minutes of this type of activity has been shown to produce a lesser fall in blood glucose levels compared with continuous moderate intensity exercise, both during and after the physical activity.[426] The participants in this study had higher heart rates and performed greater total workload during the intermittent high activity (4 seconds maximal sprint efforts every 2 minutes, in total 16 sprints). The repeated bouts of high-intensity exercise stimulated higher levels of noradrenaline that increased blood glucose levels.

In a second study, 20 minutes of moderate-intensity exercise (40% of VO_2 max, maximal oxygen uptake, on an exercise bike, equivalent to light jogging or cycling) was followed by an intense sprint at maximal intensity (cycling for as hard as possible) for 10 seconds on one occasion.[162] The fall of blood glucose during exercise was the same on both occasions, but the sprint prevented a further decline in blood glucose for at least 2 hours after the exercise. However, typical team games may last up to 90 minutes and the results may not be applicable to this length of physical activity.

Can the blood glucose level increase through exercise?

The blood glucose level will increase on account of exercise if there is not enough insulin. The cells don't "understand" that there is plenty of glucose in the bloodstream. On the contrary, they act as if the body was starving (see figures on page 25). This is caused by the muscle cells having a lack of glucose following a period of exercise in the presence of insulin deficiency. The muscle glycogen is used up, and insulin deficiency prevents new glucose from entering the cells. Hormonal signals will then tell the liver to release more glucose from its glycogen depot.

The signals to the liver are communicated by the hormones glucagon and adrenaline. The increased amount of glucose in the blood comes from both a breakdown of the liver's glycogen and a production of glucose in the liver. At the same time, when there is a lack of insulin, there will be a breakdown of fat to fatty acids which are transformed into ketones in the liver. This puts you at risk of developing ketoacidosis.[1093]

When your blood glucose level is above 14 mmol/l (250 mg/dl), and there are raised ketone levels indicating lack of insulin delivery,

Some general advice on exercise and diabetes adapted from [895]

➡ Tailor the insulin regimen to the activity. Multiple daily injections or a pump are easier to combine with active exercise.

➡ Use of detailed records of activity, insulin, food and glucose results is important for good diabetes control during exercise.

➡ Care should be taken that the meter and test strips chosen are suitable for the environment where they will be used (altitude, temperature).

➡ Any exercise is dangerous and should be avoided if pre-exercise blood glucose levels are high (> 14 mmol/l, 250 mg/dl) with elevated ketones in the urine (+ or more) or blood (> 0.5 mmol/l). Give approximately 0.05 U/kg or 5% of your TDD (total daily dose, including all meal bolus doses and basal insulin/basal rate in pump) and postpone exercise until ketones have cleared.

➡ Discuss the percentage reductions in insulin before exercise.

➡ When exercise is planned at a time of peak insulin action, a marked reduction in dose should be made.

➡ Do not inject the insulin in a site that will be heavily involved in muscular activity.

➡ A pump needs to be disconnected at least 90 minutes before starting the exercise to give a reduced basal effect during the exercise.

➡ Discuss type and amount of carbohydrate required for specific activities.

➡ Consume up 1.0–1.5 gram of carbohydrate/kg per hour of strenuous or endurance exercise when circulating insulin levels are high, if pre-exercise insulin doses are not decreased.

➡ If you drink sugar-containing fluids to keep your glucose level up, remember that dehydration is a risk unless sugar-free fluids also are consumed.

➡ Meals with high content of carbohydrates should be consumed shortly after the exercise event to take advantage of the period of heightened insulin sensitivity to help replenish liver stores of glycogen and limit post-exercise hypoglycaemia.

➡ Extra carbohydrate after the activity is often the best option to prevent hypoglycaemia for short duration and high-intensity anaerobic activities

➡ A mixture of aerobic and anaerobic exercise (soccer but also cycling, jogging and swimming with some spurts) will require extra carbohydrate before, possibly during and often after the activity.

➡ The rise in blood glucose after intense exercise may be prevented by giving a small additional dose of rapid-acting insulin at half-time or immediately after the exercise is finished, i.e. before the shower. This is especially important if you have an insulin pump that has been disconnected during the activity.

➡ Short (10 seconds) sprints added to aerobic training can decrease the risk of hypoglycaemia.

➡ Hypoglycaemia may be anticipated during or shortly after exercise, but is also possible up to 24 hours afterwards, due to increased insulin sensitivity.

➡ Alcohol inhibits the production of glucose in the liver (gluconeogenesis); hypoglycaemia is more likely if it is consumed after physical activity.

➡ Risk of post-exercise nocturnal hypoglycaemia is high, and particular care should be taken if bedtime blood glucose level is <7.0 mmol/L (125 mg/dL) with NPH basal insulin. With basal analogues (Lantus or Levemir), the bedtime glucose level can be slightly lower without a substantial risk of night time hypoglycaemia.

➡ Measure blood glucose before going to bed and decrease bedtime basal insulin (or pump basal) by 10-20% after an afternoon or evening session.

➡ Continuous glucose monitoring may have a role in helping to avoid hypoglycaemia during and after exercise.

➡ Careful advice on and planning of travel, exercise and management is essential.

➡ Snacks and hypoglycaemia remedies should always be readily available at school.

➡ Written advice on exercise and school outings should be provided for carers/teachers.

➡ Individuals who have proliferative retinopathy or nephropathy should avoid exercise likely to result in high arterial blood pressure.

➡ Professionals should take every opportunity to attend camps for children with diabetes.

exercise should be postponed while extra insulin is taken.[891] Running to lower a high blood glucose in this situation is not a good idea. It might even be dangerous. Try with half of the doses recommended in the table on page 115, and wait until your blood glucose and ketones have been lowered before exercising. If your blood glucose is high without ketones, try using half of the correction doses in the table on page 146.

Some friends of mine met a 45-year-old man when starting out on a mountain hike. He asked them if he could accompany them as he was alone, and they agreed. During the second day the man felt sick, began vomiting and appeared very tired. Then he told my friends he had diabetes. He was under the impression that exercise lowered the blood glucose level and had thought that exercise might cure his diabetes. He had left all his insulin at home. One of my friends ran 20 km (13 miles) to the nearest telephone, and called for a helicopter. But by the time it reached the camping site, the man was already dead. He died from a diabetic coma caused by a total lack of insulin, made more severe by the hard physical exercise.

This happened many years ago. Knowledge has improved since then and people with diabetes know it is dangerous to not take insulin. In spite of this, episodes of serious ketoacidosis, caused by missed insulin injections and requiring hospital treatment, are not uncommon. Many of these cases involve teenagers who do not realize how dangerous it can be to leave out insulin injections.

Hypoglycaemia after exercise

As the glycogen stores in the liver are decreased during exercise, there is a greatly increased risk of hypoglycaemia several hours after the exercise. The muscles will have increased insulin sensitivity for at least another 8-10 hours, sometimes up to 24 hours after the exercise is finished. This means that you are likely to be at risk of night time hypoglycaemia after strenu-

ous physical activity.[706] If you find yourself in this situation, you should begin by trying to refill the glycogen stores in your liver and muscles, by eating during and after the exercise. Count on needing an additional 10-15 g (1/3-1/2 ounce) of carbohydrate (15-30 g, 1/2-1 ounce, for an adult) for every 30 minutes of exercise after the initial 30 minutes,[1083] or approximately 1 g of glucose/kg body weight per hour.[363]

You might find it valuable to experiment with different amounts of carbohydrate during a game of football for example, and when you find a suitable amount, follow this up by eating the same amount of extra carbohydrate every time you play. If you start playing within 1 hour of your injection, the insulin uptake will be increased and you will probably need to

---

Research findings: Exercise and blood glucose control

♠ Controlled studies have not been able to show that physical exercise improves the management of diabetes.[1010,1093] Because of this, exercise is not considered as a treatment for diabetes.[480]

♠ However, some studies indicate that exercise in children and adolescents can have a beneficial effect on both HbA_{1c} and physical fitness. For example, a 30-minute programme of vigorous exercise three times a week was effective in lowering HbA_{1c} in children aged 5-11 years.[166]

♠ Young people (aged 10-18 years), exercising for less than one hour weekly, showed a higher HbA_{1c} level (74 mmol/mol, 8.9%) than those exercising for 2-6 hours (67 mmol/mol, 8.3%) or 6-8 hours (64 mmol/mol, 8.0%).[88]

♠ Light and moderate physical activity improved glucose control in schoolchildren, but not in teenagers, in another study.[724]

♠ Exercise capacity is not influenced by high blood glucose levels (test level 12.4 mmol/l, 225 mg/dl).[995]

To be able to run quickly your muscles need glucose. If your exercise session lasts longer than 30 minutes, you will need extra food, approximately 10-20 g of carbohydrate for every 30 minutes of exercise.

increase your carbohydrate intake again or decrease the insulin dose.[1025]

Remember that it takes more than one meal to refill the glycogen stores in your liver and muscles after heavy physical exertion. This means that even if you have eaten a substantial meal after the game you may become hypoglycaemic later in the day or evening, since the glycogen stores have not had time to be refilled completely. If you play sport in both the morning and the afternoon, you will be more likely to have problems with hypoglycaemia during the afternoon game for the same reason.

Hypoglycaemia can be minimized with appropriate reductions of the premeal doses when using multiple injection therapy with rapid-acting insulin or pumps. In addition, if you have been playing sport all afternoon, you are likely to need an extra helping at your evening snack. Your appetite may well remind you of this! However, even though you are eating more, you may still find your need for insulin has gone down, and you need to decrease the dose at the evening snack by 1-2 units. But don't decrease it too much, as the liver needs insulin to refill the glycogen stores. If you have problems with hypoglycaemia in spite of a reduced dose, you need to eat more carbohydrates. More often than not, the intermediate- or long acting insulin dose given at bedtime or before the last main meal should be decreased as well to avoid night time hypoglycaemia (decrease bedtime basal insulin or pump basal rate by 10-20%). In one hospital based study where 34% had night time hypoglycaemia using a two-dose treatment regimen NPH as basal insulin, a bedtime blood glucose of less than 7 mmol/l (125 mg/dl) suggested particular risk of nocturnal hypoglycaemia,[1103] while another study using long-acting basal analogues or pumps found a lower frequency of 13% but no threshold for nocturnal hypoglycaemia risk after exercise in the afternoon.[1043] You can try to go to sleep with a glucose level of 5-6 mmol/l (90-110 mg/dl) if the basal dose of Lantus, Levemir or a pump has been decreased. Check your blood glucose level 1-2 times during the night to know how this works for you/your child.

Research findings: Exercise and hypoglycaemia

♠ A 75-minute afternoon exercise session resulted in a drop of at least 25% from baseline blood glucose levels in most of the participants (aged 10-18 years) and 30% became hypoglycaemic (< 3.3 mmol/l, 60 mg/dl) when no extra carbohydrate was given before exercise.[1021]

♠ Children and adolescents aged 11-17 years using multiple injection treatment or pumps were found to have nearly twice the risk of night time hypoglycaemia (< 3.3 mmol/l, 60 mg/dl) after a 75-minute exercise session in the afternoon (4 × 15 minutes of exercise comparable to jogging with 5 minutes rest in between) when insulin doses were not lowered.[1043]

♠ In this study, night time hypoglycaemia was much more common in those exercising 6-7 days per week compared with < 4 days per week.

♠ Unfortunately, both low and moderate exercise can cause significant blunting of symptoms and hormonal counter-regulation (see page 33) during subsequent episodes of hypoglycaemia.[931]

♠ This effect can begin within hours of the exercise and last for 24 hours, increasing the risk of hypoglycaemia problems the next day. It is therefore very important to monitor your blood glucose frequently during exercise (every 30 minutes if needed) and afterwards (every 1-2 hours).[890]

Tips for heavy exercise

4-5 PM	Dinner/tea Decrease by 1-2 U if you are using Novo-Rapid or Humalog, preferably taking the dose at least 1 hour before the game. Take your ordinary insulin doses if you are using short-acting insulin.
	Take a blood test before the game:
< 5-6 mmol/l < 90-110 mg/dl	Take extra carbohydrates, for example lemonade
6-10 mmol/l 110-180 mg/dl	OK to get started. Many prefer no have normoglycaemia, i.e. a normal blood glucose of 4-8 mmol/l during the exercise. One way is to drink lemonade regularly to avoid hypoglycaemia. This often works better than starting high (10-12 mmol/l) so there is a margin for falling blood glucose during exercise.
10-14 mmol/l 180-250 mg/dl	Go ahead but take a blood glucose test again after 30 minutes-1 hour. Drink water when thirsty. If the glucose level is decreasing, there is insulin available and it is OK to continue. If the level is increasing, there is a lack of insulin and you should stop exercising and take extra insulin.
> 14 mmol/l > 250 mg/dl	Check for ketones in blood or urine. If positive take approximately 0.05 U/kg (0.025 U/lb) body weight of short-acting (or preferably rapid-acting) insulin and wait 1-2 hours for it to have an effect.
5-6 PM	**Game:** Eat half (or a small whole) banana at half-time.
8 PM	**Evening snack** (rich in carbohydrates): Eat more than usual. If insulin is due, take your ordinary dose but you will usually need to decrease it by 1-2 units.
10 PM	**Bedtime insulin:** Try lowering the dose by 1-2, up to 4 units, sometimes more, and have a bedtime snack. Lower the basal rate by 10-20% (0.1-0.2 units per hour) if you have a pump (use the temporary basal rate).

Tips for heavy exercise, cont.

Rule of thumb:	For every 30 minutes of heavy exercise you will need about 10-15 g (1/3-1/2 ounce) of extra carbohydrate (15-30 g, 1/2-1 ounce, for an adult). Take half as "quick-acting" carbohydrates (e.g. juice, sports drink) and half as slower carbohydrates (like a chocolate bar) or eat half to a whole banana (about 10-20 g of carbohydrate).
Hypoglycaemia:	Make sure that your coach and team-mates know how to help you should you need it. **Always carry glucose in a pocket!**
Hydration:	It is very important to prevent dehydration during exercise as this will increase the blood glucose level. In fact, a high blood glucose level prior to exercise may be partly caused by dehydration. Even a 1% decrease in body mass due to dehydration may impair performance.[841] Fluid intake should closely match sweating during exercise. Begin by drinking approximately 250 ml (~1 cup) 20 minutes before the exercise and then the same amount for every 20 minutes. of activity.[841]

It should be borne in mind that exercise can take many forms. It could include, for example, spending a full day swimming at the beach, a long bicycle ride, a day of skiing or ice skating, as well as many hours dancing or clubbing in the evening. The after effects of such aerobic exercise are all similar and often include delayed, activity-induced hypoglycaemia in the middle of the night or the next morning. Sleeping late the next morning can be especially dangerous under such circumstances. Mixing this increased activity with alcohol can cause particular problems since alcohol blocks the body's ability to respond to hypoglycaemia. Unconscious hypoglycaemic reactions or hypoglycaemic seizures may result if you forget to decrease your bedtime insulin or to have an extra snack before going to bed.

Physical education

Children and teenagers with diabetes can and should take part in physical education (P.E.) to the same extent as youngsters without diabetes. The risk of hypoglycaemia will be lower if P.E. activities can be timetabled for the second or third period following a meal if a child is using rapid-acting insulin (NovoRapid or Humalog), as the insulin level increases rapidly during the first hour after an injection (see graph on page 290). The first (or possibly the second) period in the morning, or alternatively the first (or possibly the second) period after lunch, is likely to be best when using regular short-acting insulin. The second class after lunch is less suitable for younger children as they are more likely to be active during the lunch break as well.

Talk to the P.E. teacher about the timetable well in advance to find out if it is possible to adjust the schedule. Indeed, it is important to be sure that the P.E. teacher, and any other members of staff who have regular contact with young people, is aware of any pupil with diabetes, what their particular needs are, how to recognize hypoglycaemia, what to do when it occurs and how to call others for help. The P.E. teacher and the school nurse should both have access to glucose tablets and know when and how they should be used. This should be a key part of the education plan for children with diabetes in all grades of the education system.

It would be helpful for children to have an extra snack before the P.E. lesson if their blood glucose is low. Many children need an extra snack after this sort of activity, in order to prevent delayed hypoglycaemia. Because of the risk of hypoglycaemia, a schoolchild who has diabetes should always be accompanied by a friend or teacher (who knows how to help) when climbing or balancing or on outings such as nature walks, cross country running, swimming or school trips.

In winter, most children will rush outside to play if they see snow fall, especially in areas such as southern England where global warming means this is now an exciting rarity. However, the extra exercise often makes it necessary to lower the doses by a unit or two at dinner/tea and the evening snack to avoid hypoglycaemia. If children have been out playing for many hours, it is advisable to lower the bedtime dose as well.

Top level competitive sports

You can certainly take part in competitive sports even if you have diabetes. There are many successful sportsmen and women with diabetes playing in international teams or at a professional level. A normal blood glucose level is essential if you are to achieve maximum performance. You may need to decrease the amount of insulin you take just before the physical exercise, for example a game of football or basketball. Remember that, if you have a difficult bout of hypoglycaemia, it will take you several hours to return to a level of maximum performance. Check your blood glucose level frequently to find out how your body reacts in different situations during training and competition. This will make it easier to plan food intake and insulin doses for the training sessions if they take place at regular times. For example, Sir Steve Redgrave (see page 409) has five Olympic gold medals in rowing, a tough endurance sport. While training, he needed to consume 6,000 calories a day, which he did in six meals, each accompanied by an insulin injection. And he measured his blood glucose before each meal so that he knew how much insulin to take.

High blood glucose levels may impair your performance for two reasons.[891] Firstly, if your blood glucose is high prior to the exercise, you may already be dehydrated due to increased urine volumes. Secondly, high blood glucose has been found to reduce the secretion of beta-endorphins during exercise, which has been associated with an increased rating of perceived exertion for both leg exercise [1089] and whole-body exercise.[889] A poor maximal aerobic capacity has been found in individuals with a high HbA$_{1c}$.[858] It is therefore very important

How do you take control of your blood glucose during exercise?

Sugary drink / Sugary drink
Glucose tablets

A non-diabetic person lowers the insulin level in the blood stream when exercising, to allow glucose from the liver to be released to the muscles. This is more difficult to achieve in a person with diabetes. You can instead fill up the amount of sugar that the muscles need by drinking something containing sugar, for example fruit juice or squash at regular intervals (see table on page 292). You can then begin your exercise with a slightly lower, i.e. normal, glucose level, which will boost your performance (A above). If you begin with slightly high blood glucose to leave a margin for hypoglycaemia and do not add carbohydrates during the session, you risk your blood glucose dropping so you need 'rescue glucose' resulting in a subsequent rebound phenomenon (B above).

to keep both your daily blood glucose levels and your long-term glucose control as good as possible to get the best out of your performance.

For many team sports you need your brain to take quick decisions, for example when playing ice hockey. I have had parents say that they can predict their child's blood glucose level from the stand by watching their behaviour in the game. It is then important to realize that your thinking ability and reaction time is affected both by low and high glucose levels (see page 330). A common piece of advice used to be to begin playing with a higher blood glucose level, often above

10mmol/l (180 mg/dl), to avoid hypoglycaemia when the level decreases during the exercise. However, many find that their performance improves if they begin with a normal glucose level of 5-6 mmol/l (90-110 mg/dl) and then drink a something sweet every 15-30 minutes (see table on page 292). In this way you will prevent hypoglycaemia before it occurs, and still be able to play with a normal blood glucose level. Your friends may find it strange that you who have diabetes drink something sweet while they drink water, so you may need to remind them how the insulin level decreases during exercise in a healthy person in a way that is not possible for you.

The best time to begin exercising varies slightly, depending on whether you are using regular short-acting insulin (Actrapid, Humulin S, Insuman Rapid) or rapid-acting insulin before meals (when on multiple daily injections or a pump). During the first hour after an insulin injection, the level of insulin in the blood increases quickly — particularly with Novo-Rapid or Humalog. If you were to exercise during this time, insulin would be absorbed even faster (especially if you have injected yourself in the thigh) making hypoglycaemia more likely (see illustration on page 87). You should therefore avoid injecting premeal doses in the thigh before exercising that involves leg work.[372]

① **Rapid-acting insulin**
   If you are using NovoRapid or Humalog, it may be better to decrease the dose by 1-2 units if you are going to exercise within 1-2 hours after the injection [1050] (see page 163).

② **Short-acting insulin**
   Exercise within 1 hour of the injection is usually OK.[1050] If you start your exercise 3 hours after the meal and the injection, you will probably need an extra snack before starting.

If you have problems with night time hypoglycaemia following evening training sessions, it may be better to reschedule them to the afternoon.[1093] Avoid being alone for strenuous training sessions as you may need the help of a friend if you have difficult or severe hypogly-

The blood glucose-lowering effect of exercise will last for at least 8-10 hours.
Always lower the bedtime dose by 2-4 units after heavy exertion, such as a game of football or squash.

caemia. Don't forget to decrease your bedtime insulin by 2-4 units after strenuous exercise, such as a football or rugby game. If you are using Lantus or Levemir once daily you may need to reduce the dose by 2-4 units the evening before a daytime exercise session that will last more than 2-3 hours.

If you use an insulin pump, try taking the pre-meal dose as usual (or perhaps 1-2 units less) and disconnect the pump during the period you are exercising (provided it is not for more than 1-2 hours). Another alternative is to try skipping the premeal injection before you start exercising, keeping the pump connected with the basal rate running during the exercise.

In competitive situations, your body may react a bit differently, even though you are doing the same physical work as you do during training. The stress both before and during competition will increase your blood glucose level with the help of adrenaline (by increasing the liver output of glucose).[890] This usually reduces the risk of hypoglycaemia and the need for extra carbohydrates during a competition as compared with a training session.[891] On the other hand, it will be even more important to eat extra food afterwards, so that you refill the glycogen stores in the liver and muscles. Playing sport in warm and humid environments may also increase blood glucose levels because of excessive increases in levels of counter-regulatory hormones.[890]

Physical exercise — some rules

① Plan ahead so that you have eaten and taken your premeal insulin 1-2 hours before you start exercising, otherwise you risk having the greatest blood glucose-lowering effect right at the beginning. If you are using NovoRapid or Humalog it may be better to reduce the dose by 1-2 units if you are going to exercise within 1-2 hours of the injection.[1050]

② Test your blood glucose before starting the exercise. If it is below 5-6 mmol/l (90-110 mg/dl) you should eat something before starting.[1093] If you have ketones in your blood or urine too, this is a sign that your cells are starving. You should wait until your blood glucose level has increased before you start your exercise.

③ If your blood glucose is above 14 mmol/l (250 mg/dl), you should check for ketones before starting the exercise. If your ketone levels are raised, you should not exercise until 1-2 hours after you have taken extra insulin (approximately 0.05 U/kg, 0.25 U/10 lb).

④ Eat something extra during exercise if the session lasts more than 30 minutes. Depending on your body size, a half to a whole banana (or other source of 10-20 g of glucose) is usually about right. Find out what suits you best. Take blood tests while you are exercising and note them in your logbook for future reference.

⑤ Eat a large meal after the exercise, preferably something with a high carbohydrate content, like sandwiches.

⑥ Decrease the insulin doses following exercise (evening premeal by 1-2 units and bedtime dose by 1-2, up to 4 units, or 10-20% decrease using temporary basal rate with a pump). If you exercise more than 3-4 times a week, the increased insulin sensitivity that your exercise causes will probably be effective "round the clock". You will therefore be unlikely to need to lower your insulin doses as much in this situation since they will already be adjusted for it. For seasonal sports you may need to lower your insulin 24-hour dose considerably during the active season, e.g. up to 40% when playing ice hockey.

⑦ If you exercise to lose weight, it is important to lower the premeal dose instead of eating more after exercising.

The effect of stress will often reveal itself early on in a competition. It is usually short-lived, often lasting only 10 or 20 minutes.[975] Different individuals react differently and you should find out how you react, for example by testing your

A Finnish study compared the use of Humalog and regular short-acting insulin prior to moderate exercise on a cycle exercise (comparable to jogging).[1050] This tells us that, even with relatively moderate exercise, the blood glucose level can decrease considerably if you time the exercise closely after a premeal dose of Humalog. With regular short-acting insulin you will have fewer problems with this intensity of exercise but as you see from the graph, there is still a drop in blood glucose levels which may get worse if you increase the load.

With the exercise timed late after the meal (3 hours in this study) there is a greater drop in blood glucose level with regular short-acting insulin than with Humalog.

Research findings:
exercise and carbohydrate intake

♠ Glycogen stores can be enhanced with a carbohydrate beverage approximately 1 hour before the activity (appropriate amount around 1-2 g of carb./kg (2-4 g/lb) body weight).[890]

♠ A beverage containing 6% simple sugar (i.e. sucrose, fructose, glucose) provides optimal absorption. More concentrated beverages (juice, carbonated drinks) may delay the absorption and cause stomach upset.[890]

♠ In an American study, teenage boys consumed a sports drink (Gatorade®, 6.5% sucrose/glucose) corresponding to 2 ml/kg (1.3 g of carbohydrate/10 kg, 2.8/10 lb body weight) and exercised for 10 minutes followed by 5 minutes rest.[1025]

♠ In spite of this the blood glucose level fell by on average 4.0 mmol/l (70 mg/dl) after 90 minutes (six bouts of exercise).

♠ Although the blood glucose level during exercise varies greatly between children, it does seem to be fairly constant for any given individual, as long as exercise conditions, pre-exercise insulin and carbohydrate intake are consistent.[890,1025]

♠ During heavy exercise, the total carbohydrate utilization may be as great as 1.0-1.5 g/kg per hour in adolescents both with and without diabetes.[890]

♠ By supplying this amount of carbohydrate as 6-8% glucose solution, the likelihood of hypoglycaemia was greatly reduced in a study of 20 adolescents performing 60 minutes of moderate intensity and cycling 100 minutes after an insulin injection and breakfast.[888]

♠ In another study, adolescent boys used Gatorade with glucose and fructose added to 8 or 10% carbohydrate drink.[831] When they drank ~10 ml/kg (0.9 g or 1.1 g carbohydrate/kg, 1.9 g or 2.4 g/lb respectively) there was no change in blood glucose during 60 minutes of exercise (at 55-60% of VO_2 max). During 60 minutes recovery there was a slight decrease in blood glucose when using the 8% carbohydrate drink. The high concentration did not cause any stomach distress.

♠ The only way to find out what is best for you is to experiment yourself to find out how much extra carbohydrate is needed for your type of activity.

blood glucose level during the first break of the game (like the professional soccer player Gary Mabbutt, see page 408).

If you find your blood glucose levels go up when you compete, you can try taking the insulin dose less than an hour before you start. In some team sports (such as ice hockey) you will probably be sitting on the bench for a large part of the game so there will be less physical exercise in total compared with a training session.

Very heavy exertion can cause excessive amounts of adrenaline to be secreted. This can make the blood glucose level rise even though insulin levels are adequate.[720] After a heavy bout of exercise, such as a game of football, the

Should you lower your premeal insulin doses before exercising?

A study of adults using Ultralente and Humalog, found that blood glucose was lowered approximately 3.0 mmol/l (55 mg/dl) after 60 minutes of light exercise or 30 minutes of heavy exercise.[867] This should be taken into consideration when you take your premeal insulin dose of rapid-acting insulin. If your blood glucose level is a bit high, such a drop in the level may be a good thing, but if it is lower (< 6-8 mmol/l, 110-145 mg/dl) the premeal dose can be lowered according to the table below in order to reduce the risk of hypoglycaemia. The participants in this study did not take any extra carbohydrate during the exercise. If you do eat something, the applicable reductions in insulin dose will be lower. This is very individual, of course, but after some attempts you will know which levels and doses suit your body best.

Reduction of premeal insulin dose

Intensity of exercise	30 min.	60 min.
Walking, swimming (25% of VO_2max*)	25%	50%
Jogging (50% of VO_2max)	50%	75%
Football, handball (75% of VO_2max)	75%	100% (no dose)
*Maximal oxygen uptake		

blood glucose will often be raised because of stress hormones in people who do not have diabetes. They can compensate for this by doubling the level of insulin in their blood. People with diabetes have the same reaction, but as their insulin levels are not increased, the blood glucose level will rise sharply instead.[748] Women have higher increases of blood glucose after exercise for a comparable degree of exertion.[720] The rise in blood glucose is usually transient but tends to last for up to 2 hours.[720] It is difficult to match this situation with extra insulin but if you have this reaction often, you could try taking a small dose of rapid-acting insulin at half-time or immediately after the exercise is finished.[720]

Keeping fit with diabetes

One study of teenagers with diabetes showed that those with higher HbA_{1c} had poorer capacity for physical work.[66] This means that if you want to achieve top performance you must also have an optimal HbA_{1c}. Competitive athletes risk decreasing their insulin too much in an attempt to avoid hypoglycaemia, thus resulting in higher HbA_{1c} levels compared with those doing moderate physical exercise.[314] However, in a group of young people aged 10-18 years, those taking part in a competitive sport involving at least 6 hours of exercise per week, had a lower HbA_{1c}.[88] Although physical training enhances insulin sensitivity, it improves HbA_{1c} levels only if blood glucose is carefully monitored.

Regular exercise (at least every other day) leads to a decreased insulin resistance (see page 223) that lasts between the sessions. Correspondingly, inactivity (for instance caused by being confined to bed) gives an increased resistance within days.[1083] Active athletes in training will therefore need to lower all their insulin doses considerably. When the training season is over, the doses are likely to need a considerable increase if higher blood glucose levels are to be avoided. Sometimes 30-50% more insulin is needed during the inactive season. A major ben-

efit for all young people with diabetes is that regular daily exercise of one sort or another helps to keep the weight down and also in the long term improves heart and blood vessel fitness.

However, a person with diabetes-related eye damage, kidney damage or nerve damage should consult their doctor about what type of exercise is most appropriate. It is important to be careful with strenuous physical exercise if you have pronounced complications in your eyes, kidneys or nervous system. This is because

How much extra carbohydrate is needed for exercise?

This table from reference [890] shows the estimated number of minutes that a specified activity lasts to require 15 g of extra carbohydrate to keep your blood glucose from falling. For example, a 40 kg child should consume 15 g of carbohydrate for every 15 minutes of basketball, whereas a 60 kg child should consume 15 g of carbohydrate for every 10 minutes of basketball. If you lower premeal or basal insulin doses, you will probably need less extra carbohydrate than the table shows. See reference [828] for a more complete list of sports.

Activity, minutes	Body weight		
	20 kg	40 kg	60 kg
Basketball (game)	30	15	10
Cross-country ski	40	20	15
Cycling 10 km/h	65	40	25
15 km/h	45	25	15
Figure skating	25	15	10
Ice hockey (ice time)	20	10	5
Running 8 km/h	25	15	10
12 km/h	-	10	10
Snow shoeing	30	15	10
Soccer	30	15	10
Swimming, breast stroke 30 m/min.	55	25	15
Tennis	45	25	15
Walking 4 km/h	60	40	30
6 km/h	40	30	25

vigorous exercise will increase the risk of high blood pressure or skin wounds.[1093] A cold bath after a sauna will also give a quick increase of your blood pressure. People with complicated eye damage (so called proliferative retinopathy) should avoid strenuous exercise and anyone who has loss of sensation in their feet should limit weight-bearing exercise (e.g. running or playing football).[32] People with kidney damage often have a reduced capacity for exercise, which places an automatic limit on their activity level.[32]

Camps and skiing trips

If you are physically active for a prolonged period, on a skiing trip or an outward bound camp for example, you will have an increased insulin sensitivity after 1-2 days which will probably call for substantially lower insulin doses (decreased by 20% or sometimes even 50% especially if you are not used to hard physical exercise). You must increase your food intake to compensate for the increased energy output and it is usual to be hungry after a day of vigorous activity. The increased insulin sensitivity will continue for at least a couple of days after you return home.[136] Check your blood glucose levels and you will see when it is time to increase the insulin doses again. It is important when skiing to eat extra sweet snacks before

Adventure travel

Extreme physical performance can be achieved by very careful planning, although there may still be risks. Altitude sickness is defined as headache (often severe) and one of the following symptoms: nausea, vomiting, lack of appetite, fatigue, light-headedness or sleeping difficulties.[150] The only treatment is to descend when symptoms persist. More serious symptoms are unsteady gait (indicating brain oedema) and shortness of breath when resting (indicating lung oedema). Both these are serious medical conditions that can prove fatal if left untreated. Consult a doctor with experience of altitude sickness before starting such a trip.

There appears to be no increase in the risk of altitude sickness in individuals with diabetes.[150] However, many of the symptoms may be difficult to distinguish from symptoms of hypoglycaemia. The "success rate" (rate of participants who reach the summit) seems to be almost as high as for those without diabetes.[150]

The participants with diabetes in a mountaineering expedition on Kilimanjaro decreased their insulin doses by half.[757] They had more symptoms of acute altitude sickness than the other participants. More worryingly, some experienced severe hypoglycaemia and there were two episodes of ketoacidosis. Both individuals had taken a drug called acetazolamide to prevent altitude sickness. This drug makes the blood slightly acidic and may have contributed to their ketoacidosis. However, in another report 8 out of 11 participants with diabetes used acetazolamide without side effects and

---

Exercise advice for people who have complications arising from diabetes

A careful medical history and physical examination can minimize risks associated with competitive sports for people who have long-term complications of diabetes. In many cases a formal graded exercise test will be helpful to determine the level of exercise:[533]

➠ Age > 35 years.

➠ Age > 25 years and duration of type 1 diabetes of > 15 years.

➠ Presence of any additional risk factors for heart disease (overweight, hypertension, high lipid levels).

➠ Presence of eye damage (so called proliferative retinopathy) or kidney damage (including microalbuminuria).

➠ Diabetes complications in the feet.

➠ Damage to autonomic nervous system (see page 363).

Using a sensor when exercising?

A sensor is a very practical way of getting real-time information on your glucose levels. You can try to follow the table below to find out what works for you. If your sensor glucose is < 7 mmol/l (125 mg/dl) during exercise and dropping, you need to take action:

Blood glucose	Arrows	Action
6.1-6.9 mmol/l (109-124 mg/dl)	↓ or ↓↓	8 g carbs (2 tabl.*)
5.0-6.0 mmol/l (90-108 mg/dl)	↓	16 g carbs (4 tabl.)
	↓↓	20 g carbs (5 tabl.)
<5 mmol/l (90 mg/dl)	No arrow	16 g carbs (4 tabl.)
	↓ or ↓↓	20 g carbs (5 tabl.)

*4 g glucose tablets

If your glucose is < 3.9 mmol/l (70 mg/dl), rest until your blood glucose rises. The table is adapted from reference [892]. The participants in this study aged 8-17 years and weighed approximately 40-70 kg. The amount of carbohydrate above prevented hypoglycaemia for at least 60 minutes of continued activity. There were no episodes of high glucose > 10 mmol/l (180 mg/dl) as a result of the glucose intake. Most participants had reduced their insulin administration (either basal or bolus) by 20-50% and if needed, taken a pre-exercise snack. About half of them used a pump and half used multiple daily injection therapy.

The study was done with 4 g glucose tablets, but if you only have 3 g glucose tablets available, you can try the amounts below:

Blood glucose	Arrows	Action
6.1-6.9 mmol/l (109-124 mg/dl)	↓ or ↓↓	9 g carbs (3 tabl.**)
5.0-6.0 mmol/l (90-108 mg/dl)	↓	15 g carbs (5 tabl.)
	↓↓	21 g carbs (7 tabl.)
<5 mmol/l (90 mg/dl)	No arrow	15 g carbs (5 tabl.)
	↓ or ↓↓	21 g carbs (7 tabl.)

**3 g glucose tablets

took 2 extra days of acclimatization on the way up. Seven of the 11 reached the summit at 5895 m., a similar proportion compared to those without diabetes.[584]

Meticulous planning can minimize problems, however. One father took a long-distance canoeing trip with his two sons, covering the entire coastline of Sweden (more than 2000 km, 1250 miles). One of the boys was 15 years old, and had diabetes. He managed the whole trip without severe hypoglycaemia. Talk to your doctor about how to plan insulin doses, food intake and glucose testing before you attempt any such extreme situations.

Anabolic steroids

Anabolic steroids are unfortunately used by many sportsmen and women in spite of all the warnings from the medical profession, not to mention the risk of being discovered in a doping control. How might anabolic steroids affect diabetes? They are known to disturb the glucose metabolism in people without diabetes, because they increase the body's resistance to insulin. So they are also likely to increase insulin resistance

How much energy is spent per hour? (adults)

⇨ Slow walking	100-200	kcal
⇨ Bicycling (leisure)	250-300	kcal
⇨ Table tennis, golf, tennis (doubles)	300-350	kcal
⇨ Dancing	300-400	kcal
⇨ Gymnastics	300-400	kcal
⇨ Tennis (singles)	400-500	kcal
⇨ Gym work-out	approx. 500	kcal
⇨ Jogging, downhill skiing, football	500-600	kcal
⇨ Swimming	approx. 600	kcal
⇨ Cross-country skiing	800-1000	kcal

Diving and diabetes

The diving clubs in the UK (BSAC, SAA and SSAC) allow a person with diabetes to dive if certain conditions are fulfilled.[319] These rules are also referred to by the US diving organizations DAN and UHMS.

➥ The medication regimen of the diver with diabetes should not have changed considerably during the course of the last year.

➥ No severe hypoglycaemia (requiring help from another person, glucagon treatment or hospital admission) should have occurred during the last 12 months.

➥ No hospitalization during the last 12 months for diabetes-related conditions.

➥ Satisfactory glucose control throughout the last 12 months (HbA$_{1c}$ < 75 mmol/mol (9.0%)).

➥ There should be no evidence of long-term complications of diabetes (retinopathy, nephropathy including microalbuminuria, neuropathy and heart and blood vessel disease).

➥ The physician in charge of the diver's diabetes should confirm that he/she considers the diver both mentally and physically capable of undertaking the demands of sport diving.

➥ The diver with diabetes should be prepared to give an annual lecture to his/her club on the problems associated with diabetes and diving.

➥ An SOS (MedicAlert) bracelet stating that the diver has diabetes should be worn at all times.

It is possible to dive if you have diabetes. You must be extra careful to avoid hypoglycaemia as this can be very dangerous when you are under water. However, it is not justifiable from a medical standpoint to have a standard diving certificate. The diver who has diabetes should have as their diving buddy, someone who is familiar with the problems of diabetes (but this person should not have diabetes). This can be either a regular diving partner or a trained medic/paramedic.

Diving

Diving is a fascinating sport, which places great demands on the individuals performing it. Tasks that are easy to accomplish on shore (like opening a package of dextrose) may be very difficult to do in the water even without any hypoglycaemic symptoms. Hypoglycaemia may proceed into sudden unconsciousness with the risk of drowning. It therefore implies additional risks also for the diving partner who does not have diabetes. Diving with diabetes has been much discussed and opinions on the subject differ. However, on the basis that the degree of caution called for is over and above that required of their counterparts without diabetes, most diving organizations now allow people with diabetes to dive under certain conditions (see key fact box). A continuous glucose monitoring system (CGMS worn under a dry suit) during five dives to a maximum depth of 29 metres did not show any signs of hypoglycaemia in one study.[11]

in people who have diabetes, but this has not yet been studied. There also appears to be a risk of hormonal changes, and some reports indicate problems with impotence. The long-term effects of anabolic steroids are still not very well understood, but it is likely they will prove to be very dangerous, especially for people who also have diabetes.

Tips when diving (modified from [319])

➡ To be able to experience obvious symptoms of hypoglycaemia below 4.0 mmol/l (70 mg/dl) on the day of diving, you must take care to avoid having any readings below 4-5 mmol/l (70-90 mg/dl) 1-2 weeks prior to the dive.

➡ *Never* dive if you have hypoglycaemia unawareness or if you have had any readings below 3.5 mmol/l (65 mg/dl) within 24 hours of the dive (otherwise your hypoglycaemia warning symptoms will be inadequate, see page 52).

➡ Don't drink alcohol within 24 hours of the dive.

➡ Eat more carbohydrate than usual on the day of the dive and drink enough not to be dehydrated.

➡ Dive after a meal. Leave at least 1-2 hours between your premeal insulin dose and diving if you are using rapid-acting insulin. Try decreasing the premeal dose by 1-2 units. The blood glucose level should be at least 8, preferably 10 mmol/l (145-180 mg/dl) when you start diving. Eat extra carbohydrate just before diving.

➡ Have two packets of glucose tablets or gel/liquid in the pockets of your wet suit and practise taking them out in water and under water. The nozzle of a tube of glucose gel/liquid can be placed between the mouthpiece of the demand valve and the corner of the mouth, thus avoiding the need to remove the mouthpiece from the mouth. Glucagon for injection should be readily available in the boat and on the shore, and someone should be available who can give an emergency injection.

➡ Always dive with a friend or trained medic/paramedic who is capable of giving you adequate help (such as glucose under water) if you develop hypoglycaemia. Your diving partner should *not* have diabetes.

➡ Decide on a signal in advance to indicate when you begin to feel hypoglycaemic.

➡ Measure your blood glucose after the dive and take extra food or insulin. If you deliberately keep your blood glucose level slightly high when diving, you can take extra insulin if it is still high after the dive. This will prevent your HbA$_{1c}$ from being negatively affected by frequent diving. Be aware that you are at greater risk of hypoglycaemia after heavy exertion and use only small doses of extra insulin.

Olle Sandelin, Swedish diving physician, says:[930]
— A declaration of health for a normal diving certificate is not possible when it comes to individuals having diabetes who are treated with insulin. Individuals with diabetes should dive with an instructor or with a so called handicap certificate which is only valid when they are accompanied by two people instead of one, which is the usual requirement.

Consulting physician Bengt Pergel from the Swedish Marine gives the following advice: [670]
— An ordinary diving certificate should not be issued to a person with diabetes out of consideration for both the diver and the person she/he is diving with. If a person diving has diabetes it is essential that everyone in the diving team knows about it.

— When it comes to the physical examination, the doctor issuing the certificate must be able to verify that the person doesn't have an increased risk of hypoglycaemia when doing the heavy physical work associated with diving. This may be a difficult decision even for a qualified diabetologist. It is virtually impossible to adjust blood glucose levels while diving and it is very difficult even when swimming at the surface. Divers who count on having glucose available in their life jacket pockets have probably never been diving in rapid water or a rough sea.

Christopher Edge, UK diving physician (who is referenced in the key fact boxes) says:
— Don't forget that we don't allow the vast majority of adolescents to dive with diabetes, as their control is very rarely good enough, and a lot of the time there is parental pressure on them to "dive with dad". We've only allowed one 16-year-old to dive. Certainly no-one under 16 has been considered.

While you are diving you must be able to recognize clearly symptoms of blood glucose levels below 4.0 mmol/l (70 mg/dl). If you have so-called "hypoglycaemia unawareness" (see page 52) with blood glucose levels less than 3

Limitations for the diver with diabetes [319]

➠ All members of the diving team must be informed that you have diabetes.

➠ It is advisable to dive only a maximum of two dives per day (and on not more than three consecutive days) to avoid the build-up of an excessive tissue nitrogen load.

➠ Do not dive deeper than 30 m.

➠ Remain well within the diving tables or have no more than 2 minutes no-stop time left on a dive computer.

➠ Be aware that diving sickness ("the bends") has similar symptoms to hypoglycaemia (e.g. confusion, unconsciousness, seizures). In this situation, treat as if the person has both conditions, giving both oxygen and glucose or a glucagon injection.

See references [318] and [638] for further advice.

mmol/l (55 mg/dl) without symptoms, *your life will be in danger if you dive*!

You should eat extra carbohydrates before diving, just as you would before any strenuous physical exercise, to keep your blood glucose level reasonably high (around 10-12 mmol/l, 180-215 mg/dl). This will help, as far as possible, to prevent hypoglycaemia under water. Cold water increases the body's energy consumption. If your blood glucose level is high due to an insulin deficit, you will not feel well and diving will be dangerous, even life-threatening. You should also check for ketones in your blood or urine before you dive (see page 111). The message here is that it is much better to have a higher glucose level because of eating too much, rather than because your body has too little insulin.

Hypoglycaemia in or under water is the greatest problem when diving with diabetes. Getting dextrose out of a pocket can be difficult enough even at the surface. To do it under water while experiencing hypoglycaemia may be close to impossible, as your symptoms make the task even more difficult. Practise finding dextrose both in and under water.

Stress

Stress and psychological strain affect your body and will at times increase the blood glucose level on account of the way different hormones behave. Different individuals are more or less sensitive to these reactions in their bodies.

When the body is exposed to stress, the adrenal glands secrete the hormone adrenaline which in turn increases the output of glucose from the liver. To explain this you must understand our Stone Age legacy. During this far off period, stress was usually associated with danger, for example an attacking bear. The alternatives were to stay and fight or to run away as quickly as possible. Extra fuel in the form of increased glucose in the blood is needed for both these responses.

Today, the same stress reaction can occur in front of the TV if you are watching something exciting, but you will not benefit from the increased blood glucose level. A person without diabetes will automatically release insulin from their pancreas to restore the glucose balance. In theory it is possible for a person with diabetes to take extra insulin in this situation. In practice this is often hard to accomplish since it is diffi-

cult to evaluate one's stress level, and the stress will be different from day to day. It is advisable to be careful when using extra insulin to treat high blood glucose levels caused by stress.

In one study, adults with diabetes performed a mental stress test for 20 minutes causing the blood glucose level to rise after 1 hour. It continued to be raised by about 2 mmol/l (35 mg/dl) for another 5 hours.[751] The blood pressure was increased as well and the stress induced a resistance to insulin (see page 223) via increased levels of the hormones adrenaline, cortisol and growth hormone. Patients who were able to produce some of their own insulin found the stress had less influence on their blood glucose level.

Another study used a stress-test composed of a 5-minute preparation task, a 5-minute speech task where subjects had to introduce themselves and apply for a job, and a 5-minute mental arithmetic task.[1107] Blood glucose levels were raised approximately 1.0-1.4 mmol/l (18-25 mg/dl) with a delay of 30 minutes after the test and lasted for approximately 2 hours. However, the effect of stress on blood glucose was seen only after a meal, but not if the test was performed in a fasting state. After the earthquake in Kobe, HbA$_{1c}$ levels rose in people living in the affected area. The highest increase was found in those who had experienced the death or injury of a close relative, and those whose homes had been severely damaged.[551]

Studies of heart attack victims have shown that so-called positive stress is not as dangerous as other forms of stress. Positive stress is defined as the kind of tension that is produced when you have a lot to do, but you choose to do it yourself and you are in control of the situation. The type of negative stress that increases the risk of heart attack is when the person cannot

A divorce is always stressful for a child. If, instead of cooperating, the parents engage in a "tug of war" with the child, his or her situation will become very difficult. The child will feel bad in every sense and the blood glucose levels and HbA$_{1c}$ are likely to increase as a result.

Your body is built to withstand the strenuous life of a Stone Age man or woman. In a stress situation, large amounts of adrenaline are secreted to help prepare the body for fight against, or flight away from, the danger.

Stress

➠ Stress that cannot be influenced (such as problems in the family or at work) will have the greatest effect on your health.

➠ Stress can also affect your blood glucose for the simple reason that you will not have as much time to care for your diabetes when life becomes busy and stressful.

➠ Adrenaline (stress hormone) gives

① Increased blood glucose level by:
  A) Release of glucose from the liver.
  B) Decreased uptake of glucose into the cells.

② Ketones by:
  Breakdown of fat into fatty acids that are transformed into ketones in the liver.[637]

---

influence the situation, for example, if they are having problems at work or at home within the family, such as relationship break-up or divorce. Similar situations may contribute to an increased blood glucose level as well. One of our patients was a little boy whose blood glucose level went up whenever an intravenous needle was inserted. The level remained elevated for several days in spite of increased insulin doses. It was the needle that bothered him. As soon as it was removed his blood glucose returned to normal and the insulin doses could be decreased again. In one study of adolescents, higher blood glucose levels were found after negative stress.[464]

Blood glucose readings taken at the hospital are often higher than those taken at home. Raised blood glucose levels have been observed in people with diabetes, in both outpatient [167] and inpatient [443] settings. This is also the case for blood pressure measurements, so called "white coat hypertension".

Stress in daily life

Everyday stress factors can cause a higher HbA_{1c}.[209] For example, during school exams many people find that the stress causes higher blood glucose levels. The exams also involve a change to routines and you may forget to take your insulin, or forget to bring dextrose into the

exams with you. It is not a good idea to take extra insulin before the exam, but when it is over, a small amount extra might well be justified.

Parents' stress reactions can be very important for children's psychological adjustment to diabetes. Metabolic control is better in families where the mother and, in particular, the child show initial injection anxiety and protest, but less generalized distress.[1033] This implies that distress in itself makes adaptation more difficult and that families who focused their emotional upset on the practical aspects of the disease used problem-solving coping strategies. Since the daily management of diabetes involves such a great deal of practical application, it is probably necessary to control one's feelings in order to be more problem-focused.[1033]

Learned helplessness is a phenomenon that can occur when you feel unable to control a situation and the reason for this is unrealistic expectations rather than insufficient ability on the part of the individual.[309] One example is when you follow every piece of advice given by the diabetes team and your blood glucose is still

Research findings: Stress and HbA$_{1c}$ levels

♠ One study found that individuals with higher HbA$_{1c}$ levels reported poorer quality of life, and more anxiety and depression.[730]

♠ When the HbA$_{1c}$ value was increased or decreased during the scope of the study, the scores for quality of life, anxiety and depression changed accordingly.

♠ These results suggest that you will feel better with a lower HbA$_{1c}$. However, another interpretation is that it is easier to obtain a good HbA$_{1c}$ when you feel well.

♠ Individuals who had experienced many severe stress factors (unpleasant life events, ongoing long-term problems, conflicts with other people) within the previous 3 months had higher HbA$_{1c}$ in one study.[680]

♠ Another study showed that stress causes a higher HbA$_{1c}$ but only in individuals who handle the stress in an ineffective way.[843] Anger, impatience and anxiety were examples of ineffective coping mechanisms. Stoicism (not reacting emotionally in stressful situations), pragmatism (handling stress in a problem-oriented way) and denial (disregarding the stress and thereby not letting it affect you) were effective coping mechanisms.

♠ However, in earlier studies, denial has been shown to have a correlation with impaired blood glucose control.[843] This might be explained by the fact that a problem must first be recognized before being solved. Appearing to accept a chronic disease initially, but then refusing to let it affect your daily life negatively, may be an effective form of denial.

♠ In an analysis of 24 studies (so called meta-analysis), depression in individuals with diabetes was associated with a higher HbA$_{1c}$.[700] However, it is difficult to conclude whether the elevated HbA$_{1c}$ is the result of depression or the other way around.

♠ Some data indicate that anti-depressive medication can improve HbA$_{1c}$ in people with depression.[700]

"Negative stress" is experienced when a person cannot change a stressful situation. Insurmountable problems at work, or at home within the family, may contribute to a raised blood glucose level.

much too unstable. This "teaches" you that it is not possible to control your blood glucose and, after a while, you will stop trying. The reason for this is the unrealistic expectation that you can achieve a stable blood glucose level simply by "trying hard". This has also been called "diabetes burnout".[857] An example of a realistic expectation is that your blood glucose will swing between high and low values and that you will have at least one reading above 10 mmol/l (180 mg/dl) every day. It can be realistic to try to achieve a lower average blood glucose (HbA$_{1c}$) without laying yourself open to an increase in hypoglycaemia-related problems. Realistic expectations for the long term might include being able to manage school or work, for example, without being inconvenienced to any great extent by your diabetes.

Fever and sick days

If you have an infection, especially if you are running a temperature with it, the secretion of blood glucose-raising hormones (particularly cortisol and glucagon [1081]) is increased. This effectively also increases your insulin requirements. However, it is common to eat less and rest more when you are ill, so these factors usually balance each other out. The basic rule, therefore, is to resist decreasing your insulin doses despite a drop in food intake.

Start by taking your usual dose. Measure your blood glucose level before each meal and adjust the dose before eating. If your blood glucose level is above 8 mmol/l (145 mg/dl) you should give extra insulin according to the correction factor (see page 146). The correction factor needs to be recalculated every day when the child is ill in line with how the total daily dose of insulin changes. Include extra doses given

because of high blood glucose in the total daily dose.

With temperatures above 38° C (100° F) a 25% dose increase is often needed. Sometimes up to a 50% increase of the total dose over 24 hours is needed if your temperature is above 39° C (102° F).[691] If you use a two-dose treatment it can be difficult to meet the changing needs of insulin when you are ill and it is probably best to change temporarily to four or five doses per day while you are unwell. An alternative is to give extra doses of rapid-acting insulin when the blood glucose is high (see algorithm on page 149).

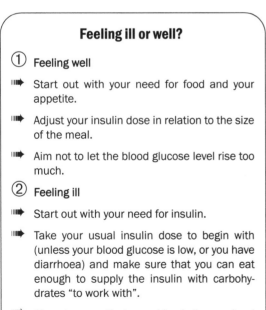

Feeling ill or well?

① **Feeling well**

⇒ Start out with your need for food and your appetite.

⇒ Adjust your insulin dose in relation to the size of the meal.

⇒ Aim not to let the blood glucose level rise too much.

② **Feeling ill**

⇒ Start out with your need for insulin.

⇒ Take your usual insulin dose to begin with (unless your blood glucose is low, or you have diarrhoea) and make sure that you can eat enough to supply the insulin with carbohydrates "to work with".

⇒ Aim at preventing your blood glucose level from falling too low by drinking something sugary if necessary.

Illness and need for insulin

⇒ Fever increases the need for insulin.

⇒ **But** — decreased appetite and food intake decrease the need for insulin.

⇒ **Thus** — you will probably have at least the same need for insulin per 24 hours as usual.

⇒ **You are likely to** need up to 25-50% more insulin when you are feverish.

⇒ You could also be at risk from **ketoacidosis** caused by insulin deficiency. Check for ketones in your blood or urine!

⇒ **But** — you may need less insulin if you have gastroenteritis with vomiting **and** diarrhoea.

IMPORTANT!

When you are ill, you need to adjust "by eye" or by changing your insulin:carb ratios to decide upon the meal doses!

➠ **Correction factor (insulin sensitivity factor):**
Begin by using your ordinary correction factor when ill. Recalculate it every day using the 100-rule for mmol/l (1800-rule for mg/dl). See page 146. Use the 200-rule for mmol/l (3600-rule for mg/dl) during the night.

➠ **Carbohydrate ratio:**
Your usual insulin doses will not suffice when you have a fever. Lower your insulin:carb ratios by 10-20% to increase your meal doses, and evaluate by checking your blood glucose 2 hours after meals. If you have problems with low glucose levels, for example when you have a tummy upset or gastroenteritis, you need to raise the insulin:carb ratios in order to decrease your insulin doses.

➠ **Measurement by eye:**
Increase or decrease your meal doses by 10-20% depending on your glucose levels.

Diabetes and illness in children

(adapted from [968])

① **Treat the current illness**
The reason for the child's illness must be diagnosed and treated in the same way as for children without diabetes.

② **Symptomatic treatment**
If the child has a fever or headache, paracetamol/acetaminophen (Calpol®, Disprol®, Panadol®) or ibuprofen (Advil®, Motrin®) can be given to relieve symptoms. The child will feel better and often have a better appetite.

③ **Staying home from school**
It is advisable to let a sick child with diabetes stay at home as blood glucose levels are affected by infection and fever.

④ **Fluid balance**
It is important to give plenty of liquids to a child who is running a temperature, especially if they also have a high blood glucose level (> 12-15 mmol/l, 215-270 mg/dl) as this will cause them to produce larger volumes of urine than usual. The risk of dehydration may increase rapidly if the child vomits or has diarrhoea.

⑤ **Nutrition**
It is important that the child gets insulin, sugar and nourishment. Serve something the child enjoys and is likely to eat.

During the remission phase (honeymoon phase, see pages 221 and 177), the insulin doses often need to be increased considerably if you are unwell. A child will usually need up to 1 U/kg per 24 hours (1 U/2.2 lb), sometimes more, an adult slightly less. The rapid increase in need for insulin is due to the fact that your own pancreas no longer contributes substantial amounts of insulin.

Good glucose control increases the body's defence against infections. Document your blood glucose and ketone readings (as well as insulin doses) in your logbook and contact your

diabetes healthcare team or the hospital if you are in the least unsure about your condition or how to handle the situation. This is equally, if not more, important advice for the parents of children with diabetes.

IMPORTANT!!

Do not adjust insulin doses "by eye" or by carbohydrate counting when you are ill!

Write down all insulin doses and test results in your logbook. You will find it easier to adjust insulin doses and food intake next time you are faced with the same situation. Make a note of how many units you have taken over 24 hours. This is the best way of measuring how the illness has affected your diabetes.

The increased insulin requirements during illness (e.g. a cold with fever) usually last for a few days, but sometimes they can last up to a week after recovery. This is due to the increased blood glucose level which, in turn, gives rise to increased insulin resistance (see page 223 and graphs on page 226). Sometimes there are increased insulin requirements during the incubation period for a few days before the onset of the illness.[967]

If the child does not feel like eating regular meals you should still try to convince him or her to eat regular amounts of carbohydrates. Offer food the child likes, such as ice cream, fruit or soup.

Nausea and vomiting

Nausea and vomiting are common symptoms of many "bugs" and illnesses, particularly in children. At the same time, nausea and vomiting in a child with diabetes can often be the first signs of insulin deficiency. This is why it is always important to check both blood glucose and ketone levels when these symptoms appear. If the blood glucose level is high and ketones are present, the child is probably feeling sick on account of insulin deficiency. The insulin level may not be high enough, despite the usual doses being taken, because an intercurrent illness can increase the body's need for insulin.

If, on the other hand, the blood glucose level is low, the illness itself is probably contributing to the nausea. Ketones may still be present in the blood or urine as a sign of a lack of food (carbohydrates) when the child has no appetite and can then contribute to the nausea.

The same principle also applies with adults. If you feel sick while you are running a temperature, and if you eat less, it is important that the food you do eat and drink contains sugar and carbohydrates, both to give your body nourishment and to lessen the risk of hypoglycaemia. The nausea will usually get worse if you drink

large amounts of liquid at one sitting. It is better to drink small amounts frequently, for example a couple of sips every 10 minutes. Oral rehydration solution (ORS), available at the pharmacy, is very useful in this situation, particularly if you are caring for a sick child with diabetes.

> **Insulin treatment during sick days (except gastroenteritis)**
>
> ⇒ Always start out by taking your usual dose (except when you have gastroenteritis).
>
> ⇒ Monitor your blood glucose before each meal and in between when needed. **Check for ketones regularly.**
>
> ⇒ Adjust insulin doses according to the results of the blood tests. Increase the premeal doses by 1-2 units or according to the correction factor. Lower the carbohydrate ratios by 10-20% to get more insulin for your meals and continue to dose according to blood glucose levels.
>
> ⇒ Give extra insulin (preferably rapid-acting NovoRapid or Humalog) 0.1 U/kg (0.5 U/10 lb) body weight if the blood glucose is more than 14 mmol/l (250 mg/dl) and you have elevated levels of ketones in the blood or urine. Repeat the dose if the blood glucose level has not decreased after 2-3 hours.
>
> ⇒ An alternative rule is to give an additional dose of 10-20% of your total daily insulin dose every 3-4 hours.
>
> ⇒ Contact your diabetes healthcare team or the hospital if you start vomiting or if your general condition is affected.

Remember to check both blood glucose and ketones in your blood or urine frequently when you are ill! Always carry on taking your insulin, and make sure you eat or drink something containing carbohydrates.

How do different illnesses affect blood glucose? (adapted from [968])

① **Not much influence at all**
Illnesses that have no significant effect on your general condition do not usually affect your insulin requirements either. Examples are common colds without fever and chickenpox with few symptoms (in children).

② **Low blood glucose levels**
These illnesses are characterized by difficulties in retaining nutrients due to nausea, vomiting and/or diarrhoea. Examples are gastroenteritis or a viral infection with abdominal pain.

③ **High blood glucose levels**
Most illnesses that give obvious distress and fever will increase the blood glucose levels, thereby increasing the need for insulin. If insulin doses are not increased when the blood glucose level rises, there may be a risk of developing ketoacidosis. Examples are colds with fever, otitis (inflammation of the ear), urinary infection with fever or pneumonia. A genital herpes infection may also result in a substantial increase in insulin requirements.[1029]

The signs that tell you when to go to hospital (adapted from [968])

⟹ Voluminous or repeated vomiting.

⟹ Increasing levels of ketones in the blood or urine, or laboured breathing.

⟹ Blood glucose levels remaining high despite extra insulin.

⟹ It is unclear what the underlying problem might be.

⟹ Severe or unusual abdominal pain.

⟹ Confusion, or a deterioration of general well-being.

⟹ The sick person is a young child (2-3 years old or under) or has another disease besides diabetes.

⟹ Exhaustion on the part of the person or their carer, for example due to repeated night time waking.

⟹ Always call if you are in the least unsure about how to manage the situation.

However, older children may not accept the taste (since it is quite salty). Try adding some juice to improve its taste. Sports drinks such as Lucozade or Gatorade can be helpful in this situation as they already contain both glucose and salts, thus helping to prevent dehydration and salt imbalance. A small dose of metoclopramide (Reglan®, Maxolon®, Pramin®, Clopamon®) or ondansetron can be helpful in preventing vomiting.

If a child with diabetes vomits and cannot keep liquids down, you should contact your diabetes healthcare team or hospital emergency department!

It is very important to give insulin, even if the child cannot eat regular meals. Give something sweet to drink, so that the blood glucose level will not fall. *Make sure that the drink contains real sugar if the blood glucose is below 10-15 mmol/l, 180-270 mg/dl.* Children usually like juice, fruit smoothies or ice cream and will take at least small helpings of these foods without problems. Sugar-free drinks should not be used at all in this situation but extra water can be given, especially with fever, once enough sugary drink has been taken to keep the blood glucose level up.

Gastroenteritis

Gastroenteritis is an infection of the intestinal tract, which usually causes both vomiting and diarrhoea. Very little nourishment will stay in the body and there are generally problems with low blood glucose levels, and you will need to

Insulin and gastroenteritis in children

Make sure that it really is gastroenteritis:

➠ Vomiting *and* diarrhoea.

➠ Low blood glucose levels.

➠ Slight or moderate elevation of levels of ketones in blood (see page 113) or urine. The blood level of starvation ketones seldom exceeds 3 mmol/l. In adults, eating 150-200 g carbohydrate daily (45-50 g every 3-4 hours) will reduce or prevent starvation ketones.[365]

① Always call the hospital if it is the first time your child has had gastroenteritis after developing diabetes or if you are in the least unsure about what to do. If your child is being very sick, you should go to the hospital. He or she might require treatment with intravenous fluids and insulin in this situation.

② Give a drink containing real sugar *(not "light" or "diet" drinks!)* in small and frequent portions (several sips every 10-15 minutes) when the child feels sick or is vomiting. Suitable drinks include fruit juice, tea with sugar, oral rehydration solution and sports drinks, such as Lucozade or Gatorade. Write down how much fluid the child has taken.

③ Measure blood glucose every other hour (every hour if at risk of hypoglycaemia) and check the blood or urine for ketones every 1-2 hours.

④ Give small boluses when the child has had something to drink containing sugar and blood glucose rises slightly. If ketones develop, that means the insulin dose has been lowered too much! The child needs both sugar and insulin.

⑤ If prolonged low blood glucose is a problem, the best approach may be to inject a small dose of glucagon, (see page 38). The dose can be repeated with good effect.

⑥ The insulin doses usually need to be lowered. There will be a balance between how much the child can eat and how much the insulin should be lowered. Low blood glucose levels will increase the insulin sensitivity (decreased insulin resistance, see page 223) and the total insulin doses may need to be lowered by 20-50%. If the child uses a two-dose treatment, start by decreasing the short-acting insulin which at times may even be omitted. The intermediate-acting insulin may need to be decreased as well.

⑦ Try with ordinary food as soon as the vomiting decreases or stops.

⑧ If the child uses a 2-dose treatment you can try to skip the meal-related part (regular or rapid-acting insulin). Often you need to cut down on the intermediate-acting part as well.

A cold with fever increases your insulin requirements, often up to 25%, sometimes even up to 50%. Begin by increasing all your doses by 1-2 units if your blood glucose levels are high. Increase further if needed, depending on results from blood glucose and ketone tests.

lower the insulin doses considerably. Gastroenteritis and food poisoning are therefore exceptions to the rule that the need for insulin will increase during illness. This reduction in need for insulin is likely to go on for some time (often 1-2 weeks) after the gastroenteritis has been cured, as the low blood glucose levels cause a drop in insulin resistance (increased insulin sensitivity, see graph on page 227).

A slower emptying of the stomach [65] contributes to a low blood glucose level when an individual has gastroenteritis. You may need to lower the insulin doses by 20-50% in order to avoid hypoglycaemia. For prolonged problems

Vomiting but no diarrhoea?

Beware! Remember that nausea and vomiting are often symptoms of insulin deficiency.

Vomiting without diarrhoea should always prompt you to suspect insulin deficiency. This also causes high blood glucose levels and elevated levels of ketones in the blood or urine. See also "What happens in the body when there is not enough insulin?" on page 28 and "Ketones" on page 109.

with low blood glucose, repeated mini-doses of glucagon can be helpful (see page 38).

Remember to drink plenty of fluids containing sugar, but take small sips at a time as long as you are being or feeling sick. Never miss a chance of giving the child something sweet to drink! Do not drink water if your blood glucose is below 15 mmol/l (270 m/dl). Even if the blood glucose is high it does not contain so much sugar. You can count about 1 gram for every mmol for an adult, and half of that for a 35 kg child. This means that the reserve of glucose in the blood will be only approximately 6 grams, i.e. 2 glucose tablets of 3 grams, at a blood glucose of 12 mmol/l (215 mg/dl).

Begin with solid food as soon as the vomiting decreases or stops. When you have stopped being sick, you can start taking ordinary food. However, we no longer recommend the diet that used to be prescribed after gastroenteritis (boiled fish, rice, toast etc.). This diet meant it was often difficult to obtain enough glucose and calories, so is rarely (if ever) used now. It is better to eat what you like. The only exception is milk for small children. If diarrhoea continues to be a problem, milk and milk products should be excluded from the child's diet for a week or two.

Be aware that vomiting can often be a symptom of insulin deficiency which should be treated with increased insulin doses.

You should check both the blood glucose and the ketone levels (in blood or urine) if you, or a child with diabetes, feels sick or vomits. If you are short of insulin, your blood glucose level will be high and the ketone test will show high readings. Extra doses of rapid-acting insulin are urgently required to prevent ketoacidosis. Talk to your diabetes doctor or nurse about the results before changing any doses if you are not sure about how to interpret them.

Wound healing

It is commonly believed that when people with diabetes injure their feet, they will heal more slowly, and because of this regular chiropody is needed. This is certainly true for individuals who have had diabetes for many years, and who are beginning to suffer from complications in the form of reduced circulation and loss of feeling in the feet and toes (see also page 363). However, if a child or young person with diabetes is injured, and the blood glucose control is good, the wound will heal just as well as it would in anyone else of the same age, provided good care is taken to prevent the wound from becoming infected.

On the other hand, the body's defence system will not work as well as it should if the diabetes is uncontrolled and the blood glucose level high. This will increase even young people's susceptibility to infection.[652]

Surgery

Your body will have a stress reaction when undergoing major surgery. Stress hormones like adrenaline, cortisol, glucagon and growth hormone will be released, all raising blood glucose by releasing and producing glucose from the liver. This will cause problems with the blood glucose level for a person having diabetes, while the person without diabetes can compensate by increasing their production of insulin. You can prepare yourself for a planned operation by eating well and fine tuning your insulin doses before admission. It is important to adjust the insulin doses carefully during and after surgery, since high blood glucose levels (over 11-13 mmol/l, 200-230 mg/dl) have been found to increase the risk of infections after surgery.[409]

People with diabetes should be taken care of in hospital if they need surgery, even if the operation is only a minor one. The operation should be scheduled for as early in the day as possible. During operations of more than 20-30 minutes under general anaesthetic, it is advisable to give insulin intravenously (see page 74).[595,844] This system is very easy to adjust and will ensure appropriate blood glucose and insulin levels throughout the operation and during the recovery phase. During shorter operations, it is better to continue with the ordinary basal insulin (or pump basal rate), which can be supplemented

with intravenous insulin, if necessary. When the person can eat and drink again, they can return to their usual method of insulin administration.

If your child is admitted to a paediatric surgical ward, you should be put in touch with a paediatric diabetes team to discuss appropriate insulin treatment. As parents of a child with diabetes, you have every right to express your own views on the treatment. Remember that your knowledge about your child's diabetes is likely to be much more extensive than that of the staff on a surgical ward.

It would also be appropriate to ensure that you, along with the anaesthetist and all members of the operating team, can contact your diabetes team in the case of any elective surgery. This will help to ensure that diabetes care and appropriate monitoring, as well as insulin adjustment, can be carried out effectively. For emergencies, it would be appropriate to insist that the diabetes doctor on emergency call be contacted, if at all possible, or the local specialists contacted, as a minimum. It is important for teenagers to be accompanied by a parent to help them keep track of their blood glucose levels.

Drugs that affect blood glucose

Drugs that contain sugar can affect blood glucose. However, the sugar content is often low enough not to raise the blood glucose appreciably. If a medication is given with a meal, 5 g (1/6 ounce) of extra sugar is unlikely to make a noticeable difference to the blood glucose level. If it does rise, however, you can give a small extra dose of insulin (0.5-1 U/10 g of sugar).

Other drugs may affect the glucose level without containing sugar. Treatment with cortisol or other steroids (e.g. prednisolone, dexamethasone) causes a marked increase in the blood glucose level, often to above 20 mmol/l (360 mg/dl). This can happen even when the steroid is given as a single dose, for example to treat asthma or croup. When taking cortisol medication for several days or longer, the insulin doses

Take care of small wounds and poor friends... (Swedish saying)

☞ Wash the wound with soap and water.

☞ Apply a clean, dry dressing.

☞ Signs of infection? See a doctor!

① Pain/throbbing from the wound after the first 1-2 days.

② Increasing redness of the skin.

③ Red streak in the skin going from the wound towards the body (infection of the lymph vessel).

④ Painful nodule in the groin or armpit (infected or inflamed lymph node).

⑤ High temperature.

Even if you eat fewer sweets than your friends, you are at risk of tooth decay. This is caused by glucose in the saliva when your blood glucose level is high. Don't forget to brush your teeth at least twice a day.

During surgery it is advisable to administer insulin intravenously. This is a convenient and safe way to obtain a stable blood glucose level without risking hypoglycaemia. When having minor surgery it often works well to continue with your ordinary basal insulin (with injections or a pump), and only give extra insulin intravenously if needed.

need to be increased considerably. The total dose for a 24-hour period often needs to be doubled, increasing both the premeal doses and the intermediate- or long-acting insulin. Steroids for inhalation affect glucose levels far less. At times, a slight increase in glucose levels is seen as a small amount of the given drug is absorbed into the bloodstream. You should try to find the lowest possible dose that is effective for the asthmatic disease. It may be advantageous to take the maintenance dose at bedtime. This will make it easier for you to increase your bedtime insulin if necessary to counteract the effect of the steroids. In acute severe asthma, the combination of beta-sympathomimetics, such as salbutamol, with prednisolone often raises the blood glucose level considerably.

Teeth

It is a good idea to see your dentist regularly, and ask for advice about your dental hygiene so that you can minimize any risk of damage. Be sure to tell your dentist that you have diabetes!

It is unusual for children with diabetes to have more tooth decay (dental caries) than other children. On the contrary, they often have fewer such problems than many children of the same age.[617] It might be seen as surprising that they have any decay at all, as they often eat fewer sweets than their friends. The explanation may be that children with diabetes eat snacks regularly. In addition, they might often need to take dextrose or something else with sugar if they become hypoglycaemic, and this contributes to an increased number of bacteria in the oral cavity. One study on adults found that the subjects who had diabetes had the same amount of caries as those in the control group who did not have diabetes.[1026]

Another contributing explanation is that glucose is excreted into the saliva when the blood glucose level is high, and this may contribute further to cavities.[1026] The saliva would not normally contain glucose but, if the blood glucose level is above a certain threshold, increased amounts of glucose will be found in the saliva. In this sense a person with very high or variable blood glucose level has a higher risk of tooth decay. Unfortunately the combination of the glucose level in blood and saliva is not very good, so it not possible to use tests on saliva to estimate the blood glucose level.[1026] Children and adolescents with higher HbA_{1c} had higher glucose levels in the saliva and more caries.[1054]

Gingivitis is an inflammation of the gums caused by bacteria accumulating in the tooth sockets. The bacterial deposits on the teeth harden into tartar. The gums go red and bleed when you brush your teeth. Gingivitis and periodontal disease (bacterial infections of the tissues surrounding and supporting the teeth) are slightly more common in people who have diabetes than in people who don't, even in young people.[851] They are also more common when the blood glucose level is high. People with diabetes may find their gingivitis progresses more rapidly, and causes more damage than it does in people who don't have diabetes. Periodontal disease is also more common in smokers. Treatment of periodontal infections in adults with diabetes has been shown to have a positive effect on HbA_{1c}.[424]

Removal of the wisdom teeth is a common procedure usually carried out on older teenagers or young adults. If the person concerned has diabetes, however, the dentist will need to take special precautions. The procedure is often carried out on a "walk in" outpatient basis, or "in the dentist's chair". The dentist or oral surgeon should have a formal protocol to follow when treating a person with diabetes as you will need intravenous glucose treatment during the procedure, and possibly insulin as well. Your insulin dose is likely to be adjusted in advance, but make sure you know what is happening and who is responsible for monitoring your blood

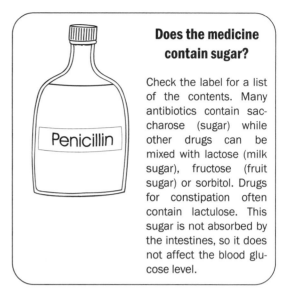

Does the medicine contain sugar?

Check the label for a list of the contents. Many antibiotics contain saccharose (sugar) while other drugs can be mixed with lactose (milk sugar), fructose (fruit sugar) or sorbitol. Drugs for constipation often contain lactulose. This sugar is not absorbed by the intestines, so it does not affect the blood glucose level.

glucose levels and making any necessary changes to your insulin dose. For a procedure such as this, it is essential that you ensure everyone involved in treating you knows well in advance that you have diabetes.

Vaccinations

Children with diabetes should have the same vaccinations as other children. See page 344 for more information about vaccinations when travelling abroad.

Smoking

Everyone knows that smoking is unhealthy. Despite this, a large number of people smoke but nobody seems to care. While we often don't seem to be very concerned about this aspect of smoking from a moral point of view, many people with diabetes feel that society at large employs double standards by disapproving of them for eating "the wrong sort of food" but completely ignoring people with all sorts of health problems who smoke. For example, if a person with diabetes stands in a queue to buy sweets, others seem to feel it is perfectly acceptable to act as "sweets police", and stare at them as if they are thinking "you are not allowed to do that". Many will even make hurtful comments. Even though smoking today is banned in all pubs, restaurants and on public transport, the smoking habits of young people have not changed much. Still, most non-smokers will not comment, despite the fact that smoking can cause even more health problems than excessive sweet-eating in a person with diabetes.

About the same number of people with diabetes smoke as do other people. And smoking results in a substantially increased risk of lung cancer, chronic bronchitis and diseases of the heart and blood vessels. Having diabetes, in itself, puts

you at increased risk of heart and blood vessel diseases such as arteriosclerosis, heart attacks and stroke. In diabetes the risks are cumulative. If you imagine diabetes as a balancing act on a slack rope, smoking may be the extra factor that tips you over. Many studies in adults confirm that the risk of premature death for a person with diabetes who smokes is 1.5-2 times that of a person with diabetes who does not smoke. But research also indicates that giving up smoking reduces this risk.[192,768]

At the 1994 World Congress on Tobacco it was established that every second smoker will die from a disease that is connected with smoking.[840] Smoking was called the greatest epidemic of the 20th century causing more deaths than both the plague and AIDS. The metaphor was made that a 14-year-old who has begun smoking should be treated like a contagious tuberculosis patient, considering the risk that such a person can influence other teenagers to start smoking too!

Nicotine from smoking affects the blood glucose level by contracting the blood vessels, resulting in a slower absorption of insulin from the injection site.[621,626] Nicotine will also cause increased insulin resistance [53,325] (a poorer

"A 14-year-old smoker is about as contagious as a patient with tuberculosis, when you consider the risk that he/she can entice other adolescents to start smoking" (message at the 1994 World Congress on Tobacco).[840]

blood glucose-lowering effect of a given dose of insulin), which makes diabetes more difficult to manage (see page 223). A larger insulin dose may therefore be needed to achieve similar glucose control in smoking patients compared to non-smokers.[326] The risk of acquiring type 2 diabetes is twice as high in both men and women who smoke compared to people who have never smoked, and 5 times higher when smoking more than 8 cigarettes/day.[362]

Smoking causes the inhalation of carbon monoxide, which binds strongly to haemoglobin in the red blood cells and prevents oxygen from binding to them. The number of red blood cells increases to compensate for this. Scientific studies show that in a person with diabetes, smoking increases the risk of renal failure, visual impairment, foot ulcers, leg amputations and heart attacks.[765,768,939] Smoking causes a decreased blood flow in the eye,[759] which will increase the risk of eye complications. In a study where smokers were compared to a group of nonsmokers with the same age, diabetes duration and HbA_{1c}, complications from the eyes and kidneys were more pronounced and more severe in the smoking group after 6 years of follow-up.[973]

Smoking increases the risk of severe hypoglycaemia (defined as unconsciousness or hospitalization) 2.6 times according to one study.[506] In this study, 15% were smokers. One explanation may be that smokers require higher insulin doses due to insulin resistance (see page 223),[712] another that smoking is a form of risk behav-

Passive smoking is dangerous to your health. Small children are often exposed to passive smoking by their parents. One woman who never had smoked developed a fatal type of lung cancer normally seen only in smokers. It was established that she had developed her cancer because people were smoking in the room where she worked. Studies show a 25% increase in the risk of lung cancer for passive smoking at home, at work or from social exposure.[145]

iour, and the same persons may take risks when dosing their insulin (like not checking blood glucose often enough).

Passive smoking

Even passive smoking will damage your health. It has been shown that children absorb nicotine into their bloodstream at twice the rate of adults through smoking passively. Smaller children are even more sensitive. Children of smoking parents also have increased levels of lead and cadmium in their blood. Smoking near an extractor fan (e.g. in the kitchen) will not prevent smoke from spreading into the house. It

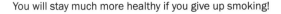

You will stay much more healthy if you give up smoking!

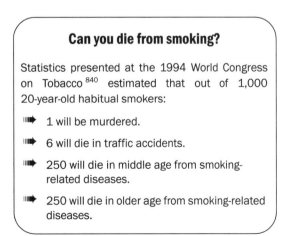

Can you die from smoking?

Statistics presented at the 1994 World Congress on Tobacco [840] estimated that out of 1,000 20-year-old habitual smokers:

⟹ 1 will be murdered.

⟹ 6 will die in traffic accidents.

⟹ 250 will die in middle age from smoking-related diseases.

⟹ 250 will die in older age from smoking-related diseases.

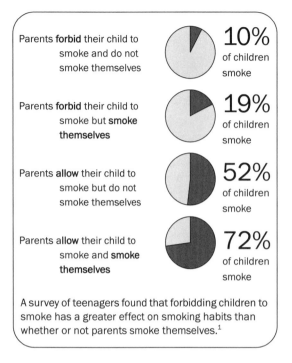

Parents **forbid** their child to smoke and do not smoke themselves

10% of children smoke

Parents **forbid** their child to smoke but **smoke themselves**

19% of children smoke

Parents **allow** their child to smoke but do not smoke themselves

52% of children smoke

Parents **allow** their child to smoke and **smoke themselves**

72% of children smoke

A survey of teenagers found that forbidding children to smoke has a greater effect on smoking habits than whether or not parents smoke themselves.[1]

It is never too late to give up smoking. For every day without a cigarette, the damaging effects of tobacco in your body are reduced.

has been claimed this is "about as effective as urinating in a corner of a swimming pool."

Giving up smoking

The easiest way to give up is never to start. Most smokers have started in their teens. It is difficult to withstand the "peer pressure" but it can save many years of your life. Besides, giving up smoking will save you a lot of money.

It may be difficult to give up smoking by yourself. Your diabetes healthcare team can help you with advice and nicotine chewing gum or patches that may be effective. However, unless you are motivated yourself, you will never succeed in giving up! In one study the HbA$_{1c}$ levels decreased from 61 to 53 mmol/mol (7.7% to 7.0%) in a group of people with diabetes who ceased smoking.[431] There is a risk that you will put on weight when you stop smoking, but this will not necessarily happen. So it may depend on how you go about trying to give up. You should talk to your diabetes healthcare team for

specific advice to maximize your chances of success while minimizing your chances of any adverse effects during the actual process of giving up. There are medical drugs available for adults that decrease the craving for smoking (Bupropion, Varenicline).

Emotional attitudes (or lack of emotions) expressed by important persons around the teenager (including the diabetes team) exerted strong influences on the smoking habits, including both initiation and motivation for quitting cigarette smoking, and were perceived as both crucial and meaningful by the teenagers with diabetes in a Swedish study.[879] So, parents and others, don't be discouraged!

Snuff

The use of snuff in the UK is almost unheard of these days, but the global picture is very different. In Sweden 30% of all men under the age of 30 use snuff and it is common in other countries as well. Nicotine from snuff is absorbed through the oral lining as quickly as from an intravenous injection. Whether you smoke it or sniff it, nicotine has strong effects on your heart, blood vessels and blood pressure. It may increase the risk of kidney damage if you have diabetes.[334] The addiction to nicotine is just as strong as that for cocaine or heroin. Because of nicotine addiction, it is just as difficult, if not more so, to give up snuff as it is to give up smoking.

Alcohol

We do not recommend a total ban on drinking alcohol if you have diabetes. However, it is important to know how alcohol works and that you take it easy, making sure you stop drinking before you get drunk. If you are not old enough to be able to drink legally, your parents should have the final say about whether or not you can drink. The age when you are allowed to buy alcohol differs from country to country (it is 18 in the UK). Your diabetes team can neither allow you to do something, nor forbid it. They can only tell you how things work, and where and why you should be particularly careful.

Alcohol and the liver

Alcohol counteracts the ability of the liver to produce new glucose (a process called gluconeogenesis) by keeping the enzymes occupied with the breakdown of alcohol.[56] The liver can still release glucose from the glycogen store (see page 34) but when this is depleted you will experience hypoglycaemia.[56] The concentration of cortisol and growth hormone in the blood will decrease after alcohol intake.[56] Both hormones have an enhancing effect on the blood glucose level, and this appears 3-4 hours after they are released into the bloodstream (see page 33). This will contribute to an increased risk of hypoglycaemia many hours after alcohol intake. The liver's ability to produce free fatty acids will also be impaired.[56] These biological factors come together, making the risk of hypoglycaemia much greater after drinking alcohol. This effect of alcohol will last the entire time it takes the liver to break down the alcohol in your body. The liver will break down 0.1 g (1.5 grains) of pure alcohol/kg body weight per hour. For example, if you weigh 70 kg (150 lb) it will take 1 hour to break down the alcohol in a bottle of light beer, 2 hours for 40 ml of liquor and 10 hours to break down the alcohol in a

bottle of wine. Therefore, if you drink during the evening you will be at risk of hypoglycaemia all night as well as part of the next day.

Why is it dangerous to drink too much if you have diabetes?

When you have diabetes you must be able to think clearly in many situations, so you can take the correct amount of insulin at the right time and be aware of feeling unwell if your insulin levels are low or you are becoming hypoglycaemic. You cannot do this if you have had too much to drink, in exactly the same way as you cannot drive a car safely after taking more than a small amount of alcohol. Severe hypoglycaemia after drinking alcohol has caused the death of young people with diabetes on rare occasions. Scientific studies show the role of alcohol in causing hypoglycaemia has more to do with losing the ability to recognize the signs of impending hypoglycaemia than with reducing the liver's ability to produce glucose.[378,605,627]

In one study, people with diabetes drank either white wine (approximately 600 ml, three average-sized glasses) or water 2-3 hours after the evening snack.[1053] The morning blood glucose

It is not dangerous for an adult person with diabetes to drink a glass or two, but if you drink too much you will find it difficult to think clearly...

was 3-4 mmol/l (55-70 mg/dl) lower after drinking wine and five of the six individuals experienced symptomatic hypoglycaemia 2-4 hours after breakfast (at this time no alcohol was detectable in the blood). Another study found twice the risk of hypoglycaemia over a 24 hour period after drinking approximately the same amounts of alcohol.[887] This suggests it is advisable to be prepared for late-morning

hypoglycaemia after an evening spent drinking, and it is advisable to lower the insulin dose both at bedtime and before breakfast.

Basic rules

Adults with diabetes can drink moderate amounts of alcohol if they eat food at the same time. For a person with diabetes, the intake should be limited to one drink (defined as a 350 ml beer, 150 ml glass of wine or 45 ml glass of distilled spirits) for women and two drinks for men in one day.[365] Make sure that your friends know you have diabetes and wear some type of diabetes ID (necklace or MedicAlert bracelet) when you are socializing. Always eat something at the same time as you are drinking alcohol. Remember that what you eat should be "long-acting" carbohydrates as the risk of hypoglycaemia extends into the next day. Alcohol containing sugar (liqueur, for example) will cause your blood glucose level to rise for a short time, but then it will drop and you will be at risk of hypoglycaemia. A glass of beer contains about the same amount of carbohydrate as a glass of milk.

It takes a long time for your liver to break down alcohol, which increases the risk of severe hypoglycaemia. Because of this, sleeping late is particularly dangerous the morning after you

Examples of alcohol and calories

Drink	Alcohol content	Kcal	Carb. g
1 bottle,300ml			
Non-alcoholic beer	< 0.5%	~60	~16
Low alcohol beer	0.5-1.2%	~40	~7
Light beer	~3-5%	~90	~5
Beer	> 4%	~160	~13
1 glass,150ml			
Red wine	9.9%	114	3.5
White wine, dry	9.5%	99	0.7
White wine, sweet	10.7%	147	9
60ml			
Sherry	16%	91	6
45ml			
Vodka	32%	100	0
Whisky	32%	100	0
Punch	20%	132	14
Liqueur	19%	150	24

If you develop severe hypoglycaemia after drinking alcohol, the person finding you is likely to assume that you are simply drunk. If you don't wear a pump, it is essential that you wear a MedicAlert necklace/bracelet. (You can also carry an ID card, but it will probably not be discovered as promptly.)

have been drinking. If you have also been especially active, playing team games or dancing at a club for example, the combined risks of extra activity with alcohol intake put you at much greater risk than usual of severe hypoglycaemia. Under such circumstances, preventing hypoglycaemia becomes imperative.

What if you've had too much to drink?

Eat extra food immediately before going to bed. You can eat potato crisps in this situation as they give a slow increase in blood glucose over several hours (see page 57). The blood glucose level should not be less than 10 mmol/l (180 mg/dl) when you go to bed. Decrease the dose of bedtime insulin by 2-4 units to avoid hypoglycaemia. Don't go to bed alone; if you have severe hypoglycaemia during the night you will need someone to help you. If you come home very late, make sure to wake a parent or partner, and let them know about your condition. Your life may actually depend upon it, even if you find the situation embarrassing. Set your alarm clock. Don't sleep in late! Be sure to eat a proper breakfast as soon as you wake up the next morning If you feel sick, check your blood glucose level. It may be caused by high glucose levels rather than a hangover.

You also need to understand that even giving a glucagon injection may be less effective in correcting severe hypoglycaemia in this situation because the liver will be "busy" breaking down the alcohol and therefore unable to respond and raise the blood glucose levels.[365] This is because

If you are under the age when it is legal for you to drink alcohol, remember that the staff at your diabetes team can neither give you permission to drink nor prohibit you from drinking alcohol. This is something to be discussed with your parents. What they can do is to tell you how alcohol affects your body if you have diabetes and what the risks might be.

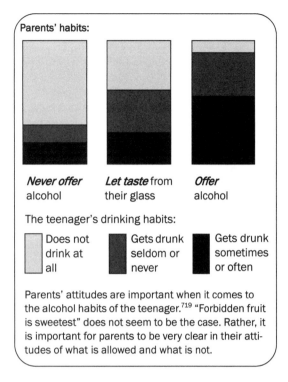

Parents' habits:

Never offer alcohol

Let taste from their glass

Offer alcohol

The teenager's drinking habits:

Does not drink at all

Gets drunk seldom or never

Gets drunk sometimes or often

Parents' attitudes are important when it comes to the alcohol habits of the teenager.[719] "Forbidden fruit is sweetest" does not seem to be the case. Rather, it is important for parents to be very clear in their attitudes of what is allowed and what is not.

alcohol counteracts glucagon's ability to increase the production of glucose in the liver. If a person becomes unconscious or has seizures due to hypoglycaemia following alcohol intake, they may need to be put on a glucose drip in hospital.

Can you drink at home?

Many assume that "stolen pleasures are sweetest", i.e. that it is better for teenagers to try alcohol at home under parental supervision than to sneak a drink on the quiet. However, studies have shown that more children start drinking alcohol if you have a permissive attitude towards trying alcohol in the home. A total prohibition of alcohol for teenagers seems to have a better preventative effect than the idea that it is advisable to test at home.[719] The same is true for smoking.[1] Whether or not parents allowed experimenting in the home had a greater impact in these studies than if the parents drank alcohol or smoked.

Illegal drugs

If you are a young person living in Britain today, sooner or later you will find you have the opportunity to try illegal drugs. In many cases, young people find they are actively pressurized by friends and schoolmates to "be like everyone else" and try the fashionable substance of the moment. This can cause problems for any young person, but if you have diabetes you face additional risks from drug use.

Drugs affect the brain and nervous systems and will make it much more difficult to manage something like diabetes. Many drugs make you forgetful and the risk of ketoacidosis will increase if you have not taken enough insulin or missed your injections. A person taking drugs is at high risk of developing hypoglycaemia since drugs make you think less clearly. If friends know about your diabetes and how to treat hypoglycaemia, they may be able to help (unless they also are too heavily affected by drugs or alcohol). Unless the drug user wears a diabetes ID, it may take some time to get appropriate help, even if the police or ambulance staff intervene.

Narcotics and other illegal drugs are likely to be very addictive, so if you start using them you will have great difficulty giving up without help. If you have diabetes, you must understand that it is completely inappropriate from a medical point of view, as well as extremely risky, to use, or even try, any type of illegal drug.

Certain drugs may have specific extra risks associated with the blood vessels. Amphetamine is known to damage the linings of blood vessels [708] thereby increasing the short-term and long-term risks of diabetes complications. Many people who are drug users would find it extremely difficult to take good care of themselves and their diabetes while continuing their drug use, because of the behavioural aspects of

Illegal drugs act as poisons on your brain, and are likely to be extremely addictive.

drug use. Casual drug users would have the same problems as those of other medications that interfere with rational self-care at the time.

In a UK study using anonymous questionnaires, 29% of young adults aged 16 to 30 years admitted that they used "street drugs", and two thirds used them at least once per month.[782] Almost half of them did warn their friends that they had diabetes and/or took extra blood glucose tests during use. Two reported hypoglycaemia after using cannabis, and 2 were admitted to hospital with ketoacidosis after using ecstasy and cannabis. A US study including teenagers with diabetes, reported that 25% had tried drugs of abuse and 5% reported ongoing use.[406]

"Uppers"

Uppers like amphetamine (speed, whizz, sulph), methamphetamine (crystal, glass, ice), ecstasy (E, pills, doves) are stimulants that give more energy and confidence. This makes them popular at clubs, parties and raves. There is a risk of dehydration when the body loses fluid through continuous dancing or other strenuous activity, which is a particular concern for anyone with diabetes. Uppers can suppress appetite, and combined with dancing there is a risk of experiencing severe hypoglycaemia. In this sense these drugs can be extremely dangerous for a person with diabetes, especially if not enough extra fluid is taken or the extra bedtime snack is forgotten. Amphetamine can raise blood glucose by stimulating adrenaline.[71] Ecstasy can make your body retain more fluid than normally, leading to water intoxication.[782] Two cases of ketoacidosis in teenagers taking ecstasy have been reported.[961]

GHB (gamma-hydroxybutyric acid) is a depressant of the central nervous system and can be dangerous if combined with similar drugs or alcohol. GHB stimulates growth hormone and cortisol, thereby causing an insulin resistance (see page 223). An increase of blood glucose to above 28 mmol/l (500 mg/dl) and production of ketones has been reported with GHB use.[79]

Cocaine (coke, charlie, snow) is also used to produce "highs" and increase confidence. The price of these drugs has come right down in recent years meaning that they are available as street drugs rather than just for the rich and famous. Cocaine is a Class A drug and, particularly in the form of crack, can be very addictive.

Benzodiazepines

This is a group of drugs that are used in a controlled way by doctors, prescribing them to people who have difficulty sleeping, or suffer from anxiety. But there is a "black market" for them too and they are used illegally as "recreational drugs".

The best known drug in this group is temazepam. This can make you feel relaxed and sleepy but, if you take a larger dose, it can have similar effects to a large amount of alcohol. It can make you very talkative or over-excited, and sometimes aggressive. It also gives you a false sense of confidence and undermines your judgement. It would certainly be very difficult

for you to be aware that your blood glucose level was too high or too low, and may even cause you to forget to take your insulin.

Cannabis

Cannabis is used for production of both marijuana and hash. Marijuana (blow, weed) is made from the green parts of the plant while hash is a kind of resin that is produced from the plant. Hash is often more potent, and gives a higher risk of over-dosing especially when eaten (brownies) or drunk (milkshake). The effect will then be delayed, which often leads to a higher dose being consumed. Use of marijuana has been viewed as less harmful than the use of "hard drugs" such as heroin, cocaine or amphetamines. In 2005, the Home Office published a new report showing that cannabis can, in fact, cause significant harm — both to physical and psychological health.[12]

In terms of making rational decisions about complex activities such as driving or diabetes self-management, cannabis is likely to impair the judgement in much the same way as too much alcohol. Combining cannabis with alcohol (as often happens) adds special risks for making diabetes-related decisions about, for example, when to wake up the next day. Many people who take cannabis find themselves becoming especially hungry and wanting to eat everything in sight, especially junk food (the "munchies") which will raise the blood glucose level considerably.

Cocaine was once a drug for the rich and famous. But falling prices mean it is much more widely available now.

Opium

Opium and opium-like drugs such as heroine and methadone can disturb the function of the hypophysis, an important gland in the brain that produces many hormones. This can lead to a decreased production of testosterone causing a decline in sexual function,[436] reduced muscle strength and decreased mental energy.[902] The function of the thyroid gland can also be affected. A cortisol failure, i.e. a decreased production of the vital hormone cortisol, can lead to a life-threatening crisis in a person who has an infection. This may explain some of the deaths of heroin addicts, that may have been blamed on an overdose or impure heroine.[902] Even the production of growth hormone can be severely disturbed, which may affect your growth patterns if you have not yet reached your full adult height.

Advice for parents from the British Government (www.homeoffice.gov.uk):

➠ **Be prepared:** Find out about drugs — the facts not the myths. Your child is more likely to listen — and talk — if she or he thinks you know what you are talking about.

➠ **Be calm:** Easier said than done but try not to shout or let the discussion become an argument.

➠ **Be open:** Listen to what your child has to say. Write it down if it helps and consider it later. Don't react to bad language or shocking stories.

➠ **Keep it broad:** Don't just focus on the drug use or your child's behaviour; look at the wider context and the good sides of the story that are always there as well.

Hallucinogenics

Hallucinogenic drugs alter your perception of the outside world. Lysergic acid or LSD (acid) found its way into the hippy culture of the 1960s and 70s. Although less widely used, it is still available now. Taking an acid tablet or "tab" can take you on a bizarre and dreamlike journey, or one that is a nightmare beyond your wildest imaginings. Even if you have taken acid before, the effects are unpredictable and trips usually last between 7 and 12 hours.

Cannabis can give you the "munchies", making you want to eat everything you can lay your hands on.

Another common hallucinogenic drug, ketamine hydrochloride (ketamine, K) was developed originally for use in hospital anaesthetics but the bizarre effects it can have means it is rarely (if ever) used in this way for humans now. Much of the ketamine that is sold on the street now was originally intended for veterinary use. As the drug was originally developed as an anaesthetic, it can lead to loss of physical sensation and even ability to move, as well as hallucinations and out of body experiences. The effects can be particularly alarming if it is mixed with alcohol and anecdotal evidence suggests that it has been used as a "date rape" drug. The combination of such effects with hypoglycaemia could well be life-threatening.

Risk-taking behaviour

Smoking, drinking alcohol and the use of drugs are all examples of risk-taking behaviour. See page 401 for more information on this topic.

Pregnancy and sexual issues

One of the first things a girl with diabetes and her family will ask is whether she will be able to have babies. Being pregnant exerts a certain strain on every woman, but there is no reason to discourage women with diabetes from having children. The mother's risk of developing diabetes complications later in life is not affected by pregnancy.[89]

Of the children born in UK and US, approximately 0.3% have a mother with diabetes.[138,474] About 70% of these mothers have type 1 diabetes.[204] Gestational diabetes (a temporary form of diabetes occurring during pregnancy) affects 3-5% of pregnancies.[984] The symptoms of diabetes usually disappear after the birth but these women have an increased risk (40-60%) of acquiring type 2 diabetes later in life.[212,812]

If the mother's blood glucose level is high, there is a risk that the unborn baby will be affected. However, if the woman has good glucose con-

If you make up your mind to achieve a good HbA_{1c} before getting pregnant (53 mmol/mol (7.0%)), you will give your growing and developing baby a better start in life.

trol with an HbA_{1c} similar to that of an individual without diabetes at the time the baby is conceived and during early pregnancy, older studies show that the risk of birth defects or miscarriage is no greater than average.[266,619,1003] This is the case even if the mother has diabetes complications.[461] The risk increases with increasing HbA_{1c} and is very great (close to 25%!) when HbA_{1c} is above 97 mmol/mol (11%).[832,1003] It is therefore very important to plan your pregnancy, if at all possible, and to ensure that your HbA_{1c} is below 53 mmol/mol (7.0%) before you get pregnant.[26,286] More recent data show that this may not be low enough.[339] A UK study found a major birth defect in 4.2% of children of diabetic mothers compared with 2.1% in the general population.[204] One quarter of the women who had a baby with a birth defect had an HbA_{1c} value of less than 53 mmol/mol (7.0%) by 13 weeks of pregnancy.[204] However, it is important to point out that even if your HbA_{1c} is high during pregnancy, this does not necessarily mean your baby will have something wrong with it. A high HbA_{1c} value is not, in itself, a reason for recommending abortion, for example.[832] Fifty per cent of all women with a high HbA_{1c}, above 86 mmol/mol (10%), have quite normal pregnancies.[90]

A Canadian meta-analysis of 1,977 pregnancies with a diabetic mother showed that if the HbA_{1c} level at the time of conception was within the range of a non-diabetic woman, the risk of birth defects was down to 2%, i.e. that of a woman without diabetes.[429] The graph above shows that there is a considerable increase in risk with higher HbA_{1c} levels.

Most major malformations can be identified by ultrasound or a blood test.[1003] The babies of women with type 2 diabetes have risks of birth defects and problems at birth comparable to those of babies of women with type 1 diabetes.[204] There is a increased risk of birth defects [635] and difficulties at delivery [834] even with diabetes that is discovered during pregnancy (gestational diabetes). However, these risks are associated with diabetes in the mother and do not apply if only the father has diabetes.

The new insulin analogues are not officially approved for the use in pregnancy. There are no reports on any negative effects of Humalog, NovoRapid or Lantus during animal pregnancies.[650] Increasing number of reports of use in humans have found them safe during pregnancy. In the individual patient, the effectiveness of the treatment with analogue insulins has to be weighed against possible risks for the unborn baby. The decision of which insulin to be used during pregnancy should be taken together with your diabetes doctor. Humalog has been on the market for the longest period of time and a report on 533 pregnancies showed a rate of major birth defects of 5.4%, which is in the same range as for women using other insulins.[1120] There has been some concern about a deterioration of diabetic eye damage when using Humalog during pregnancy, but a report from Finland shows that this is not the case.[686] A study of NovoRapid in pregnancy showed that it is at least as safe and effective as regular insulin [727] and it is now approved during pregnancy in some countries. There are now several reports of women using Lantus during pregnancy without any negative effects on the unborn baby.[387,1118] A study on Levemir in pregnant women did not show any increase in adverse outcomes for the baby.[515]

Insulin requirements may decrease early in pregnancy, especially if the woman has problems with sickness. Thereafter, the amount of insulin needed rises steadily, until close to full term (36-38 weeks), when it is often as much as twice the level it was before the pregnancy.[305,832]

Diabetes and pregnancy: risks for the unborn baby

① Early in pregnancy:

⇒ Increased risk of congenital malformations if the HbA_{1c} is increased, especially if it is higher than 75-95 mmol/mol (9-11%).

② Complications at delivery:

⇒ The baby will have the same blood glucose levels as the mother since glucose can pass freely through the placenta.
An increased amount of glucose to the infant will increase its growth, as it can produce insulin of its own.

⇒ The infant will be large in size which will increase the risk of a difficult delivery.

⇒ The infant will be at risk of developing hypoglycaemia during the first few days of life as he or she will continue to produce considerable amounts of insulin.

This increased need for insulin is partly caused by weight gain during pregnancy but also by hormones excreted from the placenta, which counteract the blood glucose-lowering effect of insulin. The average weight gain during pregnancy is around 11-12 kg (24-26 lb) but individuals vary greatly.

Although eye and kidney damage may be accelerated by pregnancy,[611] these changes have been found by the DCCT study to be reversible once the pregnancy is over.[271] However, if the mother's kidneys have been damaged by her diabetes, the risk of fetal growth retardation and premature birth will increase considerably.[90,611]

Short periods of hypoglycaemia are not dangerous to the unborn baby.[824] However, severe hypoglycaemia with seizures or unconsciousness can be dangerous.[832] Low blood glucose levels can increase "morning" sickness during pregnancy.[305] Feeling very sick may make it difficult to eat regular meals, resulting in hypogly-caemia. A vicious cycle may easily develop. The use of an insulin pump can be an effective way of minimizing these problems.

Glucose in the mother's blood will pass easily through the placenta into the blood of the unborn baby.[577] In this way, the baby is continuously consuming a large proportion of the mother's glucose, leading to a risk of hypoglycaemia when she does not eat regularly. This may result in her needing more snacks during the day and increase the risk of night time hypoglycaemia.[305]

If the mother's blood glucose level is increased, some of the glucose will be delivered via the placenta to the baby — whose own pancreas can produce enough insulin to take care of the extra sugar. However, insulin cannot pass back to the mother through the placenta. If the blood glucose level is high during a large part of the pregnancy, the baby will grow faster than it should, and will have gained excess weight by the time it is born. This may cause problems at delivery.

Even if the HbA_{1c} during pregnancy is kept well controlled, the child may have gained excess weight by the time it is born. The blood glucose level after meals seems to be most significant according to one study.[203] The recommendation in this study was to aim for a blood glucose level of approximately 7.2 mmol/l (130 mg/dl) 1 hour after the meal. With lower levels there was some risk that the baby would show a slight retardation in growth, instead of weight gain, by the time it was born.

Blood glucose levels should be as normal as possible during labour and childbirth, as high blood glucose levels cause increased insulin production in the unborn baby. This means that the baby will be less able to cope with the partial lack of oxygen that even a normal delivery entails.[89] When the umbilical cord is cut, the high insulin production by the baby's body will continue, causing the blood glucose level to drop. The child of a mother with diabetes, therefore, will be monitored carefully with

extra blood glucose tests. If the baby becomes hypoglycaemic, glucose will be given intravenously. The child will also receive extra food early on, before the mother has begun to produce breast milk.

The woman's daily insulin requirement decreases quickly after childbirth, returning to the pre-pregnant level after as little as 1 week.[771] Breast-feeding mothers usually need to decrease their insulin doses to levels lower than they were before pregnancy to avoid hypoglycaemia. If doses are not lowered considerably, there is a clear risk of experiencing severe hypoglycaemia.[1088] After a few weeks or months, the insulin doses will usually be back to the levels they were at before the pregnancy. Breast-feeding lowers blood glucose, and a high-carbohydrate snack is often needed before or during breast-feeding. Evening or late night snacks may also be necessary.[771]

Pre-pregnancy care

If you are thinking about becoming pregnant, let your diabetes team know and they will help you to get your diabetes under best control before conception. Advice and counselling will be available.

It is better for a girl to wait at least until she is in her twenties before becoming pregnant as a teenage pregnancy brings about increased medical risks both for the baby (premature birth, complications in the newborn) and the mother (anaemia, eclampsia or pre-eclampsia).

Caring for the mother

Pregnant women with diabetes are usually very highly motivated and will also receive closer attention from the maternity care services. Tell your diabetes healthcare team as soon as possible if you suspect you may be pregnant, or if you are hoping to become pregnant. They can help you get a pregnancy test (so called chorionic gonadotropin test) which will give a relia-

Estimated insulin requirements during pregnancy [305]

		U/kg	U/lb
Before pregnancy		0.6	0.27
Week	6-18	0.7	0.32
Week	18-26	0.8	0.36
Week	26-36	0.9	0.41
Week	36-delivery	1.0	0.45
During delivery		Very low	
After delivery		Below 0.6	Below 0.27
Breast-feeding		Further decrease in insulin need	

ble result within a couple of days after you have missed a period.

A general consensus is that it is a full-time job to be pregnant if you have diabetes. This means that it is quite hard work to maintain blood glucose levels at as normal a level as possible during pregnancy. The goal is for HbA_{1c} during pregnancy to be within the normal range for individuals without diabetes. Treatment with an insulin pump may be an effective way of achieving this.

During the latter part of pregnancy, it often becomes more difficult to recognize symptoms of hypoglycaemia as the threshold for developing symptoms will be lowered because of frequent low blood glucose levels [906] (see "Hypoglycaemia unawareness" on page 52). The HbA_{1c} value for women without diabetes is approximately 5-10 mmol/mol (0.5-1.0%) lower at the end of pregnancy, which is the reason for aiming for an HbA_{1c} close to 42 mmol/mol (6.0%), the upper limit for individuals without diabetes, during the later part of pregnancy.[407,462] In a Scottish study, half of the women attained an HbA_{1c} in the non-diabetic range at some point during their pregnancy.[407] Within 1 year, however, most of them increased

in HbA_{1c} to levels observed before pregnancy. This may be attributed to not having the time to take care of their diabetes in the most effective way at the same time as caring for an infant at home. Women giving birth to their second or third child had higher HbA_{1c} during pregnancy, suggesting that the amount of work to be done at home affects how easy it to care for your diabetes during pregnancy.

During pregnancy, the ketone production during periods of insulin deficiency is increased, making ketoacidosis more likely.[89] Ketoacidosis during pregnancy is very dangerous, especially for the unborn child.[305,756] You should therefore check for ketones in blood or urine regularly, especially if you are being or feeling sick, or have an infection with a raised temperature. A bedtime snack is usually necessary for pregnant women as it decreases the risk of night time hypoglycaemia and fasting ketones. Ketones will show in the urine after only 12-14 hours of fasting.[365] Urine testing every morning will show whether or not you have "starvation ketones" from inadequate carbohydrate intake in the evening. Morning ketones are present in 30% of pregnant women who do not have diabetes.[31] A slight delay in development was found in children aged 2-9 years whose mothers had raised ketone levels during pregnancy.[893]

Nearly every woman has thoughts during pregnancy about something being wrong with her child. However, most women with diabetes have a quite normal pregnancy, leading to the birth of a healthy child. If you have a low HbA_{1c} before and during pregnancy, the risks for your child are approximately the same as if you didn't have diabetes.

If you use an insulin pump, your risk of ketoacidosis will increase due to the smaller insulin depot (see page 197). If the pump infusion set fails during the night you will have high blood glucose levels and elevated levels of ketones in the morning. One method of avoiding this is to give a bedtime injection of intermediate-acting insulin (0.2 U/kg, 0.1U/lb) in addition to the normal basal dose delivered by the pump.[717] The renal threshold is usually lowered in pregnant women, causing an increased excretion of glucose via the urine. Urine tests for glucose cannot be relied upon therefore.

How will the child develop?

In a Swedish study, children of women with diabetes were seen to be developing normally at the age of 5.[89] The height and weight were also found to be normal in another study.[89] An Australian study followed children up to the age of 3 years.[959] Children of mothers having low HbA_{1c} readings were found to be developing normally, while children of mothers with high HbA_{1c} values during pregnancy had delayed language development and a smaller head circumference.

Will the child have diabetes?

If you have diabetes you may ask yourself: "Should I have a baby when there is an increased risk of the child getting diabetes?" In one study 3% of the children of mothers with diabetes went on to develop diabetes themselves by the age of 10-13 years [833] (which is about 10 times the risk of the child of a mother without diabetes). Although it is believed that half the factors contributing to diabetes are inherited, only about one in every 10 children with newly diagnosed diabetes has a parent or sibling with diabetes.[228] The hereditary disposition for developing type 1 diabetes is very common, at least 40% according to certain studies.[230] From this it follows that a person with diabetes should not in any way be discouraged from having children. See also "Heredity" on page 376.

A few people may choose adoption instead. They do this because of increased risks, both for the child acquiring diabetes and for the mother, of going through a pregnancy with diabetes, especially if she also has diabetes complications (see page 332).

It appears that the risk of a child of acquiring diabetes decreases as the mother's age increases. If a mother has diabetes and is older than 25 when she gives birth, the risk to the child of developing diabetes later in life is not significantly increased compared with mothers without diabetes.[1090] Another study showed that 8.9% of children born to fathers with diabetes, but only 3.4% of children born to mothers with diabetes, developed the disease before the age of 20.[102] If the mother was 8 years old or younger when she developed diabetes, the risk of the child was considerably higher, 13.9%, in this study.

Infertility

Women with average diabetes control have the same chances of getting pregnant as women without diabetes.[89] If you suspect problems with your fertility, contact your diabetes healthcare team who will refer you to a gynaecologist.

Will diabetes affect the menstrual periods?

Many women have noticed that their blood glucose level increases the days before they have their period.[8,699] In a Hungarian study, the premenstrual insulin doses were approximately 3 units higher than they were mid-cycle.[1018] However, during the first couple of days of menstruation, the insulin requirements may fall, predisposing to hypoglycaemia. If you notice that you have this type of problem, check your blood glucose level especially carefully the days close to menstruation. This will enable you to adjust your insulin doses upwards just before your period, and lower them again afterwards.

It is quite normal for teenage girls' menstrual periods to be irregular and unpredictable during the first 6-12 months. However, girls with diabetes seem to be twice as prone to have menstrual periods very close together in spite of a good glucose control.[384] A high HbA_{1c} increases the risk of having irregular or missed periods.[953] The risk of menstrual disturbances in adolescents in this study was increased seven times if HbA_{1c} was above 86 mmol/mol (10%) and 18 times if HbA_{1c} was above 108 mmol/mol (12%). Another study found that menstrual periods were delayed by 5 days for every increase in of HbA_{1c} with 10 mmol/mol (0.9%).[384]

Sexuality

In terms of sexual relationships, teenage boys and girls with diabetes will function in exactly the same way as their friends of the same age. The only difference is that it is particularly important to use contraceptives to avoid an unwanted pregnancy. Remember that you may encounter hypoglycaemia after having intercourse — making love can be energetic exercise! Some people find they don't function well sexually if their blood glucose level is high, but this can improve if the level is corrected.[62] According to some studies, sexual desire is negatively affected by long-standing diabetes, in both women and men.[333] Other studies, however, have not found this to be true.[333]

Impotence may be a complication of diabetes, which men who have had diabetes for many years will encounter. This can be caused by a combination of premature arteriosclerosis and a reduction in the intensity of physical response caused by disturbances in the autonomic nervous system (see page 363). In a population-based study of men who were 21 years or older, and were less than 30 years of age at diagnosis of diabetes, 20% reported erectile problems.[563] These problems increased with age, from 1.1% in those 21-30 years of age to 47.1% in those 43 years of age or older. Another study found that the risk of developing erectile problems in men with diabetes in the age group 40-69 years was 1.8 times more common compared with the general population.[620]

Impotence commonly has a psychological (rather than a physical) cause in individuals both with and without diabetes. If you have erections in the morning, it is likely that the reasons for your impotence are psychological.[62] Temporary disturbances of erection are something that all men encounter once in a while. The difficulty for a young man with diabetes is that any temporary erection problem is likely to be attributed immediately to the diabetes, when the cause may be something as simple as tiredness or feeling nervous in a new relationship. A vicious cycle may arise with negative expecta-

If you have diabetes, it is particularly important that your pregnancy be planned. Tell your diabetes team or doctor if you need contraceptives and they will refer you to the appropriate professional.

tions and the fear of continued failure. Do not hesitate to talk to your diabetes doctor or nurse about the problems.

If the impotence is a complication of diabetes, there is a good chance of getting effective treatment. In the past, injection treatment was used but the impotence drugs Viagra® and Levitra® work in around 60% of cases.[1002] If you have heart disease you should consult your doctor before using this type of drug. Part of the treatment involves lessening other risk factors such as alcohol, tobacco and drugs (for example, certain drugs for blood pressure). Unsatisfactory diabetes control with a high HbA_{1c} will increase the risk of impotence.[945] In the same way as with other complications (see page 354) the problems may be halted or even reversed if they are discovered early, and the diabetes treatment is changed, leading to a lowered HbA_{1c}.

Female sexuality is less affected by diabetes.[62] Problems with vaginal discharge and fungal infections are more common in women with diabetes and may have a negative effect on sexual desire. The vaginal mucous membranes can become temporarily dry when the blood glucose is high, and this can be troublesome during intercourse. It is not yet established whether late complications to diabetes (nerve damage) can result in the same problem.[333] A pharmacist can advise you about suitable lubricants if you have this type of problem. The ability to reach orgasm does not appear to be affected by diabe-

tes.[333] Viagra® and Levitra® can improve sexual function in women with diabetes.[173]

Contraceptives

In the past, the "minipill" (containing only progesterone) was usually recommended to women with diabetes. However, this increases the risk of "spotting" between periods, and has a narrower time margin for taking the pills (not more than 27 hours between pills). Combined contraceptives ("ordinary" pills) are more effective in preventing pregnancy. They contain two types of female sex hormone. Oestrogen prevents the egg from developing and being released from the ovary. Progesterone prevents the sperm from passing through the mucus of the neck of womb (cervix). The use of oral contraceptives does not appear to increase the risk of later complications with the eyes or kidneys.[390]

At one time, combined contraceptive pills were thought to raise the blood glucose level slightly, but recent studies show no adverse affects on glucose control.[839] If your glucose control is unpredictable during the week without pills and it is difficult to adjust your insulin doses, it might be appropriate to wait longer before interrupting, that is, take pills for 3 months without interruption.[13] Today, so called second generation combined pills are recommended to begin with.[243] Combined pills are not advisable if you smoke (due to an increased risk of thrombosis and heart attack), or if you have high blood pressure, severe migraine attacks, or complications with your eyes or kidneys.[13]

An intrauterine device (IUD, coil) is a safe contraceptive for women with diabetes according to studies.[610] Problems with infections or spotting are no more common than for women without diabetes.[612] However, they are not recommended if you have irregular or heavy menstrual periods. As there is a small risk of infection of the womb or ovary (and thus a risk of becoming infertile), intrauterine devices are not recommended for women who have never been pregnant. However, for a woman who has diabetes complications affecting the eyes or kidneys, intrauterine devices may be a good alternative to contraceptive pills. [610]

Depot injections or implants contain the same hormone (progesterone) as minipills. However, they will give a higher hormone concentration and affect the blood glucose level more than minipills. Common side effects are nausea, increased appetite or irritability, all of which make it more difficult to control the blood glucose levels. The contraceptive depot injection is not considered suitable for women with diabetes as the effects of one injection last for many months. A contraceptive implant contains the same hormone as a depot injection. It is implanted under the skin using local anaesthesia. The advantage is that it can be removed if the woman experiences serious side effects. This makes it more suitable for a woman with diabetes than the depot injection.

Remember that most contraceptive methods only prevent unwanted pregnancy. It is as important to protect yourself against sexually transmitted diseases. Some of these diseases can be life-threatening; others can have a serious effect on women's fertility. A condom is the only contraceptive that offers full protection from sexually transmitted diseases. Talk to your general practitioner or pregnancy advice service about which type of contraceptive can be suitable for you. Depending on local policies and practices, your GP can give you a prescription or refer you to a gynaecologist for further advice. Young women using oral contraceptives should have regular blood pressure monitoring and gynaecological check-up.

Forgotten to take a pill?

If you discover that you have forgotten to take your contraceptive pill, you should take an extra pill when you realize this,[147] even if it means taking two pills at the same time. If more

Contraceptive methods	
Condom	The only contraceptive that protects against sexually transmitted disease.
Ordinary pills	Sometimes result in a slight increase in blood glucose levels.
Minipills	Risk of spotting. Less margin for error when forgetting to take tablets.
Depot injection	Can affect metabolic control. Sometimes troublesome side effects.
Implant	Same as depot injection but easy to remove if side effects are not acceptable.
Diaphragm and spermicidal jelly	Not so easy to use. Risk of itching as side effect.
Intrauterine device (IUDs, coil)	Risk of pelvic infection is low but an IUD is not recommended before the first pregnancy.
"Morning-after" pills	For "emergency" situations. Needs to be taken within 72 hours.

than 36 hours have passed (more than 27 hours with minipills), you will have no protection and you must use another method when sexually active, such as condoms, during the following week.[147] If you forget this, you will need to use the "morning-after" method and take a pregnancy test. The protection effect when forgetting a pill may be different with different pills, so read the label or contact your doctor for advice. It may be easier to remember to take the first tablet after a period if you take tablets every day (28 tablets in the box). In fact, it is considerably more risky to forget the first or second tablet, compared to one of the last on the sheet.

> ## Which contraceptive should you choose if you have diabetes? [89]
>
> ① Pills (not minipills) for teenagers.
>
> ② Coil (IUD) for women who have been pregnant.
>
> ③ Using a condom is always a good alternative and, in addition, is the only way of protecting yourself from sexually transmitted diseases. Always use a condom in a temporary relationship.

> ## Morning-after methods
> ## Only for "emergency" use!
>
> ① Pills:
>
> ⟹ A new type of pill (Norlevo®, Postinor®, Levonelle®, Plan B®) give the highest security and lowest occurrence of side effects.
>
> ⟹ Two ordinary pills taken within 72 hours after unprotected intercourse and 2 pills after another 12 hours can also be used. Only special pills with high hormonal content can be used.
>
> ⟹ Contact a doctor or pregnancy advisory service as soon as possible. You will need to see your GP within 3-4 weeks to discuss which contraceptive to continue with.
>
> ② Inserting a coil:
>
> ⟹ A coil should be inserted within 72 hours, at the very latest within 5 days.
>
> ⟹ Coils are recommended only for women who have been pregnant.

Emergency contraception

Emergency contraception ("morning-after pills") is available in most countries for emergency situations, that is if you have had unprotected intercourse.[405] They can be used at any time of the menstrual cycle. The risk of getting pregnant after unprotected intercourse is 6-7% overall, and at the time of ovulation as high as 20-30%.[46] With "morning-after pills", this risk goes down to 1-3%.

This type of medication prevents the fertilized egg from implanting in the membranes of the uterus. Unfortunately, feeling or even being sick is a relatively common side effect. A new type of tablet containing only one type of hormone (progesterone, Norlevo®, Postinor®, Levonelle®, Plan B®) decreases both the risk of unwanted pregnancy and the risk of sickness. "Morning-after pills" must be taken at the very latest 72 hours after intercourse,[405] which is why you should get in touch with your pregnancy advisory service, general practitioner or local pharmacy as soon as possible. They are available as "over the counter" medication if you are above the age of 18 in the UK. The contraceptive effect is higher, the earlier the tablets are taken. Contact an emergency pharmacy, or the hospital, if the need for these arises over the weekend or after office hours.

Repeated use of emergency contraception during the same menstrual cycle will decrease the pregnancy protection effect. Emergency contraception cannot interrupt or have negative effects on an already established pregnancy.

Social issues

School

When you go back to school or work again after your diagnosis, it is important to tell your friends about your diabetes. It is very understandable not to want to talk about your diabetes at this stage and many people find this is how they feel. It takes real courage to tell your classmates and friends at home or at work. However, it really will make your life much easier if you can tell them right away and have done with it, rather than find yourself worrying about who knows and who doesn't. If it can be arranged, it is a good idea for a specialist diabetes nurse to come to your class and talk about diabetes, inviting all teachers who come into contact with you, including the physical educa-

tion teacher. Invite the diabetes nurse to come to school again when you move to a new class or change to a new school.

It is very helpful when a teacher really understands a child or teenager with diabetes. Sometimes it may be difficult for them to know if something the child does or a particular behaviour (such as tiredness or irritability) is due to a low blood glucose level or something else. Classroom attention was better in one study when glucose control was improved with an insulin pump, resulting in fewer fluctuations of blood glucose.[241] It is important for the child to be able to measure blood glucose values at school when necessary. Some parents have the impression that the school and teachers take diabetes more seriously only after the child has had a difficult hypoglycaemic reaction at school, but this is of course an unfortunate way to demonstrate how serious diabetes can be.

When a schoolchild has diabetes, it is a good idea to draw up an individualized Diabetes Healthcare Plan as a collaborative effort

Hypoglycaemia in school

☞ An emergency plan should be set up to determine who does what if a child with diabetes is unwell or develops hypoglycaemia.

☞ Your teacher or the school nurse (if there is one) should preferably be able to help you measure your blood glucose level if necessary.

☞ Make sure that your teachers and friends know where you keep your emergency glucose and when you need to take it.

☞ Snacks should be available so that you have something to eat if hypoglycaemia occurs. Eating in the classroom must be permitted.

☞ The other children must be helped to understand why you may have to eat glucose tablets, a piece of fruit or a sandwich during class to prevent or treat hypoglycaemia.

School routines (adapted from [84] and [29])

It is desirable for school routines to be adjusted in line with the needs of a child with diabetes:

⟹ Understand and recognize that the diabetes expert closest to hand is the young person and his or her parents.

⟹ Staff need to have sufficient background knowledge about diabetes, and must be made aware of the fact that type 1 diabetes in childhood is not at all the same disease as type 2 diabetes.

⟹ Reach an agreement with staff about how much help the young person needs, such as reminders to take insulin or test blood.

⟹ Appropriate help with monitoring blood glucose and ketones, taking insulin injections and managing hypoglycaemic reactions should be available, according to the age of the child, both in school and on field trips.

⟹ Understand the need for frequent trips to the bathroom when the blood glucose level is high.

⟹ Young people with diabetes should be able to test their blood and urine in an undisturbed environment when necessary. They should also be allowed to test their blood glucose during lessons.

⟹ Young people should be allowed to take their lunch time dose of insulin undisturbed.

⟹ Don't send a child who is in hypoglycaemia on their own to the school nurse. Give dextrose first and then, if necessary, send the child accompanied by a friend or an adult.

⟹ Don't send a child with diabetes home on their own from school earlier than expected (especially not after a hypoglycaemic episode) without first checking that someone is at home who can take care of him or her.

⟹ Understand that the young person's school tests and exam results can be less reliable than they should be because of hypoglycaemia. The young person should be allowed to retake the test or exam, as it is difficult to obtain full concentration for several hours after hypoglycaemia.

School routines, continued

⟹ Regular mealtimes should be established, with lunch as close to noon as possible.

⟹ The food served must be appropriate for a child with diabetes. However, it needs to be eaten if it is to do any good at all for the blood glucose level. It is important to be aware that young people with diabetes do not have the same choice as their peers to go hungry if they don't find the food appetizing. An alternative outside the regular menu must be available at all times. It may be helpful if parents check the school menu in advance, together with the young person.

⟹ Physical education should preferably be scheduled as the second or third lesson after a meal when using rapid-acting insulin (NovoRapid or Humalog), since there will be a quick increase in insulin level in your blood during the first hour (see graph on page 290). However, when using short-acting insulin physical education should preferably be scheduled as the first or second lesson in the morning or the first or second lesson after lunch. See also page 287.

⟹ Report timetable changes to parents well ahead, such as visiting a public swimming pool or a games day.

⟹ Organize a parent-teacher conference when needed, inviting the diabetes nurse or doctor to attend.

⟹ School staff can visit the diabetes healthcare team along with the child, to increase their knowledge of diabetes.

⟹ Give realistic vocational guidance.

between the child's parent or guardian, members of the diabetes care team, and the school or daycare provider — as well as with the child him or herself. This plan sets out the basic medical needs the child has while at school, and how these needs will be met. Inherent in this process are responsibilities assumed by all parties, including the parent or guardian, the school personnel, and the child. In addition to

Research findings:
Blood glucose level and learning

♠ A study on adults showed that a blood glucose higher than 15 mmol/l (270 mg/dl) was associated with poorer results on psychomotor tests, with slower reaction time and increased errors when recalling words and doing mental subtraction.[211] However, this effect was noticeable only in approximately half of the individuals, i.e there is a large individual variation. It did not seem as if it is possible to adjust to a higher blood glucose level, in that those with a higher HbA_{1c} actually performed slightly less well when their blood glucose was high.

♠ A paediatric study, including children from 6 to 11 years, found a 20% decrease in reaction time and 20% slower performance (but normal accuracy) on a mathematical test (subtraction and addition) both when blood glucose was below 3.0 mmol/l (54 mg/dl) and above 22.2 mmol/l (400 mg/dl).[411] The children noticed the difficulties in performing during hypoglycaemia, but were not aware of them when blood glucose level was high. As in the adults, there was a large individual variation, with 21% of the children having evident deterioration during hypoglycaemia and 27% during high blood glucose.

♠ From this and other work on performance when hypoglycaemic, it follows that the optimal blood glucose for school performance is between 3-4 and 15-20 mmol/l (55-70 and 270-360 mg/dl). It is then important not to overeat in an effort to avoid hypoglycaemia during a school test or exam.

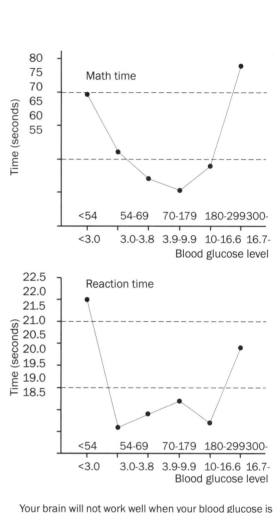

Your brain will not work well when your blood glucose is too low or too high. See the text to the left for details on this study. The graph is from reference [411].

the medical issues covered in such a healthcare plan, children with diabetes must be permitted to eat wherever and whenever they need to, even if other children are not allowed to eat (for example, in class, on the school bus, during P.E. lessons).[601]

JDRF (the Juvenile Diabetes Research Foundation, see page 337) has a special pack for schools containing brochures, a Warning Signs card, a Low Blood Sugar Emergencies card, a book list and more. ADA and CWD (www.childrenwithdiabetes.com) also have information packs and support for school issues.

Hypoglycaemia

It is important and very helpful for the child to talk to friends about diabetes and the signs of hypoglycaemia. Friends should know where to find dextrose tablets. Hypoglycaemia will affect a child's performance at school, not only when the blood glucose level is low, but also up to 3-4 hours after it has been normalized. In a study of children and adolescents between the ages of 11 and 18 years, a significant decline in mental efficiency was found at blood glucose levels of 3.3-3.6 mmol/l (60-65 mg/dl). This was most evident in measures of mental flexibility, planning, decision making, attention to detail and rapid responding.[914]

Exams

Always make sure that you have something extra to eat during an examination. Many students prefer to have a slightly higher blood glucose level during examinations to avoid hypoglycaemia. Stress before an exam may make the blood glucose levels higher (see page 299).

You should feel free to measure your blood glucose if you experience difficulties in concentrating during an examination. You will then know if you need to eat something extra. It may also be important to be able to show a low blood glucose reading to your teacher, if you feel that your results from an examination are not as

Don't send a child with diabetes home from school alone earlier than expected without checking that someone is at home. If the child experiences hypoglycaemia on his or her way home and nobody is there to help, this may easily develop into severe hypoglycaemia.

Research findings: Diabetes and school

♠ A Swedish national study involving 5.159 children with diabetes found the mean school marks to be slightly lower (3.15 vs. 3.23 on a 1-5 scale) in children with diabetes.[240] The lowest mean score was in the group of children with diabetes onset before the age of 2 years, and they also had twice the risk of not completing the 9-year compulsory school. The control group of children without diabetes were of the same age and their mothers had the same level of education.

♠ A US study in 244 children with diabetes aged 8-18 years found lower reading scores and grade point averages for children with poor glucose control (HbA$_{1c}$ > 86 mmol/mol, 10%).[733] But so did their siblings as well. As a group, children with diabetes did perform better than their siblings in maths, and better than their classmates in reading. The diabetic children had higher school absences than their siblings (7.3 days/year vs. 5.3). However, medical variables, including hospitalizations for diabetes, were not as strongly related to academic achievements as other factors like socioeconomic status and behaviour.

♠ A Canadian study looked at school attendance in 78 children with diabetes. They missed only slightly more school days (around 2-3 days a year) than their siblings and friends without diabetes.[404] This may be due to appointments with health professionals.

♠ In a study including age groups 10-17 years with an HbA$_{1c}$ of 75 mmol/mol (9.0%) or above, the school nurse measured blood glucose at lunch time, helped adjust the insulin dose and supervised the injection of both Lantus (which was given at lunch-time in this study) and NovoRapid.[783] Parents or other adult caregivers did the same at lunch time on weekends. After 3 months HbA$_{1c}$ was lowered to 60 mmol/mol (7.6%). Thus, involving the school nurse might be a very good way of improving diabetes care.

good as they should be, and you want to resit. In some cases, you might need a doctor's certificate to support this. See also page 72, 254 and 287 concerning low blood glucose levels, food and physical education in school.

Day nurseries and child care

A child with diabetes attending a day nursery will need more time and attention than children without diabetes of the same age. In some communities, children with diabetes can be counted as two in the accounting, giving the staff more time for the child. The rules and regulations differ from country to country.

In most countries, childminders or day nursery staff have no formal obligation to help with blood glucose testing. However, you will usually find someone interested enough who will help, at least if the child is not feeling well. In some places the staff will also give insulin. This may be easier to do if the child has an injection aid, such as Inject-Ease®, PenMate™, or Insuflon (see page 137) or a pump. Sometimes it may be appropriate to have glucagon available if staff members know how and when to give it.

Regular babysitters and childminders will benefit from accompanying the family on a visit to the diabetes healthcare team, or the diabetes nurse may visit the day nursery to talk to staff and children about diabetes (see also page 95).

Child care allowance

In some countries, special allowances are available for parents of a child with diabetes to compensate for the extra time and commitment that

is involved in diabetes care (e.g. Disability Living Allowance in the UK). Regulations change from time to time so it is best to obtain the current status from your diabetes clinic, especially as the forms to be filled in are often long and complicated. Special rules may also apply to healthcare insurance or benefits when you stay at home with a sick child.

Adoption

Some countries have restrictions on adoption by a parent with diabetes. Such restrictions are usually due to outdated information about life with diabetes but you may be required to get medical clearance indicating your ability to provide appropriate self-care.

Choice of job or employment

Almost all types of employment are open to people with diabetes. It is important that you, like everyone else, think first and foremost about what you would like to do. Jobs which include some type of physical work or at least not sitting still all day have the advantage of giving you regular exercise. However, considering the risk of hypoglycaemia, you should avoid jobs where your own or other people's safety depend on you *always* functioning perfectly in all situations. Particularly dangerous situations can occur for police and fire personnel while most other situations (for example a physician or other healthcare professional) would include the possibility of stopping to check blood glucose levels and making appropriate adjustments with food and/or insulin accordingly. The risk of developing hypoglycaemia will hinder someone with diabetes from becoming a policeman, pilot or airline steward, joining the armed forces, and in most countries also driving a bus, taxi or train. Professional diving or working at high altitudes is usually discouraged since these are difficult situations in which to deal with hypoglycaemic emergencies. The rules will vary in different countries.

Policemen, firemen and pilots are examples of professionals who might be putting their own or other peoples' lives at risk if they develop severe hypoglycaemia. In most countries, you are not allowed to work as a pilot or policeman if you have diabetes, but being a fire fighter or driving an ambulance may work well if you do not have problems with hypoglycaemia. However, in the UK and Canada you are allowed to pilot a commercial aircraft. In six countries (USA, UK, Canada, Australia, Israel and the Philippines) you are allowed to fly a private plane. See www.pilotswithdiabetes.com for more information.

Usually, you can adjust insulin doses to fit with most working schedules, even when irregular hours are included. When working shift patterns, or if there are frequent changes in work schedules and meal timetables, this may be more difficult to accomplish. A flexible insulin regimen or a pump with different basal rate profiles for work days and days off may help.

Examine the possibility of trying out different occupations to find out how well you can cope with your diabetes under the work situations; talking to people in different jobs may be helpful in terms of flexibility for food and snacks as well as insulin administration and blood glucose testing. People with diabetes should be individually considered for employment, based on the requirements of the specific job but this is not always the case. There are many myths about people with diabetes and what they can and cannot do, so that you may have to educate folk about diabetes in such circumstances. Ask

Diabetes UK for advice if you feel that your diabetes stops you from getting a particular job. Diabetes UK believes that a person with diabetes should be eligible for employment in any occupation for which he or she is individually qualified. They feel that a person with diabetes has the right to be assessed for specific job duties on his or her own merits based on reasonable standards applied consistently. They also believe that employers have the duty to accommodate employees with diabetes unless the employer can show it to cause undue hardship to the organization. The IRFD (International Register of Firefighters with Diabetes) is a UK organization that works to prevent diabetes discrimination in employment.

Military service

Young people in the UK do not have to do military service, but in many other countries it is still obligatory. However, young people in many parts of the world will automatically be exempt from mandatory military service if they have diabetes. In some countries non-active employment in the services are allowed, such as office or administrative work. Ask your doctor for a medical certificate if you are drafted. Your diabetes healthcare team and the military authorities can give you further information.

Licence to drive

Most countries will allow people with diabetes who are taking insulin and are free of complications to obtain a driving licence. However, regulations, restrictions and the need for a medical review vary considerably from country to country. Your diabetes clinic or Diabetes UK can tell you exactly what is applicable in Britain and other countries. People treated with insulin are able to take the driving test and obtain driving licences, but will usually need a letter from their doctor. This licence is reviewed every 3 years with respect to, for example, being able to look after diabetes competently and avoiding hypoglycaemia.

While European governments have further restricted driving licences for insulin-treated drivers with diabetes, the restrictions on drivers in the US have been relaxed. The EU driving licence directive from 1998 (91/439) prevents people who are being treated with insulin from driving lighter goods vehicles (weighing between 3.5 and 7.5 tons) and small passenger-carrying vehicles for more than eight passengers on a commercial basis.[710] Driving these vehicles on a voluntary basis is still permitted.

In the UK, if someone already has a licence for heavy goods vehicles (class C_1, 3,500-7,500 kg), and develops type 1 diabetes, that person may continue to drive subject to an annual medical examination.[401] Until recently, a person with type 1 has not been allowed to apply for a class C_1 licence. Now the DVLA (Driver and Vehicle Licensing Agency) has agreed that insulin-treated drivers with diabetes may apply for C_1 licences and be assessed individually.[401] The proposed DVLA criteria for C_1 vehicle driving include regular review by a diabetes consultant, home glucose monitoring, lack of recent severe hypoglycaemia, and also awareness of milder hypoglycaemia.

Driving and diabetes

Key safety issues with regard to driving for people with diabetes involve frequent blood glucose

testing and hypoglycaemia prevention, especially unawareness of hypoglycaemia, to maximize the individual's safety while driving and to ensure public safety as well.

The risks associated with driving while suffering from hypoglycaemia are obvious. Drivers with diabetes are generally not more prone to accidents than other drivers according to most studies.[218] However, there are case reports of serious accidents due to hypoglycaemia.[291] In the DCCT study (see page 367) hypoglycaemia was the main contributing factor in 36% of the traffic accidents that the participants encountered during the 9 years of the study.[264] In a Scottish study, 25% of the participants attributed their road accidents to hypoglycaemia.[709] Of cases reported to British authorities, 16-17% of cases of collapse at the wheel were caused by hypoglycaemia in a person with diabetes.[354] Although these studies exemplify an increased risk of traffic accidents in a small number of cases, the conclusion of a review is that, for the general population with diabetes, accident rates do not exceed the rates for drivers without diabetes.[710] As a comparison, a ban on all young male drivers would be more effective in terms of improving road safety, but would represent a totally unacceptable restriction in the freedom of individuals.[710]

You should check your blood glucose before driving and if it is below 4-5 mmol/l (70-90 mg/dl) you should eat something before beginning your trip. If you don't experience hypoglycaemic symptoms at low blood glucose levels (hypoglycaemia unawareness) you are not fit to drive. Even if you feel quite capable of driving when your blood glucose level is 2.5 mmol/l (45 mg/dl), your reaction time will be too slow for safety. This has been shown to occur below the level of approximately 2.8 mmol/l (50 mg/dl).[716] See page 52 for further information on how to treat this phenomenon, which is caused by your body becoming accustomed to low blood glucose levels. It will take a while after a hypoglycaemic episode before your reaction time is back to normal. In one study the blood glucose

Research findings:
Driving with diabetes

♠ In an American study, subjects with diabetes were tested in a driving simulator.[208] They were not told their blood glucose readings (a blind study).

♠ At a blood glucose level of 3.6 mmol/l (65 mg/dl) only 8% showed impaired driving while at 2.6 mmol/l (45 mg/dl) 35% were driving more slowly, and had steering difficulties (more swerving, spinning, time over midline, and time off road). Only half of them were aware of their impaired ability.

♠ When the same investigations were re-done 3 months later, the results were similar in that the same individuals had impaired ability to drive at lower blood glucose levels.[865]

♠ The same authors did another blinded study in a more advanced simulator where the blood glucose was lowered to 2.2 mmol/l (40 mg/dl). Driving was impaired below 4.0 mmol/l (72 mg/dl), mainly driving above speed limit and off-road driving. Below 3.3 mmol/l (60 mg/dl) many drove across the midline, showed inappropriate braking, too low speed or off-road driving.

♠ This was very individual, in that only 38% of the participants demonstrated a severe driving impairment relative to their performance at normal blood glucose level. Although 15% detected their hypoglycaemia below 4.0 mmol/l (72 mg/dl), 33% below 3.3 mmol/l (60 mg/dl) and 79% below 2.8 mmol/l (50 mg/dl), only 30% of them actually treated themselves and/or stopped driving (and then at a mean level of 2.7 mmol/l (48 mg/dl)!).

♠ In another study, the blood glucose level was reduced from 6.7 mmol/l (120 mg/dl) to 2.2 mmol/l (40 mg/dl) without the individuals being aware of their actual blood glucose level.[1096] At 6.7 mmol/l (120 mg/dl) 70% of the subjects judged they could drive safely. At 2.2 mmol/l (40 mg/dl), 22% still thought it safe to drive.

These studies illustrate the importance of checking your blood glucose before driving.

was lowered to 2.7 mmol/l (48 mg/dl). Twenty minutes after the blood glucose level had returned to normal, the reaction time was still prolonged.[338]

Insurance policies

Insurance policies for people with diabetes may differ considerably from country to country and between insurance companies as well. In countries where there is health insurance, at the time your child develops diabetes you may receive a one-off reimbursement or a monthly allowance from the insurance company. It can be difficult for a person with diabetes to get health or life insurance although some companies may have special arrangements, which allow enrolment for a higher premium (impaired risk insurance). Shop around different insurance companies to get the best deal or ask Diabetes UK for specific advice.

You may need to appeal if your health insurance conditions change after you are diagnosed as having diabetes. Unfortunately, people with diabetes don't always take as much care of themselves as they should, and the insurance companies use this information to assign higher risk to all people with diabetes. People with diabetes use hospital and emergency department

There are many situations in which one must be 100% alert when driving a car. Never drive with a blood glucose level below 4-5 mmol/l (70-90 mg/dl) even if you feel perfectly well!

To consider while driving

① Check your blood glucose level before you take your place behind the wheel. Do not start driving with a blood glucose of 4-5 mmol/l (70-90 mg/dl) without treating it. **Even if you feel quite well, your blood glucose level must never fall below** 4.0 mmol/l (70 mg/dl), **or your driving performance will be impaired.**[208]

② Don't start out on a drive or a bicycle trip if you have not eaten recently.

③ Always bring along extra food and carry dextrose tablets in your pocket or the glove compartment of the car.

④ Always pull over and stop the car if you have hypoglycaemia and wait until you feel better before continuing. Remember that your thinking and judgement will not be back to normal until several hours later.

⑤ Be extra careful when the risk of hypoglycaemia is increased, for example after playing sport or when you have recently adjusted your insulin doses.

⑥ Alcohol increases the risk of hypoglycaemia as well as making you unfit to drive. Make it a habit never to drive a car or motorcycle when you have been drinking.

⑦ Changes in your blood glucose level can result in transient blurred vision.

⑧ Refrain from driving for a week or so if you make major changes in your insulin regimen (such as changing from 2 to 4 or 5 doses per day or starting with an insulin pump) until you find out how the new treatment affects you.

⑨ No matter how good a driver you are with a normal blood glucose level, you are never a safe driver if you have hypoglycaemic unawareness (no warning symptoms until the blood glucose level is very low). See page 52 for advice on how to treat this problem.

⑩ Don't ever smoke marijuana and drive since like alcohol it can impair brain function and judgement.

You may need to appeal if your health insurance conditions change after you are diagnosed as having diabetes.

resources more than those without diabetes; people with diabetes require ongoing medications (syringes, pens, insulin, glucose and ketone testing equipment) and need more hospital or clinic visits to help manage their illness than those without chronic illnesses.

Disability insurance policies and life insurance policies are often not allowed for people with diabetes since statistically they are at higher risk of being disabled at an earlier age compared with their peers, as well as of dying prematurely. While this is clearly improved with better self-care, more self blood glucose monitoring and better insulins, this is not always apparent to individual insurance providers or even to employers. Policies may be available but with much higher premiums so that one must weigh the benefits of such policies against their costs. Travel insurance may also be available at higher premiums because of a pre-existing condition.

The present practice of increased accident insurance premiums and limited coverage is not supported by scientific evidence. A Danish study of 7,599 adult individuals with diabetes found that the risk of accidents and permanent disability was no different from that in a control group without diabetes.[726] Furthermore, the authors found an increase in average life expectancy of 15 years or more over a 40-year period (mainly because of a decreased risk of kidney damage), which should motivate and encourage insurance companies to re-evaluate their policies.[135]

Diabetes ID

It is a good idea to always carry something on your person showing that you have diabetes, such as a special necklace or bracelet (Medic-Alert® or something similar). It is not uncommon for a person with diabetes to be mistaken for being drunk when in fact he or she is hypoglycaemic. Even if you have only had a small amount to drink, people noticing the smell of alcohol are likely to pass by without helping you.

If you are travelling abroad, it is a good idea to have some kind of identification showing that you have diabetes and that you need to carry insulin and accessories. Insulin companies and Diabetes Associations often have special cards with text in different languages explaining what help you need if you become hypoglycaemic.

Juvenile Diabetes Research Foundation International

The Juvenile Diabetes Research Foundation International (JDRF) was founded in 1970 by parents of children with juvenile diabetes. JDRF volunteers have a personal connection with diabetes in the young and this translates into an unrelenting focus on the needs of all people with diabetes and a commitment to finding a cure as soon as possible.

The mission of JDRF is to find to find a cure for diabetes and its complications through the sup-

port of research. Embedded in JDRF's mission are its three core goals:

⇒ Restoring normal blood sugar levels.

⇒ Preventing and reversing complications.

⇒ Preventing type 1 diabetes.

JDRF is now leading the worldwide effort to replicate and expand upon the success of the Edmonton Protocol (see page 383), while continuing progress towards the goal of inducing tolerance to transplanted islets without the need for long-term immunosuppression. To date, JDRF has established eight centres specifically for islet transplantation, co-funded the NIH/JDRF Immune Tolerance Network, and invested or committed more than $150 million for islet transplantation worldwide.

JDRF has more than 120 Chapters, Branches and Affiliates worldwide. There are Affiliates in Australia, Canada, Chile, Greece, India, Israel, Italy, Puerto Rico and the UK. In their magazine *Countdown,* you will find in-depth analysis of cutting edge diabetes research along with information on treatments, profiles and more. *Countdown for Kids* is especially for children with diabetes and includes information and opportunities for fun, as well as access to role models and pen pals.

Children with Diabetes

The mission of Children with Diabetes is to promote understanding of the care and treatment of diabetes, especially in children; to increase awareness of the need for unrestricted diabetes care for children at school and day care; to support families living with diabetes; and to promote understanding of research into a cure. The website www.childrenwithdiabetes.com is the largest website in the world for

Most diabetes associations have journals where you can read news on diabetes research and many other helpful articles. It is a good idea to become a member of Diabetes UK or your local diabetes association.

children and adolescents with diabetes, with over 25,000 pages of content.

Diabetes Associations

In nearly every country, there is a Diabetes Association protecting the interests of people with diabetes. Local branches can be found in most towns. Find out if there is a special section for children and adolescents in your area. We strongly recommend joining your local diabetes association. You will receive valuable information including a newspaper or journal.

Diabetes UK

Diabetes UK is a charity working for people with diabetes, funding research, campaigning and helping people to live with the condition. The mission of the organization is to improve the lives of people with diabetes and to work towards a future without diabetes. Their visions include setting people free from the restrictions of diabetes, giving the highest quality care and information for all, and putting an end to discrimination and ignorance. Diabetes UK publishes magazines for people with diabetes (*Balance, On the Level* for young people, and *Link Up* for parents of children with diabetes) and for healthcare professionals (*Diabetes Update, Diabetic Medicine*). They also produce leaflets and fact sheets covering all aspects of diabetes care and some are downloadable from the www.diabetes.org.uk website.

Diabetes Federation Ireland

The aims of the Federation are:

➧ To represent people with diabetes.

➧ To help and provide information for people with diabetes, their families and the community.

➧ To create awareness and foster programmes for the early detection and prevention of diabetes.

➧ To support and encourage advances in diabetes care and research.

➧ To raise funds which will make the achievement of these aims possible.

The activities of the Federation include dissemination of non-judgmental advice and information through meetings, its magazine (*Diabetes Ireland*) and by request. The Federation provides support through its telephone helpline and regular public meetings. It raises awareness of diabetes by running campaigns and actively lobbies on behalf of people with diabetes in areas where they are being discriminated against and for national diabetes service development. All the above activities are possible only through the close collaboration of all people concerned with diabetes, whether their interest arises through their work or through living with the condition.

The International Diabetes Federation (IDF)

The International Diabetes Federation (IDF) is open to members of all countries. It promotes diabetes interests in many different areas. An international conference has been organized every third year. The 1997 conference was in Helsinki, Finland, 2000 in Mexico City and the year 2003 conference in Paris. The 2006 conference was held in Cape Town, South Africa and the 2009 conference in Montreal, Canada. The IDF conferences will from now on be held biannually and after Dubai, United Arab Emirates, 2011 the next was Melbourne, Australia in 2013. The 2015 meeting will be held in Vancouver, Canada. You can obtain further information about IDF from your local diabetes association or over the Internet.

International Society for Pediatric and Adolescent Diabetes (ISPAD)

ISPAD is the only global (professional) advocate for children and adolescents with diabetes. It is an association for diabetes teams (doctors, nurses, dietitians, educators, psychologists and all others involved in the care of children with diabetes. The society is committed to promoting the best possible health, social welfare and quality of life for *all* children and adolescents with diabetes, anywhere in the world. The aims of the society are outlined in the Declaration of Kos from 1993:

⮞ To make insulin available for *all* children and adolescents with diabetes.

⮞ To reduce the morbidity and mortality rates associated with acute metabolic complications or missed diagnosis relating to diabetes mellitus.

⮞ To increase the availability of appropriate urine and blood self-monitoring equipment for *all* children and adolescents with diabetes.

⮞ To develop and encourage research on diabetes in children and adolescents around the world.

⮞ To prepare and disseminate written guidelines and standards for the practical and realistic care and education of young patients with diabetes, and their families, emphasizing the crucial role of healthcare professionals (not just doctors) in these tasks around the world.

The National Service Framework for Diabetes (NSF)

The NSF contains a set of national standards to develop a patient-centred service, improve health outcomes for people with diabetes in England, raise the quality of services, and reduce unacceptable variations between them.[286] In the part about clinical care of children and young people with diabetes it is stated that the aim is:

⮞ To ensure that the special needs of children and young people with diabetes are recognized and met, thereby ensuring that, when they enter adulthood, they are in the best of health and able to manage their own day-to-day diabetes care effectively.

⮞ All children and young people with diabetes will receive consistently high-quality care and they, with their families and others involved in their day-to-day care, will be supported to optimise the control of their blood glucose and their physical, psychological, intellectual, educational and social development.

⮞ All young people with diabetes will experience a smooth transition of care from paediatric diabetes services to adult diabetes services, whether hospital- or community-based, either directly or via a young people's clinic. The transition will be organized in partnership with each individual and at an age appropriate to and agreed with them.

Sponsor families

Many things about diabetes are difficult to learn from a book or from the staff at the diabetes clinic. For example, few of the health professionals you come into contact with will either have diabetes themselves, or have children with diabetes. Because of this, some clinics have a system for finding a sponsor (or "befriending") family with a child of a similar age, preferably living close by. Such a family will be able to give you valuable tips and information about practical ways of handling different situations such as school, birthday parties, travel and so forth. The befriending system may be equally valuable for an adult with diabetes.

Diabetes camps and educational holidays

Participating in a diabetes camp or educational holiday gives young people the opportunity to increase their self-confidence by establishing friendships with other children with diabetes who have to abide by the same rules about insulin, diet and testing. The programme varies from camp to camp but most of these holidays emphasize improving young people's ability to manage diabetes on their own. In small groups, they can learn about correct injection technique, testing and monitoring, diet, physiology and other issues relating to diabetes.

It is more fun to take insulin and see what your blood glucose level is when your friends are doing the same thing. Children who have difficulties taking insulin or testing blood glucose levels will soon learn all about this from peers at a diabetes educational camp. The children are often relieved to find that their friends at the camp already know what diabetes is. They do not need to explain what hypoglycaemia is or why they take injections and so on, as is often the situation in daily life at home.

At diabetes camps, the children will meet friends who are "in the same boat" and understand what living with diabetes is like. Our aim is to have fun together but also to prepare the children for a life with diabetes by increasing their knowledge and ability to manage on their own.

Many will meet new friends with whom they will keep in touch for years to come. At our educational holiday for children below the age of puberty, we emphasize the importance of managing the basics of their diabetes independently. If they can handle major parts of diabetes on their own during their teenage years, they will be helped in their struggle for independence and hopefully diabetes will not play too large a role in the family conflicts associated with puberty (see also page 399). During the holiday we aim primarily for the children to be able to participate fully in all activities. From this, it follows that we will not achieve perfect control of diabetes. Some children may even have higher blood glucose levels than they managed at home. Most children will be more active than usual during the holiday and, therefore, we often lower the insulin doses, especially at bedtime, to prevent night time hypoglycaemia. Participating in a diabetes education holiday can also increase children's confidence in their own ability to manage without their mother or father. This will be especially true for children who are perhaps away from home for more than a night or two for the first time ever. Many parents find it a relief to be on their own, knowing that their child is being taken care of by professional staff. Diabetes UK runs national holidays but your own clinic might also organize holidays, weekends or other activities for children and teenagers.

Diabetes and the Internet

An increasing amount of information on diabetes is available on the Internet. Both medical companies and institutions have homepages displaying information and news. Use one of the search services to find the type of information you are looking for. Most studies and guidelines report HbA_{1c} in DCCT-units. See page 118 for conversion to IFCC units in mmol/mol or www.hba1c.nu/eng.

Diabetes and the Internet

There is a vast amount of diabetes information available on the Internet. However, you must be aware that the information on the Internet often is not reviewed by healthcare professionals and may only be the opinion of the person writing it.

Associations:

Diabetes UK	www.diabetes.org.uk
Diabetes Federation of Ireland	www.diabetes.ie
American Diabetes Association (ADA)	www.diabetes.org
Diabetes Australia	www.diabetesaustralia.com.au
International Diabetes Federation (IDF)	www.idf.org
International Society for Pediatric and Adolescent Diabetes (ISPAD)	www.ispad.org
Juvenile Diabetes Research Foundation International	www.jdrf.org
Diabetes Camping Association	www.diabetescamps.org
Diabetes Exercise & Sports Association (DESA)	www.diabetes-exercise.org

Links to patient information:

Children with Diabetes:	www.childrenwithdiabetes.com
Joslin website for persons with diabetes	www.joslin.org
Betamed — home page of this book	www.betamed.se/eng

At www.betamed.se you will find many other links of diabetes interest. Since Internet pages are constantly updated and many sites change their addresses from time to time, we have chosen not to include more links in this book.

One thing is particularly important to remember when you are reading information on the Internet. Most of what you find will not have been reviewed by healthcare professionals, and may often be only the opinion of the person writing it. However, if you judge the information somewhat critically, you may find out a lot of interesting information about diabetes and you can discuss it with your team at clinic.

There are some diabetes computer games available online over the Internet.
Try www.equalize.se/dependency (for adolescents) or http://www.diabetes.org.uk/Guide-to-diabetes/My-life/Kids/Fun-stuff/Game (for younger children)

When does a young person become an adult?

The precise age at which we enter adulthood may be difficult to determine, as most of us carry part of our childhood and adolescence with us throughout our lives. Practice and regulations about when diabetes care is transferred from paediatric to adult units differ between countries. It may also differ between centres depending on local policies. In the UK, adolescents usually start seeing an adult physician above the age of 16, although the age of transfer can vary between 13 and 22 years.[616] Systems of transition vary. One example is for the paediatrician to join the teenager for his or her first visit to the adult clinic. Another is for the diabetes nurse (and doctor) from the adult team to join the last paediatric visit before transfer. Some centres have joint adolescent or young adult clinics with both paediatric and adult physicians attending. Discuss with your care providers what is best for your individual circumstances.

Reimbursed accessories

In most countries, insulin is available free of charge for people with diabetes. Often syringes, pen injectors and needles are reimbursed as well. Sometimes the person with diabetes has to pay for blood glucose meters while the strips for testing are free or reimbursed. In the UK, meters are usually available free, but you will need a prescription from your doctor for the testing strips. Sometimes the companies producing the meters will provide them free of charge at the onset of diabetes. Insulin pumps and accessories for these are often not reimbursed, but may be available through various insurance companies or under special conditions. In the UK, a recent report from NICE (the National Institute for Health and Clinical Excellence) has recommended that pumps be made available for those in special need, in particular people who have unstable diabetes. However, funding in the NHS remains a problem.

Travel tips

Travelling is an important part of life for many people, and you should not avoid this activity just because of your diabetes. If you think things over and plan the trip ahead, no destination or means of travel is impossible. However, you must be able to measure your blood glucose during the trip, and adjust your insulin doses in line with differing conditions, if you are to manage well.

It will be necessary to test your blood glucose levels more frequently. They could be raised if you have been sitting still in the car or on a plane or eating food with more carbohydrates than usual. The excitement involved in visiting a new city or country may also increase your blood glucose level.

Remember always to take spare insulin, at least 2-3 times the amount you expect to use. Keep insulin and pens/syringes in your hand luggage but make sure that you have an extra set in another bag in case you lose one bag. Don't put insulin in the check-in luggage as there is a risk of it freezing in the aeroplane luggage hold at high altitudes. Besides, there is always the risk of your luggage being lost or arriving late. The X-ray in security controls will not affect your insulin. It is important to have some kind of ID showing that you have diabetes, as you may have to show it to the customs officer.

Usually, you will have no problem obtaining insulin from a pharmacy abroad if you can prove that you have diabetes. Take a card on which your doses, concentration and brand of insulin are documented, or bring the original pharmaceutically labelled box. It may be difficult to store your insulin in a refrigerator all the time, but usually it will not be wasted during a short trip, as long as you avoid temperatures above 25-30° C (77-86° F). Remember that it can be extremely hot (up to 50° C, 120° F) in a closed car on a sunny day. Bring a thermos flask or similar with you, containing cold water (cool it with ice before putting insulin into it) during hot days. Remember that insulin is absorbed more quickly from the injection site if you are very warm and that this can result in unexpected hypoglycaemia (see also page 90).

If you are going on a beach holiday, you need to be aware that insulin does not fare well in heat and sunshine. If you have an insulin pump, you need to cover it, and preferably the tubing as well, while you are sunbathing. When you go inside at the end of the day, you can prime the tubing with fresh insulin if you suspect that the insulin in the tubing has been exposed to sunlight. An 11-year-old girl developed ketoacidosis 48 hours after her pump was exposed to sunshine and heat (35 °C, 95° F in the air) after being left on a table in the sun while she was swimming in the pool.[862] If she had replaced the

Remember that you are never more than a phone call away from your diabetes healthcare team when on holiday or a business trip.

cartridge with fresh insulin when she came home, this could have been avoided.

Insulin that has been frozen loses its effect. Don't leave it in the car on a skiing trip, for example. Keep your insulin bottles or pen injector in an inner pocket if it is below freezing outside. Avoid storing the insulin too close to the freezing compartment in the refrigerator. A 13-year-old girl developed ketoacidosis after her insulin happened to freeze in the refrigerator during a holiday.[747] This insulin was used in the pump at a later stage by mistake. Damaged insulin will often turn cloudy or clumpy, sometimes with a brownish colour. Some blood glucose strips can give too high a reading when it is very hot outside and too low a reading when it is very cold. Many glucose meters will give you a warning if the temperature is too high or too low.

Remember that some countries use other concentrations of insulin, mostly 40 U/ml. If you use insulin of 100 U/ml in syringes designed for 40 U/ml or vice versa, you will be in trouble. The insulin concentration appropriate for each syringe is clearly printed on the side of the syringe. If you run out of insulin it is probably better to buy both insulin and syringes for 40 U/ml if 100 U/ml is not available. You can continue taking your usual doses when counting in units. The units are the same and will give just about the same insulin effect with both 40 U/ml and 100 U/ml. The only difference is that insulin of 40 U/ml may give a slightly quicker onset of action. (See also "Units and insulin concentrations" on page 78.)

Blood glucose is measured in mmol/l in some countries and mg/dl in others (see page 99 for conversion table).

1 mmol/l = 18 mg/dl   100 mg/dl = 5.6 mmol/l

Make sure that you have dextrose and glucagon when travelling, sailing or hiking. With glucagon you can treat a serious hypoglycaemia even if you are a long way from emergency care.

Make sure that your friends know how and when dextrose and glucagon should be used.

Vaccinations

There are no special restrictions for vaccinations or gamma globulin injections due to diabetes. However, it is particularly important that individuals with diabetes make sure they get the recommended vaccinations, since illness often

Names of insulin abroad

Type	UK	US
Rapid-acting analogue	NovoRapid Humalog	NovoLog Humalog
Regular insulin	Actrapid Humulin S Insuman Rapid	Novolin R Humulin R
NPH insulin	Insulatard Humulin I	Novolin Humulin N
Basal analogue	Lantus Levemir	Lantus Levemir
Lente insulin	Monotard Humulin L	Novolin L Humulin L
Ultralente	Ultratard Humulin Zn	Ultratard Humulin U
Mixed insulin (70% NPH)	Mixtard 30 Humulin M3	Novolin 70/30 Humulin 70/30
Mixed analogue (70-75% basal)	NovoMix 30 Humalog Mix 25	NovoLog Mix 70/30 Humalog Mix 75/25

Most insulins can be found under different names in different parts of the world. If you plan a longer trip, have the insulin vial and box available, or ask your doctor to write down what type of insulins you use so that you can get them from the local pharmacy if you lose your supplies. Be aware that the pre-mixed insulins have their proportions stated in opposite ways in the US from in the UK! Some insulins in the list above (Lente and Ultralente) have been withdrawn from the market in the UK or US but may be available in other countries.

Remember that insulin cannot withstand heat and sunshine as well as you can. The boot of a car or bus will be too hot for insulin in the summer and too cold in the winter.

leads to difficult consequences with problems of diabetes control. Vaccination for hepatitis A, typhoid and other diarrhoeal diseases is a sensible precaution if you travel to areas where these may be a problem. It is a good idea to have the vaccinations well ahead of the trip, as some cause an episode of fever that can affect the blood glucose for a few days after the shot.

Ill while abroad?

Remember to take documents relevant to your health insurance so that you receive compensation if you fall ill abroad. Check the small print on your insurance policy to find out whether your health insurance covers acute illness only, or whether it will also cover any deterioration of your diabetes.

If you are a citizen of the UK or another EU country, you will also need a European Health Insurance Card. Ask how to apply at your GP's surgery or go to www.dh.gov.uk/travellers. Diabetes UK offers travel insurance quotes at http://www.diabetes.co.uk/diabetic-travel-insurance.html

Always say that you have diabetes if you need to see a doctor abroad. If you become ill while in countries other than Western Europe and the US you should, if possible, try to avoid surgical intervention, blood transfusions and injections. If you need medication, ask for tablets instead of injections. If possible, also avoid dental treatment as there may be a risk of acquiring a blood infection.

Diarrhoea problems

Prophylactic antibiotic treatment aimed at avoiding diarrhoeal diseases while on holiday is a controversial issue. Since a person with diabetes will have problems with blood glucose levels and insulin adjustments when they are ill, some

Problems with travel sickness?

➠ Take travel-sickness medication: tablets or depot adhesives (e.g. scopolamine).

➠ You will be less likely to feel sick if you eat "little and often" rather than large helpings several hours apart.

➠ Avoid fizzy drinks.

➠ Sit in the front if you are in a car or bus, so you can see the road.

Avoid the following in hot climates and places with poor standards of hygiene

Tap water (even when brushing your teeth)
Ice
Milk, cream, mayonnaise
Unsealed ice cream
Diluted juice
Cold buffets
Food kept warm for a long time
Shellfish
Salad, vegetables and fruit rinsed in water
Raw food
Poorly cooked chicken

Other advice:[1113]
Wash your hands often.
Food should be freshly prepared and piping hot.
Don't eat food prepared in the street.
Drink only bottled water.
Beer, wine, coffee and tea are also safe.

doctors are more liberal about prescribing treatment for diarrhoeal diseases in advance.[172] It can be given during a short trip (3-4 weeks or less) to high-risk areas (Africa, Asia or Latin America) with a 70-90% protective effect.[1009] Without this, the risk of catching a diarrhoeal infection is 25-35%. On a longer trip, antibiotics should be given only if you actually have diarrhoea. It is best to take the antibiotics with you. Avoid buying them locally as you may not know exactly what you are getting, thereby increasing the risk of side effects.

Considering the risks of gastroenteritis, you should avoid drinking water in some countries if you cannot be sure it is entirely clean. Avoid all tap water (even frozen, i.e. ice cubes!). Bottled water and fizzy drinks (Cola, Fanta or similar) are usually safe. Oral rehydration solution (Dioralyte®, Pedialyte) is a good alternative if you feel sick or are vomiting (see "Nausea and vomiting" on page 303).

If you travel in primitive conditions, water should be disinfected by boiling it briefly or by using water purifying tablets (Chlorine®, Puritabs®, Aqua Care® or similar).[1113]

If you do not drink enough when outdoors in the heat, you will risk dehydration. This causes the insulin to be absorbed more slowly.[470] Later, when you drink properly, more insulin will be absorbed and you will risk becoming seriously hypoglycaemic. A high blood glucose level

above the renal threshold (see page 101) will also cause you to lose extra fluid as you will be passing more urine.

Passing through time zones

When you travel to other continents there will be a time difference. If you go westwards, the day will be longer, and if you go eastwards, it will be shorter. Calculate your total insulin dose for the travelling day by increasing or decreasing it by 2-4% for every hour of time shift.[593,932] You may need to increase your insulin doses slightly, depending on your regular daily physical activity, as you will be sitting down all day on the plane. If you are flying, don't order special diabetes food as this is often not very appetizing and the amount of carbohydrates served is often too small. It is better to adjust your insulin doses to the food being served on board.

Due to the pressure differences in the cabin, air bubbles easily accumulate in the pen cartridges. To avoid this, remove the needle immediately after each injection. If air bubbles are present, be sure to get rid of them before taking injections after you have landed (see page 136). It is common to feel a bit weary before adjusting to the new time zone (called jet lag) and it will usually take a couple of days before your energy levels are where they should be and your sleeping pattern returns to normal.

Multiple injection treatment

Use rapid- or short-acting insulin and eat every 4-5 hours during the trip. If you fly westwards, take 1 or 2 extra doses. If you fly eastwards, you will need fewer doses. Decrease the basal dose that you take before the flight if the day gets shorter. Take your usual bedtime insulin in

---

Oral rehydration solution

Oral rehydration solution can be found at many pharmacies, both at home and abroad. You can also mix your own rehydration solution. Remember though that the water you use must be pure! Buy bottled water if you are in any doubt.

☞ 1 litre pure water
   0.5 teaspoon of salt
   8 dextrose tablets (3 g each)
   or 2 tablespoonfuls of ordinary sugar

the evening when you arrive at your destination (at the "new" bedtime). If you take basal insulin in the morning, take this dose according to the time at your arrival. It is important to check your blood glucose before every meal when improvising like this. With an insulin pump, just let the basal rate run as usual, and adjust the clock in the pump once you arrive at your destination.

A camel can survive many days in the desert without drinking, on account of its humps. Diabetes makes you more sensitive to dehydration. Be sure always to drink plenty of fluid when you are in a hot country, especially if you have problems with diarrhoea or vomiting. If you find yourself feeling sick or vomiting, you should drink often but only a few sips at a time. (See the chapter on illness page 301.)

With short-acting insulin for meals and NPH at bedtime, you can try taking a small dose of bedtime insulin if you travel during the night and sleep for many hours on the plane. However, if you sleep less than 4-5 hours, it will probably be easier to adjust to the new time zone if you stick to only short-acting insulin during the

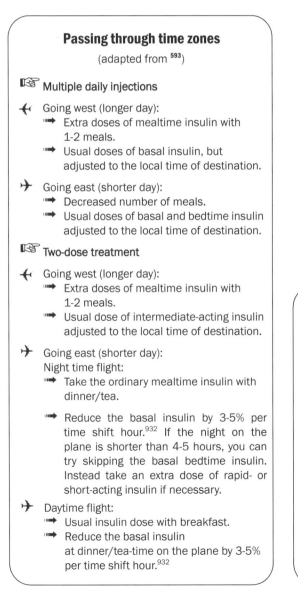

Passing through time zones

(adapted from [593])

☞ **Multiple daily injections**

✈ Going west (longer day):
→ Extra doses of mealtime insulin with 1-2 meals.
→ Usual doses of basal insulin, but adjusted to the local time of destination.

✈ Going east (shorter day):
→ Decreased number of meals.
→ Usual doses of basal and bedtime insulin adjusted to the local time of destination.

☞ Two-dose treatment

✈ Going west (longer day):
→ Extra doses of mealtime insulin with 1-2 meals.
→ Usual dose of intermediate-acting insulin adjusted to the local time of destination.

✈ Going east (shorter day):
Night time flight:
→ Take the ordinary mealtime insulin with dinner/tea.
→ Reduce the basal insulin by 3-5% per time shift hour.[932] If the night on the plane is shorter than 4-5 hours, you can try skipping the basal bedtime insulin. Instead take an extra dose of rapid- or short-acting insulin if necessary.

✈ Daytime flight:
→ Usual insulin dose with breakfast.
→ Reduce the basal insulin at dinner/tea-time on the plane by 3-5% per time shift hour.[932]

Safety rules for flying within the US

✈ Syringes or insulin delivery systems should be accompanied by the insulin in its original pharmaceutically labelled box.

✈ Capped lancets should be accompanied by a glucose meter that has the manufacturer's name embossed on the meter.

✈ An intact glucagon kit should be kept in its original preprinted, pharmaceutically labelled container.

✈ No exceptions will be made. Prescriptions and doctors' letters will not be accepted.

✈ A passenger encountering any diabetes-related difficulty because of security measures should ask to speak with a Complaints Resolution Officer (CRO) for the airline.

Travel pharmacy

✈ Glucagon.

✈ Fever-suppressing drugs.
Paracetamol/acetaminophen and/or aspirin /salicylic acid (adults only).

✈ Nose drops (flying while you have a cold can be painful).

✈ Imodium®(loperamide) for diarrhoea
(above 12 years of age).
Give if:≥ 4 loose stools a day or
≥ 2 loose stools a day and fever.
Dose: 2 tablets initially, thereafter 1 tablet
after each bout of diarrhoea.
(Maximum 8 tablets per day for 3 days.)
See a doctor if your general condition is affected,
your symptoms worsen or you do not improve
within 3 days.[1009]

✈ Oral rehydration solution, powder or tablets (Dioralyte® or similar).

✈ Antibiotics for diarrhoea when travelling to Southern Europe, Asia, Africa or Latin/South America:

✈ Lexinor®, Utinor®, norfloxacin
Not for children younger than 12
years old or pregnant women.
Dose: 200 mg twice daily for prophylactic
use or 400 mg twice daily for 3 days
if you are having acute diarrhoea.[1009]

✈ Treatment failure can be caused by resistant bacteria and azithromycin is then an alternative
(1000 mg as a single dose or 500mg once daily
for 3 days).[157]

✈ Children below the age of 12 can be given azithromycin 10 mg/kg/day once daily for up to 5
days or trimethoprim + sulphamethoxazole (Cotrimoxazole®, Colizole®).[157]

✈ Pregnant women can take Co-trimoxazole® or
Colizole®, 2 tablets twice daily for 5-10 days.[157]

✈ Travel sickness pills or scopolamine adhesives.

Always bring glucagon
wherever you go and you
will have your own emergency treatment handy.

night (see also "Staying awake all night" on page 94).

Two-dose treatment

If you use a two-dose treatment it may be difficult to adjust to a shorter or longer day. You will probably be better off if you change temporarily to premeal injections 3-4 times daily while travelling. You should have tested this regimen well in advance to know what doses are needed with different types of meals.

If you use a two-dose treatment and travel westwards (longer day) take extra premeal insulin doses on the plane and take your usual afternoon dose when you arrive, adjusting it to the night time at the destination. If you travel eastwards (shorter day) take a dose of premeal insulin for the late evening snack on the plane. If the night on the plane is shorter than 4-5 hours, you can try skipping the intermediate-acting bedtime insulin. Instead take an extra dose of rapid- or short-acting insulin if necessary. Take your usual dose of rapid- or short-acting insulin with breakfast but decrease the intermediate portion by 20-40%.[593]

Flying with a pump or sensor

✈ Change the infusion set around 12 hours before the flight, and do not fill the cartridge with more insulin than needed to last 12-24 hours after landing.

✈ There are no problems passing through the metal scan, but if you are taken out for a body scanner you should remove the pump and the CGM, if you are wearing such a device.[207]

✈ Due to laws of physics, air bubbles may appear in the insulin reservoir as the pressure in the cabin is lower than on the ground. The pressure in an aeroplane cabin is equivalent to that of being at an altitude of approximately 2,000 meters (7,600 feet). Existing air bubbles at ground level will also expand.

✈ The increased volume in the reservoir may push some insulin through the tubing, causing your blood glucose level to decrease.[613]

✈ To be on the safe side, you can disconnect the pump just before takeoff, and reconnect after removing air bubbles once you have reached cruising level after approximately 30 minutes. For young children, you can decrease this problem by not filling the reservoir with more insulin than what will be needed during the flight.

✈ If there is an emergency situation, and the oxygen masks drop down, this indicates a decrease in cabin pressure. You should immediately disconnect your pump to avoid insulin being injected into your body (as the pressure in the cartridge will be higher than the surrounding environment). Check if any air bubbles have formed, and remove them before reconnecting.

✈ After landing, the air pressure will have normalized which can cause any air bubbles in the cartridge to shrink. Disconnect and prime the pump with a few units to ensure that you can see insulin appearing at the end of the tubing.

✈ If you are wearing a subcutaneous glucose sensor, its efficacy depends on the brand. Dexcom can be worn during the whole flight, while the Navigator's signal is too strong and needs to be turned off during the entire flight.

Diabetes equipment you may need on the trip

✈ ID and necklace or bracelet indicating that you have diabetes.

✈ Extra insulin pen and/or syringes (pre-filled pens are handy for this).

✈ Keep all your insulin divided into separate items of hand-luggage.

✈ Thermometer to check the temperature of the refrigerator (for insulin).

✈ Finger-pricking device and lancets.

✈ Test strips for blood glucose, and meter (bring a spare meter).

✈ Test strips for ketones (blood and/or urine).

✈ Dextrose/glucose tablets and gel.

✈ Clinical thermometer.

✈ Telephone and fax numbers for your diabetes healthcare team at home.

✈ Enter an ICE (In Case of Emergency) number including the country prefix (+44) in your mobile to quickly reach a parent or other person for medical advice in case of accident or illness.

✈ Insurance documents.

Associated diseases

Some diseases are more common if you have diabetes. Coeliac disease and hypothyroidism are examples of so called autoimmune diseases (see page 376) where the immune system is involved. Because diabetes is, in part, a hereditary disease, it is also more common for other family members, as well as the person with diabetes, to have other autoimmune diseases. Both hypothyroidism and coeliac disease can be difficult to detect. Regular measurements with blood tests are therefore a part of annual check-ups.

The bowel lining is arranged in narrow pleats with small projections that look like fingers (called villi). In this way the absorbent surface of the intestine increases to as much as 200 square metres (250 square yards). In coeliac disease, these villi are destroyed and the surface that can absorb nourishment decreases considerably, down to as little as 2 square metres (2.5 square yards).

Coeliac disease

Coeliac disease (intolerance to gluten in wheat, oats, rye and barley) is up to 10 times more common in children and adults with diabetes. Studies have shown that 3-6% of all children with diabetes have this disease as well,[547] but a more thorough screening showed that it is closer to 10% in Sweden.[654] The risk in siblings is slightly lower, but still much higher than in the general population.[1004]

If you have untreated coeliac disease, you will have damaged bowel lining. Your body will have difficulty absorbing food and, as a result, your blood glucose levels are unlikely to be high even after meals. Your insulin requirement will tend to be low and hypoglycaemia may be more common.[547,753] Often people with this disease have no further symptoms, but some may have generalized abdominal complaints, constipation or diarrhoea and are sometimes anaemic.

In adults, infertility may be caused by coeliac disease (even if the father has the disease).[741] People with coeliac disease and people with type 1 diabetes share the same genetic background. If any of your relatives have unclear symptoms where a diagnosis is difficult to find, you should encourage them to take a blood test for coeliac disease.

Screening by a blood test for coeliac disease is recommended for both children[937] and adults[524] with diabetes. Transglutaminase (TTG) and endomysial antibodies (EMA) as well as antigliadin antibodies (used mostly in children < 2 years of age) are the names of the antibody tests used to diagnose and follow coeliac disease. The diagnosis needs to be verified by analysing a small sample (biopsy) of the intestinal mucosa, and this is often done by a so-called endoscopy. If coeliac disease is suspected, it is very important not to experiment with the diet on your own. If you do decrease the content of gluten in your diet, the antibodies will decrease, and thereby also the chance of diagnosing coeliac disease correctly. You should therefore not change anything in your diet if you suspect coeliac disease until the tests have been taken and a endoscopy performed.

The best way to manage coeliac disease is to avoid all food containing gluten. Gluten-free food may increase the blood glucose level quicker than the corresponding product containing gluten. One study showed a doubled risk of kidney complications when adolescents did not adhere to a gluten-free diet.[846]

Gluten-free products are available on prescription in the UK.

Zonulin is a substance that is produced locally in the cells of the intestinal lining. It opens the "tight junction", the binding between cells that holds them together, and lets proteins and other compounds from the intestine pass into the bloodstream.[346] When there is something poisonous in the intestine (for example bacteria or chemicals), water is passed from the blood into the intestine, resulting in diarrhoea and helping to flush the bad things out. We know that gliadin, the protein in gluten, increases the production of zonulin. This makes it possible for gliadin to pass between the cells into the blood where it is presented to the immune system. In some susceptible individuals, there will be an autoimmune reaction and the immune system will then begin harming the intestinal lining.

Increased production of zonulin and increased permeability of the intestine have been found in the pre-diabetic stage (before the onset of diabetes).[936] There may be a similar mechanism as with gliadin in the development of diabetes, although we don't currently know which substance that would be the "villain of the piece" in triggering the immune system.

Thyroid diseases

The thyroid gland in your neck, just below the Adam's apple, can be damaged by autoantibodies (called Hashimoto's thyroiditis) which lead to a decreased production of thyroid hormones (called hypothyroidism). Your body will try to compensate for this by increasing the size of the thyroid gland (called a goitre). Thyroid hor-

The thyroid gland is located in front of the windpipe and is normally not visible. When the gland cannot produce enough hormone, it will increase in size, making it clearly visible (called a goitre). A goitre can also be caused by an overproduction of hormones but is then referred to as toxic goitre.

mones regulate the metabolism in the body and a deficiency will cause tiredness, lethargy, intolerance to cold and constipation. However, there are often no symptoms at all. Hypoglycaemia may be more common in children with diabetes and hypothyroidism.[754]

Hypothyroidism is a hormone deficiency disease (as is diabetes) but the treatment is much simpler. It involves taking 1-2 tablets per day containing thyroid hormone. Your body will use the hormone from the tablets when it is needed.

Toxic goitre (also called Grave's disease or hyperthyroidism) involves increased production of thyroid hormone, and is also more common amongst people with diabetes. Frequent symptoms are weight loss, feelings of warmth and diarrhoea.

Skin diseases

When the blood glucose level is high, fluid loss via the urine may cause the skin to become dry and itchy due to a degree of dehydration.

Irregular reddish-brown skin lesions, 2-10 mm (1/10-1/2 inch) in size, may appear on the lower part of the leg and are called shin spots. Sometimes they even appear on the forearm or thighs. The cause is unclear but they can develop after an accidental trauma such as bumping the leg on the edge of a table. This type of skin lesion is fairly common, especially in men, and usually arises after the age of 30.

Another skin condition found in around 1% of people with diabetes is necrobiosis lipoidica diabeticorum (NLD).[827,1127] This shows as round or irregular red-brownish lesions with very thin skin, and sometimes ulcers. These skin changes are usually seen on the front of the lower part of the leg but can also be found on the feet, arms, hands, face or scalp.[560] They can be very distressing, especially for people who take pride in their appearance, for example when wearing shorts or a skirt. The lesions usually appear in people who are in their 30s or 40s, but can occasionally arise in people who are still only in their teens.[827] They grow slowly over many years and are not affected by blood glucose control. The cause is unknown but some data indicate an autoimmune origin.[827] There is no known effective treatment but you can try applying a stoma-type bandage (such as DuoDERM®). Skin transplants have been used successfully in more difficult cases.

Adults with diabetes can develop blisters on their fingers or toes. These look similar to burns, but the underlying skin is not irritated.[560] Usually they will dry within a week or so, but can lead to ulcers that heal slowly. The treatment of choice is to prick the blisters with a sterile needle and then apply a dry bandage.

Acanthosis nigricans is a skin disorder characterized by a dark pigmentation and insulin resistance which is sometimes found in people with type 2 diabetes (see page 13). As far as it is known, none of these skin conditions have any relationship to glucose control or HbA$_{1c}$ levels.

If you are feeling unwell or very tired, you may have another illness in addition to diabetes. It is therefore important to have a check-up with your doctor so that a number of blood samples can be taken for testing. If you have constipation you may have coeliac disease or thyroid disease. If you are tired, especially if you have a normally uncomplicated disease like a common cold, ask for your levels of cortisol and thyroid hormone to be checked.

Infections

The white blood cells that help defend the body against infections work less efficiently if the blood glucose level is above 14 mmol/l (250 mg/dl). So this makes infection more likely.[61] This is particularly true for urinary tract infections and skin infections.[652,827] It follows, therefore, that your blood glucose level should be as close to normal as possible if you are fighting off an infection. One study found bacteria in the urine without symptoms in 26% of women with type 1 diabetes.[393] With a blood glucose below 11 mmol/l (200 mg/dl), the risk of infection after surgery decreased considerably in another study.[409]

Fungal infections

Genital itching caused by fungal infections is more common in women and teenage girls with diabetes after puberty. The fungus thrives better when the blood and urine glucose level are high.[264] In the DCCT study (see page 367), the group with an HbA_{1c} of 53 mmol/mol (7.0%) had a 46% reduced rate of vaginal infection compared to the group with an HbA_{1c} 75 mmol/mol (9.0%).[264] Itching may be very intense and there may be a whitish flaky discharge. Fungal infections often arise during treatment with antibiotics that disturb the normal genital bacterial flora. The treatment of choice is improved blood glucose control and a topical antifungal cream until symptoms resolve, which may require 6-14 days of treatment.[121,827] Men can have the same type of fungal infection under the foreskin. Fungal infections in children can appear as cracks in the corner of the mouth, or sores in the cuticle or between the fingers.[827]

Diseases that can cause you to need less insulin

Cortisol deficiency:

A low cortisol production in the adrenal glands decreases the blood glucose level. This can be caused by a disease in the glands (adrenal insufficiency, Addison's disease) or disturbed function of the pituitary gland.

Growth hormone deficiency:

Low production of growth hormone (pituitary insufficiency) decreases the blood glucose level.

Gluten intolerance:

Intolerance of gluten (coeliac disease) causes reduced food absorption from the intestine.

Deficiency of thyroid hormone:

Low production of thyroid hormone (hypothyroidism) causes a slower metabolism in the body.

Renal insufficiency:

Renal insufficiency causes a decreased degradation and excretion of insulin.

Complications in blood vessels

It may be distressing to think ahead about how things will turn out in the future. Many people have relatives or friends who have had diabetes for quite a number of years. Someone might tell you about a person with diabetes who has had all kinds of complications. It is important to remember that the diabetes complications we see today are caused by 30-40 years of diabetes with the type of diabetes treatment available during that time. The result may be discouraging with serious complications in the eyes, kidneys, feet and nerves. Individuals in this age group may have had a shorter lifespan due to kidney damage or heart disease.

What causes complications?

It is well known that complications are caused by high blood glucose levels, and that high HbA$_{1c}$ values and a long duration of diabetes will increase the risk of complications. Different people are more or less susceptible to developing these complications, but the reason for this difference is not yet known. The important message is that the better the blood glucose measurements and the lower the HbA$_{1c}$, the less likely the person is to develop diabetes complications in later years.

The risk of blindness and partial sight in people with diabetes is three times higher than the general population in the UK.[473] Approximately 2.3% of all individuals with type 1 diabetes in a European study were blind.[976] It is however very important to know that the outlook for someone developing diabetes today is not at all the same as for a person who first developed the disease 30-40 years ago. Both insulin treatment and the possibilities of preventing and treating eye complications have improved considerably.

It may be very difficult to know how much one should tell children about complications. Teenagers understand more and want to know about their situation. We feel it is important that "all the cards are on the table", so you know what type of complications can occur in the long run and what the risks are. It is important to know the facts, but it is not something you need to talk about on a daily basis.

During family teaching sessions on complications in diabetes I always encourage the young person to sit in although I do not force anyone to listen. Younger children need to know as much as they can understand, but perhaps not too many details. But I will ask a question every now and then to see how interested the child is in what we are talking about. If he or she wants to go off and play after a while, probably the topic has stopped being interesting.

In the home environment, it is a good idea to bring up the subject of complications in a careful way every once in a while, preferably when the young (or not so young) person with diabetes is in the mood for talking, and there is time for thoughts and reflections. Many children and teenagers store up their questions. They sometimes don't want to raise difficult issues with their mum or dad for fear of worrying them.

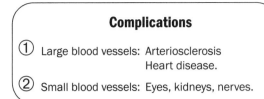

Complications

① Large blood vessels: Arteriosclerosis
                                       Heart disease.

② Small blood vessels: Eyes, kidneys, nerves.

Diabetes educational holidays provide excellent opportunities for group discussions on the dangers associated with diabetes. In the course of these, many children reveal they have thought about such issues at one time or another.

If your child has diabetes, don't threaten them with kidney damage or blindness, no matter how worried you are. Frightening your child won't do any good. On the contrary, such threats will generate feelings of hopelessness, like "drawing a blank in the lottery of life". I have all too often met children who have told me that their parents have said: "Don't eat sweets because it will make you blind!" Such statements will only cause anguish since children cannot understand the time frame involved. Try instead to explain and motivate the child to think carefully about what, and how much, they should eat.

A 13-year-old girl believed that sweets as such caused complications such as blindness (and not the high blood glucose levels that can follow from excessive sweet-eating). No wonder she was in agony whenever she ate something sweet and still she just could not resist doing it.

Diabetes is such a common disease that if we do not tell the children about complications when they are old enough to understand, then someone else will. Sooner or later, someone (with the best of intentions) will say: "Poor child, your diabetes will someday make you blind..." It is important that young people know the real facts and are able to answer: "That is how things used to be, but nowadays there are much better ways to treat diabetes!"

It used to be believed that the years before puberty were not significant when it came to the risk of developing complications. It has now been shown that the HbA_{1c} levels during the years before puberty contribute significantly to the risk of long-term complications,[194,738] although to a lesser extent than the years after puberty.[298,806]

In some patients, early signs of complications can be found on close examination after 10-20 years of diabetes, depending upon how their blood glucose levels have been over these years. In any case, signs of complications usually do not cause practical problems before 20-30 years of the disease. Some people who have had their diabetes for 60 years have still not developed signs of complications. A woman that was diag-

Heart and large blood vessel diseases: Diagnosis

① Blood pressure measurements.

② Examination of pulses in feet and lower legs, with a Doppler device if necessary.

③ Analysis of cholesterol and triglycerides in the blood.

Treatment

The same advice is given to all people with an increased risk of heart and blood vessel diseases, regardless of whether or not they have diabetes:

① Stop smoking.

② Increase the amount of physical exercise or physiotherapy.

③ Avoid putting on too much weight.

④ Avoid negative or undue stress (see page 298).

⑤ Don't drink too much alcohol.

⑥ Treat high blood pressure.

⑦ Eat foods that are rich in fibre and low in fat. Increase fruit and vegetable intake.

nosed with diabetes at age 7 in 1924, lived to be 93 and lived at home until the age of 90!

Large blood vessels

Diseases of the heart and blood vessels (cardio-vascular diseases) are more common among people with diabetes, and the large blood vessels in your body are at greater risk of developing arteriosclerosis (hardening, narrowing and eventually blocking of the blood vessels). The increased risk of arteriosclerosis and heart problems is thought to be caused in part by the

high blood glucose level. Other contributing factors are cholesterol problems and high blood pressure.

Cardiovascular diseases are the main contributors to the decreased life expectancy of a person with diabetes. Life expectancy of people with type 1 diabetes in the US improved 15 years when comparing a diabetes diagnosis between 1950-1964 with 1965-1980, and was 68.8 years compared to 72.4 in those without diabetes.[746] For patients with type 1 diabetes followed up until 1999 in the UK, the risk of dying was 4.5 times higher for men and 3.3 times

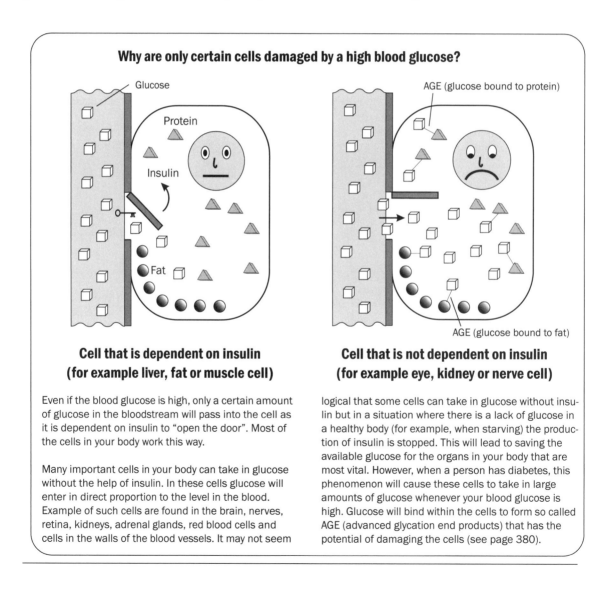

Why are only certain cells damaged by a high blood glucose?

Cell that is dependent on insulin (for example liver, fat or muscle cell)

Cell that is not dependent on insulin (for example eye, kidney or nerve cell)

Even if the blood glucose is high, only a certain amount of glucose in the bloodstream will pass into the cell as it is dependent on insulin to "open the door". Most of the cells in your body work this way.

Many important cells in your body can take in glucose without the help of insulin. In these cells glucose will enter in direct proportion to the level in the blood. Example of such cells are found in the brain, nerves, retina, kidneys, adrenal glands, red blood cells and cells in the walls of the blood vessels. It may not seem

logical that some cells can take in glucose without insulin but in a situation where there is a lack of glucose in a healthy body (for example, when starving) the production of insulin is stopped. This will lead to saving the available glucose for the organs in your body that are most vital. However, when a person has diabetes, this phenomenon will cause these cells to take in large amounts of glucose whenever your blood glucose is high. Glucose will bind within the cells to form so called AGE (advanced glycation end products) that has the potential of damaging the cells (see page 380).

higher for women compared with people without diabetes.[983] In Sweden, individuals with type 1 diabetes, diagnosed between the ages of 15 and 34 years, had a two-fold excess mortality.[1077] Remember that these investigations were done in people who had diabetes for a very long time, with the type of treatment available at that time.

If you keep your blood glucose levels under control, there is every chance that you will be able to put off the time when diseases like arteriosclerosis become a problem for you.[562,775] There is also research evidence to show that effective diabetes treatment reduces your chances of developing early heart disease.[659,775] For every mmol of decrease in blood glucose, your risk of heart disease will decrease by 11%.[609] Young people who have had diabetes for less than 8 years, and who have undergone intensive treatment using a pen or pump, showed an improved function of the blood vessels after one year, compared with those on conventional treatment with 2–3 doses/day." [364]

Some families have a history of high cholesterol levels. If this is the case, screening of lipids is recommended at diagnosis of diabetes (after blood glucose control has been established).[970] For other individuals, the first screening is recommended at 12 years of age and thereafter every 5 years. If fasting lipids are higher than they should be, the first treatment is to optimise your blood glucose control and to go through what you eat together with your dietitian to lower the intake of total and saturated fat. Weight control, exercise and quitting smoking, if you do so, are also important measures. Pharmacological treatment is strongly recommended if lipids continue to be high, i.e. if the LDL cholesterol is > 4.1 mmol/l (160 mg/dl).[970] Treatment should be considered if LDL is > 3.3 mmol/l (130 mg/dl) if you have a cardiovascular risk factor like high blood pressure or a family history of heart problems before the age of 55 years. So called statins can be given safely to

adolescents but are not approved in pregnancy.[970]

The increased risk of diseases of the heart and blood vessels is the main reason that people with diabetes are recommended not to smoke and to keep fat levels in their diet low. Fat has no direct effect on the blood glucose level other than causing the stomach to empty more slowly (see page 234). Increasing the intake of fruit and vegetables, and taking regular physical exercise, is also important in protecting against heart and blood vessel diseases.

Small blood vessels

If your blood glucose levels are high for long periods, this will lead to glucose building up in the cells in the walls of the blood vessels, causing these vessels to become more brittle.[934] The cells mainly affected by this glucose toxicity are those which don't need insulin in order to transport glucose, i.e. the eyes, kidneys, nerves and blood vessels. As glucose can pass freely into these cells, they will always be exposed to high glucose concentrations when the blood glucose level is high. Since the cells in the lining of the intestine are not dependent on insulin, they will transport glucose from the intestine (i.e. after a meal) to the bloodstream even if the blood glucose is high.[826]

If a person has diabetes, glucose binds to a protein in the wall of the red blood cells. This makes the red blood cells stiff. These stiffened cells will have difficulties passing through the finest blood vessels (capillaries) as they need to if they are to deliver oxygen to the rest of the body's tissues.[758] So it is very important from the point of view of the red blood cells that blood glucose levels can be kept under control. Normal blood glucose levels for 24 hours restore the normal texture of the blood cell walls, remedying the problem.[758]

Complications affecting the eyes (retinopathy)

The risk of eye damage has decreased considerably with modern diabetes and eye care. In 1990, the majority of people who had had diabetes for 15-20 years had some kind of retinal changes, half of which needed laser treatment.[25,1010] At that time, one in every 1,000 individuals with diabetes would sustain serious visual impairment (visual acuity 0.1 or less) each year but blindness due to diabetes was very rare in countries where modern treatment methods were available.[944] In a Swedish study from 2010, 42% of people with diabetes had some form of eye damage while 12% had a risk of affected vision.[479]

Brittle capillaries can give rise to small swellings called microaneurysms (see illustration on page 360). These are thought of as "background" problems that do not affect the sight. It is important to realize that this type of early lesion can get better if blood glucose control is improved. On the other hand, if you continue to have a high blood glucose and high HbA_{1c} the process of change in your eyes will continue, and the lesions on the retina may worsen and new blood vessels form. These new blood vessels are brittle and can easily rupture resulting in bleeding and damage to your vision. Usually, the blood will be absorbed and the sight restored. Large or repeated instances of bleeding that are left untreated can result in permanent damage to your vision and, in the worst case, blindness. Impaired colour or night vision can be a result of damage to the nervous system caused by diabetes.[796] Smoking also increases the risk of damage to your vision.[765]

Many people feel that blindness is the worst thing that can happen if they have diabetes. You may worry about this, for example if you have been eating too many sweets. However, it may be difficult to talk about this with your parents (or your partner) since they will be worried too.

If you develop diabetes today and have a good HbA_{1c} during the years to come, there is a very little risk that you will lose your sight. This is because much better methods of treatment have been developed during recent years, both for diabetes and for eye damage.

Try to talk about this at home even if it is difficult. It is important that you know all the facts and that you realize you can influence the course of events yourself. Many adults have seen what has happened to people with diabetes in the past, especially if they have older friends or relatives who have had diabetes for a long time. They may find it difficult to believe that the same need not apply to someone developing diabetes today.

Research findings: Retinopathy

♠ In an Australian study, some degree of retinopathy was present in 28% of a group of 178 children and adolescents aged 10-14 years with a diabetes duration of 4-10 years.[296]

♠ In a group of 193 older adolescents aged 15-22, retinopathy was present in 52%.[296]

♠ In a Swedish study, 14.5% of participants aged 8-25 years had retinopathy.[604]

Treatment

The most important treatment is good blood glucose control. This can reverse early changes to the retina. We inform newly diagnosed children and teenagers that they should not need to risk becoming blind as, today, we have better methods both for treating diabetes and for avoiding possible eye damage. But you need to look after your diabetes, as having high HbA_{1c} levels over a period of 20-30 years still puts you at quite high risk of becoming blind.

You may experience some worsening of eye damage if you improve your metabolic control considerably (as when starting with an insulin pump).[463,270] It is important to know that studies have shown that this situation is only temporary, even if some people need laser photocoagulation treatment. If you continue with good glucose control, the changes to your eyes will reverse. It has been suggested that people with established eye damage should try to improve their blood glucose control slowly if they are to avoid damage to their sight.[463] How-

The eye seen in cross-section. Eye damage is first noted in the retina. At check-ups, the retina is examined after dilation of the pupil. It is usually photographed (called fundus photography) and an eye specialist will have a close look at the pictures.

ever, in the DCCT study the risk was still there, even if the HbA_{1c} was gradually improved.[270] A temporary deterioration was seen in women who became pregnant during the DCCT study, and this can be attributed to the fact that their blood glucose levels improved considerably while they were pregnant. At the end of the study, the level of eye damage had decreased and was back to average level again.[271]

Laser is an effective form of treatment which can spare the sight and sometimes even improve it. In a large study of individuals with high-risk eye damage, the progression to severe visual loss decreased from 26% in untreated eyes to 11% after laser photocoagulation.[28] Some eye lesions can be operated on.

To be able to discover changes as early as possible, all individuals with diabetes should be given an eye examination annually as soon as their diabetes has 2 years' duration (5 years for those who have not yet reached puberty).[968] In addition, you may need to have your eyes examined when you apply for a driving licence. The most sensitive type of examination is photography of the retina (fundus photography). Before taking the photograph, eye drops will be applied in order to dilate the pupils, so that a larger part of the retina can be seen on the photograph. The retina can also be examined with

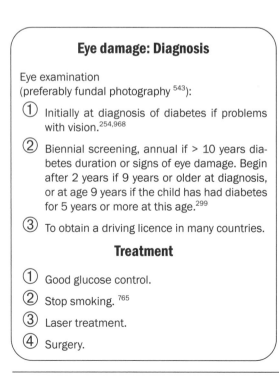

Eye damage: Diagnosis

Eye examination
(preferably fundal photography [543]):

① Initially at diagnosis of diabetes if problems with vision.[254,968]

② Biennial screening, annual if > 10 years diabetes duration or signs of eye damage. Begin after 2 years if 9 years or older at diagnosis, or at age 9 years if the child has had diabetes for 5 years or more at this age.[299]

③ To obtain a driving licence in many countries.

Treatment

① Good glucose control.

② Stop smoking. [765]

③ Laser treatment.

④ Surgery.

a special instrument (an ophthalmoscope) but this method is not as good as fundal photography in detecting changes.[764]

You should always contact your diabetes clinic if you have any kind of problems with your vision. If you have advanced eye damage, you can get a sudden onset of decreased vision, or a blurry vision due to swelling. An early sign that something is not quite right might be a perception of dark shadows over your visual field or floating spots that move.

Disturbed vision at unstable blood glucose levels

Blurred vision for a couple of hours is a common symptom of unstable blood glucose levels. It is not in any way dangerous for your vision or associated with future visual impairment. This is most likely to happen in the first week of diabetes when insulin is first started and the blood glucose levels fall considerably (see page

31). Unstable blood glucose can also cause disturbances in colour vision.

Temporarily blurred vision when blood glucose levels are high does not result in any permanent eye damage.

Sometimes the disturbed vision can continue for several weeks. This is caused by glucose being stored as sorbitol in the lens, disturbing the fluid distribution. This will have a temporary effect on the way the lens works, and make you shortsighted. However, if your blood glucose levels are high for long periods, there is some risk that permanent clouding will occur (cataract). For example, this may happen if an adolescent has had symptoms for a long time (many months) before diagnosis.[254] Cataract surgery can be performed and is usually successful.

Glasses

Your blood glucose levels should be stable when you try out new glasses. Otherwise, your vision will be affected by temporary changes in blood glucose. After the onset of diabetes, it may take 2-3 months of normal blood glucose levels before the lens has returned to its usual shape.[277] This means it is not a good idea to get glasses or replace them during this time.

Contact lenses

People with diabetes can wear contact lenses. However, you should avoid long-term lenses (that are replaced every second or third week) as the protecting cell layer of the cornea tends to be more brittle if you have diabetes.[197]

After many years of high blood glucose levels, the blood vessels of the retina will become brittle and small "bubbles" (called microaneurysms) can form. They do not affect your vision but can be seen on a photograph of the retina.

Control of blood pressure is very important to prevent and reduce kidney damage. Your blood pressure should be checked routinely at clinic visits.

Microalbuminuria is defined as more than 20 μg per min in a timed urine sample or more than 30 mg per 24 hours in two out of three consecutive tests [82,206] taken within a 2-3 month period. Macroalbuminuria (proteinuria, manifest kidney damage) is defined as more than 200 μg/min in a timed urine sample or more than 300 mg in a 24-hour period. Overnight microalbuminuria can be measured as a concentration test on early morning urine (such as Micral-Test®, with a cut-off 30 mg/l).[4] The level is lower in a morning sample as you have been lying down all night. A new and reliable method of measuring microalbuminuria in a morning spot sample is the ratio between albu-

Complications affecting the kidneys (nephropathy)

The blood vessels of the kidneys are formed into small clusters where waste products in the blood are filtered into the urine. Damage to the walls of these blood vessels causes an increased leakage of protein into the urine. Tiny amounts of protein (known as microalbuminuria) can then be detected in the urine. If the leakage continues, the person is at risk of developing high blood pressure and continuous leakage of protein into the urine (proteinuria). This may occur after 10-30 years of diabetes and, if not treated well, leads to uraemia (dangerously high levels of waste products in the blood because the body is unable to rid itself of them). If microalbuminuria is left untreated, dialysis will be necessary in a further 7-10 years.[82] Only about 30-40% of all those with diabetes will develop microalbuminuria and its associated risk of permanent kidney damage.[82,1010] Good diabetes control decreases the risk of kidney damage. It is still not known why more than half of all individuals with diabetes are not at all susceptible to kidney damage, but hereditary factors appear to play a significant part.[268]

Kidney damage: Diagnosis

① Measure blood pressure regularly.

② Check for microalbuminuria (small amounts of protein in the urine) annually:
Begin after 2 years if 9 years or older at diagnosis, or at age 9 years if the child has had diabetes for 5 years or more at this age.[299]
In adults begin after 5 years of diabetes.[31]

Check at every visit if microalbuminuria has been detected.

③ Measure kidney function when necessary.

Treatment

① Good glucose control (HbA$_{1c}$).

② Stop smoking.

③ Microalbuminuria is treated with ACE inhibitors.

④ Treatment of blood pressure above 130/80 [34,82,769] or 95th percentile for age.[968]

⑤ Treatment of urinary tract infections.

⑥ Reduction of protein and salt in your diet if you have persistent excretion of protein in the urine.[365]

⑦ Dialysis.

⑧ Transplantation.

min and creatinine (A/C ratio or ACR).[561] With this method, microalbuminuria is defined as > 2.5 mg/mmol (> 30 mg/g) [31] in men, and > 3.5 mg/mmol in women [4] because they tend to have a lower proportion of muscle to body weight. However, as pregnant women excrete more creatinine in the urine, their cut-off should be > 2.5 mg/mmol.[581] Because exercise within 24 hours, infection, fever, smoking, menstruation, a very high blood glucose level and blood in the urine may all increase the level of microalbuminuria, an abnormal value should be repeated.[33,970] Sexual activity (ejaculation) does not affect the level of microalbuminuria.[511]

The ACR microalbuminuria cut-off for a random daytime urine sample (spot urine) has been defined as more than 4.5 mg/mmol for boys and more than 5.2 mg/mmol for girls.[1055] Some adolescents have been found to have microalbuminuria although they have had diabetes for only a short time.[1055] This microalbuminuria can be caused by puberty as such and may be transient, but these individuals may also have an increased vulnerability in their kidneys leading to a greater risk of kidney damage later on if they have high HbA_{1c} values. Proteinuria can have other causes apart from diabetes.

Treatment

Just as for eye lesions, the most important treatment for nephropathy is tight insulin and blood glucose control. This is because, if microalbuminuria is discovered early, it can be reversed by lowering the blood glucose level and HbA_{1c}.[123] It is equally important to treat raised blood pressure early on. Weight control helps to keep blood pressure within target range. The average blood pressure reduction per kilogram of weight loss is 1-2 mm Hg.[365]

Research findings: Nephropathy

♠ In a Danish study of children, adolescents and young adults aged 12-27 years, 9% had microalbuminuria and 4% macroalbuminuria.[805]

♠ In one study of adults, the risk of progression to established kidney damage was increased in people whose diastolic blood pressure was higher than 80 mm Hg.[769]

♠ In another study, 53% of those smoking, 33% of those who had smoked previously, but only 11% of those who had never smoked, experienced an increase in the damage to their kidneys in the course of 1 year.[939]

♠ Young smokers (mean age 19 years, smoking five or more cigarettes per day for 1 year or longer), had a 2.8 times higher risk of microalbuminuria.[189] The microalbuminuria improved significantly in those who ceased smoking.

Treatment of albuminuria with a special type of anti-hypertensive drugs (ACE inhibitors) has shown good results even if the blood pressure is normal. This is recommended as routine treatment as soon as permanent microalbuminuria is discovered.[82,1071] However, ACE inhibitors should not be used during pregnancy since they can cause damage to the unborn child. One study showed that the risk of microalbuminuria progressing to manifest kidney damage decreased from 21.9 to 7.2% when it was treated with ACE inhibitors.[745]

The progression of renal disease can be successfully slowed by a reduction in dietary protein.[825] Renal failure can be treated with dialysis or kidney transplantation. Even advanced renal lesions can be reversed by normal glucose levels, as seen 10 years after pancreas transplantation.[353]

Nerve damage: Diagnosis

① Test of vibratory sense (tuning-fork).

② Test of sensation with a thin plastic fibre (monofilament).

③ Tests with special instruments.

Treatment

① Improved glucose control.

② Foot care, good shoes that don't hurt.

③ Treatment of foot and leg ulcers.

④ Oxygen treatment in pressurized chambers is sometimes tried if ulcers are slow to heal.

⑤ Drug treatment — ongoing research.

Complications affecting the nerves (neuropathy)

Your body's nerve fibres, which are made of very long and thin cells, can be affected after many years of diabetes. The blood vessels supplying the nerve fibres can be damaged resulting in a decreased supply of oxygen.[1030] This causes damage to the nerves' insulating covering (myelin sheath) and ultimately results in poorer nerve impulses. Sensation decreases and there can be accompanying numbing or tingling. The longest nerves are the most vulnerable; thus problems arise primarily in the feet, fingers or lower parts of the legs. Later on, a more general sensation loss can occur, starting from the toes and spreading upwards. Pain caused by nerve damage can even be felt in the hands and shoulders.

If the blood flow in your small skin capillaries is decreased, along with sensation, you will not feel the pain from small wounds and healing will be slow. Decreased perspiration in your feet can make the skin dry and cause it to crack. With inadequate foot care, small wounds get worse. If untreated, this may lead to ulcers, gangrene, and in the worst case, amputation. If you have problems with decreased sensation you should avoid sports that involve the risk of foot

The autonomic nervous system

Different organs can be affected by damage to the autonomic nervous system after many years of diabetes (modified from reference [1007]). The risk of these complications is decreased with modern diabetes care.

Organ	Problem
Heart	Dizziness when standing up.
Blood vessels	Reduced capacity for physical work.
Oesophagus	Difficulty in swallowing.
Stomach	Vomiting. Slow emptying of the stomach.
Intestines	Constipation, night time diarrhoea.
Rectum	Incontinence.
Urine bladder	Difficulties emptying the bladder. Frequent voiding.
Penis	Erection problems/impotence (see page 324). Ejaculation backwards into the bladder (can result in infertility).
Vagina	Dry mucous membranes.
Sweat glands	Profuse sweating in the face and neck after eating hot food, spices or Cheddar cheese. Decreased sweating in the feet, legs and trunk.
Skin	Increased skin temperature.
Pupils	Small pupils.

Foot care if you have nerve damage

1. Don't walk around barefoot.

2. Always use clean and dry socks. Wear them inside out (less risk of blisters from the seams).

3. Inspect your feet daily or twice daily for redness or blisters. Use a mirror to view the soles.

4. Wear shoes that fit well and don't hurt. Empty them of gravel often.

5. Wash your feet carefully and rub them with moisturizing cream in order to avoid chapping.

6. See a doctor as an emergency if you see redness, callous growth, blisters, ingrown toenails or signs of infection.

7. Ensure you have regular foot care at the diabetes clinic. Learn how to manicure your toenails to avoid sore skin.

8. If you smoke, stop!

➡ Children with diabetes have healthy feet and don't need special foot care. Ordinary hygiene is quite enough and they may very well run barefoot on the beach.

➡ Foot baths can be relieving for tired, healthy feet and there are no restrictions for children or teenagers with diabetes in this case. It is only if you already have nerve damage that foot baths with massage should be avoided. If you are in any doubt about this ask your doctor.

damage (blisters, cuts) such as running, football or squash.

If you step on a nail or splinter there is always a risk of wound infection. If you have nerve damage with diminished sensation, the risk of infection increases as you may be unaware of the wound. Impaired sensitivity to pain often means that a person with diabetes will seek medical care for such a wound later than they otherwise would (9 days after the trauma compared with 5 days for a person without diabetes in one study [657]). The infection will then have had time to spread and the risk of a complication, i.e. tissue or bone infection, becomes much greater. In the above-mentioned study, 35% of the individuals with diabetes had an infection compared with 13% of individuals without diabetes. It is also worth mentioning that 42% of those with diabetes had injured themselves

when barefoot, compared with 19% of people without diabetes.

The part of our nervous system that is self-regulatory (uncontrollable by willpower) is called the autonomic nervous system. This can also be damaged by diabetes but the symptoms will be different. They include disturbances in sweating, diarrhoea, constipation, impotence (see page 324) or delayed emptying of the stomach.

Difficulties in emptying the bladder properly may be caused by diabetes. Individuals who have had diabetes for many years should therefore empty their bladder thoroughly and often.

Delayed stomach emptying can lead to hypoglycaemia 1 or 2 hours after a meal. At that time, the insulin level will be at its highest if you are using premeal injections. However, when the peaks of glucose from the meal are delayed, the timing with premeal insulin injections will not match, especially if you are using rapid-acting insulins (NovoRapid or Humalog). One idea is to try taking insulin after rather than before the meal. Other symptoms of delayed stomach emptying are an early feeling of being full and a sense of the stomach being distended. The emptying rate of the stomach can be examined by a special type of X-ray (scintigraphy). A decreased HbA_{1c} with the avoidance of high blood glucose levels can lead to a reduction of these types of symptoms. If problems are pronounced, you should try to exclude everything that decreases the emptying rate of the stomach (fat, dietary fibre, very cold or very hot food, see page 231). Special drugs may also help.

The cells in the brain can pick up glucose directly from the blood without using insulin, but despite this they seem to be relatively immune to the long-term toxic effects of glucose.[917] This may be due to the so called blood-brain barrier that prevents substances from the blood being freely transported into the brain. The brain cells normally have much lower glucose levels than the blood.

Treatment

As with the other complications of diabetes, the most important treatment for nerve damage is improved diabetes control. Good foot care is also important. If the skin lesions are slow to heal, oxygen treatment in a pressurized chamber can be effective.[341]

Other complications

Limited joint mobility (LJM) can be a complication of diabetes.[1045] The elbow and finger exten-

---

Delayed emptying of the stomach: Diagnosis [54]

(1) Typical symptoms:
Hypoglycaemia 1 hour after a meal.
Early feeling of satiety (no more hunger).
Feeling of being full.
Distended stomach.

(2) Special X-ray (scintigraphy).

Treatment

(1) Improved glucose control.

(2) Change in diet:
Less fibre.
Less fat.
Small but frequent meals.
Temperature of food should be not less than 4°C (39°) or more than 40°C (104° F).

(3) Take insulin injection after eating.

(4) Drug treatment.

---

sion, and wrist flexion, can be decreased. Mobility can also be decreased in the feet and other joints. Mobility in the finger joints can be tested by the "prayer sign", i.e. putting the hands together in a praying position with the fingers fanned. LJM is present if there is a missing joint contact between the fingers. This is most common in the little finger.

Lowering the risk of complications

Constantly trying to achieve a good blood glucose level can be very tiresome. Many people, including teenagers, are pessimistic about the benefits of keeping the blood glucose low believing that: "Things will go to pot anyway," whatever they do.

However, there is convincing scientific evidence that good glucose control will pay off by postponing and preventing complications. While it may be impossible to avoid every type of long-term complication of diabetes completely (despite today's improved treatment methods), it is quite clear that a person with a higher HbA_{1c} risks earlier and more severe complications. The goal of intensive treatment is to postpone the beginnings of complications so far into the future that they will never cause any noticeable difficulties such as impairment of your vision. Of course there are always exceptions. Some people do have complications in spite of meticulous control while others, who have never "managed well", are spared. This may seem very unfair, but it can also be of some comfort to those individuals who do develop complications since there is no guarantee that, had they achieved better blood glucose levels, the problems would have been completely avoided.

An unusual example comes from Kuwait, where a person with kidney disease (without diabetes) received a kidney donated from a person with diabetes who was killed in a traffic accident. The kidney had been severely damaged by diabetes but no other suitable kidney was available for him. The transplanted kidney now was exposed to perfect glucose control since the person who received it as a transplant did not have diabetes. Two years later, new tests were performed on the transplanted kidney, and the diabetes lesions were found to have gone!

Many people believe that complications strike randomly among the population with diabetes. Others feel that it does not matter if you "manage well", complications will arise anyway. In fact, modern research has clearly shown that the degree of long-term complications depends directly upon the blood glucose levels over the course of the years that a person has diabetes.

If you have had a high HbA_{1c} for some years, and then decide to lower it, it will take some further years for the risk of complications to decrease.[669] This is logical if you compare to smoking, as the risk of lung cancer does not go away immediately after you have stopped smoking. In real life, you may experience that to your surprise the eye examination (fundus photography) after you have managed to lower your HbA_{1c} will show that you have developed microaneurysms (so called background retinopathy, see page 360). Sometimes this is due to a quick decrease of a rather high HbA_{1c} (see page 359), but more often it is caused by the accumulated risk caused by the elevated HbA_{1c} during the previous years. Don't panic, we have often seen that the fundus photograph after 2 to 4 years will show normal results again, as long as you maintain the lower HbA_{1c} level.

HbA$_{1c}$ in different studies

	Level of HbA$_{1c}$, %		
Linköping, Sweden [122]	5.4	7.4	9.5
Stockholm, Sweden [881]	5.0	7.1	9.2
Oslo, Norway [225]	6.6	8.3	10.1
Steno, Denmark [348]	6.7	8.7	10.8
DCCT, US [261]	6.3	8.4	10.5
IFCC, mmol/mol	46	68	91

Unfortunately HbA$_{1c}$ values have not been the same when measured at different laboratories. Remember this when you compare your own HbA$_{1c}$ with the results of studies that you find from different countries, for example, on the Internet. The table is from reference [639]. See page 368 for a comparison with the new IFCC numbers.

The DCCT study

The large US DCCT study (Diabetes Control and Complications Trial) clearly shows that a lower HbA$_{1c}$ will decrease the development of complications.[261] In the course of a 9-year period, 1,441 individuals with diabetes (aged between 13 and 39 years) were compared. They were divided into two groups, one with an average HbA$_{1c}$ of 53 mmol/mol (7.0%) using intensive treatment with insulin pumps (42% at the end of the study) or multiple daily injections, and one with a level of 75 mmol/mol (9.0%) using conventional treatment with one or two doses per day.

The insulin treatment was not the only factor that differed between the two groups. In the intensive treatment group, blood glucose was measured four times a day, and the doses of insulin adjusted if necessary. Clinic visits were scheduled once a month with telephone contacts in between on at least a weekly and often a daily basis. HbA$_{1c}$ was measured every month. The aim was specifically to attain low blood glucose readings (3.9-6.7 mmol/l, 70-120 mg/dl, before meals) and an HbA$_{1c}$ of 42

mmol/mol (6.0%), at the highest. In the group using 1-2 doses per day, the goal of treatment was to feel well including the absence of symptoms from high or low blood glucose levels. Clinic visits were scheduled every 3 months, urine or blood glucose was monitored daily and regular education was given at the visits. HbA$_{1c}$ values were taken but the results were not revealed to this group.

In the group receiving intensive treatment, the risk of developing eye damage was lowered by 76%, early kidney damage (microalbuminuria) by 39%, severe kidney damage (albuminuria) by 54% and nerve damage by 60%. The risk of severe hypoglycaemia (requiring help from another person) increased by two/threefold in the intensively treated group. Neuro-psychological tests did not show any permanent damage from the hypoglycaemic incidents.[265] The individuals in the group with intensive insulin treatment gained more weight (on average 4.6 kg, 10.1 lb). There was a 46% reduction in vaginal infections in the intensive treatment group, but no differences in the rates of other infections.[264]

Another way of presenting the data is that intensive treatment will give a person with diabetes 7.7 additional years of sight, 5.8 years of renal function, 6.0 years of limb preservation, and 5.3 additional years of life. In summary, each 10% fall in HbA$_{1c}$, for example from 80 to 72 mmol/mol (9.5 to 8.7%), decreased complications by 43-45%.[263] Neither of the two groups experienced a deterioration in the quality of their personal lives despite the increasing demands of their diabetes care and the frequency of hypoglycaemia.[267] When analysing quality of life issues and psychiatric symptoms, data showed no differences between the intensive and the conventional group despite the fact that the intensive group spent considerably more time on injections, blood glucose testing and visits to the clinic.[264] Only those individuals who had experienced repeated (three or more) episodes of severe hypoglycaemia resulting in unconsciousness or seizures scored lower on life quality. The overall conclusion was that the decreased risk of long-term complications more than compensates for the increased risk of severe hypoglycaemia.

The individual's own insulin production was better sustained in the intensive treatment group (measured by level of maintained C-peptide, see page 373) which, in turn, allowed for better glucose control, less frequent hypoglycaemia and fewer long-term complications.[269] These observations emphasize the importance of implementing intensive treatment, even during the early years of living with diabetes.

In the group of adolescents between the ages of 13 and 17 years in the DCCT study, those with 1-2 doses had an average HbA_{1c} of 84 mmol/mol (9.8%) and those with intensive treatment 65 mmol/mol, 8.1%.[262] After between 4 and 7 years of treatment, the group who had received intensive treatment had 53-70% fewer eye complications and 55% fewer kidney complications than the group on 1-2 doses of insulin per day. The intensively treated adolescents had a risk of severe hypoglycaemia with unconsciousness or seizures of 27% in 1 year.[262] The corresponding figure for adults was 16%.[264]

Many parents ask us if it is healthy for the blood glucose level to swing up and down throughout the day as often happens when multiple injections or insulin pump treatments are used to maintain an optimal HbA_{1c} value. The participants in the DCCT study with higher fluctuations in blood glucose did not have a higher risk of complications when compared with others who had the same HbA_{1c} levels.[607] People with intensive treatment had lower mean blood glucose than those taking 1-2 doses/day, when comparing at the same HbA_{1c} levels.[608] In previous editions of this book a graph was included, showing that the risk of complications was higher in the conventional group using 1-2 injections/day, even when compared with people in the intensive group having the same HbA_{1c}.[263] However, a repeated analysis has found that this was not correct, and that in fact the different HbA_{1c} levels in the 2 groups explain 96% of the difference in complica-

tions.[643] There are individual variations in the relationship between HbA_{1c} and blood glucose levels, so that some people seem to have a risk of complications at lower blood glucose levels than others (see page 119). However, your average HbA_{1c} level over the years will accurately reflect what your personal risk is.

In a follow-up of the DCCT study (the EDIC study, Epidemiology of Diabetes Interventions and Complications) it has been found that there seems to be a carry-over effect of "hyperglycaemic memory".[273,274,723] After the DCCT was finished, 75% of the former conventional group began with intensified insulin therapy and the HbA_{1c} values became almost identical to those of the former intensive group. In spite of this, the risk of eye [273], kidney [274] and nerve [723] damage was still much lower (about 50%) in the former intensive group of the DCCT during a 7-8 year follow-up. Intensive treatment with a lower HbA_{1c} during the years of the DCCT study reduced the risk of any event caused by cardiovascular disease by 42% and the risk of

Your HbA_{1c} values from 2-3 years earlier contribute most to the risk of complications. As you can see from this graph, the high blood glucose values you have had during the previous years (as measured by HbA_{1c}) will actually continue to give an increased risk for 2-3 years, but then the risk decreases substantially over the following years.[669] From this follows that the best option is of course to keep your HbA_{1c} as low as possible right from the onset of diabetes to avoid this type of accumulation of risk for complications. This analysis was done on data from the DCCT study, and explains the "hyperglycaemic memory" that was found in the follow-up (called the EDIC study, see the text).

non-fatal cardiac infarction, stroke, or death from cardiovascular disease by 57%.[776] Eighteen years after the completion of the study, the participants who had undergone intensive treatment were 46% less likely to have developed progression of eye damage and 40% lower risk of developing kidney damage (microalbuminuria). This was despite the fact that the groups continued to have the same HbA_{1c}.[427] The effect of 6-9 years of lower HbA_{1c} carries on for quite a long time afterwards, which may be worth considering if you are finding it difficult to motivate yourself to continue with a strict blood glucose control.

Among those aged 13-18 years at the start of the DCCT study, the risk of a progression of eye complications during the EDIC 4-year follow-up was approximately 75% lower in the group using multiple daily injections or pumps during the DCCT, in spite of the same HbA_{1c} of 68 mmol/mol, 8.4% in both groups.[1104] However, a higher number of the former intensive group (90% vs. 70% for former conventional group) used intensive therapy during the follow-up, which may have contributed to the results. In other words, it is really important to start caring for your diabetes as early as possible.

This is comparable with a large Swedish study of 7,454 persons with type 1 diabetes followed over 5 years, where the group with a mean HbA_{1c} of 55 mmol/mol (7.2%) had a risk reduction of 41% for coronary heart disease and 37% for cardiovascular disease compared to the group with a mean HbA_{1c} of 75 mmol/mol (9.0%).[321] Each 11 mmol/mol (1.0%) increase in HbA_{1c} gave a risk increase of

31-34% for coronary heart disease and 26-32% for cardiovascular disease.

The Oslo study

Knut Dahl-Jørgensen and collaborators in Oslo performed a long-term study comparing two-dose treatment, multiple daily treatment and pump treatment.[463] This study showed clearly that the risk of complications decreased considerably as the HbA_{1c} was lowered (see figures).

The Berlin eye study

In Berlin, 346 individuals with diabetes, aged between 8 and 35 years, were studied with a special type of X-ray displaying the vessels of the retina (fluorescence angiography). The conclusion was that if the average HbA_{1c} was lower during the previous years, retinal vessel changes developed later.[246]

Every percentage lowering of HbA_{1c} means a decreased risk of eye lesions. With an HbA_{1c}

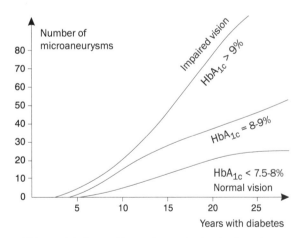

This graph is from a Norwegian study showing how the number of microaneurysms increases considerably with increased average HbA_{1c} over the course of many years.[463] With a lower HbA_{1c} the changes will probably not be severe enough to affect your vision. The HbA_{1c} levels in this study are approximately the same as in the DCCT study (see page 367).

Average HbA$_{1c}$	Years before eye changes
< 7% (< 53 mmol/l)	25
7-8% (53-64 mmol/mol)	16
8-9% (64-75 mmol/mol)	13
> 9% (> 75 mmol/l	12

HbA$_{1c}$ levels are shown in DCCT numbers (approximately 1% lower than in the Berlin study).[246]

above 53 mmol/mol (7.0%), the risk of eye damage increased considerably.

The Linköping studies

The risk of being affected by long-term complications has been studied in a series of investigations from Linköping in Sweden.[122,123,124,794] Children and adolescents whose diabetes developed during the 20 year period 1961-1980 have been studied, and a decreased risk of complications for those with onset in later years has been demonstrated, both for retinopathy and nephropathy. See their results in the figures on page 370.

Other studies

The Hvidøre Study Group on Childhood diabetes collected data from 2,269 adolescents aged 11-18 years from 19 countries in Europe, Japan, Australia and North America.[275] The patients took part in the routine care programme which at all centres had a multidisciplinary approach involving paediatric diabetologists. All tests for HbA$_{1c}$ were analysed at a central laboratory. The average HbA$_{1c}$ was 66 mmol/mol, 8.2%. However, the average HbA$_{1c}$ among the centres varied significantly, both between and within countries, from 57 mmol/mol (7.4%) to 77 mmol/mol (9.2%).

The SWEET study group included 5,749 patients from 13 countries in Europe, showing

an improvement in mean HbA$_{1c}$ from 66 mmol/mol, 8.2% in 2009 to 63 mmol/mol (7.9%) in 2012.[634] The percentage with HbA$_{1c}$

In a study of 213 individuals who had developed their diabetes before the age of 15 years (and who had had diabetes for 11-30 years), only one person with an average HbA$_{1c}$ < 65 mmol/mol (8.1%) needed laser treatment of their eyes.[124] Only two individuals with an average HbA$_{1c}$ < 77 mmol/mol (9.2%) had permanent kidney damage (so called macroalbuminuria). The conclusion is that it takes a slightly lower average blood glucose to avoid eye damage than kidney damage. However, with an HbA$_{1c}$ of 63 mmol/mol (7.9%) or less, the risk of serious long-term complications is very low.

below 58 mmol/mol (7.5%) increased from 33% in 2010 to 37% in 2012.[634]

The Swedish national pediatric diabetes register (SWEDIABKIDS) with 7,016 patients up to the age of 18 years included in 2012 shows a mean HbA_{1c} of 63 mmol/mol (7.9%) with a percentage of HbA_{1c}< 58 mmol/mol (7.5%) of 61% in the age group 0-6 years, 40% in the 7-11, and 25% in the 12-17 years old.[929]

An Australian study showed that the risk of severe hypoglycaemia increased when the average HbA_{1c} of the clinic went down from 86 to 64 mmol/mol (10 to 8%).[259] However, European studies have not shown the same increase in risk of severe hypoglycaemia when using intensive insulin treatment.[137,791,816,954] In a Swedish study of intensively treated individuals with diabetes aged 1-18 years, the risk was 15% despite a mean HbA_{1c} of 62 mmol/mol

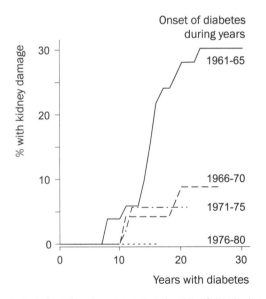

A study from Sweden shows that the risk of developing kidney damage (albuminuria) has decreased considerably in recent years.[122] Amongst those who developed diabetes before the age of 15 (between the years 1961 and 1965), 30% developed kidney damage after 25 years of diabetes. Less than 10% of those who developed diabetes from 1966 and onwards have developed kidney damage.

(7.8%).[694] See also page 50. The reason for this may lie in the fact that there is a longer tradition of using intensive treatment in Europe and that patients eventually learn, at least in part, how to avoid dangerously low blood glucose values. The frequency of hypoglycaemia in the DCCT study decreased slightly towards the end of the study,[264] an observation that supports this hypothesis. In a Swedish study on young people aged 1-18, the risk of a severe hypoglycaemia with unconsciousness or seizures was only 15% in spite of an average HbA_{1c} of 62 mmol/mol (7.8%).[694] In a more recent Swedish study, the children below age 13 had an average HbA_{1c} of 51 mmol/mol (6.8%), but had never had such severe hypoglycaemia. The teenagers who had a slightly higher HbA_{1c} of 60 mmol/mol (7.6%) had a 2% risk of severe hypoglycaemia with unconsciousness or seizures.[460] More recent studies from the US show that fewer people were affected by severe hypoglycaemia.[109,715]

In an American study, the average number of years until complications from different organs developed was calculated with different HbA_1 levels (older HbA_{1c} method). For most microvascular complications to develop, it would take, on average, 83 years with an average HbA_{1c} unit at 11 mmol/mol (1.0%) above normal (53 mmol/mol, 7.0%), 42 years at 64 mmol/mol (8.0%), 28 years at 75 mmol/mol (9.0%), 21 years at 86 mmol/mol (10%), and 18 years at 97 mmol/mol (11%).[809] From this follows that every percentage decline in HbA_{1c} is important, even if you are in the high range.

An Australian follow-up over 20 years found that the risk of retinopathy was lowered from 53% to 12% over the years as the percentage of patients being on 1 or 2 injections per day decreased from 83% to 12%.[303] Microalbuminuria also decreased from 8% to 3%. Mean HbA_{1c} did change, but not so much during these years [76 to 69 mmol/mol (9.1 to 8.5%)], indicating that the intensified insulin regimens (multiple daily injections or insulin pump) were strongly contributing to the improved outcome.

Research and new developments

Huge efforts are put into diabetes research around the world and more than 10,000 scientific studies are published every year. A large part of this is basic research, trying to throw light upon the causes of diabetes and why different things take place in the body when a person has diabetes. Even if you hear of new treatment for diabetes from newspapers or the television, you must remember that it usually takes several years before such methods become available outside the research clinics and unfortunately many new "wonder drugs" never become established treatments.

New treatments for diabetes

Implantable insulin pumps

Insulin pumps that can be implanted into the tummy (abdominal cavity) are being used as part of research programmes in some centres. These pumps are refilled with insulin by the insertion of a syringe through the skin into a membrane on the pump. Premeal bolus doses are given by using a small transmitter. Insulin from the pump is injected into the abdominal cavity (called intraperitoneal delivery) and is quickly absorbed into the bloodstream. Contrary to what one may think, the risk of hypoglycaemia is reduced by this type of insulin treatment.[774] This is because the insulin administered in this way passes through the liver *before* it reaches the other parts of the body, just like insulin secreted from a pancreas without diabetes.

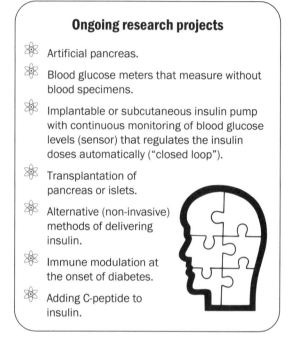

Ongoing research projects

- Artificial pancreas.
- Blood glucose meters that measure without blood specimens.
- Implantable or subcutaneous insulin pump with continuous monitoring of blood glucose levels (sensor) that regulates the insulin doses automatically ("closed loop").
- Transplantation of pancreas or islets.
- Alternative (non-invasive) methods of delivering insulin.
- Immune modulation at the onset of diabetes.
- Adding C-peptide to insulin.

Another research project involves an artificial pancreas which can be connected to a blood vessel. This device both measures blood glucose levels and injects insulin directly into the bloodstream. Such an approach is still very complicated and, at present, is found only in research laboratories.

Blood glucose meters

The possibility of measuring one's blood glucose at home has brought a revolution in diabetes treatment. We are now waiting for the next generation of blood glucose meters which can measure without obtaining a blood sample. Promising results have been shown using a ray of infrared light,[713] even during hypoglycaemic episodes.[383] It is also possible to measure the

The next step will be to let the subcutaneous sensor regulate an external insulin pump, thus creating an external artificial pancreas. Although there is a delay in the delivery of subcutaneously infused insulin into the bloodstream, the blood glucose level a couple of hours after a meal and during the night was near to normal in this study of six adults with type 1 diabetes.[991] Similar results have also been shown for children, where a small manual bolus before the meal improved the blood glucose readings even further.[1098]

glucose content of the fluid within the skin, using a needle that penetrates less than 1.5 mm (1/16 inch).[960]

Glucose sensors

A device that can measure the blood glucose levels continuously over a longer period of time is called a glucose sensor. So far such devices have only been shown to give reliable readings for a couple of days or a week at a time. Most types of sensors are implanted into the subcutaneous fat. Glucose is measured either by an enzymatic method that generates an electrical current (Medtronic MiniMed® CGMS and Guardian, Abbot Freestyle Navigator® and DexCom®, see page 107) or by a special method called microdialysis[126] that measures the glucose content in a saline solution circulating slowly through the inserted catheter. Another method (GlucoWatch®) is to measure the glucose content of fluid extracted across the skin with an electro-osmotic method (called reverse iontophoresis).[313] This device was for sale in the US for a while, but has been discontinued because of skin irritation.

With these types of devices we can measure night time blood glucose levels relatively easily, thereby gaining a better understanding of how

to adjust bedtime doses. Many parents of small children would sleep much better with an alarm for hypoglycaemia. One pump (Medtronic Veo®) that reacts on readings from the sensor, and shuts off for 2 hours when the glucose values become too low, is now available in Europe.[253] In studies, a laptop or smart phone has been used to regulate the pump in accordance with glucose readings from a subcutaneous sensor, and successful experiments with an "artificial pancreas" in the home environment are taking place in many parts of the world.[789]

Implantable sensors with a lifetime of several months have successfully been used in animal studies.[1057] The readings can be transmitted to a receiver, for example in the shape of a wrist watch.

C-peptide

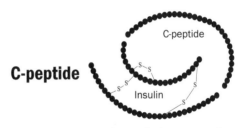

In a pancreas without diabetes, insulin is produced in the form of proinsulin. Before insulin is secreted to the bloodstream, a part called C-peptide (connecting peptide) is cut off. By measuring C-peptide, one can estimate how much a person with diabetes has left of his or her own insulin production. Early data suggested that C-peptide was of no use in the body but recently positive effects on metabolism have been shown in the form of a decreased HbA_{1c}. During a month's treatment with C-peptide, leakage of protein into the urine decreased and capillary function in the retina improved.[565] C-peptide stimulates the uptake of glucose into the muscle cells and thereby improves the effect of insulin (decreased insulin resistance). Nerve function in patients with diabetes-related nerve damage is improved as well.[566] Long-term studies have been started and it is possible that in the future C-peptide will be given along with insulin, though more research is still needed.

There is no scientific evidence that childhood vaccinations cause diabetes.

Vaccinations

Vaccinations have been proposed as one of the causes of diabetes. Some children have developed diabetes shortly after MMR vaccination (against measles, mumps and German measles/ rubella) at the age of 18 months. However, scientific studies have not been able to show a correlation between vaccination and the onset of diabetes.[337] Indeed, it appears that vaccination against measles results in a slightly lower risk of developing diabetes.[104] BCG vaccination against tuberculosis has been thought to have a protective effect but this has not been confirmed in studies.[234,819] The risk of acquiring diabetes is not affected by vaccination for pertussis (whooping cough),[475] varicella (chickenpox)[337] or other early childhood immunizations.[414] Vaccinations for hepatitis B and Haemophilus type b have not been shown to increase the risk for diabetes.[287]

Vaccination against diabetes would obviously be the ideal solution. If a virus could be identified that triggers diabetes it might be possible to vaccinate against it. If cows' milk protein plays a part in the cause of diabetes, a vaccine could perhaps prevent the onset of diabetes.[330]

Through vaccination, it may be possible to redirect the autoimmune reaction to another track so that the insulin-producing beta cells in the pancreas will not be destroyed. Animal studies vaccinating with the protein GAD (see page 381), which is found in beta cells, have been very promising and have succeeded in inducing

a tolerance to GAD. Investigations in young people aged 10-18 years have shown that when GAD vaccination (Diamyd™) was given within 18 months of diabetes onset, there was a better preservation of pancreatic ability to produce insulin (measured by C-peptide level) but no change in HbA_{1c}.[698] Intravenous treatment with so called anti-CD3 antibodies (that block the T-cells) for 2 weeks at the onset of diabetes resulted in lower HbA_{1c}, lower insulin dose and higher C-peptide after 2 years.[496] There were however considerable side effects from this treatment during the initial phase. Unfortunately both GAD vaccination and anti-CD3 trials have failed to repeat their positive results in larger recent studies.

Trials have been done where insulin is given to people with a very high risk of developing diabetes, in order to influence the immune system before all beta cells have been destroyed. In the US Diabetes Prevention Trial (DPT-1), insulin was given as twice-daily subcutaneous injections of Ultralente (total dose 0.25 U/kg per day) to close relatives of a person with diabetes (both children and adults) who themselves had a high risk of developing diabetes. Unfortunately, this type of insulin therapy over the course of 2-4 years did not succeed in preventing the development of diabetes.[290] In the other part of the DPT-1 study, insulin was given as tablets but this did not prevent the development of diabetes either.[978] However, one positive effect of participating in these studies was that diabetes was discovered earlier in its course and that therefore the risk of having ketoacidosis when diabetes was diagnosed was minimized. In a Finnish study, insulin given as nasal spray to children with a high risk of developing diabetes did not prevent or delay the onset of diabetes.[772]

Salicylic acid

Salicylic acid (aspirin, a component of many over the counter pain killers), has been used in trials to lessen the risk of heart disease as a complication of long-term diabetes.[311] The current policy is to use it for individuals with type 1 diabetes and established heart disease, but it is also recommended as a preventative measure in people with diabetes who are at increased cardiovascular risk.[35]

Amylin

Amylin is stored in the same cells as insulin in the pancreas and is produced together with insulin in a healthy person but is missing in a person with type 1 diabetes. A low level of amylin stimulates the release of insulin while a high level suppresses its release. Amylin decreases the production of glucagon and causes the stomach to empty more slowly. Amylin is registered as a drug in the US (Symlin®). A 1 year study on adults with type 1 diabetes showed a 4-8 mmol/mol (0.4-0.7%) lower HbA$_{1c}$ and also a decrease in weight of 0.5-2 kg.[874] A paediatric study found lower blood glucose after a test meal.[492]

GLP-1 (glucagon-like peptide)

GLP-1 is produced in the alpha cells in the pancreas (the same cells that produce glucagon), in the lining of the intestines and in the brain. Its

secretion is regulated both by the brain and by hormones. The release of GLP-1 is stimulated by carbohydrates and fat (especially mono-unsaturated fat) but is suppressed by insulin. The effect of GLP-1 is similar to that of amylin. GLP-1 stimulates the production and release of insulin, decreases the production of glucagon, slows down the emptying of the stomach and decreases appetite. GLP-1 may possibly also stimulate the production of new beta cells.[558] Studies have shown a lower fasting blood glucose caused by a decreased secretion of glucagon,[78] lower blood glucose after a meal caused by slower emptying of the stomach [213] and decreased calorie intake without an increase in hypoglycaemia.[558] Exendin-4 is a substance that is secreted by a lizard and that binds to the same receptor as GLP-1 but gives a longer action. It is now available as a drug for twice daily injections (Victoza®, Byetta®), and has had good effect in studies of both type 1 and type 2 diabetes.[558] Another type of drugs inhibit the breakdown of GLP-1 (DPP4-inhibitors, Januvia® and Galvus®).

Sodium transport in the kidney

A new type of drug5-minute (SGL2-inhibitors, empa- cana- and dapagliflozin) inhibit the reabsorption of glucose in the kidneys, causing an increased amount of sugar in the urine even with blood glucose levels below the normal renal threshold. This will lower blood glucose levels, and has so far been tried successfully in type 2 diabetes. It might even have some protective mechanisms for avoiding kidney damage.[398] Initial trials in type 1 diabetes have shown positive results with a reduced HbA$_{1c}$ after 8 weeks' use.[829]

What causes diabetes?

As of today we do not know what causes type 1 diabetes. However, we do know that it is not caused by eating too many sweets. A common

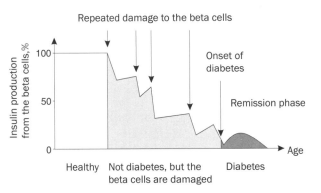

It is believed that the first attack on the beta cells in the pancreas (the cells that produce insulin) takes place several years before a person shows symptoms of diabetes. By the time diabetes is diagnosed, 80-90% of the beta cells are already damaged. The illustration is from reference [623].

view is that about 60-70% of type 1 diabetes is caused by non-hereditary factors, i.e. risk factors due to lifestyle habits, infections or being exposed to environmental factors.[230] But it is still unclear what those factors, infections or exposures are. The risk of developing diabetes is very different in different countries (see "How common is diabetes?" on page 16). The reason for this is unclear but there are many proposed theories.

Many parents feel that: "If we had only done this or that our child would probably not have developed the disease." It is important to realize that diabetes was not caused by something that you or your family have done or failed to do.

An autoimmune disease

Part of the explanation for the abnormal reaction of the body's immune defence is heredity. Certain signals or "markers" that can be measured in the blood are present in almost all children and teenagers with diabetes (such as HLA-antigens on chromosome number 6). However, these markers are also present in 20-60% of people who do not have diabetes.[230,966] Certain gene components have a protective effect in that they appear to prevent a person who has them from developing diabetes.

A viral disease is believed to induce T-cells (a type of white blood cells) that, in addition to killing the virus, in predisposed people will cross-react with and damage the insulin-producing beta cells in the pancreas. As the damage is caused by a defect in one's own immune system, diabetes is considered to be an autoimmune disease. One theory is that other agents having a structure similar to the GAD protein (see page 381) in the beta cells will react with the immune system at some time, causing the production of T-cells that also can react with GAD. Much later, perhaps many years later, when the immune system is exposed to GAD, the autoimmune "memory" will be activated, attacking the beta cell. Example of agents that have a protein structure partly similar to GAD

are viruses (enterovirus [504], rotavirus [529]) and cows' milk.[1073] Both of these viruses are common among children, and cause viral symptoms and gastroenteritis.

The beta cells will usually partly recover after some time, but if the initial attack is repeated several times, insulin production will decrease enough to raise the blood glucose level. Antibodies directed against the insulin-producing islets of Langerhans in the pancreas (GAD antibodies and ICA, islet cell antibodies), reflect the activity of immune reaction and can be detected several years prior to the onset of diabetes, and are an early sign of cell damage. However, screening for these antibodies is usually not done since, in people who do not yet have diabetes, there is at present no way of preventing the onset of the disease even if you know the risks in advance. The antibodies can even disappear spontaneously without the child developing diabetes. Most children and adolescents who develop diabetes have measurable levels of antibodies. It is common to measure ICA and GAD antibodies to determine whether an autoimmune type 1 diabetes is present, or whether it is another type of diabetes.

Heredity

At most, only 13% of children and adolescents who develop diabetes have a parent or sibling with diabetes.[228] The risk of developing diabetes by age 30 for first-degree relatives (brother/sister or parent/child) is between 3% and 10%.[301] Of children with newly diagnosed diabetes, 2-3% have a mother with type 1 diabetes, 5-6% have a father with type 1 diabetes, and 4-5% have a brother or sister with type 1 diabetes.[228] In this study only 1.5% had a first-degree relative with type 2 diabetes.[228] (See also "Will the child have diabetes?" on page 323.) Studies in identical twins have found that the risk of the other twin developing diabetes can be as high as 50-70%.[69,641]

Possible causes of diabetes

⟹ To get type 1 diabetes, you need to be genetically predisposed.

⟹ A viral disease can trigger the onset of diabetes.

⟹ If a mother has certain viral infections during pregnancy, her child may have an increased risk of developing diabetes.[233]

⟹ Impaired insulin production in the beta cells of the pancreas can be found several years before the onset of diabetes.

⟹ Drinking cows' milk during the first 6 months of life, or even later, may be a factor.

⟹ Fathers eating smoked mutton (contains nitrosamines) at the time of conception has been found to be a risk factor in Iceland.[485] High dietary intakes of nitrite and nitrate [229] and nitrate in drinking water [820] have also been shown to be risk factors.

⟹ Overweight is an important factor, but only for the development of type 2 diabetes.

⟹ Psychological stress, such as severe life events, have been found to occur more often both during the first 2 years of life [1032] and during the year before the onset of diabetes.[432,896] They are not believed to be the cause of the disease,[18] but may increase the risk by affecting the autoimmune process. [1032]

⟹ A very high standard of hygiene [628] and fewer infections [397,823] during infancy may lead to the immune defence not being "trained" correctly.

When one identical twin has type 1 diabetes, the risk of the other twin developing diabetes before the age of 35 was 70% in a Danish study.[641] The risk of diabetes in non-identical twins was 13% in this study. This indicates that more than half the explanation for the development of diabetes is inherited and the rest depends on environmental factors.

A low groundwater content of zinc, which may reflect long-term exposure through drinking water, was associated with the later development of diabetes in one study.[433] Another fact that points to an early influence is that an increased risk of diabetes has been correlated to the time and place of birth.[236] An explanation for the different ages at which diabetes occurs may be that the rate of decline in insulin production, once the disease process has started, is quite variable from one person with diabetes to another.

Sometimes children living close to each other develop diabetes at the same time which may indicate that viral infections trigger the onset (called clustering).[927] One theory is that diabetes and other autoimmune diseases are caused by so called slow viruses, i.e. viruses that can reside in the body for many years, while avoiding detection and destruction by the immune system.[139]

In countries with lower standards of hygiene, where there are more infections around, the immune system is activated to a greater degree at an earlier age. This has been shown to decrease the risk of diabetes in animal studies.[628] In Northern Ireland, the risk of diabetes was decreased in areas with a higher population

Environmental factors

Environmental factors that trigger the disease process may start early in life, many years before the onset of diabetes.[666] It is believed that the increase in the number of new cases of diabetes is caused by environmental factors as the genetic markers have not changed over time.

density, which may be explained by a higher frequency of infections early in life.[823] In a British study the risk of developing diabetes also decreased by 20% if the child had had an infection during the first year of life.[397] Preschool day care attendance (a marker for an increased number of infections) decreased the risk of developing diabetes in a European study.[337]

Infections in the newborn period seem to increase the risk of diabetes, probably due to an immature immune system.[337] Pinworm infections are very common in children but with an increased standard of hygiene, the number of infected children decreases. Pinworms can protect mice from developing diabetes, and it has been proposed that the decreased number of infected children could contribute to the rise in incidence of diabetes risk that is common in many countries.[385]

If a mother has German measles (rubella) during pregnancy, the risk of the child developing diabetes is around 20%.[666] If the mother has a particular type of virus infection (enterovirus) during pregnancy, the child will have an increased risk of developing diabetes later in life.[233,544]

There may be a link between coffee drinking during pregnancy and the baby's risk of developing diabetes. Finland has the highest incidence of type 1 diabetes in the world and the highest coffee consumption as well.[1049] Another risk factor is an increased height gain, seen mainly in boys, several years before the onset of diabetes.[105,861] Weight gain and obesity, on the other hand are not risk factors for developing type 1 diabetes.[105] However, children who developed diabetes later had a more rapid weight gain early in life (before 2-2.5 years of age) according to one study.[564] An increased birth weight is associated with an increased risk of being diagnosed with diabetes before 10 years of age.[239]

It is more common to develop diabetes during the winter months and during the years of puberty. While climate and puberty could cer-

Bring newspaper clippings to your healthcare team when you have read something interesting, such as diabetes research, so you can discuss it together. You may both learn something!

tainly not be described as the causes of diabetes, they may very well be triggering factors as both growth spurts and cold weather increase the body's insulin requirements.[666]

Environmental factors affect the individual, causing the risk of developing diabetes to change in families that have emigrated.[779] Asian children living in Great Britain and children from the Samoan Islands living in New Zealand have a higher risk of acquiring diabetes than children in their home countries.[350,1067] Most of the population of Iceland originate from Norway and have the same type of hereditary disposition.[59] Despite this, the risk of developing diabetes in Iceland is only between one third and half of what it is in Norway.[486] One might believe that this variation is caused by differences in environment and climate. However, Iceland and parts of Norway are located on the same latitude and have the same average temperature.

Cows' milk

The number of new cases of diabetes per year (incidence) in different countries coincides well with the consumption of cows' milk.[227]

Increased levels of antibodies against cows' milk have been found in children who have developed diabetes.[231,938] In the Samoan Islands where children do not drink milk at all, there is essentially no childhood diabetes. Sardinia has almost the same risk of diabetes as Finland. The consumption of milk is not as high as in Finland but on the other hand it is much higher than in the rest of Italy.[347]

Studies on rats have shown that whey protein from cows' milk increases the risk of developing diabetes.[327] When rats were fed with soya formula instead of milk they did not get diabetes. It seems that only certain types of cows (our ordinary milk cow) have the protein components which affect the risk of developing diabetes. Breast-feeding as such does not seem to affect the risk of diabetes,[926] but the time when the child is first introduced to cows' milk seems to be significant.[1067,1072] However, there are traces of cows' milk in breast milk and even children who have been fully breast-fed can have antibodies against cows' milk.[1014] This might explain why even children who have been breast-fed for a long time still can develop diabetes. In an Australian study, children who developed diabetes after the age of 9 had ingested more milk the year immediately before the onset of diabetes when compared with other children of the same age.[1067] A Finnish study showed a five-fold risk of diabetes in the siblings of children with type 1 diabetes with a high consumption (three or more glasses per day) of cows' milk during childhood.[1074] A large ongoing international research project (TRIGR) is trying to find out if a diet free from cows' milk for the first 6 months of life, in infants with a parent or sibling with diabetes, will decrease the risk of diabetes later in life. The first TRIGR results when the children were 6 years of age do not show any difference in the level of antibodies that may lead to diabetes.[624] The results regarding onset of clinical diabetes will be presented after 10 years, i.e. in 2017.

Since it is not yet proven that cows' milk causes diabetes, most authorities do not currently recommend any changes in infant diet.[692,942] How-

ever, The American Academy of Pediatrics recommends avoidance of cows' milk during the first year of life in families with a strong history of type 1 diabetes, particularly if a sibling has diabetes.[24]

Climate

There is a higher risk for diabetes in northern countries and onset is more common during the winter. A cold climate increases the need for insulin, which in turn increases the risk of triggering the onset of diabetes. Fewer hours of sunlight can lead to an increased risk of diabetes through higher turnover of calcium and reduced production of vitamin D.[232]

Insulin and cancer

In 2009, several studies were published suggesting a link between the insulin Lantus and cancer, especially breast cancer. This caused a lot of worry, but doctors did not recommend their patients to stop using Lantus as the evidence was not convincing. A later study with a follow-up of 8 years failed to show any association between breast cancer and various type of insu-

Some studies indicate an increased risk of acquiring diabetes if a child is not breast-fed at all or for only 3 months or less.[1067] Other studies indicate that it may not be the short period of breast-feeding as such, but the child's early introduction to cows' milk that increases the risk of diabetes. At the present time, however, there is insufficient data available to advise people in the general population against drinking milk during pregnancy or early infancy.[942]

lin, including both older human insulins (regular and NPH) or newer analogue insulins (NovoRapid, Humalog, Lantus).[421]

AGE

AGE stands for advanced glycation end products and represents an irreversible binding between glucose and different substances like protein, fat and nucleic acids (see illustration on page 356). Food chemists have known for a long time that a high concentration of glucose will cause protein-containing compounds to discolour and turn gluey. The proteins will become "sticky" with an increased tendency for cross-bindings. Ordinary caramel is an example of this reaction, between glucose and milk proteins or fat. The chemical structure of the compound will be altered. If this happens inside a cell, its function may change, contributing to the development of diabetes complications, for example in the eyes.[91] AGE products in food increase the level of AGE in the blood in people with diabetes [408] and may thus contribute to diabetes complications.[541] Foods of the fat group showed the highest amount of AGE content with a mean of 100 kU/g. High values were also observed for the meat and meat-substitute group (43 kU/g). The carbohydrate group contained the lowest values of AGEs (3.4 kU/g). High-temperature cooking (like broiling, grilling, frying, roasting) increases AGE levels.[408] Dietary restrictions of AGEs can significantly reduce inflammation of the blood vessels and arteriosclerosis.[541] Smokers have higher levels of AGE in the blood due to AGE-like products that are added in the processing of tobacco.[182]

In Italy [194] and Norway [85] increased levels of AGE have been measured in children and adolescents before the clinical signs of diabetes complications have started. In the Italian study, the levels decreased after 2 years of intensified diabetes treatment and lowered HbA_{1c}. An increased level of AGE has been found in the retina and in the blood vessels of eyes affected

with retinopathy.[440] An increased deposition of AGE in skin, tendons, connective tissue and joint capsules can lead to a reduced tissue flexibility. This can give rise to symptoms in the hands, hips or feet, and make problems such as foot ulcers more likely.[306]

The damage done by AGE may be counteracted at several levels by:

① Blocking the production of AGE.

② Removing AGE from the blood.

③ Breaking AGE, i.e. breaking the bond to glucose.

④ Blocking the AGE receptor on the cell surface.

Research is now being carried out to develop drugs that have these effects. So called aldose reductase inhibitors decrease AGE formation.[541] They have been shown to improve nerve conduction velocity and to improve gullet movements in people with diabetic nerve damage.[541] Promising experiments have been done with people who have kidney damage. Their blood was passed through a kind of dialysis apparatus containing a protein that binds AGE.[750] One study with pimagedine, an aminoguanide type of drug that breaks AGE bindings, showed a slowing down in the progression of both eye damage and kidney damage.[972]

Glucose may also bind to different proteins in the blood, forming AGE that can bind to receptors on the cell wall. This can cause damage to

---

Immunotherapy

In France and Canada, cell toxins (ciclosporin) have been used for experimental treatment at the onset of diabetes.

➠ Some people can do without insulin.

➠ BUT — the need for insulin always returns when the medication is stopped.

➠ These drugs carry a risk of serious side effects (such as damage to the kidneys).

the function, for example of cells in the blood vessel walls, the retina and the smooth muscle cells in our inner organs.[106] At present, it is difficult to measure AGE in blood and no routine method has yet been developed.

Blocking the immune process

At the onset of diabetes, 10-20% of the insulin-producing beta cells in the pancreas are still functioning (see illustration on page 375). If it were possible to stop the autoimmune attack on these cells it might also be possible to preserve a degree of insulin production for a long time, thereby prolonging the honeymoon phase (see page 221).

Immune treatment

Immune-modulation in the form of cell toxin drugs has been tried early in the course of diabetes. Ciclosporin (cyclosporin) is a compound that has been used successfully and has even made it possible to stop using insulin for some time.

In a study of 188 people with newly diagnosed diabetes, 25% managed without insulin after 1 year of ciclosporin treatment compared with 10% of those who had not received ciclosporin.[168] However, when ciclosporin treatment is stopped, insulin production always decreases again. Ciclosporin can have serious side effects including kidney damage and is therefore not used as a routine treatment at the present time. The International Study Group of Pediatric and Adolescent Diabetes (ISPAD) has stated that ciclosporin has no place in the treatment of diabetes in children except for clinical trials addressing questions that cannot be answered in adults.[550]

Light treatment

In a Swedish study, the white blood cells were treated with ultraviolet light (called photopheresis) at the onset of diabetes after the children and teenagers had received a special medication (psoralen).[696] The aim was to make it easier for the immune defence to recognize the cells that were causing damage to the beta cells. Patients needed less insulin but there was no difference in HbA_{1c} after 3 years.

Diazoxide

At the onset of diabetes, the immune defence attacks the body with T-cells (a special type of white blood cells) directed against a special protein (called GAD) in the beta cell. When insulin treatment is started, the beta cells do not need to work as hard and therefore the production of the protein that triggers the antibodies decreases as well, leading to a less intense immune attack. This is believed to be part of the mechanism behind the remission or honeymoon phase.

Diazoxide is a compound that puts a powerful block on the activity of the beta cells, thereby decreasing insulin production. The production of the GAD protein that is attacked by the T-cells decreases as well, therefore decreasing the damage to the beta cells. When treatment with diazoxide is stopped after a couple of months, the hope is that the immune defence will no longer react as strongly. A Swedish study of adults has shown a higher residual production of insulin up to 1.5 years after the onset of diabetes in a group with newly diagnosed diabetes that was treated with diazoxide for 3 months.[100] When the study was repeated in children, the same effect was seen after 1 year but after 2 years it was no longer so prominent.[811] However, diazoxide is not suitable for treating children with new-onset diabetes, as it is associated with a high rate of side effects.

Vitamins

Vitamin D

Vitamin D is essential for the calcium metabolism and bone strength. It needs sunlight to convert to the active vitamin and can be stored in your body. A meta-analysis (analysis of many studies) showed that vitamin D supplementation from birth gives some protection from developing type 1 diabetes later in life, especially if this was given up to 12 months of age.[1134] Eighteen months of treatment with a special form of vitamin D (calcitriol) at the onset of type 1 diabetes in adults did not affect the rate of beta cell destruction, i.e. how the body's production of insulin decreased (the honeymoon phase).[1087] There was also no difference in HbA_{1c} or insulin doses during the study.

The number of new cases in one year (called incidence) of type 1 diabetes in Finland, a northern country with long winters with low sunlight exposure, rose from 18 per 100,000 inhabitants in 1965 to 64 per 100,000 in 2005. During the same time period, the recommended daily supplementation of vitamin D was reduced in several steps from 4500 IU/day before 1964 to 400 IU/day in 1992, which may have contributed to the rise in incidence.[755]

Nicotinamide

Nicotinamide (also called vitamin PP) is a type of vitamin B that is thought to lessen the risk of developing diabetes by protecting the beta cells from attack by the immune system. In New Zealand, this substance has been given to the brothers and sisters of children who have recently been diagnosed with diabetes, for a period of couple of years, in order to prevent them from developing diabetes too.[329] It has also been given to whole classes of schoolchil-

The white blood cells are the "soldiers" in your body's army of defenders against bacteria and virus infections. When a person develops diabetes, the body thinks it is under attack, so the immune defence launches a "counter-attack" (by a special type of white blood cells called T-cells) on the insulin-producing beta cells. Immune-modulating treatment is used in research studies to influence this process.

dren, resulting in a 60-70% reduction in the risk of developing diabetes.[328]

In a large-scale study looking at parents and siblings of children with diabetes, nicotinamide was given to those with a high risk of developing diabetes indicated by a blood test (the ENDIT study). Unfortunately, the study failed to show any benefit from nicotinamide treatment.[386] The study was done with a so called double-blind technique, i.e. half of the participants were treated with nicotinamide and half with placebo (non-active tablets). Neither patients nor doctors knew who was given the nicotinamide and who the placebo. The same number of people developed diabetes in both groups.

It may seem strange that half of the people in a trial like this get medication that does not work, but this is the only scientific way to do the study to see if nicotinamide has a protective effect. It is common to conduct a double-blind study when the effect of a new drug is being tested.

Nicotinamide has been tried at the onset of diabetes to preserve the beta cell function. Only patients older than 15 years seem to be definitely affected, as their C-peptide levels did not decrease as much after 12 months as they did without the nicotinamide.[860] This indicates that residual insulin production was continued for a longer time. Nicotinamide has also been tried on a group of people who have been known to have diabetes for a period of 1-5 years, and who are still able to produce a certain amount of their own insulin.[1060] The group receiving nicotinamide had a better HbA_{1c} and a higher C-peptide level, which indicates an improved production of insulin by the beta cells.

Transplantation

Pancreas

Pancreas transplants have been performed for many years. Today most pancreas transplants are done at the same time as kidney transplants but pancreas-only transplants are also available. Kidney transplants are done on a routine basis. If a pancreas transplant works well, there is no need for further insulin injections. The individual can eat a normal diet and their HbA_{1c} will normalize.

Problems can arise after transplantation due to rejection of the transplant (the immune defence does not like "foreign" things in the body and tries to reject them). After 1 year, about 80% of the pancreas transplants function well when a kidney is transplanted at the same time.[1105] However, the results of transplanting a pancreas alone are not particularly satisfactory. The reason for this is that the rejection of a pancreas is less easy to discover than a rejection of the kidney where urine tests can be very informative. When a kidney transplant is threatened by rejection, medication can be started early, thereby protecting the pancreas transplant as well. Another problem is the possibility of tissue damage by digestive enzymes from the transplanted pancreas.

After a transplant, several drugs are needed, including cortisone which counteracts rejection. Cortisone increases the level of glucose in the blood, leading to a complicated situation. Drugs used to prevent rejection (called cytotoxic agents or immunosuppressive drugs) can

More than 10,000 articles on diabetes research are produced every year. Many small advances have resulted but so far no one has been able to solve the question of why a person develops diabetes or how to cure it. However, there is every reason to be optimistic about the future. There have been discussions about the way some of the body's own stem cells (developing stages of the beta cells) could be manipulated using gene technology to start producing insulin.

also result in numerous side effects, some of which are serious.

The beta cells in the new pancreas are susceptible to attack by the immune defence, causing diabetes to recur, especially if the transplant comes from an identical twin.[666] However, this is effectively prevented by the immune-modulating drugs that are given to prevent rejection reactions.[1008]

Even if all problems with rejection were solved, pancreas transplantation can never be the method of choice for routine treatment of diabetes because there will simply never be enough human pancreases available for transplantation.

Islet transplantation

The islets of Langerhans (see illustration on page 24) that contain insulin-producing beta cells can be extracted from a donor. These islets can be injected into the liver of the person with diabetes and will then produce a certain amount of insulin.

Previously, only 12% of patients receiving new islets have been able to manage without insulin for more than a week at a time.[1105] A breakthrough was published in 2000 from Edmonton in Canada where a cortisone-free immunosuppression programme was used (although cortisone increases blood glucose it has always been a necessary part of the immunosuppression programme).[963] A five-year follow-up of 47 people who received islets from one to three donors, and completed the transplantation process showed that they were able to manage without insulin for an average of 15 months. After 5 years, 80% still had some degree of insulin production (measured by C-peptide production) but only 10% were insulin free.[916] This "Edmonton Protocol" has been mirrored in Canada, the US and Europe, with 44% remaining insulin independent after 1 year, but only 14% after 2 years.[964]

One problem with islet transplants is that T-cells and rejection reactions can strike these islets as well as complete transplanted organs. Methods where the islets are put into small tubes or sealed within a plastic film have been tried to prevent the antibodies from attacking the islets.[990] Two patients receiving micro-encapsulated human islet cells still had insulin production in the islets after 6 months and 1 year without any immunosuppression.[165]

No islet transplantations have yet been performed on children. However, the cortisone-free immunosuppression minimizes negative effects on growth. With improved methods, islet cells from one donor may be enough for two or three children and perhaps a parent could donate part of his or her pancreatic islets to their child. With micro-encapsulation and/or safer drugs for immunosuppression, this may not be too far into the future.[467]

Engineered cells

Experiments have been conducted where so called stem cells are manipulated genetically to produce insulin.[780] The thought is very appealing because if some of your own cells were be able to produce insulin there would be no rejection problems.

Engineered rat muscle cells have been able to secrete insulin at a constant level, independent of the blood glucose level.[422] This would be an effective substitute for the night time and basal insulins used today and could produce a very stable level of insulin in the bloodstream. Cells from the pituitary gland have been engineered to recognize different levels of glucose and to produce insulin at sufficient levels to cure diabetes in mice.[345] In contrast to transplanted islet cells, these pituitary cells were resistant to autoimmune attack. Stem-like cells were collected from human womb tissue from donors in another study.[667] During two weeks, the cells were exposed to different mediums, to develop them, and they were then transplanted into diabetic mice. Levels of insulin and blood glucose were restored to normal values quickly after the transplantation.

Other ways of administering insulin

Nasal spray

Insulin given as nasal spray is absorbed more quickly through the lining of the nose than when injected subcutaneously. Many studies have been performed on humans but it is still unclear whether this can become a clinical reality.[503] Problems may arise with the insulin absorption in people who have hay fever or other allergies, or who are suffering from a cold. Also, we do not yet know how insulin might affect the nose lining in the long run. Twenty times more insulin was needed for administration via the nose than for an injection, according to one study.[503] However, 7 of the 31 participants interrupted the study prematurely due to problems with high or low blood glucose levels. HbA_{1c} increased slightly in this study, from 62 to 65 mmol/mol (7.8 to 8.1%).

Inhalation of insulin

Experiments with administering insulin as an aerosol spray (in the same way as people with asthma take their drugs) has been tried successfully in adults and children from the age of 12 years, giving the same HbA_{1c} as when using short-acting insulin for premeal injections.[979] However, there were more episodes of severe hypoglycaemia and an increased level of insulin antibodies in the inhaled insulin group. Insulin is absorbed rapidly through the thin lung lining. The onset of action of a dose of inhaled insulin is at least as quick as for Humalog, but the effect lasts for a longer time, more like that of short-acting regular insulin.[876] There may be some practical limitations to this method: in people with asthma, the absorption from inhaled insulin is decreased [491] while in smokers it is enhanced.[505] However, the long-term effects on the lungs of inhaling insulin will not be known for many years and the method is not approved for use in children and adolescents. Inhaled insulin was introduced for adult use in 2006 but has now been withdrawn from the market.

Tablets

The problem with insulin in tablet form is that it is degraded by the acid in the stomach. This can be solved by putting a capsule around the insulin tablets in order to release insulin only after the tablets reach the intestines.[534] Insulin can then be absorbed into the blood, but this is a slow process with a risk of an irregular insulin effect. One advantage is that insulin which is absorbed into the blood from the intestines, passes the liver before it enters the general blood circulation in the same way as insulin that is produced in a healthy pancreas. Insulin in tablets is extremely long-acting and one single dose can work for up to 1 week. This may cause difficulties in working out appropriate doses.

Insulin as suppositories

Insulin is absorbed from the rectum when administered as suppositories. Due to poor absorption, more than 10 times the ordinary dose is needed to obtain the appropriate blood glucose-lowering effect.[502]

Chemical alteration of the insulin molecule

Changing the composition of the insulin molecule can result in both more short-acting and more long-acting insulin. Examples of this are the rapid-acting insulin analogues, NovoRapid, Humalog and Apidra, which have a much quicker effect than regular short-acting insulin (see page 75). Another emerging method to quicken the action is to take away the zinc from the insulin preparation and change the electrical surface charge of the insulin molecule to prevent hexamer (see page 75) formation (VIAject).[993]

There is a great need for better night time and basal insulins with a more even action profile.[908] This has been achieved by replacing some of the amino acids in the insulin molecule as in insulin glargine (Lantus, see page 77). Insulin has also been made more long-acting by binding it to a protein in the bloodstream (albumin). Insulin is released slowly to maintain a steady level between meals and throughout the night. This insulin analogue is called detemir (Levemir, see page 77). Insulin degludec (Tresiba) is an even more long-acting analogue with an effect lasting for up to 42 hours in children and adolescents.[93] The prolonged effect is produced by adding an acid that causes the formation of multi-hexamers in subcutaneous tissue.

Insulin additives

The onset of insulin action of the rapid-acting analogues is not quick enough when taken just before a meal. An even more rapid onset is needed for the artificial pancreas projects (see page 373). Adding hyaluronidase [761] and EDTA [838] has given the insulin an even quicker effect. Warming the skin can also cause the insulin to have a more rapid effect, both with injections [648] and with a pump.[877]

Alternative ways of administering insulin

⇒	Nasal spray	Quick effect, good for pre-meal injections. However, unlikely to become clinical reality.
⇒	Oral insulin (tablets)	Slow effect, good for basal insulin.
⇒	Suppositories	Quick effect but large doses are needed.
⇒	Aerosol for inhalation	Quick effect but long-term side effects unknown.
⇒	Chemically bound insulin	Released only at high blood glucose levels. Technically difficult.
⇒	Altered insulin structure	Quicker or slower action.
⇒	C-peptide (see page 373)	Produced in the human pancreas but not included in today's insulin.

Psychology

The onset of diabetes

When someone develops a long-term illness, the situation for the whole family is always a difficult one. Adjusting to a new life poses challenges and takes time. Most people go through the same stages when faced with crisis. Professor Johnny Ludvigsson describes the different phases of crisis:[690]

Shock phase

During the shock phase, it is difficult to think clearly. Thoughts will whirl around in your head. Everything seems unreal. This cannot really be happening, it can't be true. Maybe it will all turn out to have been a dream. It is common to experience a sense of walking around in a kind of haze. You cannot take in information. You see your doctor, you watch the doctor's body language and see just how serious the situation is. You listen out for hope, consolation, belief in the future, but shut out all details of the disease; its likely progression and treatment, all the accompanying practicalities. You want to ask questions but find it difficult to keep your thoughts focused, or see a way forward. The doctor should listen, you think, the nurse should listen, everybody should LISTEN to your inner thoughts of what is most important right now.

"You cannot stop the birds of sorrow from flying over your head — but you can stop them from building a nest there."

Chinese saying

Reaction phase

A reaction of sorrow with tears, sleeplessness, aggression and bitterness will also take time. Consolation is important but should be honest, not hearty and unrealistic. "You need not feel sad" seems false and "You should not be sad" feels like a punch in the face. Why shouldn't one feel sad? Everybody has the right to be sad in this situation. It is only natural to feel sorrow, bitterness and disappointment. You grieve for the healthy person you used to be, and life seems unfair. It is always unfair when someone is stricken by a severe disease, but the sorrow will eventually fade away. You will feel better. You have had no part in developing the disease, it is not your fault. We must have the strength to listen, to face up to reality, to allow and acknowledge grief and fear.

The different phases of crisis

① Shock phase.
② Reaction phase.
③ Repair phase.
④ Reorientation phase.

Repair phase

After some time, you will enter the repair phase. Somebody must be able to do something about this disease. Now you need knowledge. What do you do if your blood glucose level falls too low? How do you give yourself these dreaded injections? You won't be able to relax or breathe easily again until you have got to grips with this. Now the worst part is over. You can learn more about insulin, testing, diet and hypoglycaemia. Systematically, a little bit at a time, you can absorb facts and start to rebuild your life.

Reorientation phase

It takes a long time before a crisis moves on to the reorientation phase, and a different but acceptable lifestyle is established — one where diabetes is an important part but by no means everything. At times, those around you will have difficulties in understanding that it takes time to go through the different phases of a cri-

When the first baby is born into a family, some parents feel as if there is an unexploded bomb in their midst. They never know when the baby will start crying, need their nappy changing, or get hungry. As time goes by, the parents relax, learn what to do, and become more secure in their new role. There is a parallel situation when parents first discover their child has diabetes. They thought they knew what to expect; now they find they know nothing at all. What will happen when the child becomes hypoglycaemic? What can they do as a family? But in the same way as adjusting to a new baby, parents will soon learn to accommodate their child again in this new situation.

sis, but this is inevitable when someone in a family develops diabetes. Of course it is unfair; the treatment can be difficult, life has changed, you might be afraid of dying or being different from others. But there will still be Saturday afternoons, song, laughter, dancing, good food, school or work, picnics, holidays and friends. Life will never be the same again but it can still be exciting and enjoyable even if some of the rules have changed.

There are people who come to a standstill in their grief and are unable to move on. Such people will need professional help. Continuing denial inhibits people from absorbing knowledge and adjusting life to accommodate diabetes.

Regardless of whether a crisis is caused by the death of someone near and dear, a divorce, developing diabetes or something else, there will always remain a memory of what happened, much like a scar. But when you have worked yourself through the crisis and accepted what has happened, it will be like looking at a wound that has completely healed: you can see the scar but most of the time you are unaware of its existence.

"You cannot teach a person anything — just help him or her to find it within themselves."

Galileo Galilei 1564-1642

Diabetes rules or family rules?

Diabetes can be a "thorn in the side" in different ways depending in part on the age of the person concerned. If, as a parent, you are discussing what the "rules" are at home, it is important to consider what is actually provoked by your son or daughter having diabetes, and what is a part of a normal upbringing. If you are always referring to diabetes when it comes to rules and prohibitions, the young person will hate the very thought of diabetes since it puts an end to so many nice things. However, if you think about it, most rules and methods of upbringing are influenced by other factors and

We must cooperate on equal terms when you come to see us at the diabetes clinic. If a visit feels like "a trip to the headteacher's office" something has gone badly wrong.

hold true just as much for a child with diabetes as for his or her brothers, sisters or friends without diabetes.

Many children are only allowed sweets on special occasions, such as at weekends. Most children, on the other hand, would prefer to have sweets every day if only it were allowed. This type of discussion goes on in families everywhere. However, if a child has diabetes it is very convenient just to refer to the effect on the blood glucose level when saying "No" to sweets. I often argue that it is very important to return to normal rules between children and parents as soon as possible and to refer to diabetes as little as possible when it comes to child upbringing and setting limits. In the long run it is important to be on as friendly terms as possible with your diabetes. If many rules and prohibitions are put down to diabetes, it will have the opposite effect and cause the young person to start hating the disease.

It is important, therefore, to explain to younger children that most rules or limitations relating to food or treats are not caused by their diabetes, but would have applied anyway. The child will otherwise associate all prohibitions with diabetes.

Remember that there were both rules and limitations in the child's life even before diabetes entered the scene. Diabetes brings with it many restrictions, resulting in a lot of "not this and not that's". Try instead to encourage your child to do the things he or she still can — this will still include most aspects of everyday life. Give encouragement and praise. The praise is well-deserved, as a child with diabetes has to do many things on a daily basis that most adults would not be very keen to do. Praise the child for doing the necessary blood tests, and give due credit for giving injections. Encourage the child when he or she chooses to eat in a way appropriate for diabetes, show your appreciation when the child does not eat sweets behind your back. (How many parents have not taken out their own sweets from the cupboard when the children have gone to bed?) Praise and encouragement help everything to run so much more smoothly.

Even as a parent or an adult with diabetes, you will naturally need encouragement, praise and "positive reinforcement" when you visit the diabetes clinic. If it feels like "being called in to see the headteacher" something is wrong. You don't come to pass or fail a test. It is our job to cooperate and help you, in the best way possi-

"We learn by our own mistakes", as the saying goes. But does one always have to invent the wheel again? You can learn a lot by discussing with other parents or friends who have diabetes. They can give you tips about day-to-day practicalities that the staff at the diabetes clinic are less familiar with, since most of us don't live with diabetes at home.

ble, to cope with diabetes as part of your family life.

How far would a football team advance without encouragement and praise? Any person, be they child or adult, who has diabetes needs a coach to motivate them, assess their abilities and potential, and adjust their diabetes training on a continuous basis. Let the young person know that you recognize just how difficult things are — often it is much more difficult for children or teenagers to manage life with diabetes well than it would be for their parents to give up smoking, for example. On the other hand, it is important not to embarrass the young person with an overload of praise and encouragement at times when everything is going smoothly. It is far too easy to be overprotective of children with diabetes. Sympathy is fine but pity is less helpful.

Making friends with your diabetes

Your diabetes will be with you 24 hours a day. So it is important that you find a way to make friends with it, or at least to avoid seeing it as an enemy. If you allow yourself to hate the illness, it will be difficult to get on with your life without being negatively affected by it. There are three common ways in which people view their diabetes:

It may be a good idea to be apprenticed to someone who has had diabetes for many years and has had time to learn how to live with it in a positive way.

Yin and yang are conceptions in the Chinese philosophy for two principles that are in balance and harmony. Try to see your diabetes as a part of yourself which can melt into balance and harmony with the rest of your personality. Your attitude is a very important part of diabetes treatment. Those who hate their illness will soon begin fighting against it.

① Ignoring it, eating what they like and only taking enough insulin to avoid feeling bad at that moment.

Many teenagers will go through this phase for a shorter or longer period of time, and some will never be able to leave it because they hate their illness. If you have this attitude when you enter adulthood, there is a risk that you will never be able to change it. Try instead to see the end of the teenage years as an opportunity when you dare to take action, and can do something about your lifestyle and your diabetes.

② Becoming absorbed and obsessed by diabetes, living only to take care of the illness as effectively as possible.

"Regulating illness" or "regulopathy" is the term used when you give up your ordinary life and your goals for the future.[359] Initially, both parents and caregivers at the clinic are under the impression that everything is going along very well. However, if the efforts to obtain a perfect glucose level prevent the young person from enjoying social activities, parties, being with friends or staying overnight with friends or at camps, things have gone too far. If this applies to you, it is high time to give yourself a break and allow yourself to start living life again.

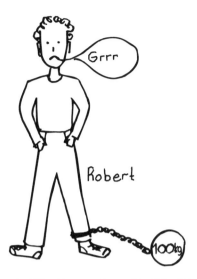

One may feel like this many times. It is difficult to live with diabetes, often very difficult. But if you hate your diabetes it will be difficult to make friends with it... It is important not to let diabetes take control. Decide instead what kind of life you want to live, and your diabetes team will help you to adjust your treatment according to your wishes.

If your diabetes is too strictly regulated, you are likely to end up having too many hypoglycaemic episodes or hypoglycaemia unawareness (see page 52), which is far from healthy.

③ Making diabetes a natural part of everyday life.

This is easier said than done, as everyone knows who has tried. But it is possible to accept your illness without letting it take control of your life completely. If taking insulin becomes like brushing your teeth, something you do daily without really thinking about it but that you would absolutely not want to be without, then you have come a long way.

How do you go about making diabetes a part of your daily life? Learn from your friends, observe others with diabetes and you will probably find someone who has an attitude worth learning from. Just as young people used to have a period of apprenticeship when learning a profession, so you now may need to "be apprenticed" to someone who manages their diabetes in a good way.

Diabetes affects the whole family

Different people will feel differently about the relative difficulty of various aspects of diabetes. For a small child, the injections are often the hardest part. Older children and teenagers often find the need to be punctual, and explaining diabetes to others more bothersome. Adults often find food issues and weight control to be the most difficult thing.

TIGER

Teaching something to someone is not the same as the other person learning it...

"Treatment of insulin-dependent diabetes — art or science?" was the title of a lecture by the British physician, Robert Tattersall, from Nottingham.[1024] He described what happens in a family when a child develops diabetes:

— A good recipe for putting the "thumb-screws" on someone is to let a family member, preferably a child, develop a chronic disease.

— The disease should have an unclear cause but with a hereditary component so that family members are forced to check the family tree to find a "scapegoat", Robert Tattersall continues. The treatment should be an important part of the disease, time consuming and preferably painful.

— To put further pressure on the family, the management of the disease should affect the life of all other family members. Self-control and self-management should be important components.

— The future outlook completes the picture. Terrible results of an unwise lifestyle can be indicated perhaps by sitting the family members in a waiting room together with other sufferers from the same disease who are showing obvious and drastic consequences such as amputations. Better still, if health professionals are uncertain about treatment goals and regimes, they will give contradictory information which of course will make the situation even worse. Don't forget, says Professor Tattersall, that a family where someone has developed diabetes will be in exactly this situation.

Being a relative or friend of someone with diabetes

People close to you only want what is best for you but it may not always look like this. It is important to know what kind of help individuals with diabetes want, and what they can manage on their own. At the same time a child, a teenager or a partner must understand how

Diabetes is an invisible handicap, and can't be seen from the outside. You may sometimes feel better if nobody knows. However, both you and your friends will find it easier in the long run if you let everyone know. If, for instance, you become hypoglycaemic, everyone will understand what is going on and what to do if you have informed them beforehand. Many people have described how embarrassing and troublesome they found it, having to explain their diabetes for the first time when they became hypoglycaemic and needed help.

much those closest to them need to know about their everyday life, for them to feel secure and confident.

It can be easy for parents to become overprotective, and the young person can then react by wanting to manage too much by themselves, or rebel by, for example, eating too many sweets. Try to be as open as possible about each others' needs in the family. A "family council", where you put aside time to sit down together, can be an ideal forum to discuss how to come to agreement on different subjects within the family.

Friends need to know how they can help, otherwise they may turn into "sweets policemen" who, with the best of intentions, will go on about this or that being unhealthy to eat. It becomes a balance between saying: "I don't care about your diabetes, it is your problem" and "Are you really going to eat that bag of sweets?" It is a good idea to talk things over and decide upon "how much or how little" help and support you want from those close to you.

Family and friends must also be sufficiently knowledgeable about diabetes if they are to offer any help or understanding. Treatment of hypoglycaemia is an obvious example, and it would be useful if they could also give an injection of glucagon. The more your friends know, the more help you will be able to receive from them. Try to explain what you are doing and why. Explain how insulin works, how exercise works, why sometimes you can eat sugar and sometimes you can't.

Telling your friends

Many people do not want to talk about their diabetes since it is not visible from the outside. At the same time it is evident that you have not accepted your diabetes if you do not want to tell your friends. It is important your friends understand why you might be feeling unwell, and what they can do about it. It is best to tell everybody as soon as possible after you have been diagnosed. Then it is over with and things will not feel so strange any more. It is much worse to walk around wondering to yourself what or how much any individual knows.

My earliest memory of diabetes is when I was 8 years old. The girl living next door was my age and had diabetes. The only thing I knew about

You may drift away from your friends if they do not understand why you must do certain things at particular times. Try to make diabetes a natural part of your life by telling friends at school or work about it. It is important that they know what to do if you need help, for example if you have a difficult hypoglycaemic episode.

it was that she was not allowed to eat sugar. But I also observed sugar lumps in her pocket that she would eat from time to time. It was very difficult for me to understand this and, as nobody explained to me why she did it, I thought she was cheating.

How do you change your lifestyle?

Many people ask themselves this question. It is not easy to persuade someone that they must change their habits to feel better. Persuasion may not even be the best way of getting a person to do what is best for his or her health. And what is really "best", from the person's own perspective?

Elisabeth Arborelius, Ph.D. in Psychology, has studied how to change people's life habits.[171]

— It is all about concentrating the information on behaviour instead of knowledge. It is not always true that knowledge will affect attitudes which in turn will affect behaviour. We assume that human beings are rational but they are not, she claims. Something that is disadvantageous to a person's health, from an objective point of view, will not necessarily be experienced that way by the person concerned.

— I once heard a nurse say: "I am not a fanatic, but I see no reasons why people should smoke!" Of course she was right if she disregarded the patient's point of view. If the objective is to change behaviour, the person with diabetes must have the opportunity to explain the advantages and disadvantages he or she will experience on account of a change of habits.

— We have come to believe that the balance between an individual's experienced advantages and disadvantages is very important in whether or not that person will change his or her behaviour. If the disadvantages seem to outweigh the advantages, it will not help that there is a threat of worsening health. The person with diabetes will not change his or her lifestyle habits anyway.

Diabetes at different developmental stages

The psychological effect of diabetes in the family will be different at different ages and depends very much on the child's development and basic needs for that age. Naturally, parents will often feel unsure about how to handle specific situations, and may on occasion need expert help to address particular issues. Sometimes the help of a child psychologist will be appropriate. It is a good idea to let all children and adolescents see the psychologist at least once during the early months after diagnosis. That way, if parents feel psychological help is necessary at a later date, the initial contact will already have been made.

Marianne Helgesson who is a psychologist at the Department of Paediatrics in Linköping, Sweden, lectures on psychology and diabetes in individuals at different ages. She teaches the following: [671]

— It is not always easy to accommodate three people in a marriage. The first crack between spouses often appears when the first child is born. Discussions and disputes begin to focus on how to organize time, something that may not have been an issue before.

— It will become a question of balance as to how much time and care one should devote to the child, to one's partner and to oneself. The parents must come to an agreement on how work at home should be divided, and whether one of them or both will be able to pursue a career.

— Child raising is for the most part a repetition of how you were brought up yourself, since this is the only model you are familiar with. But usually there are two parents, both with their own upbringing behind them. Conflicts are inevitable and the result will be a combination of both parents' previous experiences.

— However, if the child has a chronic illness, there is usually a lack of role models and this will make parents feel insecure. The balance between dependency and responsibility is difficult to establish and the question arises as to how much to help the child without being over-protective.

Infants (0-1.5 years)

This period is characterized by a so called symbiosis, at first between mother and child. Later on the father is also included. During this time it is very important that the parent subordinates his or her own needs in favour of the child's needs. The child, after all, is not in any position to give priority to the parent's needs. When the child is able to move around unaided, after about 1 year of age, he or she will begin to explore the world.

Risks from diabetes

Diabetes at this age will inevitably bring stress into the family. If parents find it difficult to handle this without feeling tense and uncertain towards the child, they will also find it difficult to communicate security and confidence to the child. Security and confidence have a close relationship with the issue of food and diabetes. Young children do not understand why they should eat if they are not hungry and vice versa, so there is considerable risk of feeding problems at this age. Multiple injections or pump therapy can help to address such problems.

Children need to feel their parents display trust and confidence in various situations, but clearly this may be difficult when a child has diabetes. Over-protectiveness may lead to a child anxiously staying by the parent's side instead of looking outwards to the world beyond. Young children cannot understand injections and blood testing, or the pain, anger and anxiety that go with them. We cannot explain to them why they must be hurt in this way. Usually, the best approach is to get the injection out of the way as quickly as possible, and then comfort the child. Injection aids may be very helpful for this age group (see page 137).

Toddlers (1.5-3 years)

Toddlers start to explore the world more actively. Around the age of 2, the child will often take a step "backwards", becoming more attached to the mother again. This is quite normal and is not due to inappropriate parental attitudes towards the child.

The "obstinate age" (the age of practising one's own free will) begins between 2 and 3 years of age. Children will first test the parents' and then their own ability to set limits. All children will show quite a lot of anger and frustration during this time. They must experience their own limitations which can be unpleasant. It is important that parents engage in such "battles of will" as it is through these that children learn how to stand up for something, to compromise and to give in.

Risks from diabetes

It can be difficult to know whether or not a child's bad temper is caused by a low or high blood glucose level. Should the child be given something to eat every time he or she is angry? It may be difficult to take a blood test every time. A child with diabetes will have more limitations than other children due to injections, mealtimes and monitoring. There is always a

tendency with a chronic illness that parents will want to compensate for the restrictions caused by the illness by letting the child decide about everything else. In doing this the parent shows pity for the child and becomes less effective in setting limits in other areas. The child then becomes insecure and disorderly, continuously testing the limits in order to provoke a parental reaction. However, if the parents do not have enough strength to deal with such aggressiveness the child may turn inwards, becoming passive and insecure, with a low feeling of self-confidence. Parents, too, need understanding, as this period may be very challenging. But they also need encouragement because a child with diabetes needs a normal upbringing just as much as any other child.

A fear of strange environments (such as the hospital) can be even greater than the fear of injections. Some children of this age will become very anxious if they feel they are being restrained. Try to give injections and take blood tests in as secure an environment as possible.

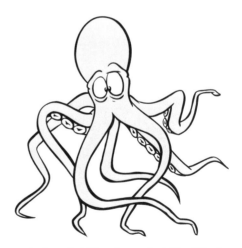

Any parent of small children knows that it is difficult enough to find time for everything. But when there is diabetes to cope with as well, parents can feel they need as many arms as an octopus in order to cope with blood glucose monitoring, injections, meal planning and all the other adjustments of daily life that have to be made.

Preschool children (3-6 years)

The child in this age group begins to understand more about the outside world and will be conscious of the fact that his or her body can experience both desire and pain. The child will role play and have a very rich imaginative life.

During this period the differentiation of sex roles takes place. The child wants to imitate the parent of the same sex and falls in love, often wanting to marry the parent of the opposite sex. A child of 4-5 years will be "the king of the universe", knowing and being able to do everything, especially knowing what he or she wants and does not want. Children feel powerful when they discover how to control others. A 6-year-old is usually more willing to fit in with what the parent wants.

Plant the tree of knowledge early within children. Children who have grown up with diabetes often find it easier to manage during puberty compared with those developing diabetes in prepubertal or pubertal years. As children grow up, they will be trained by their parents to take responsibility for themselves. The goal should be that they will be able to take responsibility for important aspects of their diabetes before entering puberty.

Children begin to develop a conscience, thinking about crime and punishment in a "primitive way" in terms of "an eye for an eye and a tooth for a tooth". They become aware of the boundaries of the body. Plasters have a magic ability to restore and heal. See also "Children and blood glucose tests" on page 106.

Risks from diabetes

Children in this age group may believe they have developed diabetes as a punishment for doing something wrong, or that a blood glucose test is a punishment. This must be brought up and into the open with the child even if he or she does not ask about it. After all, even adults ask themselves "What have I done to deserve this?" when something unpleasant or unfortunate occurs. We all try to find a logical connection between things that have happened.

Children can be limited in the amount of freedom they have on account of the parents' fear of hypoglycaemia. It may be difficult to give insulin and take tests when children refuse to cooperate. They will have definite views on what they do and don't want to eat. It may be very difficult to know in advance how much of the meal a child will eat. Try letting him or her decide about some other details of daily life instead. Multiple injections or an insulin pump give children more freedom over what they eat and how much.

Don't tell a child in this age group too far in advance about injections, testing or other unpleasant things. They can easily build this up to unrealistic proportions in their imagination.

In a family where the children are of different sexes, diabetes may be linked to gender in the child's mind. For example, a girl might believe it would be better to be a boy since her brother does not have diabetes (or vice versa).

"Consider what the restrictions may cost in terms of development before you say no ..."
Marianne Helgesson, child psychologist

Primary school children

Starting school is stressful for all children, and many will find it difficult to adjust in the beginning. Primary school children are occupied with understanding and exploring the world. They like to take things apart and understand how everything works. They will also be interested in understanding how their diabetes works. Friends become increasingly important and it is important to do the same sort of things as they do. Children in this age group like to keep track of how long an activity takes, such as running an errand. They are interested when they know something is going to happen but really cannot yet understand how long it will take. They expand their relationships from parents to other adults, including teachers and other caregivers at school. During the primary school years, children learn how to control their impulses, and to behave within acceptable limits and guidelines.[41]

Stealing sweets from the cupboard behind the parent's back is not uncommon behaviour for preschool children. It is important to avoid over dramatizing this — even children who do not have diabetes will do it. I think it is important that the result is not a total ban on sweets. It is often more practical to give some extra sweets once in a while, perhaps with the afternoon snack for 1-2 weeks, and give some extra insulin as well (see page 264). Explain that you are making an exception and that you expect the child to be able to choose more wisely about sweet-eating as he or she grows older. The child will usually get over the craving for sweets after a while.

Risks from diabetes

The fear of the unknown is still there even if the child seems interested in exploring. It is important to adapt the information to the age of the child. "Normalize", i.e. tell the child that it is quite normal and fully understandable ("Other children would feel the same way") to feel the

Being a good parent for a toddler is not the same as being a good parent for a teenager. The important, but difficult issue is to adjust the demands to the child's age in order to promote maturity. Children of all ages need lots of love, but it must be adapted to the age of the child. "Toddler love" to a teenager is experienced as over-protection and prevents liberation.

way he or she does in different situations, such as taking an injection or a blood test. Keeping track of time will often help, for instance when administering an injection. Food at school does not taste the same as it does at home, and sometimes the child will not eat at all. It is important to find someone at school who is able and willing to help the child take insulin at lunchtime. At first you may feel very insecure — what happens if my child becomes hypoglycaemic at school? Try to ensure that one parent is always contactable by telephone and can come to school if necessary, especially early on. It is important that school teachers know how to deal with hypoglycaemia. They will often take the child's illness more seriously after seeing a hypoglycaemic episode.

Intermediate-level children

This part of life is referred to as the latency phase in psychological terms. Children are usually very receptive towards all types of education, including diabetes. They want to expand their views but at the same time they have learned to stay within the limits their parents have set. During this time a social role develops: "Can I join in?", "Will I be accepted?" There is also competition with peers as to "who is the greatest, cleverest and most beautiful". Peers become increasingly important. Children will benefit from meeting others with diabetes in the same age group with whom they can identify, for instance at a diabetes education camp or holiday. Encouragement is important at this age as children need confirmation that they have done things correctly.

Risks from diabetes

All children wonder about their role in life during this period. At the age of 9 or 10, a child

with a chronic disease will usually start to reflect upon and react to their illness in a new way. "Why did this happen to me?" is a common question. There will often be a time when the child experiences everything that has to do with diabetes as difficult and strenuous. For the first time the child understands that having diabetes means having it for the rest of his or her life. It will take some time to accept this.

During this time it is important to talk openly and often to the child about what diabetes entails, as this will help him or her to move towards acceptance. Show that you as a parent also feel concerned, and confirm that life with diabetes is both difficult and unfair. Children usually pass through this phase after a while but some may, on occasion, need help from a psychologist or counsellor.

As children in this age group are very receptive to learning without defying their parents' authority, it is important to make diabetes management a natural part of daily life during the years leading up to puberty. Children who are confident about managing their diabetes before the onset of puberty will be less likely to feel their diabetes prevents their growth and independence.

When should children take over responsibility for diabetes control?

During the early school years, all children expand their skills across a wide range of areas: athletic, artistic, academic and self-control. As a natural part of this generalized increased ability in many fields, children will also gradually increase their participation in, and responsibility for, various diabetes-related tasks. However, current research indicates that parents should continue to take part in diabetes tasks throughout these years.[41] It is helpful if the expectation for continued parental involvement throughout the primary school years and into adolescence is introduced to children and families by the diabetes team as early as possible.[41] Don't hand over responsibility too early!

Puberty

During puberty, the teenager should begin the development of an adult identity, having independence and an equal standing with other adults. This increasing independence is fragile, which is why teenagers need to defend their integrity so strongly.

In a way, earlier stages of development are repeated. Teenagers often vacillate between behaving like children and being grown up. It is important to realize that they have the chance to "revisit" areas that have not been completed during earlier phases of development. Many parents look upon the teenage period with horror, but if you try instead to see puberty as a "final run through" of the childhood and adolescent years before embarking upon adulthood, your view may be more positive.

Friends are very important, and as it is only natural to want to be able to do the same things as everyone else. Teenagers like to go out in the evening to have a hamburger or pizza with their friends, instead of staying at home to eat the usual evening meal. It is important that young people are given both the freedom and responsibility to experiment with insulin doses on such occasions. Teenagers are very interested in their own body, especially during early adolescence, and are well aware just who that body belongs to. They want to be well informed about the way diabetes affects their body. At the same time they are often shy about exposing their body and, in this sense, are not at all as open-minded as might be expected.

We encourage older teenagers to come to some of the visits without their mother or father. An alternative is to let the parent enter the room at the end of the consultation and then only raise issues that the teenager has consented to. It is important for teenagers to understand that the professional confidentiality also applies to parents. If a young person wants to raise personal issues, he or she should be able to do so without fear of the information being passed on.

Teenagers often bring a buddy or a boyfriend/girlfriend to the visits. They appreciate someone's support but feel too old to bring their mother or father. It may be a difficult for parents to know just how much involvement with the teenager's diabetes is appropriate. It can be difficult to remain sufficiently well informed as you are less and less involved with your child's diabetes and clinic visits. Most teenagers prefer to manage without their parents' input but at the same time want them to be informed. One 18-year-old girl said: "Of course I want them to know how my diabetes is managed — who else can jump in and help me if I fail?"

Research shows that teenagers need their parents on board,[42] although they may feel like they are "nagging". Try to explain to the teenager that he or she still needs a "coach" for their diabetes, in the same way as for any sporting activity. Young people need to do the job themselves but, as in most sports, the good results come only with a good relationship with, and good tutoring by a coach. Of course, life in other areas must go on as usual, with increasing independence. But many parents find it difficult to allow young people to take full control of their diabetes.

Risks from diabetes

The teenage years are a difficult period in which to develop diabetes. Teenagers are not mature enough to take sole responsibility for their diabetes but find it hard to let their parents do it. Children who are younger at the onset of diabetes find it easier for the parents to take full control, and then gradually let go as the child matures. Children who develop diabetes early in life are likely therefore to have better diabetes control and adherence to the treatment during the years of puberty than those developing it in the early teens.[554]

Learning to stand on their own two feet will be more difficult for a teenager with diabetes. They feel that they will never quite become an adult and will never have complete control over their own body. Just when it is time to cut the umbilical cord, it is securely tied again. In addition, their body will be inspected on regular visits to the clinic.

"Teenagers are impossible to raise, but it doesn't matter as long as parents do not stop trying."

Ackerman

Of course, teenagers with diabetes will be concerned about the future. They will worry about what sort of job they can do, how to find a partner, whether they will be able to have children, as well as about complications of diabetes and so on. It is quite natural to become depressed about these things if you look towards the future in a negative way. It is not uncommon to have existential thoughts in general, but it is important to be on the lookout for suicidal thoughts as well.

At the same time, teenagers will often not think beyond the next few days. The risk of having

Friends are very important in the teenage years. When you start seeing your diabetes healthcare team without your parents it is a good idea to bring a buddy or girl/boyfriend instead.

eye damage or renal complications at the age of 40 if their blood glucose level continues to be high, matters less: "Then I will be so old that it will not matter anyway". But it may help to explain like this: When you are 25 or 30, and complications begin showing up, we don't want you to say: "Why didn't you stop me or do something more when I was not taking care of myself?"

Most teenagers want to take injections in an adult way, that is to say without showing emotions. They hate it if this can't be managed and they are forced to be "a baby" again by crying or being unable to take the injection by themselves. It is just as important to "normalize" for teens as it is for younger children, that is to reassure them that many adults also find injections difficult. Teenagers who can feel their behaviour is accepted are likely to grow in self-confidence.

Remember that being a good parent to a teenager is not the same as being a good parent to a younger child. Inappropriate adjustment by the teenager to diabetes has been found to be related to inappropriate adjustment on the part of the parents to the child's increasing need for independence during the years leading up to puberty.

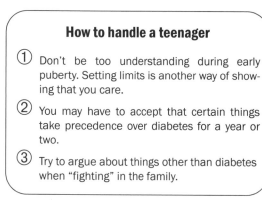

How to handle a teenager

① Don't be too understanding during early puberty. Setting limits is another way of showing that you care.

② You may have to accept that certain things take precedence over diabetes for a year or two.

③ Try to argue about things other than diabetes when "fighting" in the family.

When teenagers have control over their diabetes, other subjects can be brought up as they grow in independence.

Let your teenager practise as much as possible on his or her own. However, it is equally important to discuss afterwards how things went and why. Although the onset of puberty marks a dramatic change in a child's development and level of independence, children with diabetes and their parents must protect diabetes responsibilities (for example, the task of remembering blood glucose tests and injections) from excessive independence, handing over responsibility in a very gradual manner.[41]

In the interplay between children and parents, negotiation and agreement are essential. When young people say they want to assume the responsibility for something, let them give it a try. It is natural for parents always to want to know where their children are when they are away from home. If a young person has diabetes it is even more important. It is a good idea therefore to come to some agreement about having contact at certain times. A mobile phone may be a practical and popular way of keeping in touch with a child or teenager with diabetes.

Many teenagers demonstrate so called risk-taking behaviour" in that they like to do things that are slightly (or very) risky to test their ability. This is often more pronounced in boys than in girls. If this is the case, try connecting this behaviour with the diabetes treatment and encourage experimenting with insulin dosages for example. There may very well be an element of risk included (such as how to dose insulin when staying up all night) but it is equally

important that there be a "protective network" in the form of friends or adults whom the teenager can trust if something goes wrong.

A serious type of risk-taking behaviour is forgetting or skipping insulin injections. In an American interview study, 25% of the teenagers (11-19 years of age) stated that they had missed one or more insulin injections during the last 10 days, mainly due to forgetfulness.[1100] Of these, 29% missed taking blood glucose tests which had been previously agreed upon and a further 29% had entered a lower blood glucose reading in their logbook than was actually registered. The adolescents who had missed insulin injections had a higher HbA_{1c} value. If insulin doses are missed, blood glucose levels will start swinging around and the diabetes will become difficult to regulate.[760]

An Italian self-report study with anonymous questionnaires answered by 215 teenagers aged 12-18 years found that the teenagers with diabetes were as likely to engage in risk-taking behaviour as their healthy peers.[941] The males with diabetes used contraceptives more often than their non-diabetic peers (87% vs. 70%), while the diabetic girls used contraceptives less often (60% vs. 79%). Daily smoking was recorded by 47% of the boys with diabetes, and 25% of the girls (compared to 38% and 55% of their peers). Only 18% of the boys and 13% of the girls with diabetes reported never having been drunk (similar numbers were reported by their peers). Cannabis smoking had been tried by 39% of the boys and 41% of the girls with diabetes (compared to 39% and 32% of their peers). HbA_{1c} was higher in the group reporting one or more risk-taking behaviours (68 vs. 62 mmol/mol, 8.4 vs. 7.8%). This group also reported more management problems like missing injections on purpose (34%), reporting false blood glucose readings (69%) and skipping meals or snacks (41%).

This may seem like very high numbers, and will certainly be different in different cultures. A large German study with 27,561 participants found only 5% smokers in 11 to 15-year-old young people with diabetes, and 28.4% in the 15 to 20-year-old age group.[519] In a Norwegian study with 1,658 participants, only 3% of those 12 years of age or older reported smoking.[718] Boys smoked more often than girls in both these studies.

"Puberty is a necessary good. A person that does not pass through all the phases of puberty will risk becoming a bad copy of their parents."

Torsten Tuvemo, paediatric diabetologist

Healthy siblings

Being a healthy brother or sister to a child with a chronic disease can be difficult at times. Siblings often see many of the "advantages" that the ill child has, not to mention all the increased attention from the parents. At the same time it is difficult for a brother or sister totally to understand the situation of the child with diabetes. They will need help in answering some questions even if they don't bring them up by themselves:

— Is it my fault that my brother/sister has developed diabetes?

— Is it contagious? Will I get it as well?

— Who will take care of me when my parents are busy with my brother's/sister's diabetes?

It is important to listen to healthy siblings and accept that they can sometimes feel that "It is difficult to be the one not ill". Parents may find it easy to say: "You should be grateful that you are healthy" or "Would you want to be in that position?" Often it will be enough just to confirm the feelings of the child not having diabetes by saying: "I understand that it can be difficult at times".

Take it seriously when a sibling complains for instance about a headache or abdominal pain, even if you as a parent have the impression that it is not so serious. The brother or sister may benefit from seeing a doctor of his or her own.

They may certainly benefit from being able to discuss stress and worry, and how these can cause headaches and other physical symptoms.

You can give a healthy sibling some extra attention. For example, the two of you could do something together on your own. It will not matter much what you do. Being alone with a parent is always something special. Take the opportunity to eat something tasty together and keep it "a secret" from the other family members. Do something else secretly together with the child with diabetes, like visiting a special playground, or, if the child is older, a theatre or exhibition. The purpose of keeping it "a secret" is to avoid envy between the siblings (regardless of whether they have diabetes or not).

It is difficult for siblings always having to hear that they cannot eat this or that because their brother or sister has diabetes and must not be tempted. One method, practised in most families, is to allow something special to be eaten when the child with diabetes is not at home. As the child with diabetes gets older, he or she must become accustomed to not having the same arrangements as everyone else. Children with other diseases or problems (such as coeliac disease, allergies or a tendency to put on weight) must learn that they cannot eat like their friends. Try to find something else that is desirable for the child with diabetes in order to avoid unfair treatment within the family. The goal is that, as children get older, they become increasingly able to withstand temptation on their own, for instance at school or during leisure times.

When a healthy brother or sister has a birthday party, parents should make an exception and let this child make all the decisions about what the treats should be. The child with diabetes can take some extra insulin that day in order to be able to join the party.

As brothers and sisters grow older, a strong feeling of friendship often develops. In many instances a good relationship develops between older teenagers with diabetes and their siblings,

As a teenager you want to spend time with your friends. It is important that your diabetes doesn't stop you from doing this. Practise taking responsibility for adjusting your insulin doses and mealtimes so they will fit with the type of life you want to live.

providing a springboard from which they can take the step towards adulthood, assuming responsibility for their diabetes. This can be particularly helpful, for example, in situations where parents are caught up in divorce, other conflict or are too over-protective, leading to difficulties in letting a maturing teenager take over responsibility and control.

A report from Australia did not find any increased behavioural or emotional problems in siblings aged 11 to 17 years relative to children in the general population.[980] According to their parents, the siblings were even better adjusted compared to their peers with fewer conduct problems and less hyperactive behaviour and peer-related problems. However, younger siblings were more likely to have emotional and behavioural problems, indicating that they lack the coping strategies attained at adolescence. A longer diabetes duration was associated with better sibling functioning, showing that most families adjust well in the long run.

Divorced families

More and more children these days do not live with both their parents. About one quarter of all children and teenagers in the UK and US live with only one biological parent. Divorced parents often have difficulties communicating and the children can end up delivering messages between them.

When a child develops a chronic illness, great demands are put on both parents to cooperate and trust each other. If the parents are divorced, the best approach is for both to obtain the same information from the very onset of diabetes. If they have new partners, these partners will also need information. The situation between the parents may be tense, but it will always be better for children if the parents can remain on speaking terms and cooperate with regard to the child's diabetes as much as possible.

Fathers' involvement

In a Swedish study, different factors were investigated characterizing families where the children had varying levels of diabetes adjustment (high/low HbA_{1c} and psychological adjustment to disease).[919] In families with poorer adjustment, the fathers were more impulsive and dependent. The children were also more impulsive. In families with better adjustment, the fathers were more independent and because of this, in a better position to support the mother and the child in coping with the diabetes. Children, especially boys, will find it easier to identify with their father and be inspired to take a greater responsibility for their diabetes. Fathers who took an active part in their child's diabetes care were more likely to have been at home with their children on parental leave when they were very young: "I was engaged in my child when it was young, so of course I will be so now as well".[132]

It is difficult to generalize from a single study. However, from a clinical point of view it is clear that things work best in families where both mother and father are engaged with the child and his or her diabetes. Two people can usually find it easier to deal with a problem than one person alone, especially if they are able to discuss how different situations can be managed. If the father is not involved, but lets the mother take care of diabetes, it does appear that boys, in particular, are likely to have problems in their teens. It is important that fathers be with their child as much as possible at the time of diagnosis and that both parents be allowed to take an active part in the diabetes management from the very beginning.

The above applies also to divorced families where it is still important for both parents to cooperate and share the care of their child's diabetes (see above) as far as possible. Sometimes this is impossible for practical reasons and a single parent will have to take full responsibility for the child. This is of course an extra stress for that parent, and they may need additional support from extended family networks or friends. But in the overwhelming majority of cases it works very well.

"One cannot be cautious enough when choosing one's parents."

Henrik Pontoppidan

Brittle diabetes

Brittle diabetes can be caused by many different factors. It is defined as a diabetes that is so difficult to control "that life is constantly being disrupted by episodes of high or low blood glucose levels, whatever their cause".[1022] In spite of great efforts from everyone, the swinging blood glucose levels continue. Swinging unstable blood glucose levels happen in all young people but "brittleness" may have contributing physical causes (such as insulin antibodies, decreased insulin sensitivity, puberty, delayed emptying of the stomach, missed insulin doses, incorrect injection technique) and also psychological factors where chronic stress (as in a divorce situation) may create a high or swinging blood glucose level.

When a person has brittle diabetes, the insulin doses will often be very large, even if the sensitivity for intravenously administered insulin is normal.[570] Ketones may be produced even when

the levels of counter-regulatory hormones are normal, and these patients will often have ketoacidosis.[570]

Sometimes a person with "brittle" diabetes deliberately manipulates the insulin doses for various reasons, creating widely varying blood glucose levels. This can create a vicious cycle which is difficult both to understand and to break. Afterwards, when looking back at this behaviour, people often find it hard to believe that they really did this. If you think about it as a temporary coping response when the world is difficult to live in, it is not all that strange. Most adults have done things in their younger years that they are not all that proud of.

If this sort of behaviour continues, however, it can lead to dangerously unstable glucose control and repeated episodes of hypoglycaemia and/or ketoacidosis. Anyone in this situation needs help to straighten things out. The most important starting point is "to put the cards on the table" by beginning to enter correct readings in your logbook, take your insulin doses regularly, and note in your logbook when you miss or forget an insulin dose. Otherwise your diabetes team has no way of knowing what is going on in your body and, because of this, may give you quite incorrect advice. For example, if you have a lot of high blood glucose readings, and give no indication that you have missed a lot of doses, your doctor is likely to advise you to increase your doses. But if you take these higher doses, you may end up with severe hypoglycaemia.

It may not be necessary at this point to actually state that you have been "forgetting" doses — we all find it difficult "to lose face" and the most important thing right now is to get a new start. Just one little wish: if you do tell your doctor or nurse what really happened (perhaps many years later), they will have a better chance of finding clues and helping someone else in your situation to get out of that vicious cycle.

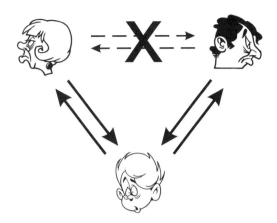

If the parents cannot agree, after a divorce for example, there is a risk that the child will act as a "messenger" between them. "Tell your Father that..." or "Ask your Mother about...". This is a role that will put the child in an awkward situation, causing distress and ultimately a high HbA$_{1c}$ value.

Occasionally, sexual abuse from an adult in the child's or teenager's close surroundings, sometimes even by their father, can be the reason for a "brittle diabetes".[781] Remember that if something like this happens it is NEVER the young person's fault. Sexual abuse is always the fault of the adult and it is illegal. Something like this is very difficult to think about and even more difficult to reveal to anyone else. However, if you recognize yourself when reading this you must confide in someone whom you trust. This is the only way to make it stop, the only way to start over again and to have the opportunity once again to feel safe.

All doctors and nurses at your family surgery or diabetes clinic are sworn to professional secrecy. This means that anything you tell your doctor or nurse stays between you, in confidence. Wherever you live, your diabetes team is under professional and legal obligation to guard every secret disclosed. Another alternative may be to speak to a priest, counsellor or teacher who you feel you can trust.

Quality of life

Diabetes is an illness that affects you 24 hours of every day, and will therefore have a substantial influence on your quality of life. In an international study from 17 countries, including 2,101 adolescents aged 10-18 years, the main conclusion was that a lower HbA$_{1c}$ was associated with a better quality of life (as judged by the young people themselves).[518] Parents also found the family burden of diabetes to be lower. Teenagers from single-parent families and ethnic minority groups showed both higher HbA$_{1c}$ and poorer quality of life. Teenage girls had more difficulties with diabetes control than boys from the same age group. The message is that young people who try hard to improve their diabetic control also find that their overall quality of life is better, not worse.

Needle phobia

Phobia for injections and blood tests will show up in different ways at different ages (see page 394). Injection aids (such as i-port or Insuflon, see page 137) or a pump can help many children take injections, though blood tests are still impossible to avoid. If you "get stuck" in these matters it is important to see a psychologist as quickly as possible to prevent needle phobia from becoming a permanent problem for you, your child or your family. See also page 106 and 125.

Topical anaesthetic cream (EMLA®, Ametop®) gives effective pain relief and can be used to make some blood tests less unpleasant. It can be used for insulin injections on isolated occasions but, in practice, it is impossible to use for every insulin injection. Creams like this do not work on the fingertips as the skin there is too thick.

Children who are asked how they feel about injections often say they wonder why adults look so happy when they stick needles in children. "Do they enjoy hurting us?" It is easy to misinterpret an adult's smile, which is meant to comfort the child, as something else.

Needle phobia: general advice

(adapted from Marianne Helgesson)

① Parents' attitudes to needle stabs are very important. You must be sure the finger prick or needle stab is necessary, otherwise you can never convey this to the child. If you, as a parent, have a needle phobia of your own, it will be difficult to stick a needle into your child.

② The child must know exactly what is going to happen and why. Many children (even older ones) may believe that the injection or blood test is a punishment for something done wrong. You must state clearly that the needle is necessary, and not because anyone has behaved badly. Remember that the person sticking the needle in is not "being mean". He or she is only doing what has to be done.

③ Be honest about the pain. A needle prick can be painful, no matter how much we would like it not to be.

④ Indicate the acceptable limits of protest, such as: "You can cry if you feel like it, but you must not pull your hand away."

Needle phobia, cont.

⑤ Offer realistic choices. They lessen the child's feeling of being a victim. But do not offer to give the injection another time as you cannot do that. The child will only remember being tricked and things will be even more difficult the next time around.

⑥ Suggest diverting activities, such as choosing a plaster.

⑦ The phase of persuasion should be short. When dealing with smaller children it is best to hold them firmly, do the needle prick and then comfort. If inserting the needle takes time, the child will suffer for longer. Use a firm grip if you must hold the child, so that the injection is over quickly.

⑧ Don't smile to encourage. The child may believe that you are laughing.

⑨ **Afterwards:** Comfort, praise and talk to the child. Dealing with what has been difficult through drawing or play may help. Stay with the child when playing in order to be able to correct misunderstandings and help the child come to terms with the experience.

It need not always be difficult to start taking injections. Elin was 5 years old when she was diagnosed with diabetes. She did not mind the nurse giving her injections as she had an injection aid (Insuflon) inserted subcu- taneously in her tummy (see page 137). Her mother does not seem to be upset by this either.

Well-known people with diabetes

People with diabetes can be found in most professions. You probably know prominent people with diabetes in your home town or country. Below are some examples of how successful people cope with their diabetes.

Nick Jonas

The singer-songwriter Nick Jonas was diagnosed with type 1 diabetes at age 12. The day after Nick left the hospital, he performed in a concert and jumped right back into the flow of doing shows and touring.[289] He started out taking multiple daily injections, checking his blood sugar about twelve times a day, but is now using an insulin pump.

In March 2007, about a year and a half after his diagnosis, Nick publicly announced that he has diabetes at Carnival For a Cure. He had known from the start that he wanted to go public with his diabetes; it was simply a matter of when. He waited until he felt comfortable with managing his diabetes before telling everyone about it. Of course, he didn't test in public until after his announcement, but now he tests wherever he is.

He knows that diabetes "is a huge part of my life and I can't just forget about it, obviously. I have to keep taking care of it and managing it, and learning more things about it. I have this passion to be able to share with young people my age and be a positive light in a situation that might not be so positive." Being on tour adds a dimension of difficulty to managing his diabetes because the schedule is "kind of insane".

To newly diagnosed kids with diabetes, Nick would say: "At first, I was worried that diabetes would keep me from performing and recording and doing everything a teenager likes to do. I want to let kids know that it doesn't have to be

so hard. The most important thing is to never ever let yourself get down about having diabetes, because you can live a really great life as a kid with diabetes."

Gary Mabbutt

In his professional footballing days, Gary Mabbutt played for Tottenham Hotspur for 16 years (11 of them as Captain). He also played for England. He developed diabetes when he was 17 years old, but did not let this stand in his way. The doctor gave his parents the following advice: "Let the boy try a suitable regimen, let him continue his previous life and we will see what happens".[170] And things went quite well! When playing professionally, Gary used to have four injections every day.

"A match day starts with a blood glucose test, insulin injection and then breakfast. I have now learned in detail what signals the tests give and from that I find out how much I can eat for lunch. Before warming up I take another test to find out how much sports drink I need before the first half. The same procedure takes place in the break before the second half. If the match goes into extra time, a few tablets of dextrose is enough to take me through it. If I follow this schedule I feel certain that nothing will happen."

Gary campaigns for sporting charities, and to help people with chronic health problems lead a normal life and enjoy exercise. He advises young people with diabetes to:

"Live as usual but keep an eye on insulin and mealtimes. Don't let the disease control you. Get control of it instead with the help of regular hours. No matter if it is about sports, studying or working, you have the same great chances as others without diabetes. You make your own possibilities!"

Tara Moran

Tara Moran grew up in Yorkshire and has been acting since she was 6 years old. In fact she is rarely far from our television screens. Her career to date includes appearances in Coronation Street, EastEnders, Casualty, A Touch of Frost, Heartbeat, The Bill, Doctors, Shameless and Scott and Bailey – and that is just a selection! "I think it's like any job — you get to a certain age and you realize what your strengths and weaknesses are and I'm better at soap acting." [220]

She's also very up front about her diabetes, which she's also had since she was six. Not for her the denials and embarrassed injections in toilets. When she was young Tara went on several Diabetes UK children's holidays. She has worked closely with Diabetes UK and was a

judge of the Diabetes UK Young Achievers Awards

Tara makes a point of telling cast and crew she has diabetes, always carries glucose tablets with her and on one occasion called "cut" on a scene as she needed her lunch. "I have to look after myself otherwise I wouldn't work and I've never wanted to be a diabetes martyr. I really knuckled down and took care as I never wanted to be off stage for even one night because of diabetes. It would be a very bad advert for the condition." She continues: "I don't see why I have to give myself exactly the same dose of insulin every day because not every day is exactly the same."

Steve Redgrave

Sir Steve Redgrave won gold medals for rowing at five consecutive Olympics. He was diagnosed with type 2 diabetes at the age of 35. He immediately went on an insulin regimen with rapid-acting insulin with each meal, and is now using an insulin pump.

He admits that he had considered giving up competition after being told he had diabetes 6 months before the Sydney Olympics in 2000. "My first thought was that my rowing career was at an end. But I spoke to my GP and my specialist, and both said that I should be aware that the path to success was not going to be easy. However, there is very little known about endurance sports and diabetes, so it has been a steep learning curve for all of us. But I felt I had to give it a go.

But let's not be blasé about it. At first I went into a denial phase – you do not want to accept that this thing is happening to you – and took as little insulin as possible. But after some months, I ended up taking as much as I could, always keeping in mind the maximum permitted dosage. It isn't rocket science – frankly, it's pretty straightforward."

Although he no longer takes part in competitive rowing, Sir Steve remains a strong and positive role model with a high profile He is also an honorary vice president of Diabetes UK. "Kids are my special concern, so I want to do all I can to help them. It's vital to dispel some of the myths surrounding the condition, and show them that people with diabetes can achieve great things."

He explains how coping with diabetes is as much about controlling your lifestyle as it is about health. "As an athlete you have to be tremendously disciplined, and I test six or seven times a day. I'll help spread the message, on a national and international basis, stressing that regular testing is vital for people with the condition. This is an area where I can use my status as a sportsman to project a positive message and get people to think about the issues associated with testing."

There are many other famous people in the world who take insulin for their diabetes. They include sportsmen and women, film stars, professors, captains of industry. All of them prove how you can live with diabetes successfully with a bit of courage and motivation.

Ostrich strategy, i.e. not caring about diabetes and not taking any responsibility for its management, is among the most dangerous things a person with diabetes can do. Your diabetes team can contribute with knowledge, tips and advice — but living with your diabetes is something only YOU can do.

"If you become a teacher, by your pupils you will be taught."

Hammerstein and Rogers, 1951 [439]

Epilogue

When diabetes occurs in a family, life will naturally become difficult. If the person with diabetes is a child or teenager, issues of dependence and independence will be heightened. Parents will find themselves facing the dilemma of how to be sufficiently supportive without being over-protective.

When one family member has a chronic disease, extra demands fall on every other family member, and conflicts can result. When a child is sick, parents may find it extremely difficult to find enough time, as well as to balance the time needed for the child and his or her illness, time for other siblings, time for the individual parent as well as time to have an adult relationship with a spouse or partner. Try to remember though, that all families have problems, especially if the children are in their teen years. Diabetes is not the only reason for stress. It can be helpful to try to think through how you might have handled the situation if the family member concerned had not had diabetes.

Artwork and other credits

In addition to the acknowledgments made at the beginning of this book, I wish to express my gratitude to the following authors and medical journals (© owners) who kindly gave me permission to print their illustrations (the full credit line is in the reference list on page 423):

Acta Paediatrica Scandinavia
(Scandinavian University Press):
Cedermark et al. 1990 (p. 270)

American Journal of Medicine
(Elsevier Science)
Weinger et al. 1995 (p. 103)

Land ahead! As an adult, one will often continue with the same attitude towards diabetes as one had when leaving the teens. But don't forget that "today is the first day of the rest of your life". It is never too late to decide to do something radical about your diabetes if you have high HbA_{1c} values. Every percentage decrease in HbA_{1c} will reduce your risk of complications in the future!

Archives of Diseases in Childhood
(BMJ Publishing Group):
Sackey et al. 1994 (p. 83)

Clinical Science (The Biochemical Society and Medical Research Society):
Welch et al. 1987 (p. 236)

Diabetologia (Springer-Verlag GmbH & Co. KG):
Amiel et al. 1998 (p. 47)
Lind et al. 2010 (p. 368)
Malherbe et al. 1969 (p. 23)
Maran et al. 1995 (p. 53)
Tuominen et al. 1995 (p. 290)
Wahren et al. 1978 (p. 281)

Diabetes (American Diabetes Association):
Steil et al. 2004 (p. 373)

Diabetes Care (American Diabetes Association):
Bantle et al. 1993 (p. 127)
Bussau et al. 2006 (p. 282)
Frid et al. 1988 (p. 87)
Gonder-Frederick et al. 2009 (p. 330)
Guelfi et al. 2005 (p. 282)
Guerci et al. 2003 (p. 201)
Guerin et al. 2007 (p. 319)
Linde 1986 (p. 88)
Schiffrin et al. 1982 (p. 123)

Diabetic Medicine (John Wiley & Sons Ltd):
Hanssen et al. 1992 (p. 369)
Bojestig et al. 1998 (p. 370)

Endocrine Reviews
(The Endocrine Society):
Yki-Järvinen 1992 (p. 225)

European Journal of Paediatrics
(Springer-Verlag GmbH & Co. KG):
Cedermark et al. 1993 (p. 270)

JAMA (American Medical Association):
Brodows et al. 1984 (p. 71)
Nathan et al. 1984 (p. 266)

Journal of Pediatrics (Mosby, Inc)
Hanas et al. 2002 (p. 140)

New England Journal of Medicine
(Massachusetts Medical Society):
Bojestig et al. 1994 (p. 371)

Nordic Medicine (Nordisk Medicin):
Knip M 1992 (p. 375)

Scandinavian Journal of Nutrition
(The Swedish Nutrition Foundation):
Andersson et al. 1986 (p. 232)

I am also thankful to the following authors and
medical publications (© owners) for letting me
adapt their tables for use in the book:

APEG handbook on childhood and adolescent
diabetes (Australian Paediatric Endocrine
Group):
Silink M. 1996 (p. 304)

Diabetes Reviews International (Macmillan):
Kassianos G. 1992 (p. 347)

Diabetes Care (American Diabetes Association):
Hirsch IB et al. 1990 (p. 151)
Kullberg CE et al. 1996 (p. 367)
McCrimmon RJ et al. 1995 (p. 45)
Holzmeister LA 2000 (p. 238)

Pediatric Diabetes (Blackwell Munksgaard)
Riddell et al. (p. 292)

SPRI and Swedish Medical Society 1989:
Berg K. (p. 329)
Sundkvist G. (p. 363)

The Insulin Pump Therapy Book (MiniMed):
Tanenberg RJ, Bode BW, Davidson PC, Sonnenberg GE (pp. 184, 188, 202)

Diving and Subaquatic Medicine (Arnold)
Edge C. 2002 (p. 295)

Dietetic Management of Diabetes (John Wiley)
Waldron S. (p. 251)

Special thanks to Diabetes, the official journal
of the Swedish Diabetes Association, for letting
me print quotations from their journal.

Drawings are reproduced with the permission
of the individual artist. Comic strips are reproduced with the permission of the respective ven-
dor. The clip art is published with permission
from the following vendors (© owners):
3 G Graphics Inc., BeeLine ArtProfile, Corel
Corporation, Image Club Graphics Inc., One
Mile Up Inc. and Totem Graphics Inc. LifeART
Images Copyright © 1989-1997 by TechPool
Studios Inc. US.

Every effort has been made to trace all the copyright holders, but if any have been inadvertently
overlooked, the author and publishers will be
pleased to make the necessary additions at the
earliest opportunity.

When using multiple injections or an insulin pump you will have increased freedom — but only if you take the responsibility that goes with it. One should not confuse this with an "anything goes" mentality where everything is allowed. It is a question of quantity as well — exceptions must be exceptions. If you make the exception every day it becomes a habit instead.

It is important to remember that it is not your blood glucose level today or tomorrow that counts in the long run, but your average blood glucose level over a long period of time to come, years and tens of years. As a parent (or teenager or adult with diabetes) you need to make some exceptions to learn and get used to the guidelines you should continue with in the future.

Today, Camilla is a young adult using an insulin pump and takes good care of her diabetes. As a teenager, she had strong support from her parents when she chose to make exceptions, but also clear limits on how much and how many exceptions she could allow herself. In my opinion this is a very good start of a long and well-managed life with diabetes. Thank you Camilla, for all the observations and good points about living with diabetes that you have given me throughout the years.

Glossary

< Less than
> More than
≥ Equal to or more than
≤ Equal to or less than
[28] The references where the text is taken from are shown as small, superscript numbers. See page 423.

Italic type indicates a separate glossary entry.

Units

Weight
1 kg (kilogram) = 2.2 pounds (lb)
1 g = 1 gram   = 15.4 grains = 0.035 ounces
1 ounce   = 28.35 grams = 1/16 pound

Length
1 cm (centimetre) = 0.4 inches
1 inch   = 2.54 cm

Capacity
1 litre = 1.76 UK pints = 0.22 UK gallons
250 ml = ¼ litre ≈ 1 cup
(1 UK cup = 280 ml, 1 US cup = 240 ml)
1 UK fluid oz. = 28 ml, 1 US fluid oz. = 30 ml
1 tablespoon = 15 ml
1 teaspoon = 5 ml

Temperature
$° F = (9/5 \times °C) + 32$

Time
14 = 2 PM
02 = 2 AM

Terms

ACE inhibitors
Drugs that inhibit an *enzyme* (ACE, angiotensin converting enzyme) in the kidneys that increases the blood pressure.

Acesulfam K
Sweetener that provides negligible energy.

Acetone
Is produced when there is an excess of *ketones* in the blood. Acetone can be smelt on the breath when the level of ketones is raised.

Acidosis
Shifting of the pH in the blood towards being acidic.

Adrenal glands
Small organs situated above the kidneys that produce a number of different hormones, including adrenaline and cortisol.

Adrenaline
Stress hormone from the *adrenal glands* that increases the blood glucose level.

Adrenergic symptoms
Bodily symptoms of hypoglycaemia caused mainly by adrenaline.

Albuminuria
A larger amount of albumin in the urine than the traces of albumin found with *microalbuminuria*. A sign of permanent kidney damage.

Aldose reductase inhibitors
Drugs that can affect nerve damage caused by diabetes.

Alpha cells
Cells in the *islets of Langerhans* of the pancreas that produce the hormone *glucagon*.

Amino acid
Protein building blocks.

Amnesia
Loss of memory.

Amylase
An enzyme that is produced in the saliva and the pancreas. Amylase breaks down the starch in the food.

Anaesthetic cream
Cream that numbs the skin (EMLA®, Ametop®). Can be used to reduce pain when inserting a pump catheter or Insuflon.

Analogue insulin
Human insulin preparations contain exactly the same insulin as is produced in a human pancreas. Analogue insulins have a slightly different chemical structure that makes them either faster or slower than human insulin.

Anorexia
Lack of appetite. Also commonly used to mean anorexia nervosa, an eating disorder in which a person starves him or herself.

Antibiotics
Drugs that kill bacteria. Penicillin is one type of antibiotic.

Antibody
A substance, produced by the *immune defence* to destroy viruses and bacteria.

Arteriosclerosis
Hardening, narrowing and eventual blocking of the blood vessels.

Aspartame
Sweetener that provides negligible energy.

Autoimmune
Sometimes things go wrong with the *immune defence*, causing it to attack the cells of your own body. This is referred to as an autoimmune response or autoimmune disorder.

Autonomic nervous system
The "independent" part of the nervous system that is operated without one having to give it a

thought, includes such aspects as breathing and the movements of the intestines.

Basal insulin
A low level of insulin that covers the body's need for insulin between meals and during the night. This insulin is given as *intermediate-* or *long-acting insulin* or in a pump.

Basal rate
With an *insulin pump*, a low dose of basal insulin is infused every hour of the day and night.

Beta cells
Cells in the *islets of Langerhans* of the pancreas that produce the hormone *insulin*.

Blood glucose level
The level of *glucose* in the blood. It is measured in mmol/l (SI units) or mg/dl (mg%). For conversion table see page 99. Can be measured as *plasma glucose* or whole blood glucose. Earlier meters showed values in whole blood glucose but today, patient meters in most countries display *plasma glucose*. Unless otherwise mentioned, values in this book refer to plasma glucose (whole blood glucose values were used in the first edition of this book).

Brittle diabetes
Diabetes with very unstable blood glucose (rapid swings up and down) that prevents the person from living a normal life.

Bulimia
Eating disorder involving binge eating, i.e. sometimes eating huge amounts of food followed by purge (induced) vomiting or use of laxatives.

Capillary blood
The capillaries are the very fine blood vessels between arteries and veins where the blood delivers oxygen to the tissues. Blood tests from fingers contain capillary blood.

Carbohydrate
All compounds that are made up of different types of sugar, such as cane and beet sugar,

grape sugar, syrup, starch, cellulose.

Cataract
Clouding of the lens in the eye.

Cellulose
Glucose molecules in long chains, present in all plants. Cannot be broken down in the intestines.

Chylomicrones
Small drops of fat that are transported from the blood into the lymph drainage system.

Ciclosporin
A *cytotoxic drug* that has been used to stop the immune process at the onset of diabetes.

Coeliac disease
Illness where the person cannot tolerate *gluten,* a substance found in wheat, oats, barley and rye.

Coma
Unconsciousness. Can occur in people with diabetes when the blood glucose is very low (*insulin coma*) or very high (*diabetic coma*).

Cortisol
Stress hormone that is produced in the adrenal gland.

Counter-regulation
The body's defence against low levels of blood glucose. The excretion of the counter-regulating hormones (glucagon, adrenaline, growth hormone and cortisol) increases when the blood glucose level falls too low.

C-peptide
"Connecting peptide", a protein produced together with insulin in the *beta cells*. By measuring C-peptide, the residual insulin production of the pancreas can be estimated.

CSII
Continuous subcutaneous insulin infusion, treatment with an insulin pump.

Cyclamate
Sweetener that does not provide any energy.

Cyclosporin
See *ciclosporin.*

Cytotoxic drugs
Drugs that affect the ability of cells to divide. Often used for cancer therapy.

Dawn phenomenon
The growth hormone level rises during the night, causing the blood glucose level to rise early in the morning.

Depot effect
Part of the insulin that is injected is stored in the fat tissue as a depot (a "spare tank" of insulin). The longer the action of the insulin, the larger the depot will be.

Dextrose
Pure glucose.

Diabetes ketones
Ketones that are produced when the cells in the body are starving due to a lack of insulin. The blood glucose level is high. See *ketones.*

Diabetic coma
Severe *ketoacidosis* that has led to unconsciousness.

Dialysis
The process of extracting harmful substances from the blood when the kidneys do not work properly.
See *uraemia.*

Direct-acting insulin
Term for *rapid-acting insulin* used in some countries. Used in the first edition of this book.

DNA
The genetic code inside the chromosomes is made of DNA.

Double-blind study
Technique to perform a study where neither the

participant nor the investigator knows who is treated with which type of medication or intervention.

EEG
Electroencephalography ("brain-wave"), a method for measuring the very weak electrical currents in the brain.

Enzyme
Protein compound that cleaves chemical bonds.

Fasting glucose
Plasma glucose test taken before eating in the morning. In a person without diabetes, the plasma glucose result would not normally be higher than 5.6 mmol/l (100 mg/dl).

Fat pad
See *lipohypertrophy*.

Fatty acids
Substances produced when fat is broken down in the body.

Fluorescein angiography
Special type of X-ray technique to visualize the retinal blood vessels in the back of the eye.

Fructosamine
Blood test that measures how much glucose that is bound to proteins (mainly albumin) in the blood. Gives a measure of the average blood glucose level during the last 2-3 weeks.

Fructose
Fruit sugar.

Galactose
Sugar molecule. *Lactose* consists of galactose and *glucose*.

Gastroparesis
Slower stomach emptying caused by diabetes complications (*neuropathy*).

Gestational diabetes
Diabetes discovered during pregnancy. The symptoms usually disappear after childbirth but the woman has an increased risk of acquiring type 2 diabetes later on in life.

Glucagon
Hormone that raises the blood glucose level. It is produced in the *alpha cells* in the *islets of Langerhans* of the *pancreas*.

Gluconeogenesis
Production of sugar (*glucose*) in the liver.

Glucose
Simple carbohydrate, *dextrose*, grape sugar, corn sugar.

Glucose tolerance test
Test to diagnosis early stages of diabetes. Tells how much the blood glucose level rises after orally ingested (OGTT) or intravenously given (IVGTT) glucose.

Gluten
Compound that makes dough sticky. Found in wheat, oats, rye and barley.

Glycaemic index
A method to classify *carbohydrates* and foods according to how they affect the blood glucose level. Abbreviates to GI.

Glycogen
Glucose is stored as glycogen in the liver and muscles. The glucose molecules are connected in long chains. See illustration on page 232.

Glycogenolysis
The breakdown of the *glycogen* store in liver or muscles.

Glycosylated haemoglobin
See HbA_{1c}.

Goitre
Enlarged thyroid gland.

Grape sugar
Glucose.

Growth hormone
Hormone that is produced in the pituitary gland. Increased growth is the most important effect. Increases the blood glucose level.

HbA$_1$
Older method of measuring HbA$_{1c}$. Gives values approximately 2% higher than HbA$_{1c}$.

HbA$_{1c}$
Blood test that measures how much glucose binds to red blood cells. Gives a measure of the average blood glucose level during the last 2-3 months.

HLA antigens
Genetic markers on chromosome 6 that are important when transplanting organs and for studying the heredity of different diseases.

Honeymoon phase
See *remission phase*.

Hormone
Chemical compound that is produced in one of the glands in the body and that attains its target organ or tissue through the blood. Hormones work as "keys" to influence the cells in the body to perform different functions.

Hyperglycaemia
High blood glucose level.

Hyperinsulinism
High level of insulin in the blood.

Hyperthyroidism
Excessively elevated levels of thyroid hormone in the blood. The thyroid gland is enlarged (toxic goitre).

Hypoglycaemia
Too low a level of blood glucose. Usually defined as a blood glucose level below 3-3.5 mmol/l (55-65 mg/dl).

Hypophysis
See *pituitary gland*.

Hypothyroidism
Too low a level of thyroid hormone in the blood. The thyroid gland is often enlarged (goitre).

ICA
Islet cell antibodies. Antibodies directed against the *islets of Langerhans*. Indicates an attack of the immune defence on the islets.

IDDM
Insulin-dependent diabetes mellitus, former name for type 1 diabetes.

Immune defence
The defence in the body against foreign substances, such as bacteria and virus.

Implantable insulin pump
Insulin pump that is implanted under the skin in the subcutaneous tissue. Infuses insulin through a thin tubing into the abdominal (intra-peritoneal) cavity.

Incidence
The number of diagnosed cases per year of a particular disease.

Incubation time
The time between when you have been infected with a contagious disease and when you show the first symptoms of the disease.

Indwelling catheter
An aid to lessen the pain when injecting insulin, such as Insuflon® and i-port®. It consists of a soft Teflon catheter which is inserted into the subcutaneous tissue, and you inject into a silicon membrane instead of the skin.

Insulin
Hormone produced in the pancreatic *beta cells*. Lowers the blood glucose level by "opening the door" of the cells.

Insulin analogues
Newer types of insulin where the structure of the insulin molecule has been changed to make the insulin action quicker (NovoRapid, Huma-

log, Apidra) or slower (Lantus, Levemir).

Insulin antibodies
Antibodies in the blood that bind insulin. The insulin that is bound has no function, but can be released at a later time when the concentration of insulin in the blood is lower (e.g. during the night).

Insulin coma
Unconsciousness caused by severe *hypoglycaemia*.

Insulin depot
See *depot effect*.

Insulin pump
An alternative to injections. Insulin is infused continuously into the *subcutaneous* tissue through thin tubing during day and night. Pre-meal doses are taken by pressing buttons on the pump.

Insulin receptor
Structure on the cell surface to which insulin binds. Initiates the signal that opens the cell membrane for glucose transport.

Insulin resistance
Decreased insulin sensitivity. A higher level of insulin than normal is needed to obtain the same blood glucose-lowering effect.

Intermediate-acting insulin
Insulin that has an effective time action of 8-12 hours, corresponding to a normal night.

Intracutaneous injection
A very superficial injection into the skin that often leaves a small nodule (bubble) and is likely to hurt.

Intramuscular injection
Injection into a muscle.

Intraperitoneal delivery of insulin
Insulin is administered into the abdominal (intraperitoneal) cavity where it is absorbed into the bloodstream leading to the liver.

Intravenous injection
Injection directly into a vein.

Islets of Langerhans
Small islets in the pancreas with cells that produce insulin (*beta cells*) and glucagon (*alpha cells*).

Isophane insulin
Same as *NPH insulin*.

Jet injector
Injection without a needle. A thin jet of liquid is propelled using a very high pressure and penetrates the skin.

Jet-lag
Tiredness after long-distance flights when the day gets longer or shorter.

Joule
Unit for energy. 1 Joule = 0.24 calories.

Juvenile diabetes
Diabetes in childhood and adolescence.

Ketoacidosis
A state in which the blood turns acidic from a high level of *ketones* when there is a deficiency of insulin. Can develop into *diabetic coma*.

Ketones
Fat is broken down to fatty acids when the cells are starving due to a lack of *glucose*. The fatty acids are transformed into ketones in the liver. This can occur when there is a lack of insulin ("high blood glucose, diabetes ketones") or when there is a lack of food (low blood glucose, "starvation ketones").

Ketosis
Increased amounts of ketones in the blood.

Kg
Kilogram, unit of weight. 1 kg = 2.2 lb.

Lactose
Milk sugar.

LADA
Latent autoimmune diabetes in the adult. Onset of type 1 diabetes after the age of 35, usually with less dramatic symptoms.

Langerhans
The scientist who discovered the *islets of Langerhans* (in the pancreas) in 1869.

Latency phase
Psychological term for describing the years before puberty.

Lente insulin
Insulin made *intermediate-* or *long-acting* with a mixture of zinc.

Lipoatrophy
Cavity in the *subcutaneous* tissue that can be caused by an immunological reaction towards insulin.

Lipohypertrophy
Tissue build-up ("fatty lump") that develops when you inject many times into the same area.

Long-acting insulin
Insulin with a very prolonged action, up to 24 hours.

Macroangiopathy
Diabetes complications in the large blood vessels (arteriosclerosis, cardiovascular disease).

Meta-analysis
An analysis of several studies that are combined to get a better basis for statistical calculations with a larger number of subjects included.

Microalbuminuria
Small amounts of protein in the urine. The first sign of kidney damage (*nephropathy*) caused by many years of high blood glucose levels. Microalbuminuria is reversible if the blood glucose control is improved.

Microaneurysm
Small protuberances on the retinal blood vessels (see illustration on page 360). The first sign of eye damage caused by many years of high blood glucose levels. Microaneurysms are reversible if the blood glucose control is improved.

Microangiopathy
Diabetes complications in the small blood vessels (eyes, kidneys, nerves).

MODY
Maturity-onset diabetes of the young. A special kind of diabetes that is inherited.

Monocomponent insulin
Purified porcine (pig) insulin. Gives fewer problems with antibody formation than older types of insulin.

Multiple injection treatment
Treatment with injections of *short-* or *rapid-acting insulin* before meals and *intermediate-* or *long-acting insulin* to cover the night. When using rapid-acting insulin for meals you will need *basal insulin* during the day as well.

Nasal insulin
Insulin in aerosol form that is given via the nose.

Necrobiosis lipoidica diabeticorum
A special type of skin lesion that can be seen in individuals with diabetes.

Nephropathy
Kidney damage caused by many years of high blood glucose levels.

Neuroglycopenic symptoms
Symptoms of brain dysfunction caused by a low blood glucose level.

Neuropathy
Nerve damage caused by many years of high blood glucose levels.

Nicotinamide
A vitamin B compound that has been shown to lower the risk of acquiring diabetes in some studies but a larger study showed no effect.

NIDDM
Non-insulin-dependent diabetes mellitus, a former name for type 2 diabetes.

NPH (Neutral Protamine Hagedorn) **insulin**
Insulin made *intermediate-acting* by adding a protein (protamine).

Pancreas
An organ in the abdominal cavity that produces digestive *enzymes* (released into the intestines) and different *hormones* (released directly into the blood).

Pituitary gland
Small gland situated in the brain where many of the most important hormones in the body are produced.

Plasma glucose
A way of measuring the glucose content in the bloodstream. Plasma is the fluid that remains in the blood when the blood cells have been removed. Plasma glucose values are approximately 11-15% higher than whole blood glucose values. Check which type of readings your meter displays. In this book "blood glucose" refers to plasma glucose values.

Premeal injection
Injection with *short-* or *rapid-acting insulin* prior to a meal.

Prevalence
The total number of existing cases of a disease at a given time.

Prospective study
A study that investigates what happens from now and onwards when giving a certain treatment. This is the best method of conducting a study of the effect of a new treatment.

Protamine
A protein from salmon that is added to protract the action time of insulin. *NPH insulin* is based on this method.

Proteinuria
Protein in the urine due to permanent kidney damage (*nephropathy*) from having high blood glucose levels for many years.

Pylorus
The lower sphincter (opening) of the stomach into the small intestine.

Randomize
A common procedure in scientific studies to prove the effect of a treatment or medication. Participants are randomized to either of two treatment groups by a random procedure, often like a type of lottery.

Rapid-acting insulin
Insulin *analogues* (NovoRapid, Humalog, Apidra) with a much quicker action than regular short-acting insulin. In some countries these are called ultra-rapid insulins, in others, direct-acting insulins.

Rebound phenomenon
After a hypoglycaemic episode, the blood glucose may rise to high levels. This is caused both by the secretion of counteracting hormones (see *counter-regulation*) and by eating too much when feeling hypoglycaemic.

Receptor
A special structure on the cell surface that fits with a hormone. The hormone ("the key") must fit into the receptor for it to mediate its effect to the cell.

Regression
Psychological term to describe when a person temporarily regresses to an earlier stage of psychological development. An independent teenager who is hospitalized will often become more dependent and react as if he or she were several years younger.

Regular insulin
Also called soluble or *short-acting insulin*. This is the type of insulin that is produced in the human pancreas.

Remission phase
Also called honeymoon phase. The need for insulin will often be lowered during the months after the onset of diabetes due to an increase of the residual insulin production in the pancreas.

Renal threshold
If the blood glucose level is above this level, glucose will show up in the urine when you test it.

Retinopathy
Eye damage caused by many years of high blood glucose levels.

Retrospective study
A study that investigates what happened when a certain treatment was given by looking backwards in time at treated individuals. Compare with *prospective* study.

Saccharin
Sweetener that does not provide any energy.

Sensor
Device to measure blood glucose continuously.

Short-acting insulin
Soluble insulin without additives.

Somogyi phenomenon
A special type of night time rebound phenomenon with high blood glucose level in the morning.

Sorbitol
Sugar alcohol, a sweetener that gives energy.

Starch
Complex *carbohydrates* found for example in potatoes, corn, rice and wheat.

Starvation ketones
Ketones that are produced when the cells starve due to a low blood glucose level. Caused by not eating enough food containing *carbohydrates*.

Subcutaneous
In the fatty tissue under the skin.

Sucrose
Cane or beet sugar, brown sugar, table sugar, powdered sugar, invert sugar, saccharose.

Transplantation
The implantation of a new organ into the body by surgery.

T-cells
T-cells belong to a group of white blood cells known as lymphocytes. They play a central role in the type of immune response that does not involve antibodies.

Type 1 diabetes
Previously called insulin-dependent diabetes (IDDM). Diabetes that needs to be treated with insulin from the onset. Is caused by a failure of the pancreas to produce insulin.

Type 2 diabetes
Previously called non-insulin-dependent diabetes (NIDDM). Diabetes that initially can be treated with diet and oral drugs. Is caused by an increased resistance to the insulin produced by the pancreas.

U
Short for international units of insulin.

Unawareness of hypoglycaemia
A hypoglycaemic episode without having had warning symptoms associated with decreasing blood glucose.

Uraemia
Urine poisoning when the body cannot get rid of its waste products. End stage of *nephropathy*.

Venous blood test
Test taken by puncturing a blood vessel (vein).

References

1) Aarø LE. Hauknes R, Berglund E-L. Smoking among Norwegian schoolchildren 1975-1980. II. The influence of the social environment. Scand J Psychology 1981;22:297-309.
2) Acerini CL, Patton CM, Savage MO, Kernell A, Westphal O, Dunger DB. Randomised placebo-controlled trial of human recombinant insulin-like growth factor I plus intensive insulin therapy in adolescents with insulin-dependent diabetes mellitus. Lancet 1997;350:1199-204.
3) Acerini CL, Cheetham TD, Edge JA, Dunger DB. Both insulin sensitivity and insulin clearance in children and young adults with type I (insulin-dependent) diabetes vary with growth hormone concentrations and with age. Diabetologia 2000;43:61-8.
4) Acerini C, Craig M, de Beaufort C, Maahs D, Hanas R. (Eds). ISPAD Clinical Practice Consensus Guidelines 2014 Compendium. Pediatric Diabetes 2014;15 (Suppl. 20)::1-290.
5) Ackerman MJ, Tester DJ, Driscoll DJ. Molecular autopsy of sudden unexplained death in the young. Am J Forensic Med Pathol 2001;22:105-11.
6) Adamsson U, Lins PE. Hormonal counterregulation of hypoglycaemia in insulin treated diabetics. Lakartidningen 1985;40:3369-70.
7) Adamsson U. Hypoglycaemia. In the book: Diabetes. SPRI and Swedish Medical Society 1989: 238-47.
8) Adamsson U, Lins P-E. Clinical views on insulin resistance in type 1-diabetes. In the book: Agardh C-D, Berne C, Östman J. Diabetes. Almqvist & Wiksell, Stockholm 1992: 142-50.
9) Adlersberg MA, Fernando S, Spollett GR, Inzucchi SE. Glargine and lispro: two cases of mistaken identity. Diabetes Care 2002;25:404-5.
10) Admon G, Weinstein Y, Falk B, Weintrob N, Benzaquen H, Ofan R, Fayman G, Zigel L, Constantini N, Phillip M. Exercise with and without an insulin pump among children and adolescents with type 1 diabetes mellitus. Pediatrics 2005;116:e348-55.
11) Adolfsson P, Örnhagen H, Jendle J. The Benefits of Continuous Glucose Monitoring and a Glucose Monitoring Schedule in Individuals with Type 1 Diabetes during Recreational Diving. J Diab Science Tech 2008;2:778-84.
12) Advisory Council on the Misuse of Drugs (2005) Further Consideration of the Classification of Cannabis under the Misuse of Drugs Act 1971. London, The Home Office.
13) Ahlqvist J, Andersson K, Anzén B, von Bahr C, Endresen L, Hagenfeldt K et al. Contraception. Recommendations from a group of experts. Lakartidningen 40/1993;90:3456-64.
14) Ahmed AB, Home PD. The effect of the insulin analog lispro on nighttime blood glucose control in type 1 diabetic patients. Diabetes Care 1998;21:32-7.
15) Ahmed AB, Mallias J, Home PD. Optimization of evening insulin dose in patients using the short-acting insulin analog lispro. Diabetes Care 1998;21:1162-6.
16) Ahmed AM. Islamic pillars: possible adverse effects on diabetic patients. Pract Diab Internat 1997:96-97.
17) Airaghi L, Lorini M, Tedeschi A. The insulin analog aspart: a safe alternative in insulin allergy. Diabetes Care 2001;24:2000.
18) Åkerblom HK. Aetiological factors in type 1 diabetes. Nord Med 1992;107:204-6,230.
19) Alemzadeh R, Parton EA, Holzum MK. Feasibility of continuous subcutaneous insulin infusion and daily supplemental insulin glargine injection in children with type 1 diabetes. Diabetes Technol Ther 2009;11:481-6.
20) Al-Khawari M, Al-Ruwayeh A, Al-Doub K, Allgrove J. Adolescents on basal-bolus insulin can fast during Ramadan. Pediatr Diabetes 2010;11:96-100.
21) Åman J, Wranne L. Treatment of hypoglycaemia in diabetes: Failure of absorption of glucose through rectal mucosa. Acta Ped Scand 1984;73:560-61.
22) Åman J, Wranne L. Hypoglycaemia in childhood diabetes: I. Clinical signs and hormonal counterregulation. Acta Ped Scand 1988;77:542-7.
23) Åman J, Wranne L. Hypoglycaemia in childhood diabetes: II. Effect of subcutaneous or intramuscular injection of different doses of glucagon. Acta Ped Scand 1988;77:548-53.
24) American Academy of Pediatrics Work Group on Cows' Milk Protein and Diabetes Mellitus. Infant feeding practices and their possible relationship to the etiology of diabetes mellitus (RE9430). Pediatrics 1994/5;94:752-54.
25) American Diabetes Association. Diabetic retinopathy. Clinical Practice Recommendations 2003. Diabetes Care 2003;26(Suppl 1):S99-102.
26) American Diabetes Association. Clinical Practice Recommendations 2003. Diabetes Care 2003;26:Suppl 1.
27) American Diabetes Association. Report of the expert committe on the diagnosis and classification of diabetes mellitus. Diabetes Care 2003;26(Suppl 1):S5-20.
28) American Diabetes Association. Diabetic Retinopathy. Diabetes Care 1998;21:157-59.
29) American Diabetes Association. Care of children with diabetes in the school and day care setting. Clinical Practice Recommendations 2003. Diabetes Care 2003;26 (suppl 1):S131-135.
30) American Diabetes Association: Hyperglycemic crisis in patients with diabetes. Diabetes Care 2001;24:154-161.
31) American Diabetes Association: Tests of glycemia in diabetes. Clinical Practice Recommendations 2003. Diabetes Care 2003;26(Suppl 1):S106-108.
32) American Diabetes Association: Physical Activity/Exercise and Diabetes Mellitus. Clinical Practice Recommendations 2003. Diabetes Care 2003;26(Suppl 1):S73-77.
33) American Diabetes Association: Diabetic Nephropathy. Clinical Practice recommendations 2003. Diabetes Care 2003;26(Suppl 1):S94-98.
34) American Diabetes Association: Standards of Medical Care for Patients With Diabetes Mellitus. Clinical Practice recommendations 2003. Diabetes Care 2003;26(Suppl 1):S33-50.
35) American Diabetes Association. Standards of Medical Care in Diabetes—2010. Clinical Practice Recommendations 2003. Diabetes Care 2010;33 (Suppl 1):S11-S61.
36) Amiel SA, Pottinger RC, Archibald HR, Chusney G. Effect of antecedent glucose control on cerebral function during hypoglycaemia. Diabetes Care 1991;14: 109-118.
37) Amiel S. Gale E. Physiological responses to hypoglycaemia. Counterregulation and cognitive function. Diabetes Care 1993;16, suppl 3:48-55.
38) Amiel SA, Maran A, Powrie JK et al. Gender differences in counterregulation to hypoglycaemia. Diabetologia 1993;36:460-64.
39) Amiel SA. Hypoglycaemia in diabetes mellitus - protecting the brain. Diabetologia 1997;40:S62-S68.
40) Amiel SA. Cognitive function testing in studies of acute hypoglycaemia: rights and wrongs? Diabetologia 1998;41:713-9.
41) Anderson B, Laffel L. Behavioral and psychosocial research with school-aged children with type 1 diabetes. Diabetes Spectrum 1997;10:277-81.
42) Anderson BJ, Brackett J, Ho J, Laffel LM. An office-based intervention to maintain parent-adolescent teamwork in diabetes management. Impact on parent involvement, family conflict, and subsequent glycemic control. Diabetes Care. 1999 May;22(5):713-21.
43) Anderson JH, Brunelle RL, Koivisto VA, Pfützner A, Trautmann ME, Vignati L, DiMarchi R et al. Reduction of postprandial hyperglycemia and frequency of hypoglycemia in IDDM patients on insulin-analog treatment. Diabetes 1997;46:265-70.
44) Andersson H, Asp N-G, Hallmans G. Diet and diabetes. Scand J Nutrition 1986;30:78-90.
45) Annersten M, Frid A. Insulin pens dribble from the tip of the needle after injection. Pract Diab Int 2000;17:109-111.
46) Anzén B, Zetterström J. Postcoital contraception, a forgotten and unused resource? Lakartidningen 1992;89:2948-2950.
47) Apelqvist, J. Personal communication 1996.
48) Arbelaez AM, Semenkovich K, Hershey T. Glycemic extremes in youth with T1DM: The structural and functional integrity of the developing brain. Pediatr Diabetes 2013;14:541-53.
49) Ashwell SG, Amiel SA, Bilous RW, Dashora U, Heller SR, Hepburn DA, Shutler SD, Stephens JW, Home PD. Improved glycaemic control with insulin glargine plus insulin lispro: a multicentre, randomized, cross-over trial in people with Type 1 diabetes. Diabet Med 2006;23:285-92.
50) Asp NG. Nutritional classification and analysis of food carbohydrates. Am J Clin Nutr 1994;59:679S-681S.
51) Attia N, Jones TW, Holcombe J, Tamborlane WV. Comparison of human regular and lispro insulins after interruption of continuous subcutaneous insulin infusion and in the treatment of acutely decompensated IDDM. Diabetes Care 1998;21:817-21.
52) Attvall S, Lager I, Smith U. Rectal glucose administration cannot be used to treat hypoglycemia. Diabetes Care 1985;8:412-13.
53) Attvall S, Fowelin J, Lager I, Schenck H, Smith U. Smoking induces insulin resistance - a potential link with the insulin resistance syndrome. J Intern Med 1993;233:327-32.
54) Attvall S, Abrahamsson H, Schvarcz E, Berne C. Gastric emptying is important for the patients with diabetes. Lakartidningen 1995;92(45):4166-72.
55) Austin A, Warty V, Janosky J, Arslanian S. The relationship of physical fitness to lipid and lipoprotein(a) levels in adolescents with IDDM. Diabetes Care 1993;16:421-5.
56) Avogaro A, Beltramello P, Gnudi L, Maran A, Valerio A, Miola M, Marin N, Crepaldi C, Confortin L, Costa F, Macdonald I, Tiengo A. Alcohol intake impairs glucose counterregulation during acute insulin-induced hypoglycemia in IDDM patients. Diabetes 1993;42:1626-34.
57) Axelsen M, Wesslau C, Lonnroth P, Arvidsson Lenner R, Smith U. Bedtime uncooked cornstarch supplement prevents nocturnal hypoglycaemia in intensively treated type 1 diabetes subjects. J Intern Med 1999;245:229-36.
58) Aye T, Barnea-Goraly N, Ambler C, Hoang S, Schleifer K, Park Y, Drobny J, Wilson DM, Reiss AL, Buckingham BA. White matter structural differences in young children with type 1 diabetes: a diffusion tensor imaging study. Diabetes Care 2012;35:2167-73.
59) Backman VM, Thorsson AV, Fasquel A, Andrason HS, Kristjansson K, Gulcher JR, Stefansson K. HLA class II alleles and haplotypes in Icelandic Type I diabetic patients: comparison of Icelandic and Norwegian populations. Diabetologia 2002;45:452-3.
60) Baechle C, Castillo K, Strassburger K, Stahl-Pehe A, Meissner T, Holl RW, Giani G, Rosenbauer J, In Cooperation with the German Paediatric Surveillance U, the DPVSI. Is disordered eating behavior more prevalent in adolescents with early-onset type 1 diabetes than in their representative peers? Int J Eat Disord 2013;

61) Bagdade JD, Root RK, Bulger RJ. Impaired leukocyte function in patients with poorly controlled diabetes. Diabetes 1974;23:9-15.

62) Bancroft J. Sexual problems in diabetes. Diabetes Reviews International 1995;3:2-5.

63) Bantle JP, Weber MS, Rao SMS, Chattopadhyay MK, Robertson RP. Rotation of the anatomic regions used for insulin injections and day-to-day variability of plasma glucose in type 1 diabetic subjects. JAMA 1990;263: 1802-6.

64) Bantle JP, Neal L, Frankamp LM. Effects of the anatomical region used for insulin injections on glycemia in type 1 diabetes subjects. Diabetes Care 12/1993;16:1592-97.

65) Bardhan PK, Salam MA, Molla AM. Gastric emptying of liquid in children suffering from acute rotavirus gastroenteritis. Gut 1992;33:26-29.

66) Barkai L, Peja M. Impaired work capacity in diabetic children with autonomic dysfunction. Lecture, ISPAD, Atami, Japan 1994.

67) Barkai L, Vámosi I, Lukács K. Prospective assessment of severe hypoglycemia in diabetic children and adolsescents with impaired and normal awareness of hypoglycemia. Diabetologia 1998;41:898-903.

68) Barnea-Goraly N, Raman M, Mazaika P, Marzelli M, Hershey T, Weinzimer SA, Aye T, Buckingham B, Mauras N, White NH, et al. Alterations in white matter structure in young children with type 1 diabetes. Diabetes Care 2014;37:332-40.

69) Barnett AH, Eff C, Leslie RDG, Pyke DA. Diabetes in identical twins. Diabetologia 1981;20:87-93.

70) Bastyr III EJ, Holcombe JH, Anderson JH, Clore JN. Mixing insulin lispro and ultralente insulin. Diabetes Care 1997;20:1047-8.

71) Baudrie V, Chaouloff F. Mechanisms involved in the hyperglycemic effect of the 5-HT1C/5-HT2 receptor agonist, DOI. Eur J Pharmacol 1992;213:41-6.

72) Beaser R. Fine-tuning insulin therapy. Postgraduate Medicine 1992;91:4.

73) Beck RW, Buckingham B, Miller K, Wolpert H, Xing D, Block JM, Chase HP, Hirsch I, Kollman C, Laffel L, et al. Factors predictive of use and of benefit from continuous glucose monitoring in type 1 diabetes. Diabetes Care 2009;32:1947-53.

74) Becker DJ. Management of insulin-dependent diabetes mellitus in children and adolescents. Curr Opinion Ped 1991;3:710-23.

75) Becker RH, Frick AD, Burger F, Scholtz H, Potgieter JH. A comparison of the steady-state pharmacokinetics and pharmacodynamics of a novel rapid-acting insulin analog, insulin glulisine, and regular human insulin in healthy volunteers using the euglycemic clamp technique. Exp Clin Endocrinol Diabetes 2005;113(5):292-7.

76) Becker RH, Frick AD, Nosek L, Heinemann L, Rave K. Dose-response relationship of insulin glulisine in subjects with type 1 diabetes. Diabetes Care 2007;30:2506-7.

77) Beer SF, Lawson C, Watkins PJ. Neurosis induced by home monitoring of blood glucose concentrations. BMJ;298:362.

78) Behme MT, Dupre J, McDonald TJ. Glucagon-like peptide 1 improved glycemic control in type 1 diabetes. BMC Endocr Disord 2003;3:3.

79) Bell DS. Hyperglycaemia and ketosis induced by gamma hydroxybutyrate (GHB). Diabetologia 2010;53:1539-40.

80) Bendtson I, Gade J, Theilgaard A, Binder C. Cognitive function in Type 1 (insulin-dependent) diabetic patients after nocturnal hypoglycemia. Diabetologia 1992;35:898-903.

81) Bendtson I, Kverneland A, Pramming S, Binder C. Incidence of nocturnal hypoglycemia in insulin-dependent diabetic patients on intensive therapy. Acta Med Scand 1988;223:453-548.

82) Bennett PH, Haffner S, Kasiske BL, Keane WF, Mogensen CE, Parving HH, Steffes MW, Striker GE. Screening and management of microalbuminuria in patients with diabetes mellitus: Recommendations to the Scientific Advisory Board of the National Kidney Foundation from an Ad Hoc Committee of the Council on Diabetes Mellitus of the National Kidney Foundation. Am J Kidney Dis 1995;25:107-12.

83) Beregszàszi M, Tubiana-Rufi N, Benali K, Noel M, Bloch J, Czernichow P. Nocturnal hypoglycemia in children and adolescents with insulin- dependent diabetes mellitus: prevalence and risk factors. J Pediatr 1997;131:27-33.

84) Berg Kelly K. Living with diabetes. In the book: Diabetes. SPRI and Swedish Medical Society 1989: 285-90.

85) Berg TJ, Clausen JT, Torjesen PA, Dahl-Jørgensen K, Bangstad HJ Hanssen KF. The advanced glycation end product Nepsilon-(carboxymethyl)lysine is increased in serum from children and adolescents with type 1 diabetes. Diabetes Care 1998;21:1997-2002.

86) Berg TJ. Advanced glycation end products. Thesis, Aker University Hospital 1998.

87) Berger M, Cüppers J, Hegner H, Jörgens V, Berchthold P, Absorption kinetics and biologic effects of subcutaneously injected insulin preparations. Diabetes Care 1982;5:77-91.

88) Bernardini AL, Vanelli M, Chiari G, Iovane B, Gelmetti C, Vitale R, Errico MK. Adherence to physical activity in young people with type 1 diabetes. Acta Biomed Ateneo Parmense 2004;75:153-7.

89) Berne C, Hansson, Persson B. Pregnancy and diabetes. In the book: Diabetes. SPRI and Swedish Medical Society 1989: 119-134.

90) Berne C, Persson B. Pregnancy. In the book: Agardh C-D, Berne C, Östman J. Diabetes. Almqvist & Wiksell, Stockholm, 1992: 226-41.

91) Bierhaus A, Ziegler R Nawroth PP. Molecular mechanisms of diabetic angiopathy - clues for innovative therapeutic interventions. Horm Res 1998;50: 1-5.

92) Biessels GJ, Kappele AC, Bravenboer B, Erkelens DW, Gispen WH. Cerebral function in diabetes mellitus. Diabetologia 1994;37:643-50.

93) Biester T, Blaesig S, Remus K, Aschemeier B, Kordonouri O, Granhall C, Sondergaard F, Kristensen NR, Haahr H, Danne T. Insulin degludec's ultra-long pharmacokinetic properties observed in adults are retained in children and adolescents with type 1 diabetes. Pediatr Diabetes 2014;15:27-33.

94) Binder C, Lauritzen T, Faber O, Pramming S. Insulin pharmacokinetics. Diabetes Care 1984;7:188-199.

95) Bingham EM, Dunn JT, Smith D, Sutcliffe-Goulden J, Reed LJ, Marsden PK, Amiel SA. Differential changes in brain glucose metabolism during hypoglycaemia accompany loss of hypoglycaemia awareness in men with type 1 diabetes mellitus. An [11C]-3-O-methyl-D-glucose PET study. Diabetologia 2005;48:2080-9.

96) Birke G (Ed.) Drug Handbook. US English Pharmaceutical Company 1991-92, p 324.

97) Birkebaek NH, Johansen A, Solvig J. Cutis/subcutis thickness at insulin injection sites and localization of simulated insulin boluses in children with type 1 diabetes mellitus: need for individualization of injection technique? Diabet Med 1998;15:965-71.

98) Birkebaek NH, Solvig J, Hansen B, Jorgensen C, Smedegaard J, Christiansen JS. A 4-mm needle reduces the risk of intramuscular injections without increasing backflow to skin surface in lean diabetic children and adults. Diabetes Care 2008;31:e65.

99) Bjørgaas M, Sand T, Vik T, Jorde R. Quantitative EEG during controlled hypoglycaemia in diabetic and non-diabetic children. Diabet Med 1998;15: 30-7.

100) Björk E, Berne C, Kämpe O, Wibell L, Oskarsson P, Karlsson FA. Diazoxide treatment at onset preserves residual insulin secretion in adults with autoimmune diabetes. Diabetes 1996;45:1427-30.

101) Blackett PR. Insulin pump treatment for recurrent ketoacidosis in adolescence. Diabetes Care 1995;18:881-2.

102) Bleich D, Polak M, Eisenbarth GS, Jackson RA. Decreased risk of type 1 diabetes in offspring of mothers who acquire diabetes during adrenarchy. Diabetes 1993;42:1433-39.

103) Blohmé G. Insulin treatment - possibilities and limitations. Swedish Diabetes Association, Booklet no. 6, 1987.

104) Blom L, Nyström L, Dahlquist G. The Swedish childhood diabetes study. Vaccinations and infections as risk determinants for diabetes in childhood. Diabetologia 1991;34/3: 176-81.

105) Blom L, Persson LÅ, Dahlquist G. A high linear growth is associated with an increased risk of childhood diabetes mellitus. Diabetologia 1992;35:528-33.

106) Bloomgarden ZT. The 32nd annual meeting of the European Association for the Study of Diabetes. Neuropathy, health care, and glycation. Diabetes Care 1997;20:1037-9.

107) Blumer IR. Severe injection site reaction to insulin detemir. Diabetes Care 2006;29:946.

108) Bodansky HJ, Staines A, Stephenson C, Haigh D, Cartwright R. Evidence for an environmental effect in the aetiology of insulin dependent diabetes in a transmigratory population. Bmj 1992;304:1020-2.

109) Bode B, Steed D, Davidson P. Long-term pump use and SMBG in 205 patients. Diabetes 1994;43 (Suppl 1):220A.

110) Bode BW. Establishing & Veryfying Basal Rates. In the book: Fredrickson L (Ed.). The Insulin Pump Therapy Book. Insights from the experts. MiniMed, Los Angeles 1995.

111) Bode BW, Steed RD, Davidson PC. Reduction in severe hypoglycemia with long-term continuous subcutaneous insulin infusion in type 1 diabetes. Diabetes Care 1996;19:324-27.

112) Bode BW, Strange P. Efficacy, safety, and pump compatibility of insulin aspart used in continuous subcutaneous insulin infusion therapy in patients with type 1 diabetes. Diabetes Care 2001;24:69-72.

113) Bode BW, Gross TM, Thornton KR, Mastrototaro JJ. Continuous glucose monitoring used to adjust diabetes therapy improves glycosylated hemoglobin: a pilot study. Diabetes Res Clin Pract 1999;46:183-90.

114) Bode BW, Gross TM, Ghegan MB, Davidson PC. Factors Affecting the Reduction of Starting Insulin Dose in Continuous Subcutaneous Insulin Infusion (CSII): A Review of 389 Pump Initiations. Diabetes 2000;48(suppl. 1):abstract 264.

115) Bode BW, Strange P. Efficacy, safety, and pump compatibility of insulin aspart used in continuous subcutaneous insulin infusion therapy in patients with type 1 diabetes. Diabetes Care 2001;24:69-72.

116) Bode BW, Weinstein R, Bell D, McGill J, Nadeau D, Raskin P, Davidson J, Henry R, Huang WC, Reinhardt RR. Comparison of insulin aspart with buffered regular insulin and insulin lispro in continuous subcutaneous insulin infusion: a randomized study in type 1 diabetes. Diabetes Care 2002;25: 439-44.

117) Bode BW, Steed RD, Schleusener DS, Strange P. Switch to multiple daily injections with insulin glargine and insulin lispro from continuous subcutaneous insulin infusion with insulin lispro: a randomized, open-label study using a continuous glucose monitoring system. Endocr Pract 2005;11:157-64.

118) Bode B, Gross K, Rikalo N, Schwartz S, Wahl T, Page C, Gross T, Mastrototaro J. Alarms based on real-time sensor glucose values alert patients to hypo- and hyperglycemia: the guardian continuous monitoring system. Diabetes Technol Ther 2004;6:105-13.

119) Boëthius G, Gilljam H. Out of 1000 youngsters who smoke today 500 will die from smoking. Is further documentation necessary? Lakartidningen 119;92:375.

120) Bohannon N. Benefits of lispro insulin: control of postprandial glucose levels is within reach. Postgrad Med 1997 ;101/2:73-6, 79-80. (http://www.postgradmed.com/issues/1997/02_97/bohannon.htm).

121) Bohannon NJV. Treatment of vulvovaginal candidiasis in patients with diabetes. Diabetes Care 1998;21:451-56.

122) Bojestig M, Arnqvist H, Hermansson G, Karlberg B, Ludvigsson J. Declining incidence of nephropathy in insulin-dependent diabetes mellitus. New Engl J of Medicine 1994;330:15-18.

123) Bojestig M, Arnqvist H, Karlberg B, Ludvigsson J. Glycemic control and prognosis in type 1 diabetic patients with microalbuminuria. Diabetes Care 1996;19:313-17.

124) Bojestig M, Arnqvist HJ, Karlberg BE, Ludvigsson J. Unchanged incidence of severe retinopathy in a population of Type 1 diabetic patients with marked reduction of nephropathy. Diabet Med 1998;15:863-9.

125) Boland E, Ahern J, Ahern J, Vincent M. Pumps and kids: basal requirements for excellent metabolic control. Diabetes 2002:51(Suppl 2):A3 (abstract).

126) Bolinder J, Hagström-Toft E, Ungerstedt U, Arner P. Self-monitoring of blood glucose in type 1 diabetic patients: Comparison with continous microdialysis measurements of glucose in subcutaneous adipose tissue during ordinary life conditions. Diabetes Care 1997;20:64-70.

127) Bolli G, de Feo P, Compagnucci P, Cartechini MG, Angeletti G, Santeusanio F, Brunetti P, Gerich JE. Abnormal glucose counterregulation in insulin-dependent diabetes mellitus. Interaction of anti-insulin antibodies and impaired glucagon and epinephrine secretion. Diabetes 1983;32:134-41.

128) Bolli GB, De Feo P, De Cosmo S, Perriello G, Ventura MM, Calcinaro F, Lolli C, Campbell P, Brunetti P, Gerich JE. Demonstration of a dawn phenomenon in normal human volunteers. Diabetes 1984;33:1150-3.

129) Bolli G, Fanelli C, Perriello G, De Feo P. Nocturnal blood glucose control in type 1 diabetes mellitus. Diabetes Care 1993;16:suppl 3, 71-89.

130) Bolli GB, Di Marchi RD, Park GD, Pramming S, Koivisto VA. Insulin analogues and their potential in the management of diabetes mellitus. Diabetologia 1999;42:1151-67.

131) Boman A, Povlsen L, Dahlborg-Lyckhage E, Hanas R, Borup I. Fathers' encounter of support from paediatric diabetes teams; the tension between general recommendations and personal experience. Health Soc Care Community 2013;21:263-70.

132) Boman A, Povlsen L, Dahlborg-Lyckhage E, Hanas R, Borup IK. Fathers of Children With Type 1 Diabetes: Perceptions of a Father's Involvement From a Health Promotion Perspective. J Fam Nurs 2014;20:337-354.

133) Bondia J, Dassau E, Zisser H, Calm R, Vehi J, Jovanovic L, Doyle FJ. Coordinated Basal-bolus infusion for tighter postprandial glucose control in insulin pump therapy. J Diabetes Sci Technol 2009;3:89-97.

134) Bonfanti R, Bazzigaluppi E, Calori G, Riva MC, Viscardi M, Bognetti E, Meschi F, Bosi E, Chiumello G, Bonifacio E. Parameters associated with residual insulin secretion during the first year of disease in children and adolescents with Type 1 diabetes mellitus. Diabet Med 1998;15:844-50.

135) Borch-Johnsen K. Improving prognosis of type 1 diabetes. Mortality, accidents, and impact on insurance. Diabetes Care 1999;22 Suppl 2:B1-3.

136) Borghouts LB, Keizer HA. Exercise and insulin sensitivity: a review. Int J Sports Med 2000;21:1-12.

137) Bott S, Bott U, Berger M, Mühlhauser I. Intensified insulin therapy and the risk of severe hypoglycaemia. Diabetologia 1997;40:926-32.

138) Bottalico JN. Diabetes in pregnancy. J Am Osteopath Assoc 2001;101:S10-3.

139) Bottazo, GF. On the honey disease. Diabetes 1993;42:778-800.

140) Boyle PJ, Schwartz NS, Shah SD, Clutter WE, Cryer PE. Plasma glucose concentrations at the onset of hypoglycemic symtoms in patients with poorly controlled diabetes and in nondiabetes. N Engl J Med 1988;318:1487-92.

141) Boyle PJ, Kempers SF, O'Connor AM, Nagy RJ. Brain glucose uptake and unawareness of hypoglycemia in patients with insulin-dependent diabetes mellitus. N Engl J Med 1995;333:1726-31.

142) Braatvedt GD, Mildenhall L, Patten C, Harris G. Insulin requirements and metabolic control in children with diabetes mellitus attending a summer camp. Diabet Med 1997;14:258-61.

143) Brand-Miller J, Hayne S, Petocz P, Colagiuri S. Low-glycemic index diets in the management of diabetes: a meta-analysis of randomized controlled trials. Diabetes Care 2003;26(8):2261-7.

144) Braun D, Konrad D, Lang-Muritano M, Schoenle E. Improved glycemic control and lower frequency of severe hypoglycemia with insulin detemir; long-term experience in 105 children and adolescents with type 1 diabetes. Pediatr Diabetes 2008;9:382-7.

145) Brennan P, Buffler PA, Reynolds P, Wu AH, Wichmann HE, Agudo A, Pershagen G, Jockel KH, Benhamou S, Greenberg RS, et al. Secondhand smoke exposure in adulthood and risk of lung cancer among never smokers: a pooled analysis of two large studies. Int J Cancer 2004;109:125-31.

146) Brink SJ, Miller M, Moltz KC. Education and multidisciplinary team care concepts for pediatric and adolescent diabetes mellitus. J Pediatr Endocrinol Metab 2002;15:1113-30.

147) British Medical Association and Royal Pharmaceutical Society of Great Britain. British National Formulary. London, UK 2002.

148) Brodows G, Williams C, Amatruda J. Treatment of insulin reactions in diabetics. JAMA 24/1984;252:3378-3381.

149) Brown B. The effects of exercise on gastric emptying. Motility 1995/31:4-6.

150) Brubaker PL. Adventure travel and type 1 diabetes: the complicating effects of high altitude. Diabetes Care 2005;28:2563-72.

151) Brunelle BL, Llewelyn J, Anderson JH, Jr., Gale EA, Koivisto VA. Meta-analysis of the effect of insulin lispro on severe hypoglycemia in patients with type 1 diabetes. Diabetes Care 1998;21:1726-31.

152) Brunner GA, Hirschberger S, Sendlhofer G, Wutte A, Ellmerer M, Balent B, Schaupp L, Krejs GJ, Pieber TR. Post-prandial administration of the insulin analogue insulin aspart in patients with Type 1 diabetes mellitus. Diabet Med 2000;17:371-5.

153) Bryden KS, Neil A, Mayou RA, Peveler RC, Fairburn CG, Dunger DB. Eating habits, body weight, and insulin misuse: A longitudinal study of teenagers and young adults with type 1 diabetes. Diabetes Care 1999;22:1956-60.

154) Buckingham B, Beck RW, Tamborlane WV, Xing D, Kollman C, Fiallo-Scharer R, Mauras N, Ruedy KJ, Tansey M, Weinzimer SA, et al. Continuous glucose monitoring in children with type 1 diabetes. J Pediatr 2007;151: 388-93, 393 e1-2.

155) Buckingham B, Wilson DM, Lecher T, Hanas R, Kaiserman K, Cameron F. Duration of nocturnal hypoglycemia before seizures. Diabetes Care 2008; 31:2110-2.

156) Buckingham B, Xing D, Weinzimer S, Fiallo-Scharer R, Kollman C, Mauras N, Tsalikian E, Tamborlane W, Wysocki T, Ruedy K, et al. Use of the Direc-Net Applied Treatment Algorithm (DATA) for diabetes management with a real-time continuous glucose monitor (the FreeStyle Navigator). Pediatr Diabetes 2008;9:142-7.

157) Buhl M, Falck B, Norén T. Travel Medicine Handbook 2005. Travel Medicine Publishers, Aarhus, Danmark.

158) Bulsara MK, Holman CD, van Bockxmeer FM, Davis EA, Gallego PH, Beilby JP, Palmer LJ, Choong C, Jones TW. The relationship between ACE genotype and risk of severe hypoglycaemia in a large population-based cohort of children and adolescents with type 1 diabetes. Diabetologia 2007;50:965-71.

159) Burdick J, Chase HP, Slover RH, Knievel K, Scrimgeour L, Maniatis AK, Klingensmith GJ. Missed insulin meal boluses and elevated hemoglobin A1c levels in children receiving insulin pump therapy. Pediatrics 2004;113: e221-4.

160) Burdick P, Cooper S, Horner B, Cobry E, McFann K, Chase HP. Use of a subcutaneous injection port to improve glycemic control in children with type 1 diabetes. Pediatr Diabetes 2009;10:116-9.

161) Burge MK, Castillo KR, Schade DS. Meal composition is a determinant of Lispro-induced hypoglycemia in IDDM. Diabetes Care 1997;20/2:152-55.

162) Bussau VA, Ferreira LD, Jones TW, Fournier PA. The 10-s maximal sprint: a novel approach to counter an exercise-mediated fall in glycemia in individuals with type 1 diabetes. Diabetes Care 2006;29(3):601-6.

163) Buyken AE, Toeller M, Heitkamp G, Vitelli F, Stehle P, Scherbaum WA, Fuller JH and the EURODIAB IDDM Complications Study Group. Relation of fibre intake to HbA1c and the prevalence of severe ketoacidosis and severe hypoglycaemia. Diabetologia 1998;41(8):882-90.

164) Byrne HA, Tieszen KL, Hollis S, Dornan TL, New JP. Evaluation of an electrochemical sensor for measuring blood ketones. Diabetes Care 2000;23: 500-3.

165) Calafiore R, Basta G, Luca G, Lemmi A, Montanucci MP, Calabrese G, Racanicchi L, Mancuso F, Brunetti P. Microencapsulated pancreatic islet allografts into nonimmunosuppressed patients with type 1 diabetes: first two cases. Diabetes Care 2006;29:137-8.

166) Campaigne BN, Gilliam TB, Spencer ML, Lampman RM, Schork MA. Effects of a physical activity program on metabolic control and cardiovascular fitness in children with insulin-dependent diabetes mellitus. Diabetes Care 1984;7:57-62.

167) Campbell LV, Ashwell SM, Borkman M, Chrisholm DJ. White coat hyperglycemia: disparity between diabetes clinic and home blood glucose concentrations. BMJ 1992;305:1194-6.

168) The Canadian-European Randomized Control Trial Group. Cyclosporin-induced remission of IDDM after early intervention: association of 1 year of cyclosporin treatment with enhanced insulin secretion. Diabetes 1988; 37: 1574-82.

169) Canadian Diabetes Association. Clinical Practice Guidelines for the prevention and management of diabetes in Canada. Can J Diab 2008;32(suppl 1):S151.

170) Carlsson O. Against all odds. Diabetes (Swed. Diab. Ass.) 1994/3:30-31.

171) Carpelan C. Why don't they change lifestyle? Diabetes (Swed. Diab. Ass.) 3/93:34

172) Cars O, Uhnoo I, Linglöf T, Svenungsson B, Burman L. Self administration of antibiotics in traveller's diarrhea. Advantages are not in balance with the risk. Lakartidningen 36/1990;87:2751-52.

173) Caruso S, Rugolo S, Agnello C, Intelisano G, Di Mari L, Cianci A. Sildenafil improves sexual functioning in premenopausal women with type 1 diabetes who are affected by sexual arousal disorder: a double-blind, crossover, placebo-controlled pilot study. Fertil Steril. 2006 May;85(5):1496-501.

174) Casella SJ, Mongilio MK, Plotnick LP, Hesterberg MP, Long CA. Accuracy and precision of low-dose insulin administration. Pediatrics 1993;91/6: 1155-57.

175) CDC Clinical Reminders 2012: Insulin pens must never be used for more than one person. www.cdc.gov/injectionsafety/PDF/Clinical-Reminder-insulin-pen.pdf

176) Cedermark G. Selenius M. Tullus K. The postprandial blood glucose response to sucrose/glucose intake in a mixed snack in diabetic teenagers. Acta Pediatr Scand 1990;79: 473-474.

177) Cedermark G. Selenius M. Tullus K. Glycaemic effect and satiating capacity of potato chips and milk chocolate bar as snacks in teenagers with diabetes. Eur J Pediatr 1993;152:635-39.

178) Cengiz E, Tamborlane WV, Martin-Fredericksen M, Dziura J, Weinzimer SA. Early pharmacokinetic and pharmacodynamic effects of mixing lispro with glargine insulin: results of glucose clamp studies in youth with type 1 diabetes. Diabetes Care 2010;33:1009-12.

179) Cengiz E, Swan KL, Tamborlane WV, Sherr JL, Martin M, Weinzimer SA. The alteration of aspart insulin pharmacodynamics when mixed with detemir insulin. Diabetes Care 2012;35:690-2.

180) Cengiz E, Weinzimer SA, Sherr JL, Tichy E, Martin M, Carria L, Steffen A, Tamborlane WV. Acceleration of insulin pharmacodynamic profile by a novel insulin infusion site warming device. Pediatr Diabetes 2013;14:168-73.

181) Cengiz E, Xing D, Wong JC, Wolfsdorf JI, Haymond MW, Rewers A, Shanmugham S, Tamborlane WV, Willi SM, Seiple DL, et al. Severe hypoglycemia and diabetic ketoacidosis among youth with type 1 diabetes in the T1D Exchange clinic registry. Pediatr Diabetes 2013;14:447-54.

182) Cerami C, Founds H, Nicholl I, Mitsuhashi T, Giordano D, Vanpatten S, Lee A, Al-Abed Y, Vlassara H, Bucala R, et al. Tobacco smoke is a source of toxic reactive glycation products. Proc Natl Acad Sci U S A 1997;94:13915-20.

183) Cersosimo E, Garlick P, Ferretti J. Renal glucose production during insulin-induced hypoglycemia in humans. Diabetes 1999;48:261-6.

184) Chalew SA, Gomez R, Butler A, Hempe J, Compton T, Mercante D, Rao J, Vargas A. Predictors of glycemic control in children with type 1 diabetes: the importance of race. J Diabetes Complications 2000;14:71-7.

185) Chantelau E, Heinemann L, Ross D. Air bubbles in insulin pens. Lancet 1989;336:387-88.

186) Chantelau E, Lee DM, Hemmann DM, Zipfel U, Echterhoff S. What makes insulin injections painful? BMJ 1991;303:26-7.

187) Charron-Prochownik D, Maihle T, Siminerio L, Songer T. Outpatient versus inpatient care of children newly diagnosed with IDDM. Diabetes Care 1997; 20:657-60.

188) Chase HP, Crews KR, Garg S, Crews MJ, Cruickshanks KJ, Klingensmith G, Gay E, Hamman, RF. Outpatient management vs in-hospital management of children with new-onset diabetes. Clinical Ped 1990:29:450-56.

189) Chase HP, Garg SK, Marshall G, Berg CL, Harris S, Jackson WE, Hamman RE. Cigarette smoking increases the risk of albuminuria among subjects with type I diabetes. Jama 1991;265:614-7.

190) Chase HP, Saib SZ, MacKenzie T, Hansen MM, Garg SK. Post-prandial glucose excursions following four methods of bolus insulin administration in subjects with Type 1 diabetes. Diabet Med 2002;19:317-21.

191) Chase HP, Beck R, Tamborlane W, Buckingham B, Mauras N, Tsalikian E, Wysocki T, Weinzimer S, Kollman C, Ruedy K, Xing D. A randomized multicenter trial comparing the GlucoWatch Biographer with standard glucose monitoring in children with type 1 diabetes. Diabetes Care 2005: 28: 1101-1106.

192) Chaturvedi N, Stevens L, Fuller JH, WHO Multinational Study Group. Which features of smoking determine mortality risk in former cigarette smokers with diabetes? Diabetes Care 1997;20:1266-72.

193) Chew I, Brand JC, Thorburn AW, Truswell AS. Application of glycemic index to mixed meals. Am J Clin Nutr 1988;47:53-6.

194) Chiarelli F, de Martino M, Mezzetti A, Catino M, Morgese G, Cuccurullo F, Verrotti A. Advanced glycation end products in children and adolescents with diabetes: relation to glycemic control and early microvascular complications. J Pediatr 1999;134:486-91.

195) Chiasson, J L. Ducros, F. Poliquin-Hamet, M. Lopez, D. Lecavalier, L. Hamet, P. Continous subcutaneous insulin infusion (Mill-Hill Infuser) versus multiple injections (Medi-Jector) in the treatment of insulindependent diabetes mellitus and the effect of metabolic control on microangiopathy. Diabetes Care 1984 ;4: 331-37.

196) Chng HH, Leong KP, Loh. Primary systemic allergy to human insulin: recurrence of generalized urticaria after successful desensitization. Allergy 1995;50/12:984-87.

197) Christiansson J. The diabetic eye. Swedish Diabetes Association, Booklet no. 1, 1992.

198) Chlup R, Marsálek E, Bruns W. A prospective study of multiple use of disposable syringes and needles in intensified insulin therapy. Diabet Med 1990;7:624-7.

199) Ciofetta M, Lalli C, Del Sindaco P, Torlone E, Pampanelli S, Mauro L, Chiara DL, Brunetti P, Bolli GB. Contribution of postprandial versus interprandial blood glucose to HbA1c in type 1 diabetes on physiologic intensive therapy with lispro insulin at mealtime. Diabetes Care 1999;22:795-800.

200) Clarke W, Jones T, Rewers A, Dunger D, Klingensmith GJ. Assessment and management of hypoglycemia in children and adolescents with diabetes. Pediatr Diabetes 2009;10 Suppl 12:134-45.

201) Cohen M. Changing from regular to lispro insulin: Lessons after 2 years. Diabetes 1999;48(Suppl 1):abstract 1562.

202) Colquitt J, Royle P, Waugh N. Are analogue insulins better than soluble in continuous subcutaneous insulin infusion? Results of a meta-analysis. Diabet Med 2003;20:863-6.

203) Combs CA, Gavin AL, Gunderson E, Main EK, Kitzmiller JL. Relationship of fetal macrosomia to maternal postprandial glucose control during pregnancy. Diabetes Care 1992;15:1251-57.

204) Confidential Enquiry into Maternal and Child Health: Pregnancy in Women with Type 1 and Type 2 Diabetes in 2002–03, England,Wales and Northern Ireland. London: CEMACH; 2005.

205) Conrad SC, McGrath MT, Gitelman SE. Transition from multiple daily injections to continuous subcutaneous insulin infusion in type 1 diabetes mellitus. J Pediatr 2002;140:235-40.

206) Consensus Guidelines for the Management of Insulin-dependent (Type 1) Diabetes. Implementing the St Vincent Declaration. European IDDM Policy Group, Medicom Europe BV, Bussum, The Netherlands 1993.

207) Cornish A, Chase HP. Navigating airport security with an insulin pump and/ or sensor. Diabetes Technol Ther 2012;14:984-5.

208) Cox DJ. Gonder-Frederick L, Clarke W. Driving decrements in type 1 diabetes during moderate hypoglycemia. Diabetes 1993;42:239-43.

209) Cox D, Taylor A, Nowdeek G, Holley-Wilcox P, Pohl SN. The relationship between psychological stress and insulin-dependent diabetic blood glucose control: preliminary investigations. Health Psychol 1984;63-75.

210) Cox D, Gonder-Frederick L, Polonsky W, Schlundt D, Julian D, Clarke W. A multicenter evaluation of blood glucose awareness training-II. Diabetes Care 1995;18:523-28.

211) Cox DJ, Kovatchev BP, Gonder-Frederick LA, Summers KH, McCall A, Grimm KJ, Clarke WL. Relationships between hyperglycemia and cognitive performance among adults with type 1 and type 2 diabetes. Diabetes Care 2005;28:71-7.

212) Coustan DR. Gestational Diabetes. Diabetes Care 1993;16 (Suppl 3):8-15.

213) Creutzfeldt WO, Kleine N, Willms B, Orskov C, Holst JJ, Nauck MA. Glucagonostatic actions and reduction of fasting hyperglycemia by exogenous glucagon-like peptide I(7-36) amide in type I diabetic patients. Diabetes Care 1996;19:580-6.

214) Cryer P, Gerich J. Hypoglycemia in insulin-dependent diabetes mellitus. In the book: Rifkin H, Porte D. Diabetes Mellitus, Theory and Practice. Elsevier 1990:526-46.

215) Cryer P. Iatrogenic hypoglycemia as a cause of hypoglycemia-associated autonomic failure in IDDM. Diabetes 1992;41:255-60.

216) Cryer P. Perspectives in Diabetes. Hypoglycemia begets hypoglycemia in IDDM. Diabetes 1993;42:1691-93.

217) Cryer PE. Hypoglycemia unawareness in IDDM. Diabetes Care 1993;16, suppl 3:40-47.

218) Cryer P, Fisher J, Shamoon H. Hypoglycemia. Diabetes Care 1994;17:734-55.

219) Cuenca-Garcia M, Jago R, Shield JP, Burren CP. How does physical activity and fitness influence glycaemic control in young people with Type 1 diabetes? Diabet Med 2012;29:e369-76.

220) Cullen M. A life less ordinary. Balance 2000/178.

221) Cutfield WS, Peart JM, Thompson JMD, Holt J, Jefferies CA, Lawton SA, Hofman P. Prepubertal children are at high risk of intramuscular insulin administration based upon subcutaneous fat thickness. JPEM 2002;15(Suppl 4): 1076(abstract).

222) The DAFNE study group. Training in flexible, intensive insulin management to enable dietary freedom in people with type 1 diabetes: dose adjustment for normal eating (DAFNE) randomised controlled trial. BMJ 2002;325:746.

223) Dagogo-Jack S, Craft S, Cryer P. Hypoglycemia-associated autonomic failure in insulin-dependent diabetes mellitus. J Clin Invest. 1993;91:819-28.

224) Dahl-Jørgensen K, Brinchmann-Hansen O, Hanssen KF, Sandvik L, Aagenaes O. Rapid tightening of blood glucose control leads to transient deterioration of retinopathy in insulin dependent diabetes mellitus: the Oslo study. Br Med J (Clin Res Ed) 1985;290:811-5.

225) Dahl-Jørgensen K, Brinchmann-Hansen O, Hanssen K, Ganes T, Kierulf P, Smeland E. Effect of near normoglycaemia for two years on progression of early diabetic retinopathy, nephropathy and neuropathy: the Oslo study. BMJ 1986; 293: 1195-9.

226) Dahl-Jørgensen K, Torjesen P, Hanssen KF, Sandvik L, Aagenaes O. Increase in insulin antibodies during continuous subcutaneous insulin infusion and multiple-injection therapy in contrast to conventional treatment. Diabetes 1987;36:1-5.

227) Dahl-Jørgensen K, Joner G, Hanssen KF. Relationship between cows' milk consumption and incidence of IDDM in childhood. Diabetes Care 1991;14: 1081-83.

228) Dahlquist G, Blom L, Holmgren G, Hägglöf B, Wall S. Epidemiology of diabetes in Swedish children 0-14 years of age. A six year prospective study. Diabetologia 1985; 28:802-8.

229) Dahlquist G, Blom L, Persson LÅ, Sandström A, Wall S. Dietary factors and the risk of developing insulin dependent diabetes in childhood. BMJ 1990; 300:1302-6.

230) Dahlquist G. Epidemiology of type 1-diabetes. In the book: Agardh C-D, Berne C, Östman J. Diabetes. Almqvist & Wiksell, Stockholm 1992:50-55.

231) Dahlquist G, Savilahti E, Landin-Olsson M. An increased level of antibodies to β-lactoglobulin is a risk determinant for early-onset type-I (insulin dependent) diabetes mellitus independently of islet cell antibodies and early introduction of cows' milk. Diabetologia 1992;35:980-84.

232) Dahlquist GG, Mustonen LR. Clinical onset characteristics of familial versus nonfamilial cases in a large population-based cohort of childhood-onset diabetes patients. Diabetes Care, 1995;18/6,:852-4.

233) Dahlquist G, Frisk G, Ivarsson SA, Svanberg L, Forsgren M, Diderholm H. Indications that maternal coxsachie B virus infection during pregnancy is a risk factor for childhood-onset IDDM. Diabetologia 1995;38:1371-73.

234) Dahlquist G, Gothefors L. The cumulative incidence of childhood diabetes mellitus in Sweden unaffected by BCG-vaccination. Diabetologia 1995;38: 7, 873-4.

235) Dahlquist G, Frisk G, Ivarsson SA et al. Indications that maternal Coxsackie B virus infection during pregnancy is a risk factor for childhood-onset IDDM. Diabetologia 1995;38:1371-3.

236) Dahlquist GG, Kallen BAJ. Time-space clustering of date at birth in childhood-onset diabetes. Diabetes Care 1996;19:328-32.

237) Dahlquist G, Mustonen L. Analysis of 20 years of prospective registration of childhood onset diabetes time trends and birth cohort effects. Swedish Childhood Diabetes Study Group. Acta Paediatr 2000;89:1231-7.

238) Dahlquist G, Kallen B. Mortality in childhood-onset type 1 diabetes: a population-based study. Diabetes Care 2005;28:2384-7.

239) Dahlquist GG, Pundziute-Lycka A, Nystrom L. Birthweight and risk of type 1 diabetes in children and young adults: a population-based register study. Diabetologia 2005;48:1114-7.

240) Dahlquist G, Kallen B. School performance in children with type 1 diabetes–a population-based register study. Diabetologia 2007;50:957-64.

241) Daley KB, Wodrich DL, Hasan K. Classroom attention in children with type 1 diabetes mellitus: the effect of stabilizing serum glucose. J Pediatr 2006; 148:201-6.

242) Daly ME, Vale C, Littlefield A, Walker M, Alberti KGMM. Altering food preparation decreases glycemic response with a greater decrease in insulin response. Diab Med 2000;17(Suppl 1):Abstract P132.

243) Damm P, Mathiesen E, Clausen TD, Petersen KR. Contraception for women with diabetes mellitus. Metab Syndr Relat Disord 2005;3:244-9.

244) Dammacco F, Torelli C, Frezza E, Piccinno F Tansella F. Problems of hypoglycemia arising in children and adolescents with insulin-dependent diabetes mellitus. The Diabetes Study Group of The Italian Society of Pediatric Endocrinology & Diabetes. J Pediatr Endocrinol Metab 1998;11 Suppl 1:167-76.

245) Daneman D, Olmsted M, Rydall A, Maharaj S, Rodin G. Eating disorders in young women with type 1 diabetes. Prevalence, problems and prevention. Horm Res 1998;50:79-86.

246) Danne T, Weber B, Hartmann R, Enders I, Burger W, Hovener G. Long-term glycemic control has a nonlinear association to the frequency of background retinopathy in adolescents with diabetes. Diabetes Care 1994;17: 1390-96.

247) Danne T, Mortensen HB, Hougaard P, Lynggaard H, Aanstoot HJ, Chiarelli F, Daneman D, Dorchy H, Garandeau P, Greene SA, et al. Persistent differences among centers over 3 years in glycemic control and hypoglycemia in a study of 3,805 children and adolescents with type 1 diabetes from the Hvidore Study Group. Diabetes Care 2001;24:1342-7.

248) Danne T, Aman J, Schober E, Deiss D, Jacobsen JL, Friberg HH, Jensen LH. A comparison of postprandial and preprandial administration of insulin aspart in children and adolescents with type 1 diabetes. Diabetes Care 2003;26:2359-64.

249) Danne T, Lupke K, Walte K, Von Schuetz W, Gall MA. Insulin detemir is characterized by a consistent pharmacokinetic profile across age-groups in

children, adolescents, and adults with type 1 diabetes. Diabetes Care 2003;26:3087-92.

250) Danne T, Becker RH, Heise T, Bittner C, Frick AD, Rave K. Pharmacokinetics, prandial glucose control, and safety of insulin glulisine in children and adolescents with type 1 diabetes. Diabetes Care 2005;28:2100-5.

251) Danne T, Endahl L, Haahr H, Datz N, Nestoris C, Westergaard L, Kordonouri O. Lower within-subject variability in pharmacokinetic profiles of insulin detemir in comparison to insulin glargine in children and adolescents with type 1 diabetes. Diabetologia 2007;50(Suppl 1):S84(abstract).

252) Danne T, Battelino T, Jarosz-Chobot P, Kordonouri O, Pankowska E, Ludvigsson J, Schober E, Kaprio E, Saukkonen T, Nicolino M, Tubiana-Rufi N, Klinkert C, Haberland H, Vazeou A, Madacsy L, Zangen D, Cherubini V, Rabbone I, Toni S, de Beaufort C, Bakker-van Waarde W, van den Berg N, Volkov I, Barrio R, Hanas R, Zumsteg U, Kuhlmann B, Aebi C, Schumacher U, Gschwend S, Hindmarsh P, Torres M, Shehadeh N, Phillip M. Establishing glycaemic control with continuous subcutaneous insulin infusion in children and adolescents with type 1 diabetes: experience of the PedPump Study in 17 countries. Diabetologia 2008;51:1594-601.

253) Danne T, Kordonouri O, Holder M, Haberland H, Golembowski S, Remus K, Blasig S, Wadien T, Zierow S, Hartmann R, et al. Prevention of hypoglycemia by using low glucose suspend function in sensor-augmented pump therapy. Diabetes Technol Ther 2011;13:1129-34.

254) Datta V, Swift PG, Woodruff GH, Harris RF. Metabolic cataracts in newly diagnosed diabetes. Arch Dis Child 1997;76:118-120.

255) Davidson PC, Hebblewhite HR, Steed RD, Bode BW. Analysis of guidelines for basal-bolus insulin dosing: basal insulin, correction factor, and carbohydrate-to-insulin ratio. Endocr Pract 2008;14:1095-101.

256) Davis EA, Soong SA, Byrne GC, Jones TW. Acute hyperglycaemia impairs cognitive function in children with IDDM. J Pediatr Endocrinol Metab 1996; 9:455-61.

257) Davis EA, Jones TW. Hypoglycemia in children with diabetes: incidence, counterregulation and cognitive dysfunction. J Pediatr Endocrinol Metab 1998;11 Suppl 1:177-82.

258) Davis EA, Keating B, Byrne GC, Russel M, Jones TW. Hypoglycemic incidence and clinical predictors in a large population-based sample of children and adolescents with IDDM. Diabetes Care 1997;20:22-25.

259) Davis EA, Keating B, Byrne GC, Russell M, Jones TW. Impact of improved glycaemic control on rates of hypoglycaemia in insulin dependent diabetes mellitus. Arch Dis Child 1998;78:111-5.

260) The DCCT Research group. Diabetes control and complications study (DCCT): Results of feasibility study. Diabetes Care 1987;10:1-19.

261) The DCCT Research Group. The effect of intensive treatment of diabetes on the development and progression of long-term complications in insulindependent diabetes mellitus. N Engl J Med 1993;329:977-986.

262) The DCCT Research Group. Effect of intensive diabetes treatment on the development and progression of long-term complications in adolescents with insulin-dependent diabetes mellitus: Diabetes Control and Complications Trial. J Ped 1994;125:177-88.

263) The DCCT Research Group. The relationship of glycemic exposure (HbA$_{1c}$) to the risk of development and progression of retinopathy in the Diabetes Control and Complications Trial. Diabetes 1995;44:968-83.

264) The DCCT Research Group. Adverse events and their association with treatment regimens in the Diabetes Control and Complications Trial. Diabetes Care 1995;18:1415-27.

265) The DCCT Research Group. Effects of intensive diabetes therapy on neuropsychological function in adults in the Diabetes Control and Complications Trial. Ann Intern Med 1996;124:379-88.

266) The DCCT Study Group. Pregnancy outcomes in the Diabetes Control And Complications Trial. Am J Obstet 1996;174/4;1343-53.

267) The DCCT Study Group. Influence of intensive diabetes treatment on quality-of-life outcomes in the Diabetes Control and Complications Study. Diabetes Care 1996;19:195-203.

268) The DCCT Research Group. Clustering of long-term complications in families with diabetes in the diabetes control and complications trial. The Diabetes Control and Complications Trial Research Group. Diabetes 1997;46: 1829-39.

269) The DCCT Research Group. Effect of intensive therapy on residual beta-cell function in patients with type 1 diabetes in the diabetes control and complications trial. A randomized, controlled trial. Ann Intern Med 1998;128: 517-23.

270) The DCCT Research Group. Early worsening of diabetic retinopathy in the Diabetes Control and Complications Trial. Arch Ophtalmol 1998;116:874-76.

271) The DCCT Research Group. Effect of pregnancy on microvascular complications in the diabetes control and complications trial. Diabetes Care 2000; 23:1084-91.

272) The DCCT Research Group. Summary of revisions for the 2006 Clinical Practice Recommendations. Diabetes Care 2006;29 Suppl 1:S3.

273) The DCCT/EDIC writing team. Effect of intensive therapy on the microvascular complications of type 1 diabetes mellitus. Jama 2002;287:2563-9.

274) The DCCT/EDIC writing team. Sustained effect of intensive treatment of type 1 diabetes mellitus on development and progression of diabetic nephropathy: the Epidemiology of Diabetes Interventions and Complications (EDIC) study. Jama 2003;290(16):2159-67.

275) de Beaufort CE, Swift PG, Skinner CT, Aanstoot HJ, Aman J, Cameron F, Martul P, Chiarelli F, Daneman D, Danne T, et al. Continuing stability of center differences in pediatric diabetes care: do advances in diabetes treatment improve outcome? The Hvidoere Study Group on Childhood Diabetes. Diabetes Care 2007;30:2245-50.

276) Debrah K, Sherwin RS, Murphy J, Kerr D. Effect of caffeine on recognition of and physiological responses to hypoglycaemia in insulin-dependent diabetes. Lancet 1996;347:19-24.

277) Dedorsson I, Eye complications. In the book: Diabetes. SPRI and Swedish Medical Society 1989:135 - 42.

278) Deeb LC, Holcombe JH, Brunelle R, Zalani S, Brink S, Jenner M, Kitson H, Perlman K, Spencer M. Insulin lispro lowers postprandial glucose in prepubertal children with diabetes. Pediatrics 2001;108:1175-9.

279) DeFronzo RA, Hendler R, Christensen N. Stimulation of counterregulatory hormonal response in diabetic man by a fall in glucose concentration. Diabetes 1980;29:125-131.

280) DeFronzo RA, Matsuda M, Barret EJ. Diabetic ketoacidosis. A combined metabolic-nephrologic approach to therapy. Diabetes Reviews 1994;2:209-38.

281) Deiss D, Bolinder J, Riveline JP, Battelino T, Bosi E, Tubiana-Rufi N, et al. Improved glycemic control in poorly controlled patients with type 1 diabetes using real-time continuous glucose monitoring. Diabetes Care 2006; 29(12):2730-2.

282) Deiss D, Kordonouri O, Hartmann R, Hopfenmuller W, Lupke K, Danne T. Treatment with insulin glargine reduces asymptomatic hypoglycemia detected by continuous subcutaneous glucose monitoring in children and adolescents with type 1 diabetes. Pediatric diabetes. 2007; 8:157-62.

283) Del Sindaco P, Ciofetta M, Lalli C, Perriello G, Pampanelli S, Torlone E, Brunetti P, Bolli GB. Use of the short-acting insulin analogue lispro in intensive treatment of type 1 diabetes mellitus: importance of appropriate replacement of basal insulin and time-interval injection-meal. Diabet Med 1998; 15:592-600.

284) Delahanty LM, Halford BN. The role of diet behaviors in achieving improved glycemic control in intensively treated patients in the Diabetes Control and Complications Trial. Diabetes Care 1993;16:1453-8.

285) Denker P, Leonard D, DiMarco P, Maleski P. An easy sliding scale formula. Diabetes Care 1995;18:278.

286) Department of Health. National Service Framework for Diabetes (England) Standards. London: The Stationery Office; 2001 [www.dh.gov.uk/PublicationsAndStatistics/Publications/PublicationsPolicyAndGuidance/PublicationsPolicyAndGuidanceArticle/fs/en?CONTENT ID=4002951&chk=09Kkz1].

287) DeStefano F, Mullooly JP, Okoro CA, Chen RT, Marcy SM, Ward JI, Vadheim CM, Black SB, Shinefield HR, Davis RL, et al. Childhood vaccinations, vaccination timing, and risk of type 1 diabetes mellitus. Pediatrics 2001;108: E112.

288) Detlofsson I, Kroon M, Aman J. Oral bedtime cornstarch supplementation reduces the risk for nocturnal hypoglycaemia in young children with type 1 diabetes. Acta Paediatr 1999;88:595-7.

289) Diabetes Health 2007: http://www.diabeteshealth.com/read/2007/04/26/5150/type-1-pop-star-nick-jonas-tells-his-story/

290) Diabetes Prevention Trial. Effects of insulin in relatives of patients with type 1 diabetes mellitus. N Engl J Med 2002;346:1685-91.

291) DiaMond Project Group on Social Issues. Global regulations on diabetics treated witn insulin and their operation of commercial motor vehicles. BMJ 1993;307:250-53.

292) Dinneen S, Alzaid D, Rizza. Failure of glucagon suppression contributes to postprandial hyperglycemia in IDDM. Diabetologia 1995;38:337-43.

293) Dixon B, Peter Chase H, Burdick J, Fiallo-Scharer R, Walravens P, Klingensmith G, et al. Use of insulin glargine in children under age 6 with type 1 diabetes. Pediatric Diabetes 2005;6(3):150-4.

294) Dixon AN, Bain SC. Nausea and vomiting due to insulin glargine in patient with type 1 diabetes mellitus. Bmj 2005;330:455.

295) Domargard A, Sarnblad S, Kroon M, Karlsson I, Skeppner G, Aman J. Increased prevalence of overweight in adolescent girls with type 1 diabetes mellitus. Acta Paediatr 1999;88:1223-8.

296) Donaghue KC, King J, Fung ATW, Chan A, Hing S, Howard NJ, Fairchild J, Silink M. The effect of prepubertal diabetes duration on diabetes microvascular complications in early and late adolescence. Diabetes Care 1997;20: 77-80.

297) Donaghue KC, Pena MM, Chan AK, Blades BL, King J, Storlien LH, et al. Beneficial effects of increasing monounsaturated fat intake in adolescents with type 1 diabetes. Diabetes Res Clin Pract 2000;48:193-9.

298) Donaghue KC, Fairchild JM, Craig ME, Chan AK, Hing S, Cutler LR, Howard NJ, Silink M. Do all prepubertal years of diabetes duration contribute equally to diabetes complications? Diabetes Care 2003;26:1224-9.

299) Donaghue KC, Chiarelli F, Trotta D, Allgrove J, Dahl-Jorgensen K. Microvascular and macrovascular complications associated with diabetes in children and adolescents. Pediatric Diabetes 2009;10:195–203.

300) Dorchy H. What level of HbA$_{1c}$ can be achieved in young patients beyond the honeymoon period? Diabetes Care 1993;16:1311-13.

301) Dorman JS, O'Leary LA, Koehler AN. Epidemiology of childhood diabetes. In the book: Childhood and adolescent diabetes. Chapman & Hall Medical, London 1995.

302) Douvin C, Zinelabine H, Wirquin V, Perlemuter C, Dhumeaux D. An outbreak of hepatitis B in an endocrinology unit traced to an capillary-blood-sampling device. N Engl J Med 1991;322:57.

303) Downie E, Craig ME, Hing S, Cusumano J, Chan AK, Donaghue KC. Continued reduction in the prevalence of retinopathy in adolescents with type 1 diabetes: role of insulin therapy and glycemic control. Diabetes Care 2011; 34:2368-73.

304) Draelos MT, Jacobson AM, Weinger K, Widom B, Ryan CM, Finkelstein DM, Simonson DC. Cognitive function in patients with insulin-dependent diabetes mellitus during hyperglycemia and hypoglycemia. Am J Med 1995;98: 135-144.

305) Drexler AJ. Pump therapy in preconception and pregnancy. In the book: Fredrickson L (Ed.). The Insulin Pump Therapy Book. Insights from the experts. MiniMed, Los Angeles 1995.

306) Duffin AC, Donaghue KC, Potter M, McInnes A, Chan AK, King J, Howard NJ, Silink M. Limited joint mobility in the hands and feet of adolescents with Type 1 diabetes mellitus. Diabet Med 1999;16:125-30.

307) Dunger DB, Edge JA. Diabetes and endocrine changes of puberty. Pract Diab Internat 1995;12:63-66.

308) Dunger DB, Sperling MA, Acerini CL, Bohn DJ, Daneman D, Danne TP, Glaser NS, Hanas R, Hintz RL, Levitsky LL, et al. ESPE/LWPES consensus

statement on diabetic ketoacidosis in children and adolescents. Arch Dis Child 2004;89:188-94.

309) Dunn SM. Psychological issues in diabetes management: (I) Blood glucose monitoring and learned helplessness. Practical Diabetes 1987;4:108-10.

310) Eapen SS, Connor EL, Gern JE. Insulin desensitization with insulin lispro and an insulin pump in a 5-year-old child. Ann Allergy Asthma Immunol 2000;85:395-7.

311) Early Treatment Diabetic Retinopathy Study Group: Aspirin effects on mortality and morbidity in patients with diabetes mellitus. JAMA 1992;268: 1292-300.

312) EASD, The Diabetes and Nutrition Study Group(DNSG). Recommendations for the nutritional management for patients with diabetes mellitus. Euro J Clin Nutr 2000;54:353-56.

313) Eastman RC, Chase HP, Buckingham B, Hathout EH, Fuller-Byk L, Leptien A, Wyhe MMV, Davis TL, Fermi SJ, Pechler H, et al. Use of the GlucoWatch biographer in children and adolescents with diabetes. Pediatric Diabetes 2002;3:127-134.

314) Ebeling P, Tuominen JA, Bourey R, Koranyi L, Koivisto VA. Athletes with IDDM exhibit impaired metabolic control and increased lipid utilization with no increase in insulin sensitivity. Diabetes 1995;44:471-7.

315) Ebeling P, Jansson PA, Smith U, Lalli C, Bolli GB, Koivisto VA. Strategies toward improved control during insulin lispro therapy in IDDM. Importance of basal insulin. Diabetes Care 1997;20:1287-9.

316) Eckert B, Ryding E, Agardh CD. The cerebral vascular response to a rapid decrease in blood glucose to values above normal in poorly controlled type 1 (insulin-dependent) diabetes mellitus. Diabetes Res Clin Pract, 1995; 27/3:221-7.

317) Eckert B, Rosén I, Stenberg G, Agardh CD. The recovery of brain function after hypoglycemia in normal man. Diabetologia 1992;35 (Suppl 1): abstract 161.

318) Edge C. Diving and diabetes. UK Sports Diving Medical Committee. http://www.ukdiving.co.uk/ukdiving/info/medicine/diabetes.htm

319) Edge C, Bryson P. Insulin-dependent diabetes mellitus. In the book: Edmonds C, Lowry C, Pennefather J, Walker R (Eds). Diving and Subaquatic Medicine. Arnold, London, 2002.

320) Edge JA, Ford-Adams ME, Dunger DB. Causes of death in children with insulin dependent diabetes 1990-96. Arch Dis Child 1999;81:318-23.

321) Eeg-Olofsson K, Cederholm J, Nilsson PM, Zethelius B, Svensson AM, Gudbjornsdottir S, Eliasson B. Glycemic control and cardiovascular disease in 7,454 patients with type 1 diabetes: an observational study from the Swedish National Diabetes Register (NDR). Diabetes Care 2010;33:1640-6.

322) Ehtisham S, Barrett TG, Shaw NJ. Type 2 diabetes mellitus in UK children--an emerging problem. Diabet Med 2000;17:867-71.

323) Eizirik D. Damage and repair in human islet cells. Diabetes in the XXI century; Part II. 1995:21-22.

324) Ekholm L, Björk E, Åman J. Insulin pens have the best precision when injecting small dosages of insulin. Lakartidningen 22/1991;88:2050.

325) Eliasson B, Attvall S, Taskinen MR, Smith U. The insulin resistance syndrome in smokers is related to smoking habits. Arterioscler Thromb, 1994 Dec, 14:12, 1946-50.

326) Eliasson B. Cigarette smoking and diabetes. Prog Cardiovasc Dis 2003;45: 405-13.

327) Elliott RB, Martin JB. Dietary protein: A trigger of insulin-dependent diabetes in the BB rat? Diabetologia 1984;26:297-9.

328) Elliott RB, Pilcher CC. Prevention of diabetes in normal school children. Diab Res Clin Pract 1991;14, suppl 1:85.

329) Elliott RB, Chase HP. Prevention or delay of Type I (insulin-dependent) diabetes mellitus in children using nicotinamide. Diabetologia 1991;34:362-5.

330) Elliott RB. Lecture, ISPAD Annual Meeting, Greece 1993.

331) Ellison JM, Stegmann JM, Colner SL, Michael RH, Sharma MK, Ervin KR, Horwitz DL. Rapid changes in postprandial blood glucose produce concentration differences at finger, forearm, and thigh sampling sites. Diabetes Care 2002;25:961-4.

332) Enander R, Gundevall C, Stromgren A, Chaplin J, Hanas R. Carbohydrate counting with a bolus calculator improves post-prandial blood glucose levels in children and adolescents with type 1 diabetes using insulin pumps. Pediatr Diabetes 2012;13:545-551.

333) Enzlin P, Mathieu C, Vanderschueren D, Demyttenaere K. Diabetes mellitus and female sexuality: a review of 25 years' research. Diabet Med 1998; 15:809-15.

334) Ernström U. High price for a pinch of snuff. Diabetes (Swed. Diab. Ass.) 4/91:32-33.

335) Engström I, Kroon M, Arvidsson CG, Segnestam K, Snellman K, Aman J. Eating disorders in adolescent girls with insulin-dependent diabetes mellitus: a population-based case-control study. Acta Paediatr 1999;88:175-80.

336) Escalante D, Davidson J, Garber A. Maximizing glycemic control. How to achieve normal glycemia while minimizing hyperinsulinemia in insulin-requiring patients with diabetes mellitus. Clinical Diabetes Jan/Feb 1993: 3-6.

337) EURODIAB Substudy 2 Study Group. Infections and vaccinations as risk factors for childhood type I (insulin-dependent) diabetes mellitus: a multi-centre case-control investigation. Diabetologia 2000;43:47-53.

338) Evans ML, Pernet A, Lomas J, Jones J, Amiel SA. Delay in onset of awareness of acute hypoglycemia and of restoration of cognitive performance during recovery. Diabetes Care 2000;23:893-7.

339) Evers IM, de Valk HW, Visser GH. Risk of complications of pregnancy in women with type 1 diabetes: nationwide prospective study in the Netherlands.BMJ. 2004 Apr 17;328(7445):915.

340) Ewing FME, Deary IJ, McCrimmon RJ, Strachan MWJ, Frier BM. Auditory information processing during acute hypoglycaemia in IDDM. Diab Med 1998 (Suppl 1):S36 (abstract).

341) Faglia E, Favales F, Aldeghi A et al. Adjunctive systemic hyperbaric oxygen therapy in treatment of severe prevalently ischemic diabetic foot ulcer: a randomized study. Diabetes Care 1996;19/12:1338-43.

342) Fanelli CG, Epifano L, Rambotti AM, Pampanelli S, DiVincenzo A, Modarelli F, Lepore M, Annibale B, Ciofetta M, Bottini P, Porcellati F, Scionti L, Santeusanio F, Brunetti P, Bolli GB. Meticulous prevention of hypoglycemia normalizes the glycemic thresholds and magnitude of most neuroendocrine responses to, symptoms of and cognitive function during hypoglycemia in intensively treated patients with short-term IDDM. Diabetes 1993;42: 1683-89.

343) Fanelli C, Pampanelli S, CalderoneS, Lepore M, Annibale B, Compagnucci P, Brunetti P, Bolli GB. Effects of recent, short-term hyperglycemia on responses to hypoglycemia in humans. Relevance to the pathogenesis of hypoglycemia unawareness and hyperglycemia-induced insulin resistance. Diabetes 1995;44:513-19.

344) Fanelli CG, Paramore DS, Hershey T, Terkamp C, Ovalle F, Craft S, Cryer PE. Impact of nocturnal hypoglycemia on hypoglycemic cognitive dysfunction in type 1 diabetes. Diabetes 1998;47:1920-7.

345) Faradji RN, Havari E, Chen Q, Gray J, Tornheim K, Corkey BE, Mulligan RC, Lipes MA. Glucose-induced toxicity in insulin-producing pituitary cells that coexpress GLUT2 and glucokinase. Implications for metabolic engineering. J Biol Chem 2001;276:695-702.

346) Fasano A. Intestinal zonulin: open sesame! Gut 2001;49:159-162.

347) Fava D, Leslie D, Pozzilli P. Relationship between dairy product consumption and incidence of IDDM in childhood in Italy. Diabetes Care 1994;17: 1488-90.

348) Feldt-Rasmussen B, Mathiesen ER, Jensen T, Lauritzen T, Deckert T. Effect of improved metabolic control on loss of kidney function in type 1 (insulin-dependent) diabetic patients: an update of the Steno studies. Diabetologia 1991;34:164-70.

349) Felig P, Bergman M. Integrated physiology of carbohydrate metabolism. In the book: Rifkin H, Porte D. Diabetes Mellitus, Theory and Practice. Elsevier 1990:51-60.

350) Feltbower RG, Bodansky HJ, McKinney PA, Houghton J, Stephenson CR, Haigh D. Trends in the incidence of childhood diabetes in south Asians and other children in Bradford, UK. Diabet Med 2002;19:162-6.

351) Feltbower RG, McKinney PA, Parslow RC, Stephenson CR, Bodansky HJ. Type 1 diabetes in Yorkshire, UK: time trends in 0-14 and 15-29-year-olds, age at onset and age-period-cohort modelling. Diabet Med 2003;20:437-41.

352) Fiallo-Scharer R, Horner B, McFann K, Walravens P, Chase HP. Mixing rapid-acting insulin analogues with insulin glargine in children with type 1 diabetes mellitus. J Pediatr 2006: 148: 481-484.

353) Fioretto P, Steffes MW, Sutherland DE, Goetz FC, Mauer M. Reversal of lesions of diabetic nephropathy after pancreas transplantation. N Engl J Med 1998;339:69-75.

354) Flanagan DE, Watson J, Everett J, Cavan D, Kerr D. Driving and insulin--consensus, conflict or confusion? Diabet Med 2000;17:316-20.

355) Flanagan SE, Edghill EL, Gloyn AL, Ellard S, Hattersley AT. Mutations in KCNJ11, which encodes Kir6.2, are a common cause of diabetes diagnosed in the first 6 months of life, with the phenotype determined by genotype. Diabetologia 2006;49:1190-7.

356) Fleming DR, Jacober SJ, Vandenberg MA, Fitzgerald JT, Grunberger G. The safety of injecting through clothing. Diabetes Care 1997;20:244-47.

357) Fogh-Andersen N, D'Orazio P. Proposal for standardizing direct-reading biosensors for blood glucose. Clin Chem 1998;44:655-9.

358) Fort P, Waters S, Lifshitz F. Low-dose insulin infusion in the treatment of diabetic ketoacidosis: Bolus versus no bolus. Journal of Pediatrics 1980; 96:36-40.

359) Fortunat W, Binter E. Do young diabetic patients benefit from functional insulin therapy in the long run? Wien Med Wochenschr 1991;141:53-5.

360) Foster-Powell K, Holt SH, Brand-Miller JC. International table of glycemic index and glycemic load values: 2002. Am J Clin Nutr 2002;76:5-56.

361) Fowelin J, Attvall S, v Schenck H, Bengtsson BÅ, Smith U, Lager I. Effect of prolonged hyperglycemia on growth hormone levels and insulin sensitivity in Insulin-dependent diabetes mellitus. Metabolism 1993;42:387-94.

362) Foy CG, Bell RA, Farmer DF, Goff DC, Jr., Wagenknecht LE. Smoking and incidence of diabetes among U.S. adults: findings from the Insulin Resistance Atherosclerosis Study. Diabetes Care 2005;28:2501-7.

363) Francescato MP, Geat M, Fusi S, Stupar G, Noacco C, Cattin L. Carbohydrate requirement and insulin concentration during moderate exercise in type 1 diabetic patients. Metabolism 2004;53:1126-30.

364) Franklin VL, Khan F, Kennedy G, Belch JJ, Greene SA. Intensive insulin therapy improves endothelial function and microvascular reactivity in young people with type 1 diabetes. Diabetologia 2008;51:353-60.

365) Franz MJ, Bantle JP, Beebe CA, Brunzell JD, Chiasson JL, Garg A, Holzmeister LA, Hoogwerf B, Mayer-Davis E, Mooradian AD, et al. Evidence-based nutrition principles and recommendations for the treatment and prevention of diabetes and related complications. Diabetes Care 2002;25: 148-98.

366) Franz MJ, Bantle JP. Response to Wolever. Diabetes Care 2002;25:1264-5.

367) Franzén I, Ludvigsson J. Specific instructions gave reduction of lipomas and improved metabolic control in diabetic children. Diabetologia 1997;40 (Suppl 1):A615, abstract 2421.

368) Frayn K. Metabolic Regulation. A human perspective. In the book: Snell K. (Ed.). Frontiers in Metabolism. Portland Press Ltd, London 1996, p 229-36.

369) Fredrickson DD, Guthrie DW, Nehrling JK, Guthrie R. Effects of DKA and severe hypoglycemia on cognitive functioning: a prospective study. Diabetes 1995;44(suppl. 1) abstract 97.

370) Freeman SL, O'Brien PC, Rizza RA. Use of human ultralente as the basal insulin component in the treatment of patients with IDDM. Diab Res Clin Pract 1991;12:187-92.r

371) Frid A, Gunnarsson R, Günther P, Linde B. Effects of accidental intramuscular injections on insulin absorption in IDDM. Diabetes Care 1988;11:41-45.

372) Frid A, Östman J, Linde B. Hypoglycemia risk during exercise after intra-muscular injection of insulin in thigh in IDDM. Diabetes Care 1990;13:473-77.

373) Frid A. Injection and absorption of insulin. Thesis, Lund, Sweden 1992.

374) Frid A, Linde B. Intraregional differences in the absorption of unmodified insulin from the abdominal wall. Diabetic Med 1992;9:236-39.

375) Frid A, L. H, Gaspar R, Hicks D, Kreugel G, J. L, Letondeur C, Sauvanet J, Tubiana-Rufi N, Strauss K. New injection recommendations for patients with diabetes. Diabet Metab 2010;36:S3-S18.

376) Friedrich I, Levy Y. Diabetic ketoacidosis during the Ramadan fast. Hare-fuah 2000;138:19-21, 86.

377) Frier BM. Morbidity of hypoglycemia in type 1 diabetes. Diabetes Res Clin Pract 2004;65 Suppl 1:S47-52.

378) Fritsche A, Schnauder G, Eggstein M, Schmülling RM. Blood glucose per-ception (BGP) in type 1 diabetic patients during exercise and after con-sumption of alcohol. Diabetologia 1993;36 (Suppl 1):abstract 582.

379) Frohnauer MK, Liu K, Devlin JT. Adjustment of Basal Lispro insulin in CSII to minimize glycemic fluctuations caused by exercise. Diab Res Clin Pract 2000;50(suppl 1): S80(abstract).

380) Frost G. Is carbohydrate a complex problem? Pract Diab Internat 1995;12:160-63.

381) Fruhstorfer H. Pain and diabetes monitoring. Diabetes NEWS 1998;19:7-8.

382) Fujikura J, Fujimoto M, Yasue S, Noguchi M, Masuzaki H, Hosoda K, Tachibana T, Sugihara H, Nakao K. Insulin-induced lipohypertrophy: report of a case with histopathology. Endocr J 2005;52:623-8.

383) Gabriely I, Wozniak R, Mevorach M, Kaplan J, Aharon Y, Shamoon H. Trans-cutaneous glucose measurement using near-infrared spectroscopy during hypoglycemia. Diabetes Care 1999;22:2026-32.

384) Gaete X, Vivanco M, Eyzaguirre FC, Lopez P, Rhumie HK, Unanue N, Cod-ner E. Menstrual cycle irregularities and their relationship with HbA1c and insulin dose in adolescents with type 1 diabetes mellitus. Fertil Steril 2010;94:1822-6.

385) Gale EA. A missing link in the hygiene hypothesis? Diabetologia 2002;45:588-94.

386) Gale EA. Intervening before the onset of Type 1 diabetes: baseline data from the European Nicotinamide Diabetes Intervention Trial (ENDIT). Dia-betologia 2003;46:339-46.

387) Gallen IW, Jaap A, Roland JM, Chirayath HH. Survey of glargine use in 115 pregnant women with Type 1 diabetes. Diabet Med 2008;25:165-9.

388) Ganrot PO. Insulin resistance syndrome: posiible key role of blood flow in resting muscle. Diabetologia 1993;36:876-79.

389) Gardner SG, Pingley PJ, Sawtell PA et al. Rising incidence of insulin dependent diabetes in children aged under 5 years in the Oxford region: time trend analysis. The Bart's-Oxford Study Group. Br Med J (Clin Res Ed) 1997;315/7110:713-17.

390) Garg SK, Chase PH, Marshall G, Hoops SL, Holmes DL, Jackson WE. Oral contraceptives and renal and retinal complications in young women with insulindependent diabetes mellitus. J Am Med Assoc. 1994;271:1099-102.

391) Garg S, Zisser H, Schwartz S, Bailey T, Kaplan R, Ellis S, Jovanovic L. Improvement in glycemic excursions with a transcutaneous, real-time con-tinuous glucose sensor: a randomized controlled trial. Diabetes Care 2006;29:44-50.

392) Gaudieri PA, Chen R, Greer TF, Holmes CS. Cognitive function in children with type 1 diabetes: a meta-analysis. Diabetes Care 2008;31:1892-7.

393) Geerlings SE, Stolk RP, Camps MJ, Netten PM, Hoekstra JB, Bouter PK, Braveboer B, Collet TJ, Jansz AR, Hoepelman AM. Asymptomatic bacteriuria can be considered a diabetic complication in women with diabetes melli-tus. Adv Exp Med Biol 2000;485:309-14.

394) George E, Marques JL, Harris ND, Macdonald IA, Hardisty CA, Heller SR. Preservation of physiological responses to hypoglycemia 2 days after ante-decent hypoglycemia in patients with IDDM. Diabetes Care 1997;20:1293-98.

395) Georgakopoulos K, Katsilambros N, Fragaki M, Poulopoulou Z, Kimbouris J, Sfikakis P, Raptis S. Recovery from insulin-induced hypoglycemia after saccharose or glucose administration. Clin Physiol Biochem 1990;8:267-72.

396) Giacco R, Parillo M, Rivellese AA, Lasorella G, Giacco A, D'Episcopo L, Ric-cardi G. Long-term dietary treatment with increased amounts of fiber-rich low-glycemic index natural foods improves blood glucose control and reduces the number of hypoglycemic events in type 1 diabetic patients. Diabetes Care 2000;23:1461-6.

397) Gibbon C, Smith T, Egger P, Betts P Phillips D. Early infection and subse-quent insulin dependent diabetes. Arch Dis Child 1997;77:384-5.

398) Gilbert RE. Sodium-glucose linked transporter-2 inhibitors: potential for renoprotection beyond blood glucose lowering? Kidney Int 2013;

399) Gilbertson HR, Brand-Miller JC, Thorburn AW, Evans S, Chondros P, Wer-ther GA. The effect of flexible low glycemic index dietary advice versus measured carbohydrate exchange diets on glycemic control in children with type 1 diabetes. Diabetes Care 2001;24:1137-43.

400) Gill GV, Redmond S, Garratt F, Paisey R. Diabetes and alternative medi-cine: cause for concern. Diabetic Med. 1994;11:210-13.

401) Gill G, Durston J, Johnston R, MacLeod K, Watkins P. Insulin-treated diabe-tes and driving in the UK. Diabet Med 2002;19:435-9.

402) Gillespie SJ, Kulkarni KD, Daly AE. Using carbohydrate counting in diabetes clinical practice. J Am Diet Assoc 1998;98:897-905.

403) Ginsberg BH, Parkes JL, Sparacino C. The kinetics of insulin administration by insulin pens. Horm Metab Research 1994;26:584-87.

404) Glaab LA, Brown R, Daneman D. School attendance in children with Type 1 diabetes. Diabet Med 2005;22:421-6.

405) Glasier A, Thong KJ, Dewar M, Mackie M, Baird DT. Mifepristone (RU 486) compared with high-dose estrogen and progesterone for emergency post-coital contraception. N Engl J Med 1992;327:1041-4.

406) Glasgow AM, Tynan D, Schwartz R, Hicks JM, Turek J, Driscol C, O'Donnell RM, Getson PR. Alcohol and drug use in teenagers with diabetes mellitus. J Adolesc Health 1991;12:11-4.

407) Gold AE, Reilly C, Walker JD. Transient improvement in glycemic control. The impact of pregnancy in women with IDDM. Diabetes Care 1998;21:374-8.

408) Goldberg T, Cai W, Peppa M, Dardaine V, Baliga BS, Uribarri J, Vlassara H. Advanced glycoxidation end products in commonly consumed foods. J Am Diet Assoc 2004;104:1287-91.

409) Golden SH, Peart-Vigilance C, Kao WH, Brancati FL. Perioperative glycemic control and the risk of infectious complications in a cohort of adults with diabetes. Diabetes Care 1999;22:1408-14.

410) Goldstein DE, Little RR, Lorenz RA, Malone JI, Nathan D, Peterson CM. Tests of glycemia in diabetes. Diabetes Care 1995;18:896-909.

411) Gonder-Frederick LA, Zrebiec JF, Bauchowitz AU, Ritterband LM, Magee JC, Cox DJ, Clarke WL. Cognitive function is disrupted by both hypo- and hyper-glycemia in school-aged children with type 1 diabetes: a field study. Diabe-tes Care 2009;32:1001-6.

412) Graff MR, Rubin RR, Walker EA. How diabetes specialists treat their own diabetes: findings from a study of the AADE and ADA membership. Diabe-tes Educ 2000;26:460-7.

413) Grajower MM, Fraser CG, Holcombe JH, Daugherty ML, Harris WC, De Felip-pis MR, Santiago OM, Clark NG. How long should insulin be used once a vial is started? Diabetes Care 2003;26:2665-6; discussion 266-9.

414) Graves PM, Barriga KJ, Norris JM, Hoffman MR, Yu L, Eisenbarth GS, Rew-ers M. Lack of association between early childhood immunizations and beta-cell autoimmunity. Diabetes Care 1999;22:1694-7.

415) Gray RO, Butler PC, Beers TR, Kryshak EJ, Rizza RA. Comparison of the ability of bread versus bread plus meat to treat and prevent subsequent hypoglycemia in patients with insulin-dependent diabetes mellitus. J Clin Endocrinol Metab 1996;81:1508-11.

416) Green A, Gale EAM, Patterson CC, the EURODIAB ACE Study Group. Inci-dence of childhood-onset insulin-dependent diabetes mellitus: the EURO-DIAB ACE Study. Lancet 1992;339:905-909.

417) Green A, Patterson CC. Trends in the incidence of childhood-onset diabetes in Europe 1989-1998. Diabetologia 2001;44 Suppl 3:B3-8.

418) Gregory R, Edwards S, Yateman NA. Demonstration of insulin transforma-tion products in insulin vials by High-performance liquid chromatography. Diabetes Care 1991;14:42-48.

419) Grey M, Boland EA, Tamborlane WV. Use of lispro insulin and quality of life in adolescents on intensive therapy. Diabetes Educ 1999;25:934-41.

420) Griffin ME, Feder A, Tamborlane WV. Lipoatrophy associated with lispro insulin in insulin pump therapy: an old complication, a new cause? Diabe-tes Care 2001;24:174.

421) Grimaldi-Bensouda L. Risk of Breast Cancer by Individual Insulin Use: An International Multicenter Study. Diabetes Care 2014;37:134–143.

422) Gros L, Riu E, Montoliu L, Ontiveros M, Lebrigand L, Bosch F. Insulin pro-duction by engineered muscle cells. Hum Gene Ther 1999;10:1207-17.

423) Gross TM, Kayne D, King A, Rother C, Juth S. A bolus calculator is an effec-tive means of controlling postprandial glycemia in patients on insulin pump therapy. Diabetes Technol Ther 2003;5:365-9.

424) Grossi SG, Skrepcinski FB, DeCaro T, Robertson DC, Ho AW, Dunford RG, Genco RJ. Treatment of periodontal disease in diabetics reduces glycated hemoglobin. J Periodontol 1997;68:713-9.

425) Gscwend S, Ryan C, Atchinson J, Arslanian S, Becker D. Effects of acute hyperglycemia on mental efficiency and counterregulatory hormones in adolescents with insulin-dependent diabetes mellitus. J Pediatrics 1995;126:178-184.

426) Guelfi KJ, Jones TW, Fournier PA. The decline in blood glucose levels is less with intermittent high-intensity compared with moderate exercise in individ-uals with type 1 diabetes. Diabetes Care 2005;28:1289-94.

427) Gubitosi-Klug R. The Diabetes Control and Complications Trial/Epidemiolo-gyof Diabetes Interventions and Complications Study at 30 Years: Sum-mary and Future Directions. Diabetes Care 2014;37:44–49.

428) Guerci B, Benichou M, Floriot M, Bohme P, Fougnot S, Franck P, Drouin P. Accuracy of an electrochemical sensor for measuring capillary blood ketones by fingerstick samples during metabolic deterioration after contin-uous subcutaneous insulin infusion interruption in type 1 diabetic patients. Diabetes Care 2003;26:1137-41.

429) Guerin A, Nisenbaum R, Ray JG. Use of maternal GHb concentration to estimate the risk of congenital anomalies in the offspring of women with prepregnancy diabetes. Diabetes Care 2007;30:1920-5.

430) Gunning R, Garber A. Bioactivity of Instant Glucose - Failure of absorption through oral mucosa. JAMA 1978;240:1611-12.

431) Gunton JE, Davies L, Wilmshurst E, Fulcher G, McElduff A. Cigarette smok-ing affects glycemic control in diabetes. Diabetes Care 2002;25:796-7.

432) Hägglöf B, Blom L, Dahlquist G, Lönnberg G, Sahlin B. The Swedish Child-hood Diabetes Study: Indications of severe psychological stress as a risk factor for type 1 (insulin-dependent) diabetes mellitus in childhood. Diabet-ologia 1991;34:579-83.

433) Haglund B, Ryckenberg K, Selenius O, Dahlquist G. Evidence of a relation-ship between childhood-onset type 1 diabetes and low groundwater con-centration of zinc. Diabetes Care 1996;19:873-75.

434) Halberg IB, Jacobsen LV, Dahl UL. A study on self-mixing insulin aspart with NPH insulin in the syringe before injection. Diabetes 1999;48(Suppl 1): abstract 448.

435) Halfon P, Belkhadir J, Slama G. Correlation between amount of carbohy-drate in mixed meals and insulin delivery by artificial pancreas in seven IDDM subjects. Diabetes Care 1989;12:427-9.

436) Hallinan R, Byrne A, Agho K, McMahon CG, Tynan P, Attia J. Hypogonadism in men receiving methadone and buprenorphine maintenance treatment. Int J Androl 2009;32:131-9.

437) Ham MR, Okada P, White PC. Bedside ketone determination in diabetic children with hyperglycemia and ketosis in the acute care setting. Pediatr Diabetes 2004;5:39-43.

438) Hamann A, Matthaei S, Rosak C, Silvestre L. A randomized clinical trial comparing breakfast, dinner, or bedtime administration of insulin glargine in patients with type 1 diabetes. Diabetes Care 2003;26:1738-44.

439) Hammerstein O, Rogers R. The King and I. Williams music, Hel Leonard Publications, Milwaukee 1951.

440) Hammes HP, Alt A, Niwa T, Clausen JT, Bretzel RG, Brownlee M, Schleicher ED. Differential accumulation of advanced glycation end products in the course of diabetic retinopathy. Diabetologia 1999;42:728-36.

441) Hanaire-Broutin H, Schumicki D, Hoogma R, Souhami E. Safety of Insulin Glulisine C ompared with Insulin Aspart Administered by Continuous Subcutaneous Insulin Infusion (CSII). Diabetes 2004;53(Suppl 2):A4(abstract).

442) Hanas R, Ludvigsson J. Side effects and indwelling times of subcutaneous catheters for insulin injections: A new device for injecting insulin with a minimum of pain in the treatment of insulin-dependent diabetes mellitus. Diabetes Res Clin Pract 1990; 10:73-83.

443) Hanas R, Ludvigsson J. Metabolic control is not altered when using indwelling catheters for insulin injections. Diabetes Care 1994;17:716-18.

444) Hanas R, Ludvigsson J. Experience of pain from insulin injections and needle-phobia in young patients with IDDM. Practical Diabetes 1997;14:95-99.

445) Hanas, R. Carlsson S, Frid A, Ludvigsson J. Unchanged insulin absorption after 4 days' use of subcutaneous indwelling catheters for insulin injectons. Diabetes Care 1997;20:487-90.

446) Hanas R. Dead-in-bed syndrome in diabetes mellitus and hypoglycemic unawareness. Lancet 1997;350:492-3 (letter). Lancet 1997;350:1032-33 (reply).

447) Hanas R, Stanke CG, Ostberg H. Diagnosis of the cause of malfunction of indwelling catheters for insulin injections by the use of digital fluoroscopy. Pediatr Radiol 2000;30:674-6.

448) Hanas R, Lytzen L, Ludvigsson J. Thinner needles do not influence injection pain, insulin leakage or bleeding in children and adolescents with type 1 diabetes. Pediatric Diabetes 2000;1:142-49.

449) Hanas R. Low Risk of Hypoglycemia Despite Metabolic Control at DCCT Level in a Population of Children and Adolescents Using Intensified Insulin Treatment. Diabetes 2000;49 (Suppl 1):Abstract 540.

450) Hanas R. Reducing injection pain in children and adolescents with diabetes. Studies on indwelling catheters and injection needles. Linköpings Universty Medical Dissertations # 700, UniTryck, Linköping 2001.

451) Hanas R, Adolfsson P, Elfvin-Akesson K, Hammaren L, Ilvered R, Jansson I, Johansson C, Kroon M, Lindgren J, Lindh A, Ludvigsson J, Sigstrom L, Wiik A, Aman J. Indwelling catheters used from the onset of diabetes decrease injection pain and pre-injection anxiety. J Pediatr 2002;140:315-20.

452) Hanas R. Psychological impact of changing the scale of reported HbA(1c) results affects metabolic control. Diabetes Care 2002;25:2110-1.

453) Hanas R, Adolfsson P. Insulin pumps in pediatric routine care improve long-term metabolic control without increasing the risk of hypoglycemia. Pediatric Diabetes 2006;7:25-31.

454) Hanas R, Lundqvist K, Windell L. Blood glucose and beta-hydroxybutyrate responses when the insulin pump is stopped in children and adolescents. Pediatric Diabetes 2006;7(suppl 5):35(abstract).

455) Hanas R, Lindgren F, Lindblad B. A 2-yr national population study of pediatric ketoacidosis in Sweden: predisposing conditions and insulin pump use. Pediatr Diabetes 2009;10:33-7.

456) Hanas R, de Beaufort C, Hoey H, Anderson B. Insulin delivery by injection in children and adolescents with diabetes. Pediatr Diabetes 2011;12:518-26.

457) Hanas R, Lundqvist K, Sjöstrand A, Windell L. The Duration of Insulin Action setting in young prepubertal pumpers with good metabolic control does not match published pharmacodynamic data on insulin action time. Pediatric Diabetes 2013;14 (Suppl s18), abstract P239.

458) Hanas R, John WG. 2013 update on the worldwide standardization of the hemoglobin A(1)c measurement. Diabetes Res Clin Pract 2013;100:e64-5.

459) Hanas R, Lundqvist K, Windell L. The American Diabetes Association's HbA1c goals for young children are not realistic Diabetes Res Clin Pract 2013;(abstract PD-863).

460) Hanas R, Lundqvist K, Windell L, Sjöstrand A. Which HbA1c Goals Are Attainable in Children and Adolescents? Diabetes 2014;63:A625 (abstract).

461) Hanson U, Persson B, Thunell S. Relationship between haemoglobin A$_{Ic}$ in early type 1 (insulin-dependent) diabetic pregnancy and the occurrence of spontaneous abortion and fetal malformation in Sweden. Diabetologia 1990;33:100-4.

462) Hanssen KF. Pregnancy in insulin-dependent diabetes. Nord Med 8-9/ 1992;107:211-12.

463) Hanssen KF, Bangstad HJ, Brinchmann-Hansen O, Dahl-Jørgensen K. Blood glucose control and diabetic microvascular complications. Long term effects of near-normoglycaemia. Diabetic Medicine 1992;9:697-705.

464) Hansson SL, Pichert JW. Perceived stress and diabetes control in adolescents. Health Psychol 1986;5:439-52.

465) Harris S, Ng R, Syed H, Hillson R. Near patient blood ketone measurements and their utility in predicting diabetic ketoacidosis. Diabet Med 2005;22:221-4.

466) Hartley M, Thomsett MJ, Cotterill AM. Mini-dose glucagon rescue for mild hypoglycaemia in children with type 1 diabetes: the Brisbane experience. J Paediatr Child Health 2006;42:108-11.

467) Hathout E, Lakey J, Shapiro J. Islet transplant: an option for childhood diabetes? Arch Dis Child 2003;88:591-4.

468) Hattersley AT, Ashcroft FM. Activating mutations in Kir6.2 and neonatal diabetes: new clinical syndromes, new scientific insights, and new therapy. Diabetes 2005;54:2503-13.

469) Hauner H, Stockamp B, Haastert B. Prevalence of lipohypertrophy in insulin-treated diabetic patients and predisposing factors. Exp Clin Endocrinol Diabetes 1996;104:106-10.

470) Haycock P. Insulin Absorption: Understanding the Variables. Clinical Diabetes Sept/Oct 1986:98-118.

471) Haymond MW, Karl IE, Clarke WL, Pagliara AS, Santiago JV. Differences in circulating gluconeogenic substrates during short-term fasting in men, women, and children. Metabolism 1982;31:33-42.

472) Haymond MW, Schreiner B. Mini-dose glucagon rescue for hypoglycemia in children with type 1 diabetes. Diabetes Care 2001;24:643-5.

473) Hayward LM, Burden ML, Burden AC, Blackledge H, Raymond NT, Botha JL, Karwatowski WS, Duke T, Chang YF. What is the prevalence of visual impairment in the general and diabetic populations: are there ethnic and gender differences? Diabet Med 2002;19:27-34.

474) Hawthorne G, Irgens LM, Lie RT. Outcome of pregnancy in diabetic women in northeast England and in Norway, 1994-7. BMJ 2000;321:730-1.

475) Heijbel H, Chen RT, Dahlquist G. Cumulative incidence of childhood-onset IDDM is unaffected by pertussis immunization. Diabetes Care 1997;20: 173-5.

476) Heine RJ, Bilo HJG, Fonk T, Van der Veen EA, Van der Meer J. Absorption kinetics and action profiles of mixtures of short- and intermediate acting insulins. Diabetologia 1984; 27:558-62.

477) Heinemann L, Sinha K, Weyer C, Loftager M, Hirschberger S, Heise T. Time-action profile of the soluble, fatty acid acylated, long-acting insulin analogue NN304. Diabet Med 1999;16:332-8.

478) Heinemann L, Nosek L, Kapitza C, Schweitzer MA, Krinelke L. Changes in basal insulin infusion rates with subcutaneous insulin infusion: time until a change in metabolic effect is induced in patients with type 1 diabetes. Diabetes Care 2009;32:1437-9.

479) Heintz E, Wirehn AB, Peebo BB, Rosenqvist U, Levin LA. Prevalence and healthcare costs of diabetic retinopathy: a population-based register study in Sweden. Diabetologia 2010;53:2147-54.

480) Heise T, Berger M Sawicki PT. Non-evidence-based concepts are still established in the treatment of IDDM. Horm Res 1998;50:74-8.

481) Heise T, Bott S, Rave K, Dressler A, Rosskamp R, Heinemann L. No evidence for accumulation of insulin glargine (LANTUS): a multiple injection study in patients with Type 1 diabetes. Diabet Med 2002;19(6):490-5.

482) Heise T, Nosek L, Ronn BB, Endahl L, Heinemann L, Kapitza C, et al. Lower within-subject variability of insulin detemir in comparison to NPH insulin and insulin glargine in people with type 1 diabetes. Diabetes 2004;53: 1614-20.

483) Heise T, Pieber TR. Towards peakless, reproducible and long-acting insulins. An assessment of the basal analogues based on isoglycaemic clamp studies. Diabetes Obes Metab 2007;9:648-59.

484) Heise T, Nosek L, Spitzer H, Heinemann L, Niemoller E, Frick AD, Becker RH. Insulin glulisine: a faster onset of action compared with insulin lispro. Diabetes Obes Metab 2007;9:746-53.

485) Helgasson T, Jobnasson MR, Evidence for a food additive as cause of ketosis-prone diabetes. Lancet 1981;11:716-20.

486) Helgasson T, Danielsen R, Thorsson AV. Incidence and prevalence of Type 1 (insulin-dependent) diabetes mellitus in Icelandic children 1970-89. Diabetologia 1992;35:880-3.

487) Heller SR, Amiel SA, Mansell P. Effect of the fast-acting insulin analog lispro on the risk of nocturnal hypoglycemia during intensified insulin therapy. U.K. Lispro Study Group. Diabetes Care 1999;22:1607-11.

488) Heller SR. Abnormalities of the electrocardiogram during hypoglycaemia: the cause of the dead in bed syndrome? Int J Clin Pract Suppl 2002(129): 27-32.

489) Henriksen JE, Djurhuus MS, Vaag A, Thye-Rønn P, Knudsen D, Hother-Nielsen O, Beck-Nielsen H. Impact of injection sites for soluble insulin on glycaemic control in Type 1 (insulin-dependent) diabetic patients treated with a multiple insulin injection regimen. Diabetologia 1993;36:752-58.

490) Henriksen JE, Vaag A, Ramsgaard Hansen I, Lauritzen M, Djurhuus MS, Beck-Nielsen H. Absorption of NPH (Isophane) insulin in resting diabetic patients: evidence for subcutaneous injection on the thigh as the preferred site. Diabetic Medicine 1991;8:453-57.

491) Henry RR, Mudaliar SR, Howland IW, Chu N, Kim D, An B, Reinhardt RR. Inhaled Insulin Using the AERx Insulin Diabetes Management System in Healthy and Asthmatic Subjects. Diabetes Care 2003;26;764-9.

492) Heptulla RA, Rodriguez LM, Bomgaars L, Haymond MW. The role of amylin and glucagon in the dampening of glycemic excursions in children with type 1 diabetes. Diabetes 2005;54:1100-7.

493) Herbst A, Bachran R, Kapellen T, Holl RW. Effects of regular physical activity on control of glycemia in pediatric patients with type 1 diabetes mellitus. Arch Pediatr Adolesc Med. 2006;160(6):573-7

494) Hermansen K, Fontaine P, Kukolja KK, Peterkova V, Leth G, Gall MA. Insulin analogues (insulin detemir and insulin aspart) versus traditional human insulins (NPH insulin and regular insulin) in basal-bolus therapy for patients with type 1 diabetes. Diabetologia 2004;47:622-9.

495) Herold KC, Polonsky KS, Cohen RM, Levy J, Douglas F. Variable deterioration in cortical function during insulin-induced hypoglycaemia. Diabetes 1985;34:677-85.

496) Herold KC, Gitelman SE, Masharani U, Hagopian W, Bisikirska B, Donaldson D, Rother K, Diamond B, Harlan DM, Bluestone JA. A single course of anti-CD3 monoclonal antibody hOKT3gamma1(Ala-Ala) results in improvement in C-peptide responses and clinical parameters for at least 2 years after onset of type 1 diabetes. Diabetes 2005;54:1763-9.

497) Hershey T, Bhargava N, Sadler M, White NH, Craft S. Conventional versus intensive diabetes therapy in children with type 1 diabetes: effects on memory and motor speed. Diabetes Care 1999;22:1318-24.

498) Hildebrandt P, Sestoft L, Nielson RL. The absorption of subcutaneously injected short-acting soluble insulin:influence of injection-technique and concentration. Diabetes Care 1983;6:459-62.

499) Hildebrandt P, Birch K. Subcutaneous insulin infusion: Change in basal rate infusion has no immediate effect on insulin absorption rate. Diabetes Care 1986;9:561-64.

500) Hildebrandt P. Skinfold thickness, local subcutaneous blood flow and insulin absorption in diabetic patients. Acta Physiol Scand. 1991;143 (Suppl. 603):41-45.

501) Hildebrandt P, Vaag A. Local skin-fold thickness as a clinical predictor of depot size during basal rate infusion. Diabetes Care 1993;16:1-3.

502) Hildebrandt R, Ilius U, Schliack V. Effect of insulin suppositories in type 1 diabetic patients (preliminary communication). Exp Clin Endocrinol 1984; 83(2):168-72.

503) Hilsted J, Madsbad S, Hvidberg AM, Rasmussen MH, Krarup T, Ipsen H, Hansen B, Pedersen M, Djurup R, Oxenbøll. Intranasal insulin therapy: The clinical realities. Diabetologia 1995;38:680-84.

504) Hiltunen M, Hyoty H, Knip M, Ilonen J, Reijonen H, Vahasalo P, Roivainen M, Lonnrot M, Leinikki P, Hovi T, et al. Islet cell antibody seroconversion in children is temporally associated with enterovirus infections. Childhood Diabetes in Finland (DiMe) Study Group. J Infect Dis 1997;175:554-60.

505) Himmelmann A, Jendle J, Mellen A, Petersen AH, Dahl UL, Wollmer P. The impact of smoking on inhaled insulin. Diabetes Care 2003;26:677-82.

506) Hirai FE, Moss SE, Klein BE, Klein R. Severe hypoglycemia and smoking in a long-term type 1 diabetic population: Wisconsin Epidemiologic Study of Diabetic Retinopathy. Diabetes Care 2007;30:1437-41.

507) Hirsch IB, Farkas-Hirsch R, Skyler JS. Intensive insulin therapy for treatment of type 1 diabetes. Diabetes Care 12/1990;13:1265-1283.

508) Hirsch IB, Boyle PJ, Craft S, Cryer PE. Higher glycemic thresholds for symptoms during ß-adrenergic blockade in IDDM. Diabetes 1991;40:1177-88.

509) Hirsch IB, Farkas-Hirsch R, Cryer PE. Continuous subcutaneous insulin infusion for the treatment of diabetic patients with hypoglycemia unawareness. Diab Nutr Metab 1991;4:41-43.

510) Hirsch IB, Heller SR, Cryer PE. Increased symptoms of hypoglycaemia in the standing position in insulin-dependent diabetes mellitus. Clinical Science 1991;80:583-86.

511) Hirsch IB, Farkas-Hirsch R, Herbst JS, Skyler JS. The effect of ejaculation on albumin excretion rate. J Diabetes Complications 1992;6:163-5.

512) Hirsch IB, Paauw DS, Brunzell J. Inpatient management of adults with diabetes. Diabetes Care 1995;18:870-78.

513) Hirsch IB, Polonsky WH. Hypoglycemia and its prevention. In the book: Fredrickson L (Ed.). The Insulin Pump Therapy Book. Insights from the experts. MiniMed, Los Angeles 1995.

514) Hirsch LJ, Gibney MA, Albanese J, Qu S, Kassler-Taub K, Klaff LJ, Bailey TS. Comparative glycemic control, safety and patient ratings for a new 4 mm x 32G insulin pen needle in adults with diabetes. Curr Med Res Opin 2010; 26:1531-41.

515) Hod M, Mathiesen ER, Jovanovic L, McCance DR, Ivanisevic M, Duran-Garcia S, Brondsted L, Nazeri A, Damm P. A randomized trial comparing perinatal outcomes using insulin detemir or neutral protamine Hagedorn in type 1 diabetes. J Matern Fetal Neonatal Med 2014;27:7-13.

516) Hoelzel W, Miedema K. Development of a reference system for the international standardization of HbA1c/Glycohemoglobin determinations. J Internat Fed Clin Chem 1996;9:62-67.

517) Hoelzel W, Weykamp C, Jeppsson JO, Miedema K, Barr JR, Goodall I, Hoshino T, John WG, Kobold U, Little R, et al. IFCC reference system for measurement of hemoglobin A1c in human blood and the national standardization schemes in the United States, Japan, and Sweden: a method-comparison study. Clin Chem 2004;50:166-74.

518) Hoey H, Aanstoot HJ, Chiarelli F, Daneman D, Danne T, Dorchy H, Fitzgerald M, Garandeau P, Greene S, Holl R, et al. Good metabolic control is associated with better quality of life in 2,101 adolescents with type 1 diabetes. Diabetes Care 2001;24:1923-8.

519) Hofer SE, Rosenbauer J, Grulich-Henn J, Naeke A, Frohlich-Reiterer E, Holl RW. Smoking and metabolic control in adolescents with type 1 diabetes. J Pediatr 2009;154:20-23 e1.

520) Hofman PL, Lawton SA, Peart JM, Holt JA, Jefferies CA, Robinson E, Cutfield WS. An angled insertion technique using 6-mm needles markedly reduces the risk of intramuscular injections in children and adolescents. Diabet Med 2007;24:1400-5.

521) Hollander P, Pi-Sunyer X, Conif R. Acarbose in the treatment of type 1 diabetes. Diabetes Care 1995;20:248-253.

522) Holleman F, van den Brand JJ, Hoven RA, van der Linden JM, van der Tweel I, Hoekstra JB, Erkelens DW. Comparison of LysB28, ProB29-human insulin analog and regular human insulin in the correction of incidental hyperglycemia. Diabetes Care 1996;19/12,:1426-9.

523) Holm J, Koellreutter B, Wursch P. Influence of sterilization, drying and oat bran enrichment of pasta on glucose and insulin responses in healthy subjects and on the rate and extent of in vitro starch digestion. Eur J Clin Nutr 1992;46:629-40.

524) Holmes GK. Coeliac disease and Type 1 diabetes mellitus - the case for screening. Diabet Med 2001;18:169-77.

525) Holzmeister, LA. The Diabetes Carbohydrate and Fat Gram Guide. The American Diabetes Association, Alexandria, Virginia 2000.

526) Home P. Potency of insulin. Diabetes Care 1988;11:604.

527) Home PD, Lindholm A, Hylleberg B, Round P. Improved glycemic control with insulin aspart: a multicenter randomized double-blind crossover trial in type 1 diabetic patients. UK Insulin Aspart Study Group. Diabetes Care 1998;21:1904-9.

528) Home PD, Lindholm A, Riis A. Insulin aspart vs. human insulin in the management of long-term blood glucose control in Type 1 diabetes mellitus: a randomized controlled trial. European Insulin Aspart Study Group. Diabet Med 2000;17:762-70.

529) Honeyman MC, Coulson BS, Stone NL, Gellert SA, Goldwater PN, Steele CE, Couper JJ, Tait BD, Colman PG, Harrison LC. Association between rotavirus infection and pancreatic islet autoimmunity in children at risk of developing type 1 diabetes. Diabetes 2000;49:1319-24.

530) Hoogma RP, Schumicki D. Safety of insulin glulisine when given by continuous subcutaneous infusion using an external pump in patients with type 1 diabetes. Horm Metab Res 2006;38:429-33.

531) Hopkins DFC, Cotton, SJ, Williams G. Effective treatment of insulin-induced edema using ephedrine. Diabetes Care 1993;16:1026-28.

532) Hordern SV, Wright JE, Umpleby AM, Shojaee-Moradie F, Amiss J, Russell-Jones DL. Comparison of the effects on glucose and lipid metabolism of equipotent doses of insulin detemir and NPH insulin with a 16-h euglycaemic clamp. Diabetologia 2005;48:420-6.

533) Hornsby W, Chetlin R. Management of competitive athletes with diabetes. Diabetes Spectr 2005;18:102-107.

534) Hosny EA, Ghilzai NM, al-Najar TA, Elmazar MM. Hypoglycemic effect of oral insulin in diabetic rabbits using pH- dependent coated capsules containing sodium salicylate without and with sodium cholate. Drug Dev Ind Pharm 1998;24:307-11.

535) Houghton LA, Magnall YF, Read NW. Effect on incorporating fat into a liquid test meal on the relation between intragastric distribution and gastric emptying in human volunteers. Gut 1990;31:1126-29.

536) Houtzagers CMGJ, Visser AP, Berntzen PA, Heine RJ, van der Veen EA. The Medi-Jector II: Efficacy and acceptability in insulin dependent diabetic patient with and without needle-phobia. Diabet Med 1988;5:135-8.

537) Houtzagers CMGJ, Berntzen PA, van der Stap H, et al. Efficacy and acceptance of two intensified conventional insulin therapy regimens: a long-term crossover comparison. Diabetic Med 1989; 6:416-21.

538) Houtzagers CMGJ, Visser AP, Berntzen PA, et al. Multiple daily insulin injections improve self-confidence. Diabetic Med 1989; 6:512-519.

539) Houtzagers CMGJ. Subcutaneous insulin delivery: Present status. Diabetic Med 1989;6:754-61.

540) Howey DC, Bowsher RR, Brunelle RL,Woodworth JR. [Lys(B28,Pro(B29)]-human insulin: a rapidly absorbed analogue of human insulin. Diabetes 1994;43:396-402.

541) Huebschmann AG, Regensteiner JG, Vlassara H, Reusch JE. Diabetes and advanced glycoxidation end products. Diabetes Care 2006;29:1420-32.

542) Husband AC, Crawford S, McCoy LA, Pacaud D. The effectiveness of glucose, sucrose, and fructose in treating hypoglycemia in children with type 1 diabetes. Pediatr Diabetes 2010;11:154-8.

543) Hutchinson A, McIntosh A, Peters J, O'Keeffe C, Khunti K, Baker R, Booth A. Effectiveness of screening and monitoring tests for diabetic retinopathy - a systematic review. Diabet Med 2000;17:495-506.

544) Hyoety H, Hiltunen M, Knip M, Laakkonen M, Uaehaesalo P, Karjalainen J, Koskela P, Roivainen M, Lenikki P; Hovi T et al. A prospective study of the role of coxsackie B and other enterovirus infections in the pathogenesis of IDDM. Diabetes 1995;16:652-7.

545) Hyllienmark L, Ludvigsson J. Insulin pump - a realistic alternative for treatment of diabetes in children and adolescents. Lakartidningen 13/1992; 89:1057-62.

546) Iafusco D, Angius E, Prisco F. Early preprandial hypoglycemia after administration of insulin lispro. Diabetes Care 1998;21:1777-8.

547) Iafusco D, Rea F, Prisco F. Hypoglycemia and reduction of the insulin requirement as a sign of celiac disease in children with IDDM. Diabetes Care 1998;21:1379-81.

548) International Diabetes Federation. Diabetes Atlas 2003.

549) International Diabetes Federation. Diabetes Atlas 2013, sixth edition.

550) International Study Group for Diabetes in Children (now ISPAD). Position statement, Diabetes in the Young 1989.

551) Inui A, Kitaoka H, Majima M, Takamiya S, Uemoto M, Yonenaga C, Honda M, Shirakawa K, Ueno N, Amano K, et al. Effect of the Kobe earthquake on stress and glycemic control in patients with diabetes mellitus. Arch Intern Med 1998;158:274-8.

552) Jackson A, Ternand C, Brunzell C, Kleinschmidt T, Dew D, Milla C, Moran A. Insulin glargine improves hemoglobin A1c in children and adolescents with poorly controlled type 1 diabetes. Pediatr Diabetes 2003;4:64-69.

553) Jackson RL, Hardin RC, Walker GL, Hendricks AB, Kelly HG. Degenerative changes in young diabetic patients in relationship to level of control. Pediatrics 1950;5:959-71.

554) Jacobson AM, Hauser ST, Lavori P, Wolfsdorf JI, Herskowitz RD, Milley JE, Bliss R, Gelfand E, Wertlieb D, Stein J. Adherence among children and adolescents with insulin-dependent diabetes mellitus over a four-year longitudinal follow-up: I. The influence of patient coping and adjustment. J Pediatr Psychol 1990;15:511-26.

555) Janssen MM, Casteleijn S, Devillé W, Popp Snijders C, Roach P, Heine RJ. Nighttime insulin kinetics and glycemic control in type 1 diabetes patients following administration of an intermediate-acting lispro preparation. Diabetes Care 1997;20(12):1870-73.

556) JDRF Continuous Glucose Monitoring Study Group. Bode B, Beck RW, Xing D, Gilliam L, Hirsch I, Kollman C, Laffel L, Ruedy KJ, Tamborlane WV, et al. Sustained benefit of continuous glucose monitoring on A1C, glucose profiles, and hypoglycemia in adults with type 1 diabetes. Diabetes Care 2009;32:2047-9.

557) Jefferson IG, Swift PG, Skinner TC, Hood GK. Diabetes services in the UK: third national survey confirms continuing deficiencies. Arch Dis Child 2003; 88:53-6.

558) Jeha GS, Heptulla RA. Newer therapeutic options for children with diabetes mellitus: theoretical and practical considerations. Pediatr Diabetes 2006; 7:122-38.

559) Jehle PM, Micheler C, Jehle DR, Breitig D, Boehm BO. Inadequate suspension of neutral protamine Hagedorn (NPH) insulin in pens. Lancet 1999; 354:1604-7.

560) Jelinek J. Skin disorders associated with diabetes mellitus. In the book: Rifkin H, Porte D. Diabetes Mellitus, Theory and Practice. Elsevier 1990: 838-49.

561) Jensen JS, Clausen P, Borch-Johnsen K, Jensen G, Feldt-Rasmussen B. Detecting microalbuminuria by urinary albumin/creatinine concentration ratio. Nephrol Dial Transplant 1997;12 Suppl 2:6-9.

562) Jensen-Urstadt KJ, Reichard PG, Rosfors JS et al. Early atherosclerosis is retarded by improved long-term blood glucose control in patients with IDDM. Diabetes 1996;45/9:1253-8.

563) Johannes CB, Araujo AB, Feldman HA, Derby CA, Kleinman KP, McKinlay JB. Incidence of erectile dysfunction in men 40 to 69 years old: longitudinal results from the Massachusetts male aging study. J Urol 2000;163:460-3.

564) Johansson C, Samuelsson U, Ludvigsson J. A high weight gain early in life is associated with an increased risk of Type 1 (insulin-dependent) diabetes mellitus. Diabetologia 1994;37:91-94.

565) Johansson BL, Kernell A, Sjoeberg S, Wahren J. Influence of combined C-peptide and insulin administration on renal function and metabolic control in diabetes type 1. J Clin. Endocrinol. Metab. 1993;77:976-81.

566) Johansson BL, Borg K, Fernqvist-Forbes E, Kernell A, Odergren T, Wahren J. Beneficial effects of C-peptide on incipient nephropathy and neuropathy in patients with Type 1 diabetes mellitus. Diabet Med 2000;17:181-9.

567) Johansson UB, Amsberg S, Hannerz L, Wredling R, Adamson U, Arnqvist HJ, Lins PE. Impaired absorption of insulin aspart from lipohypertrophic injection sites. Diabetes Care 2005;28:2025-7.

568) Johnsson S. Retinopathy and nephropathy in diabetes mellitus: comparison of the effects of two forms of treatment. Diabetes 1960;9:1-8.

569) Johnston A. Diabetes and Food. Yorkhill Diabetes Service 1998.

570) Johnston DG, Alberti KGMM. Hormonal control of ketone body metabolism in the normal and diabetic state. Clin Endocrin Met 1982;11:329-361.

571) Jones KL, Horowitz M, Berry M, Wishart JM, Guha S. Blood glucose concentration influences postprandial fullness in IDDM. Diabetes Care 1997;20: 1141-6.

572) Jones KL, Arslanian S, Peterokova VA, Park JS, Tomlinson MJ. Effect of metformin in pediatric patients with type 2 diabetes: a randomized controlled trial. Diabetes Care 2002;25:89-94.

573) Jones SM, Quarry JL, Caldwell-McMillan M, Mauger DT, Gabbay RA. Optimal insulin pump dosing and postprandial glycemia following a pizza meal using the continuous glucose monitoring system. Diabetes Technol Ther 2005;7:233-40.

574) Jones TW, Boulware SD, Kraemer DT, Caprio S, Sherwin RS, Tamborlane WV. Independent effects of youth and poor diabetes control on responses to hypoglycemia in children. Diabetes 1991;40:358-63.

575) Jones TW, Porter P, Sherwin RS, Davis EA, O'Leary P, Frazer F, Byrne G, Stick S, Tamborlane WV. Decreased epinephrine responses to hypoglycemia during sleep. N Engl J Med 1998;338:1657-62.

576) Jorgensen D, Solbeck H. Dilution of insulin aspart with NPH medium for small dose use in continuous subcutaneous insulin infusion does not affect in vitro stability. Diabetes 2005;54(suppl 1):A102(abstract).

577) Jornsay DL. Continous subcutaneous insulin infusion (CSII) during pregnancy. Diabetes Spectrum 1998;11:26-32.

578) Joseph SE, Korzon-Burakowska A, Woodworth JR, Evans M, Hopkins D, Janes JM, Amiel SA. The action profile of lispro is not blunted by mixing in the syringe with NPH insulin. Diabetes Care 1998;21:2098-102.

579) Joslin Diabetes Center 2003. Correcting Internet Myths About Aspartame. http://www.joslin.harvard.edu/education/library/aspartame.shtml

580) Jungheim K, Koschinsky T. Glucose Monitoring at the Arm: Risky delays of hypoglycemia and hyperglycemia detection. Diabetes Care 2002;25:956-60.

581) Justesen TI, Petersen JL, Ekbom P, Damm P, Mathiesen ER. Albumin-to-creatinine ratio in random urine samples might replace 24-h urine collections in screening for micro- and macroalbuminuria in pregnant woman with type 1 diabetes. Diabetes Care 2006;29:924-5.

582) Käär ML, Mäenpää J, Knip M. Insulin administration via a subcutaneous catheter. Diabetes Care 1993;16:1412-13.

583) Kadiri A, Al-Nakhi A, El-Ghazali S, Jabbar A, Al Arouj M, Akram J, Wyatt J, Assem A, Ristic S. Treatment of type 1 diabetes with insulin lispro during Ramadan. Diabetes Metab 2001;27:482-6.

584) Kalson NS, Davies AJ, Stokes S, Frost H, Whitehead AG, Tyrrell-Marsh I, Earl MD. Climbers with diabetes do well on Mount Kilimanjaro. Diabet Med 2007;24:1496.

585) Kamps JL, Hempe JM, Chalew SA. Racial disparity in A1C independent of mean blood glucose in children with type 1 diabetes. Diabetes Care 2010; 33:1025-7.

586) Kanc K, Janssen MM, Keulen ET, Jacobs MA, Popp-Snijders C, Snoek FJ, Heine RJ. Substitution of night-time continuous subcutaneous insulin infusion therapy for bedtime NPH insulin in a multiple injection regimen improves counterregulatory hormonal responses and warning symptoms of hypoglycaemia in IDDM. Diabetologia 1998;41:322-9.

587) Kaneto H, Ikeda M, Kishimoto M, Iida M, Hoshi A, Watari T, Kubota M, Kajimoto Y, Yamasaki Y, Hori M. Dramatic recovery of counter-regulatory hormone response to hypoglycemia after intensive therapy in poorly controlled type 1 diabetes mellitus. Diabetologia 1998;41:982-83.

588) Kaplan W, Rodriguez LM, Smith OE, Haymond MW, Heptulla RA. Effects of mixing glargine and short-acting insulin analogs on glucose control. Diabetes Care 2004;27:2739-40.

589) Karaguzel G, Satilmis A, Akcurin S, Bircan I. Comparison of breakfast and bedtime administration of insulin glargine in children and adolescents with Type 1 diabetes. Diabetes Res Clin Pract 2006;74:15-20.

590) Karges B, Boehm BO, Karges W. Early hypoglycaemia after accidental intramuscular injection of insulin glargine. Diabet Med 2005;22:1444-5.

591) Karlander S, Efendic S. Rapid and slow carbohydrates in the diabetic diet - time for a reevaluation? Lakartidningen 39/1984;81:3463-64.

592) Karvonen M, Viik-Kajander M, Moltchanova E, Libman I, LaPorte R, Tuomilehto J. Incidence of childhood type 1 diabetes worldwide. Diabetes Mondiale (DiaMond) Project Group. Diabetes Care 2000;23:1516-26.

593) Kassianos G. Some aspects of diabetes and travel. Diabetes Reviews International 2/1992;3:11-13.

594) Katahira M, Hara I, Nishizaki T. Insulin allergy decreased by Humulin S (Humulin R) and not by insulin aspart or Actrapid Penfill (Penfill R). Diabet Med 2005;22:1455-7.

595) Kaufman FR, Devgan S, Roe TF, Costin G. Perioperative management with prolonged intravenous insulin infusion versus subcutaneous insulin in children with type 1 diabetes mellitus. J Diabetes Complications 1996;10/1: 6-11.

596) Kaufman FR, Devgan S. Use of uncooked cornstarch to avert nocturnal hypoglycemia in children and adolescents with type 1 diabetes. J Diabetes Complications 1996;10/2:84-7.

597) Kaufman FR, Epport K, Engilman R, Halvorson M. Neurocognitive functioning in children diagnosed with diabetes before age 10 years. J Diabetes Complications 1999;13:31-8.

598) Kaufman FR, Halvorson M, Miller D, Mackenzie M, Fisher LK, Pitukcheewanont P. Insulin pump therapy in type 1 pediatric patients: now and into the year 2000. Diabetes Metab Res Rev 1999;15:338-52.

599) Kaufmann FR, Halvorson M, Kim C, Pitukcheewanont P. Use of insulin pump therapy at nighttime only for children 7-10 years of age with type 1 diabetes. Diabetes Care 2000;23:579-82.

600) Kaufman FR, Gibson LC, Halvorson M, Carpenter S, Fisher LK, Pitukcheewanont P. A pilot study of the continuous glucose monitoring system: clinical decisions and glycemic control after its use in pediatric type 1 diabetic subjects. Diabetes Care 2001;24:2030-4.

601) Kaufman FR. Diabetes at school: What a child's health care team needs to know about federal disability law. Clin Diab 2002;20:91-92.

602) Kawasaki E, Matsuura N, Eguchi K. Type 1 diabetes in Japan. Diabetologia 2006;49:828-36.

603) Kemp P, Staberg B. Smoking reduces insulin absorption from subcutaneous tissue. BMJ 1982;284:237.

604) Kernell A, Dedorsson I, Johansson B, Wickström CP, Ludvigsson J, Tuvemo T, Neiderud J, Sjöström K, Malmgren K, Kanulf P, Mellvig L, Gjötterberg M, Sule J, Persson LÅ, Larsson LI, Åman J, Dahlquist G. Prevalence of diabetic retinopathy in children and adolescents with IDDM. A population-based study. Diabetologia 1997;40:307-10.

605) Kerr D, Macdonald IA, Heller SR, Tattersall RB. Alcohol causes hypoglycaemic unawareness in healthy volunteers and patients with type 1 (insulin-dependent) diabetes. Diabetologia 1990;33:216-21.

606) Kida K, Mimura G, Ito T, Murakami K, Ashkenazi I, Laron Z. Incidence of Type 1 diabetes mellitus in children aged 0-14 in Japan, 1986-1990, including an analysis for seasonality of onset and month of birth: JDS study. The Data Committee for Childhood Diabetes of the Japan Diabetes Society (JDS). Diabet Med 2000;17:59-63.

607) Kilpatrick ES, Rigby AS, Atkin SL. The effect of glucose variability on the risk of microvascular complications in type 1 diabetes. Diabetes Care 2006;29:1486-90.

608) Kilpatrick ES, Rigby AS, Atkin SL. Variability in the relationship between mean plasma glucose and HbA1c: implications for the assessment of glycemic control. Clin Chem 2007;53:897-901.

609) Kilpatrick ES, Rigby AS, Atkin SL. Mean blood glucose compared with HbA(1c) in the prediction of cardiovascular disease in patients with type 1 diabetes. Diabetologia 2008;51:365-71.

610) Kimmerle R, Weiss R, Berger M, Kurz K. Effectiveness, safety, and acceptance of a copper intrauterine device (CU Safe 300) in type 1 diabetic women. Diabetes Care 1993;16:1227-30.

611) Kimmerle R, Zass RP, Cupisti S, Somville T, Bender R, Pawlowski B, Berger M. Pregnancies in women with diabetic nephropathy: long-term outcome for mother and child. Diabetologia 1995;38:227-35.

612) Kimmerle R, Heinemann L, Berger M. Intrauterine devices are safe and effective contraceptives for type 1 diabetic women [letter]. Diabetes Care 1995;18:1506-7.

613) King B, Goss P, Paterson M, Crock P, Anderson D. Changes in Atmospheric Pressure Alters Insulin Delivery From Insulin Pumps. Diab Tech Ther 2011; 13:241 (abstract 119).

614) King P, Kong MF, Parkin H, Macdonald IA, Tattersall RB. Well-being, cerebral function and physical fatigue after nocturnal hypoglycaemia in IDDM. Diabetes Care 1998;21:341-45.

615) King AB. Continuous glucose monitoring-guided insulin dosing in pump-treated patients with type 1 diabetes: a clinical guide. J Diabetes Sci Technol 2012;6:191-203.

616) Kipps S, Bahu T, Ong K, Ackland FM, Brown RS, Fox CT, Griffin NK, Knight AH, Mann NP, Neil HA, et al. Current methods of transfer of young people with Type 1 diabetes to adult services. Diabet Med 2002;19:649-54.

617) Kirk JM, Kinirons MJ. Dental health of young insulin dependent diabetic subjects in Northern Ireland. Community Dent Health 1991;8:335-41.

618) Kitabchi AE, Umpierrez GE, Murphy MB, Barrett EJ, Kreisberg RA, Malone JI, Wall BM. Management of hyperglycemic crises in patients with diabetes. Diabetes Care 2001;24:131-53.

619) Kitzmiller JL, Gavin LA, Gin GD, Jovanovic-Peterson L, Main EK, Zigrang WD. Preconception care of diabetes. Glycemic contol prevents congenital anomalies. JAMA 1991;265:731-36.

620) Klein R, Klein BE, Lee KE, Moss SE, Cruickshanks KJ. Prevalence of self-reported erectile dysfunction in people with long-term IDDM. Diabetes Care 1996;19:135-41.

621) Klemp P, Staberg B. Smoking reduces insulin absorption from subcutaneous tissue. BMJ 1982;284:237.

622) Klupa T, Benbenek-Klupa T, Malecki M, Szalecki M, Sieradzki J. Clinical usefulness of a bolus calculator in maintaining normoglycaemia in active professional patients with type 1 diabetes treated with continuous subcutaneous insulin infusion. J Int Med Res 2008;36:1112-6.

623) Knip M. Prevention of Childhood type 1 diabetes. Nord Med 8-9/1992; 107:207-210.

624) Knip M, Akerblom HK, Becker D, Dosch HM, Dupre J, Fraser W, Howard N, Ilonen J, Krischer JP, Kordonouri O, et al. Hydrolyzed infant formula and early beta-cell autoimmunity: a randomized clinical trial. JAMA 2014;311: 2279-87.

625) Kobold U, Jeppsson JO, Dülffer T, Finke A, Hoelzel W, Miedema K. Candidate reference methods for hemoglobin A$_{1c}$ based on peptide mapping. Clin Chem, 1997;43:1944-51.

626) Koivisto VA. Various influences on insulin absorption. Neth J Med 1985;28 suppl 1:25-28.

627) Koivisto VA, Haapa E, Tulokas S, Pelkonen R, Toivonen M. Alcohol with a meal has no adverse effect on postprandial glucose homeostasis in diabetic patients. Diabetes Care 12/1993;16:1612-14.

628) Kolb H, Elliot RB. Increasing incidence of IDDM a consequence of improving hygiene? Diabetologia 1994;37:729.

629) Kollind M. Lins P-E. Adamsson U. The man behind the phenomenon. Michael Somogyi and blood glucose regulation in unstable diabetes. A controversial hypothesis still discussed. Lakartidningen 10/1991;88:878-879.

630) Kong MF, King P, Macdonald IA, Blackshaw PE, Horowitz M, Perkins AC, Armstrong E, Buchanan KD, Tattersall RB. Euglycaemic hyperinsulinaemia does not affect gastric emptying in type I and type II diabetes mellitus. Diabetologia 1999;42:365-72.

631) Kong N, Ryder RE. What is the role of between meal snacks with intensive basal bolus regimens using preprandial lispro? Diabet Med 1999;16:325-31.

632) Kordonouri O, Lauterborn R, Deiss D. Lipohypertrophy in young patients with type 1 diabetes. Diabetes Care 2002;25:634.

633) Kordonouri O, Hartmann R, Remus K, Blasig S, Sadeghian E, Danne T. Benefit of supplementary fat plus protein counting as compared with conventional carbohydrate counting for insulin bolus calculation in children with pump therapy. Pediatr Diabetes. 2012; 13:540-4.

634) Kordonouri O, Witsch M, Sumník J, Veeze H, Danne T, de Beaufort C, Robert J, Forsander G, Szypowska A, Allgrove J, et al. The SWEET-Project 2006–2012: data analysis from 741 to 5749 patients per year – improving average glycemic control and completeness of monitoring. Pediatric Diabetes 2013;14 (Suppl 18):29 (abstract).

635) Kousseff BG. Gestational diabetes mellitus (class A): a human teratogen? Am J Med Genet 1999;83:402-8.

636) Kramer L, Fasching P, Madl C, Schneider B, Damjancic P, Waldhausl W, Irsigler K, Grimm G. Previous episodes of hypoglycemic coma are not associated with permanent cognitive brain dysfunction in IDDM patients on intensive insulin treatment. Diabetes 1998;47:1909-14.

637) Krane E. Diabetic Ketoacidosis. Biochemistry, physiology, treatment and prevention. Ped Clin North Am 4/1987;34:935-60.

638) Kruger D, Owen S, Whitehouse F. Scuba diving and diabetes. Practical guidelines. Diabetes Care 1995;18:1074.

639) Kullberg CE, Bergström A, Dinesen B, Larsson L, Little RR, Goldstein DE, Arnqvist HJ. Comparisons of studies on diabetic complications hampered by differences in GHb measurements. Diabetes Care 1996;7:726-29.

640) Kumar D. Lispro analog for treatment of generalized allergy to human insulin. Diabetes Care 1997;20:1357-59.

641) Kyvik KO, Gren A, Beck-Nilsen H. Concordance rates of insulin dependent diabetes mellitus: A population based study of young Danish twins. BMJ 1995;311:913-17.

642) Kølendorf K, Bojsen J, Deckert T. Clinical factors influencing the absorption of 125 I-NPH insulin in diabetic patients. Horm Metabol Res 1983;15: 274-8.

643) Lachin JM, Genuth S, Nathan DM, Zinman B, Rutledge BN. Effect of glycemic exposure on the risk of microvascular complications in the diabetes control and complications trial–revisited. Diabetes 2008;57:995-1001.

644) Laffel L. Ketone bodies: a review of physiology, pathophysiology and application of monitoring to diabetes. Diabetes Metab Res Rev 1999;15:412-26.

645) Laffel LM, Wentzell K, Loughlin C, Tovar A, Moltz K, Brink S. Sick day management using blood 3-hydroxybutyrate (3-OHB) compared with urine ketone monitoring reduces hospital visits in young people with T1DM: a randomized clinical trial. Diabet Med 2006;23:278-84.

646) Lager I. Metabolic disturbances in diabetes. In the book: Agardh C-D, Berne C, Östman J. Diabetes. Almqvist & Wiksell, Stockholm 1992:205-25.

647) Lahtela JT, Knip M, Paul R, Antonen J, Salmi J. Severe antibody-mediated insulin resistance: Successful treatment with the insulin analog Lispro. Diabetes Care 1997;20:71-73.

648) Landau Z, Klonoff D, Nayberg I, Feldman D, Levit SB, Lender D, Mosenzon O, Raz I, Wainstein J. Improved pharmacokinetic and pharmacodynamic profile of insulin analogs using InsuPatch, a local heating device. Diabetes Metab Res Rev 2014;

649) Landin-Olsson M, Öhlin AC, Agardh CD. Blood glucose: influence of different methods for analysis and procedures for sampling. Pract Diab 1997; 14:47-50.

650) Lapolla A, Dalfra MG, Fedele D. Insulin therapy in pregnancy complicated by diabetes: are insulin analogs a new tool? Diabetes Metab Res Rev 2005;21:241-52.

651) Larger E. Weight gain and insulin treatment. Diabetes Metab 2005;31: 4S51-4S56.

652) Larkin J. Typical infections in diabetes and their treatment. In the book: Pharmacology of Diabetes. Walter de Greyter, Berlin 1991:325-42.

653) Larsen ML, Hørder M, Mogensen EF. Effect of long-term monitoring of glycosylated Hemoglobin levels in insulin-dependent IDDM. N Engl J Med 1990;323:1021-25.

654) Larsson K, Carlsson A, Cederwall E, Jonsson B, Neiderud J, Lernmark A, et al. Annual screening detects celiac disease in children with type 1 diabetes. Pediatr Diabetes. 2008; 9:354-9.

655) Lauritzen T, Pramming S, Deckert T. Pharmacokinetics of continous subcutaneous insulin infusion. Diabetologia 1983;24:326-29.

656) Lauritzen T. Pharmacokinetic and clinical aspects of intensified subcutaneous insulin therapy. Dan Med Bull 1985;32:104-18.

657) Lavery LA, Harkless LB, Walker SC, Felder-Johnson K. Infected puncture wounds in diabetic and nondiabetic adults. Diabetes Care 1995;18:1588-1591.

658) Lawler-Heavner J, Cruickshanks KJ, Hay WW, Gay EC, Hamman RF. Birth size and risk of IDDM. Diabetes Res Clin Pract 1994;24:153-9.

659) Lawson ML, Gerstein HC, Tsui E, Zinman B. Effect of intensive therapy on early macrovascular disease in young individuals with type 1 diabetes. A systematic review and meta-analysis. Diabetes Care 1999;22 Suppl 2:B35-9.

660) Leahy JL, Cooper HE, Deal DA, Weir GC. Chronic hyperglycemia is associated with impaired glucose influence on insulin secretion. A study in normal rats using chronic in vivo glucose infusions. J Clin Invest 1986;77:908-15.

661) Lebovitz HE. Diabetic ketoacidosis. Lancet 1995;345:767-71.

662) Lehmann R, Kaplan V, Bingisser R, Bloch KE, Spinas GA. Impact of physical activity on cardiovascular risk factors in IDDM. Diabetes Care 1997;20: 1603-11.

663) Leiker, M. Kara Neumann, spiritual healing, and the law. Wisconstin Med J. 2009;108:415.

664) Lepore M, Pampanelli S, Fanelli C, Porcellati F, Bartocci L, Di Vincenzo A, Cordoni C, Costa E, Brunetti P, Bolli GB. Pharmacokinetics and pharmacodynamics of subcutaneous injection of long-acting human insulin analog glargine, NPH insulin, and ultralente human insulin and continuous subcutaneous infusion of insulin lispro. Diabetes 2000;49:2142-8.

665) Lernmark Å, Sundkvist G. Etiology of type 1-diabetes. In the book: Agardh C-D, Berne C, Östman J. Diabetes. Almqvist & Wiksell, Stockholm 1992:56-64.

666) Leslie RD, Elliot RB. Early environmental events as a cause of IDDM. Diabetes 1994;43:843-50.

667) Li HY, Chen YJ, Chen SJ, Kao CL, Tseng LM, Lo WL, Chang CM, Yang DM, Ku HH, Twu NF, et al. Induction of insulin-producing cells derived from endometrial mesenchymal stem-like cells. J Pharmacol Exp Ther 2010; 335:817-29.

668) Liese AD, D'Agostino RB, Jr., Hamman RF, Kilgo PD, Lawrence JM, Liu LL, Loots B, Linder B, Marcovina S, Rodriguez B, et al. The burden of diabetes mellitus among US youth: prevalence estimates from the SEARCH for Diabetes in Youth Study. Pediatrics 2006;118:1510-8.

669) Lind M, Oden A, Fahlen M, Eliasson B. The shape of the metabolic memory of HbA1c: re-analysing the DCCT with respect to time-dependent effects. Diabetologia 53:1093-8.

670) Lindberg A-S. Diving into the depth of prejudice - or ignorance? Diabetes (Swed. Diab. Ass.) 2/1990:22-25.

671) Lindberg A-S. Even children with diabetes need an upbringing. Diabetes (Swed. Diab. Ass.)2/1993:14-15.

672) Lindberg A-S. Adolescents breaking up. One must chop the umbilical cord. Diabetes (Swed. Diab. Ass.) 6/1990:18-20.

673) Lindblad B. Data from the National Swedish Childhood Diabetes Registry 2001.

674) Linde B. Dissociation of insulin absorption and blood flow during massage of a subcutaneous injection site. Diabetes Care 1986;9:570-74.

675) Lindholm A, McEwen J, Riis AP. Improved postprandial glycemic control with insulin aspart. A randomized double-blind cross-over trial in type 1 diabetes. Diabetes Care 1999;22:801-5.

676) Lingenfelser T, Renn W, Buettner U, Kaschel R, Martin J, Jakober B, Tobis M. Improvement of impaired counterregulatory hormone response and symtom perception by short-term avoidance of hypoglycemia in IDDM. Diabetes Care 1995;18:321-5.

677) Little RR, Goldstein DE. Measurements of glycated haemoglobin and other circulating glycated proteins. In the book: Research Methodologies in Human Diabetes. Walter de Greyter, Berlin 1994.

678) Litton J, Rice A, Friedman N, Oden J, Lee MM, Freemark M. Insulin pump therapy in toddlers and preschool children with type 1 diabetes mellitus. J Pediatr 2002;141(4):490-5.

679) Liu D, Moberg E, Wredling R, Lins PE, Adamson U. Insulin absorption is faster when keeping the injection site in use for three days during continuous subcutaneous insulin infusion. Diabetes Res Clin Pract 1991;12:19-24.

680) Lloyd CE, Dyer PH, Lancashire RJ, Harris T, Daniels JE, Barnett AH. Association between stress and glycemic control in adults with type 1 (insulin-dependent) diabetes. Diabetes Care 1999;22:1278-83.

681) Lodefalk M, Aman J, Bang P. Effects of fat supplementation on glycaemic response and gastric emptying in adolescents with Type 1 diabetes. Diabet Med 2008;25:1030-5.

682) Loeb J, Herold K, Barton K, Robinson L, Jaspan J. Systematic approach to diagnosis and managment of biphasic insulin allergy with local anti-inflammatory agents. Diabetes Care 6/1989;12:421-23.

683) Loghmani E, Rickard K, Washburne L, Vandagriff J, Fineberg N, Golden M. Glycemic response to sucrose-containing mixed meals in diets of children with insulin dependent diabetes mellitus. J Pediatrics 1991;119:531-537.

684) Lönnroth P. Insulin's effects. In the book: Agardh C-D, Berne C, Östman J. Diabetes. Almqvist & Wiksell, Stockholm 1992:29-37.

685) Look D, Strauss K. Reuse of sharps in diabetic patients: is it completely safe? Diabetes Journal 1998;10:31-34.

686) Loukovaara S, Immonen I, Teramo KA, Kaaja R. Progression of retinopathy during pregnancy in type 1 diabetic women treated with insulin lispro. Diabetes Care 2003;26:1193-8.

687) Lteif AN, Schwenk WF. Accuracy of pen injectors versus insulin syringes in children with type 1 diabetes. Diabetes Care 1999;22:137-40.

688) Lucidarme N, Alberti C, Zaccaria I, Claude E, Tubiana-Rufi N. Alternate-site testing is reliable in children and adolescents with type 1 diabetes, except at the forearm for hypoglycemia detection. Diabetes Care 2005;28:710-11.

689) Ludvigsson J, Hermansson G, Häger A, Kernell A, Nordenskjöld K. Adequate substitution of insulin deficiency is a base in the treatment of diabetes in young people. Lakartidningen 22/1988;85:2004-08.

690) Ludvigsson J. Insulin, love & care. Horm Res 1989;31:204-09.

691) Ludvigsson J, Tuvemo T. Diabetes in children. In the book Agardh C-D, Berne C, Östman J. Diabetes. Liber, Stockholm 2005:196-215 (Swedish text).

692) Ludvigsson J. Is diabetes in children caused by cows' milk? Lakartidningen 16/1993;90:1529-1531.

693) Ludvigsson J. Measurement of HbA_{1c} with a rapid method. Improved handling of patients with diabetes. Lakartidningen 21/1994;91:2135-36.

694) Ludvigsson J, Nordfeldt S. Hypoglycemia during intensified insulin therapy of children and adolescents. J Ped Endo & Met 1998;11(suppl 1):159-166.

695) Ludvigsson J. Pain and diabetes monitoring in children and teenagers. Diabetes NEWS 1998;19:3-5.

696) Ludvigsson J, Samuelsson U, Ernerudh J, Johansson C, Stenhammar L, Berlin G. Photopheresis at onset of type 1 diabetes: a randomised, double blind, placebo controlled trial. Arch Dis Child 2001;85:149-54.

697) Ludvigsson J, Hanas R. Continuous Subcutaneous Glucose Monitoring improved metabolic control in pediatric patients with type 1 diabetes: A controlled cross-over study. Pediatrics 2003;111:933-38.

698) Ludvigsson J, Casas R, Vaarala O, Forsander G, Ivarsson S, Johansson C, Lindh A, Nilsson N, Åman J, Örtqvist E, et al. The Swedish GAD-vaccination Trial: outcomes of a phase II safety and efficacy trial with Diamyd™ for preservation of beta cell function in children with T1D. Diabetologia 2006; 49 (suppl 1):149 (abstract).

699) Lunt H, Brown JLJ. Self-reported changes in capillary glucose and insulin requirements during the menstrual cycle. Diabetic Med 1996;13/6:525-30.

700) Lustman PJ, Anderson RJ, Freedland KE, de Groot M, Carney RM, Clouse RE. Depression and poor glycemic control: a meta-analytic review of the literature. Diabetes Care 2000;23:934-42.

701) Luzi L, Barrett EJ, Groop LC, Ferrannini E, DeFronzo RA. Metabolic effects of low-dose insulin therapy on glucose metabolism in diabetic ketoacidosis. Diabetes 1988;37:1470-7.

702) Ly TT, Nicholas JA, Retterath A, Lim EM, Davis EA, Jones TW. Effect of sensor-augmented insulin pump therapy and automated insulin suspension vs standard insulin pump therapy on hypoglycemia in patients with type 1 diabetes: a randomized clinical trial. JAMA 2013;310:1240-7.

703) Lytzen L, Hansen B, Sørensen JP. Pain perception and frequency of bleeding. A single-blind, randomized investigation comparing NovoPen Needle gauge 27/12mm, 28/12mm and 30/12mm. Abstract, AIDSPIT, Igls, January 1993.

704) Maahs D, Hermann J, DuBose S, Miller K, Heidtmann B, DiMeglio L, Rami-Merhar B, Beck R, Schober E, Tamborlane W, Kapellen T, Holl R. Contrasting the clinical care and outcomes of 2,622 children with type 1 diabetes less than 6 years of age in the United States T1D Exchange and German/Austrian DPV Registries. Diabetologia 2014:in press.

705) MacCuish AC. Treatment of hypoglycemia. In the book: Frier B, Fisher M. Hypoglycemia and diabetes: Clinical and physiological aspects. Edward Arnold, London 1993:212-21.

706) MacDonald MJ. Postexercise late-onset hypoglycemia in insulin-dependent diabetic patients. Diabetes Care 1987;10:584-8.

707) Macfarlane PE, Walters M, Stutchfield P. A prospective study of symtomatic hypoglycemia in childhood diabetes. Diabetic Med 1989;6:627-30.

708) MacKenzie RG. A practical approach to the drug-using adolescent and young adult. Ped Clin N Am 1973;20:1035-45.

709) MacLeod KM, Hepburn DA, Frier BM. Frequency and morbidity of severe hypoglycaemia in insulin-treated diabetic patients. Diabet Med 1993;10: 238-45.

710) MacLeod KM. Diabetes and driving: towards equitable, evidence-based decision-making. Diabet Med 1999;16:282-90.

711) Madero MF, Sastre J, Carnes J, Quirce S, Herrera-Pombo JL. IgG(4)-mediated allergic reaction to glargine insulin. Allergy 2006;61:1022-3.

712) Madsbad S, McNair P, Christensen MS, Christiansen C, Faber OK, Binder C, Transbol I. Influence of smoking on insulin requirement and metbolic status in diabetes mellitus. Diabetes Care 1980;3:41-3.

713) Malchoff CD, Shoukri K, Landau JI, and Buchert JM. A Novel Noninvasive Blood Glucose Monitor. Diabetes Care 2002;25: 2268-2275.

714) Malherbe C, de Gasparo M, de Hertogh R, Hoet J: Circadian variations of blood sugar and plasma insulin. Diabetologia 1969;5:397-404.

715) Maniatis AK, Klingensmith GJ, Slover RH, Mowry CJ, Chase HP. Continuous subcutaneous insulin infusion therapy for children and adolescents: an option for routine diabetes care. Pediatrics 2001;107:351-6.

716) Maran A, Lomas J, Macdonald IA, Amiel SA. Lack of preservation of higher brain function during hypoglycaemia in patients with intensively-treated IDDM. Diabetologia 1995;38:1412-18.

717) Marcus AO, Fernandez MP. Insulin pump therapy: acceptable alternative to injection therapy. Postgraduate Medicine 1996;99/3:125-32.

718) Margeirsdottir HD, Larsen JR, Brunborg C, Overby NC, Dahl-Jorgensen K. High prevalence of cardiovascular risk factors in children and adolescents with type 1 diabetes: a population-based study. Diabetologia 2008;51:554-61.

719) Marklund U. Drugs and Influence. Pupil analysis as starting-point for drug education. Thesis, Göteborg Studies in Educational Science 42, 1983. Göteborgs University, Dept. of Pedagogics, Sweden.

720) Marliss EB, Vranic M. Intense exercise has unique effects on both insulin release and its roles in glucoregulation: implications for diabetes. Diabetes 2002;51 Suppl 1:S271-83.

721) Marran K, Segal D. Exponential increase in postprandial blood-glucose exposure with increasing carbohydrate loads using a linear carbohydrate-to-insulin ratio. S Afr Med J 2013;103:

722) Marshall SM, Barth JH. Standardization of HbA1c measurements - a consensus statement. Diabet Med 2000;17:5-6.

723) Martin CL, Albers J, Herman WH, Cleary P, Waberski B, Greene DA, Stevens MJ, Feldman EL. Neuropathy among the diabetes control and complications trial cohort 8 years after trial completion. Diabetes Care 2006;29: 340-4.

724) Massin MM, Lebrethon MC, Rocour D, Gerard P, Bourguignon JP. Patterns of physical activity determined by heart rate monitoring among diabetic children. Arch Dis Child 2005;90:1223-6.

725) Mastrototaro JJ, Cooper KW, Soundararajan G, Sanders JB, Shah RV. Clinical experience with an integrated continuous glucose sensor/insulin pump platform: a feasibility study. Adv Ther 2006;23(5):725-32.

726) Mathiesen B, Borch-Johnsen K. Diabetes and accident insurance. A 3-year follow-up of 7,599 insured diabetic individuals. Diabetes Care 1997;20: 1781-84.

727) Mathiesen ER, Kinsley B, Amiel SA, Heller S, McCance D, Duran S, Bellaire S, Raben A. Maternal glycemic control and hypoglycemia in type 1 diabetic pregnancy: a randomized trial of insulin aspart versus human insulin in 322 pregnant women. Diabetes Care 2007;30:771-6.

728) Matyka KA, Wigg L, Pramming S, Stores G, Dunger DB. Cognitive function and mood after profound nocturnal hypoglycaemia in prepubertal children with conventional insulin treatment for diabetes. Arch Dis Child 1999;81: 138-42.

729) Mawby M (editorial). Time for law to catch up with life. Diabetes Care 1997; 20:1640-41.

730) Mazze RS, Lucido D, Shamoon H. Psychological and social correlates of glycemic control. Diabetes Care 1984;7:360-66.

731) McCarter RJ, Hempe JM, Gomez R, Chalew SA. Biological variation in HbA1c predicts risk of retinopathy and nephropathy in type 1 diabetes. Diabetes Care 2004;27:1259-64.

732) McCarter RJ, Hempe JM, Chalew SA. Mean blood glucose and biological variation have greater influence on HbA1c levels than glucose instability: an analysis of data from the Diabetes Control and Complications Trial. Diabetes Care 2006;29:352-5.

733) McCarthy AM, Lindgren S, Mengeling MA, Tsalikian E, Engvall J. Factors associated with academic achievement in children with type 1 diabetes. Diabetes Care 2003;26:112-7.

734) McCarthy JA, Covarrubias B, Sink P. Is the traditional alcohol wipe necessary before an insulin injection? Diabetes care 1993;16/1:402.

735) McCrimmon RJ, Gold AE, Deary IJ, Kelnar CJH, Frier BM. Symptoms of hypoglycemia in children with IDDM. Diabetes Care 1995;18:858-61.

736) McCullough D, Kurtz A, Tattersall R. A new approach to the treatment of nocturnal hypoglycemia using alpha-glucosidase inhibition. Diabetes Care 5/1993;6:483-87.

737) McHugh PR, Moran TH. Calories and gastric emptying: a regulatory capacity with implications for feeding. Am J Physiology 1979;236:R254-60.

738) McNally PG, Raymond NT, Swift PGF, Hearnshaw JR, Burden AC. Does the prepubertal duration of diabetes influence the onset of microvascular complications? Diab Med 1993;10:906-8.

739) Mecklenburg RS, Benson EA, Benson W, Fredlund PN, Cuinn T, Metz RJ, Nielsen RL, Sannar CA. Acute complications associated with insulin infusion pump therapy. Report of experience with 161 patients. JAMA 1984; 252:3265-69.

740) Melki V, Renard E, Lassmann-Vague V, Boivin S, Guerci B, Hanaire-Broutin H, Bringer J, Belicar P, Jeandidier N, Meyer L, Blin P, Augendre-Ferrante B, Tauber JP. Improvement of HbA$_{1c}$ and blood glucose stability in IDDM patients treated with lispro insulin analog in external pumps. Diabetes Care 1998; 21:977-86.

741) Meloni GF, Dessole S, Vargiu N, Tomasi PA, Musumeci S. The prevalence of coeliac disease in infertility. Hum Reprod 1999;14:2759-61.

742) Mendosa R. On-line Resources for Diabetics. Glycemic Index Lists. 1997 (http://www.mendosa.com/gilists.htm)

743) Mendosa R. The GI factor. 1997 (http://www.mendosa.com/gifactor.htm)

744) Mettenburg J. Role Models: Nicole Johnson, Miss America 1999. Countdown for Kids Spring 1999.

745) The Microalbuminuria Captopril Study Group. Captopril reduces the risk of nephropathy in IDDM patients with microalbuminuria. Diabetologia 1996; 39:587-93.

746) Miller RG, Secrest AM, Sharma RK, Songer TJ, Orchard TJ. Improvements in the life expectancy of type 1 diabetes: the Pittsburgh Epidemiology of Diabetes Complications study cohort. Diabetes 2012;61:2987-92.

747) Minuto N, Tambroni B, Vannati M, Emmanuele V, Russo C, Lorini R, d'Annunzio G. Diabetic ketoacidosis caused by exposure of insulin to low temperature. Diabetes Technol Ther 2010;12:745-6.

748) Mitchell TH, Abraham G, Schiffrin A, Leiter LA, Marliss EB. Hyperglycemia after intense exercise in IDDM subjects during continuous subcutaneous insulin infusion. Diabetes Care 1988;11:311-7.

749) Mitrakou A, Platanisiotis D, Partheniou C, Kytelis E, Livadas S, Raptis SA. Glucose fall from hyper- to normoglycemia triggers norepinephrine secretion in type 1 diabetes. Diabetologia 1993;36 (Suppl 1):abstract 575.

750) Mitsuhashi T, Li YM, Fishbane S, Vlassara H. Depletion of reactive advanced glycation endproducts from diabetic uremic sera using a lysozyme-linked matrix. J Clin Invest 1997;100:847-54.

751) Moberg E, Kollind M, Lins P-E, Adamsson U. Acute mental stress impairs insulin sensitivity in IDDM patients. Diabetologia 1994;37:247-251.

752) Mohn A, Strang S, Wernicke-Panten K, Lang AM, Edge JA, Dunger DB. Nocturnal glucose control and free insulin levels in children with type 1 diabetes by use of the long-acting insulin HOE 901 as part of a three-injection regimen. Diabetes Care 2000;23:557-9.

753) Mohn A, Cerruto M, Iafusco D, Prisco F, Tumini S, Stoppoloni O, Chiarelli F. Celiac Disease in Children and Adolescents with Type I Diabetes: Importance of Hypoglycemia. J Pediatr Gastroenterol Nutr 2001;32:37-40.

754) Mohn A, Di Michele S, Di Luzio R, Tumini S, Chiarelli F. The effect of subclinical hypothyroidism on metabolic control in children and adolescents with Type 1 diabetes mellitus. Diabet Med 2002;19:70-3.

755) Mohr SB, Garland FC, Garland CF, Gorham ED, Ricordi C. Is there a role of vitamin D deficiency in type 1 diabetes of children? Am J Prev Med 2010; 39:189-90.

756) Montoro MN, Myers VP, Mestman JH, Xu Y, Anderson BG, Golde SH. Outcome of pregnancy in diabetic ketoacidosis. Am J Perinatology 1993;10:17-20.

757) Moore K, Vizzard N, Coleman C, McMahon J, Hayes R, Thompson CJ. Extreme altitude mountaineering and Type 1 diabetes; the Diabetes Federation of Ireland Kilimanjaro Expedition. Diabet Med 2001: 18: 749-755.

758) Morain WD, Colen BC. Wound healing in diabetes. Clin Plast Surg 1990;17: 493-501.

759) Morgado PB, Chen HC, Patel V, Herbert L, Kohner EM. The acute effect of smoking on retinal blood flow in subjects with and without diabetes. Ophthalmology 1994;101:1220-6.

760) Morris AD, Boyle DI, McMahon AD, Greene SA, MacDonald TM, Newton RW. Adherence to insulin treatment, glycaemic control, and ketoacidosis in insulin-dependent diabetes mellitus. Lancet 1997;350:1505-10.

761) Morrow L, Muchmore DB, Hompesch M, Ludington EA, Vaughn DE. Comparative pharmacokinetics and insulin action for three rapid-acting insulin analogs injected subcutaneously with and without hyaluronidase. Diabetes Care 2013;36:273-5.

762) Mortensen HB, Hougaard P and the Hvidøre Study Group on Childhood Diabetes. Comparison of metabolic control in a cross-sectional study of 2,873 children and adolescents with IDDM from 18 countries. Diabetes Care 1997;20:714-720.

763) Mortensen HB, Lindholm A, Olsen BS, Hylleberg B. Rapid appearance and onset of action of insulin aspart in paediatric subjects with type 1 diabetes. Eur J Pediatr 2000;159:483-8.

764) Moss SE, Klein R, Kessler SD, Richie KA. Comparison between ophthalmoscopy and fundus photography in determining severity of diabetic retinopathy. Ophthalmology 1985;92:62-7.

765) Moss SE, Klein R, Klein BE. Ten-year incidence of visual loss in a diabetic population. Ophthalmology 1994;106:1061-70.

766) Mudaliar SR, Lindberg FA, Joyce M, Beerdsen P, Strange P, Lin A, Henry RR. Insulin aspart (B28 asp-insulin): a fast-acting analog of human insulin: absorption kinetics and action profile compared with regular human insulin in healthy nondiabetic subjects. Diabetes Care 1999;22:1501-6.

767) Mühlhauser I, Koch J, Berger M. Pharmacokinetics and bioavailability of injected glucagon: differences between intramuscular, subcutaneous, and intravenous administration. Diabetes Care 1985;8:39-42.

768) Mühlhauser I. Cigarette smoking and diabetes: An update. Diabetes 1994; 11:336-43.

769) Mulec H, Blohmé G, Grände B, Björck S. The effect on metabolic control on rate of decline in renal function in insulin dependent diabetes mellitus with overt diabetic nephropathy. Nephrol Dial Transplant 1998;13:651-5.

770) Murphy NP, Keane KK, Ford-Adams ME, Edge JA, Dunger DB. A Randomized Cross-Over Trial Comparing Insulin Glargine Plus Lispro with NPH Insulin Plus Soluble Insulin in Adolescents with Type 1 Diabetes. Diabetes 2002;51(suppl2):A54(abstract 218).

771) Murtaugh MA, Ferris AM, Capacchione CM, Reece EA. Energy intake and glycemia in lactating women with type 1 diabetes. J Am Diet Assoc 1998; 98:642-8.

772) Nanto-Salonen K, Kupila A, Simell S, Siljander H, Salonsaari T, Hekkala A, Korhonen S, Erkkola R, Sipila JI, Haavisto L, Siltala M, Tuominen J, Hakalax J, Hyoty H, Ilonen J, Veijola R, Simell T, Knip M, Simell O. Nasal insulin to prevent type 1 diabetes in children with HLA genotypes and autoantibodies conferring increased risk of disease: a double-blind, randomised controlled trial. Lancet 2008;372:1746-55.

773) Nathan DM, Godine JE, Guthier-Kelley C, Kawahara D, Grinvalsky M. Ice cream in the diet of insulin-dependent diabetes. JAMA 1984;251:2825-27.

774) Nathan DM, Dunn FL, Bruch J et al. Postprandial insulin profiles with implantable pump therapy may explain decreased frequency of severe hypoglycemia, compared with intensive subcutaneous regimens, in insulin-dependent diabetes mellitus patients. Am J Med 1996;100/4:412-17.

775) Nathan DM, Lachin J, Cleary P, Orchard T, Brillon DJ, Backlund JY, O'Leary DH, Genuth S. Intensive diabetes treatment and carotid intima-media thickness in type 1 diabetes mellitus. N Engl J Med 2003;348:2294-303.

776) Nathan DM, Cleary PA, Backlund JY, Genuth SM, Lachin JM, Orchard TJ, Raskin P, Zinman B. Intensive diabetes treatment and cardiovascular disease in patients with type 1 diabetes. N Engl J Med 2005;353:2643-53.

777) Nathan DM, Kuenen J, Borg R, Zheng H, Schoenfeld D, Heine RJ. Translating the A1C assay into estimated average glucose values. Diabetes Care 2008;31:1473-8.

778) Nayak B, Clement S. Insulin Pen Delivery Systems: Comparison of Dosage Accuracy of OptiClik and FlexPen Insulin Pens. Diabetes 2007;56(Suppl 1): A533(abstract 2106-PO).

779) Neu A, Willasch A, Ehehalt S, Kehrer M, Hub R, Ranke MB. Diabetes incidence in children of different nationalities: an epidemiological approach to the pathogenesis of diabetes. Diabetologia 2001;44 Suppl 3:B21-6.

780) Newgard C. Cellular treatment and gene therapy for insulin replacement in diabetes. Diabetes 1994;43:341-350.

781) Newton RW, Greene SA. Diabetes in the adolescent. In the book: Kelnar CJH (Ed.). Childhood and Adolescent Diabetes. Chapman & Hall 1995:367-74.

782) Ng RS, Darko DA, Hillson RM. Street drug use among young patients with Type 1 diabetes in the UK. Diabet Med 2004;21:295-6.

783) Nguyen TM, Mason KJ, Sanders CG, Yazdani P, Heptulla RA. Targeting blood glucose management in school improves glycemic control in children with poorly controlled type 1 diabetes mellitus. J Pediatr 2008;153:575-8.

784) Nguyen TM, Renukuntla VS, Heptulla RA. Mixing insulin with detemir does not affect glucose excursion in children with type 1 diabetes. Diabetes Care 2010;33(11):2-5.

785) NICE Guidelines. Type 1 Diabetes: Diagnosis and Management of Type 1 Diabetes in Children and Young People. National Institute for Clinical Excellence, UK 2004.

786) NICE Guidelines 2014

787) Nicolajsen T, Samuelsson A, Hanas R. Insulin Doses before and One Year after Pump Start: Children Have a Reversed Dawn Phenomenon. J Diab Sci Tech 2012;6:589-94.

788) Nielsen S, Emborg C, Molbak AG. Mortality in concurrent type 1 diabetes and anorexia nervosa. Diabetes Care 2002;25:309-12.

789) Nimri R, Danne T, Kordonouri O, Atlas E, Bratina N, Biester T, Avbelj M, Miller S, Muller I, Phillip M, et al. The "Glucositter" overnight automated closed loop system for type 1 diabetes: a randomized crossover trial. Pediatr Diabetes 2013;14:159-67.

790) Nimri R, Lebenthal Y, Shalitin S, Benzaquen H, Demol S, Phillip M. Metabolic control by insulin detemir in basal-bolus therapy: treat-to-target study in children and adolescents with type 1 diabetes. Pediatr Diabetes 2013; 14:196-202.

791) Nordfeldt S, Ludvigsson J. Severe hypoglycemia in children with IDDM. A prospective population study, 1992-94. Diabetes Care 1997;20:497-503.

792) Nordfeldt S, Ludvigsson J. Seasonal variation of HbA1c in intensive treatment of children with type 1 diabetes. J Pediatr Endocrinol Metab 2000; 13:529-35.

793) Nordfeldt S, Samuelsson U. Serum ACE predicts severe hypoglycemia in children and adolescents with type 1 diabetes. Diabetes Care 2003;26: 274-8.

794) Nordwall M, Bojestig M, Arnqvist HJ, Ludvigsson J. Declining incidence of severe retinopathy and persisting decrease of nephropathy in an unselected population of Type 1 diabetes-the Linkoping Diabetes Complications Study. Diabetologia 2004;47:1266-72.

795) Nordin G, Dybkaer R. Recommendation for term and measurement unit for "HbA1c". Clin Chem Lab Med 2007;45:1081-2.

796) North RV, Farell U, Banford D, Jones C, Gregory JW, Butler, Ownes DR. Visual function in young IDDM patients over 8 years of age. Diabetes Care 1997;20:1724-30.

797) Northam EA, Anderson PJ, Werther GA, Warne GL, Andrewes D. Predictors of change in the neuropsychological profiles of children with type 1 diabetes 2 years after disease onset. Diabetes Care 1999;22:1438-44.

798) Northam EA, Anderson PJ, Jacobs R, Hughes M, Warne GL, Werther GA. Neuropsychological profiles of children with type 1 diabetes 6 years after disease onset. Diabetes Care 2001;24:1541-6.

799) Nosek L, Heinemann L, Kaiser M, et al. No increase in the duration of action with rising doses of insulin aspart. Diabetes 2003 Jun; 52 Suppl. 1: 128-9 (abstract).

800) Nutall F. Dietary fibers in the management of Diabetes. Diabetes 1993;42: 503-508.

801) Nyström L, Dahlquist G, Rewers M, Wall S. The Swedish childhood diabetes study. An analysis of the temporal variation in diabetes incidence 1978-87. Int J Epidemiol 1990;19:141-46.

802) Nyström L, Ostman J, Wall S, Wibell L. Mortality of all incident cases of diabetes mellitus in Sweden diagnosed 1983-87 at age 15-34 years. Diabetes incidence Study in Sweden (DISS) Group. Diabetic Med. 1992;9:422-7.

803) Olinder AL, Kernell A, Smide B. Missed bolus doses: devastating for metabolic control in CSII-treated adolescents with type 1 diabetes. Pediatr Diabetes 2009;10:142-8.

804) Öberg D, Östenson CG. Performance of glucose dehydrogenase-and glucose oxidase-based blood glucose meters at high altitude and low temperature. Diabetes Care 2005;28:1261.

805) Olsen BS, Johannesen J, Sjolie AK, Borch-Johnsen K, Hougarrdss P, Thorsteinsson B, Prammingss S, Marinelli K, Mortensen HB. Metabolic control and prevalence of microvascular complications in young Danish patients with Type 1 diabetes mellitus. Danish Study Group of Diabetes in Childhood. Diabet Med 1999;16:79-85.

806) Olsen BS, Sjolie AK, Hougaard P, Johannesen J, Marinelli K, Jacobsen BB, Mortensen HB. The significance of the prepubertal diabetes duration for the development of retinopathy and nephropathy in patients with type 1 diabetes. J Diabetes Complications 2004;18:160-4.

807) Olsson PO. Insulin treatment. In the book: Diabetes. SPRI and Swedish Medical Society 1989:226-32.

808) Olsson PO, Arnqvist H, Asplund J. No pharmacokinetic effect of retaining the infusion site up to four days during continuous subcutaneous insulin infusion therapy. Diabet Med 6/1993;10:477-80.

809) Orchard TJ, Forrest KY, Ellis D, Becker DJ. Cumulative glycemic exposure and microvascular complications in insulin- dependent diabetes mellitus. The glycemic threshold revisited. Arch Intern Med 1997;157:1851-6.

810) Östman J, Andersson D. Diabetes mellitus. In the book: Drugs. Swedish Pharmaceutical Company 1993-94:474.

811) Örtqvist E, Björk E, Wallensteen M, Ludvigsson J, Åman J, Forsander G, Lindgren F, Berne C, Persson B, Karlsson FA. Diazoxide treatment at onset in childhood type 1 diabetes. JPEM 2001;14(Suppl 3):1044(abstract).

812) O'Sullivan JB. Subsequent morbidity among gestational diabetic women. In the book: Sutherland HW, Stowers JM (Eds) Carbohydrate Metabolism in Pregnancy and the Newborn. New York: Churchill Livingstone 1984;174-80.

813) Owens DR, Coates PA, Luzio SD, Tinbergen JP, Kurzhals R. Pharmacokinetics of ^{125}I-labeled insulin glargine (HOE 901) in healthy men: comparison with NPH insulin and the influence of different subcutaneous injection sites. Diabetes Care 2000;23:813-9.

814) Packer SC, Dornhorst A, Frost GS. The glycaemic index of a range of gluten-free foods. Diabet Med 2000;17:657-60.

815) Pampanelli S, Torlone E, Lalli C, Sindaco PD, Ciofetta M, Lepore M, Bartocci L, Brunetti P, Bolli GB. Improved postprandial metabolic control after subcutaneous injection of a short-acting insulin analog in IDDM of short duration with residual pancreatic β-cell function. Diabetes Care 1995; 18(11):1452-59.

816) Pampanelli S, Fanelli C, Lalli C, Ciofetta M, Sindaco PD, Lepore M, Modarelli F, Rambotti AM, Epifano L, Di Vincenzo A, et al. Long-term intensive insulin therapy in IDDM: effects on HbA$_{1c}$, risk for severe and mild hypoglycaemia, status of counterregulation and awareness of hypoglycaemia. Diabetologia 1996;39:677-86.

817) Pampanelli S, Lepore M, Fanelli C, Del Sindaco P, Lalli C, Ciofetta M, Calabrese G, Brunetti P, Bolli GB. Intensive treatment maintains normal glucagon response to hypoglycemia in short-term IDDM. Diabetologia 1998; 41(Suppl 1):A68.

818) Pankowska E, Szypowska A, Lipka M, Skorka A. Sustained metabolic control and low rates of severe hypoglycaemic episodes in preschool diabetic children treated with continuous subcutaneous insulin infusion. Acta Paediatr 2007;96:881-4.

819) Parent ME, Siemiatycki J, Menzies R, Fritschi L, Colle E. Bacille Calmette-Guérin vaccination and incidence of IDDM in Montreal, Canada. Diabetes Care 1997;20:767.

820) Parslow RC, McKinney PA, Law GR, Staines A, Williams R, Bodansky HJ. Incidence of childhood diabetes mellitus in Yorkshire, northern England, is associated with nitrate in drinking water: an ecological analysis. Dabetologia 1997;40:550-56.

821) Partanen TM, Rissanen A. Insulin injection practices. Pract Diab Int 2000; 17:252-54.

822) Patino-Fernandez AM, Delamater AM, Applegate EB, Brady E, Eidson M, Nemery R, Gonzalez-Mendoza L, Richton S. Neurocognitive functioning in

preschool-age children with type 1 diabetes mellitus. Pediatr Diabetes 2010;11:424-30.

823) Patterson CC, Carson DJ and the Northern Ireland Diabetes Study Group. Epidemiology of childhood IDDM in Northern Ireland 1989-1994: Low incidence in areas with highest population density and most household crowding. Diabetologia 1996;39:1063-69.

824) Pedersen M. Lecture EASD 1993. In: Madsbad S, Dejgaard A. Highlights of the 29th EASD meeting, Istanbul 6-9 September 1993. NovoCare.

825) Pedrini MT, Levey AS, Lau J et al. The effect of dietary protein restriction on the progression of diabetic and nondiabetic renal diseases: a meta-analysis. Ann Intern Med 1996;124/7:627-32.

826) Pennant ME, Bluck LJ, Marcovecchio ML, Salgin B, Hovorka R, Dunger DB. Insulin administration and rate of glucose appearance in people with type 1 diabetes. Diabetes Care 2008;31:2183-7.

827) Perez M, Kohn S. Cutaneous manifestations of diabetes mellitus. J Amer Acad Derm 1994;30:519-531.

828) Perkins B, Riddell M. Type 1 diabetes and exercise: Using the insulin pump to maximum advantage. Can J Diab 2006;30:72-80.

829) Perkins BA, Cherney DZ, Partridge H, Soleymanlou N, Tschirhart H, Zinman B, Fagan NM, Kaspers S, Woerle HJ, Broedl UC, et al. Sodium-glucose cotransporter 2 inhibition and glycemic control in type 1 diabetes: results of an 8-week open-label proof-of-concept trial. Diabetes Care 2014;37:1480-3.

830) Perriello G, Torlone E, Di Santo S, Fanwelli C, De Feo P, Santeusanio F, brunett P, Bolli GB. Effect of storage temperature of insulin on pharmacokinetics and pharmacodynamics of insulin mixtures injected subcutaneously in subjects with type 1 (insulin-dependent) diabetes mellitus. Diabetologia 1988;31/11:811-15.

831) Perrone C, Laitano O, Meyer F. Effect of carbohydrate ingestion on the glycemic response of type 1 diabetic adolescents during exercise. Diabetes Care 2005;28:2537-8.

832) Persson B, Hansson U. Diabetes and pregnancy. Swedish Diabetes Association, Booklet no. 5, 1987.

833) Persson B. Long term morbidity in infants of diabetic mothers. Acta Endocrinol 1986;suppl 1:156.

834) Persson B, Hanson U. Neonatal morbidities in gestational diabetes mellitus. Diabetes Care 1998;21 Suppl 2:B79-84.

835) Peter R, Luzio SD, Dunseath G, Miles A, Hare B, Backx K, Pauvaday V, Owens DR. Effects of exercise on the absorption of insulin glargine in patients with type 1 diabetes. Diabetes Care 2005;28:560-5.

836) Peters A, Klose O, Hefty R, Keck F, Kerner W. The influence of insulin antibodies on the pharmacokinetics of NPH insulin in patients with type 1 diabetes treated with human insulin. Diabet Med 1995;12:925-30.

837) Peters AL, Davidson MB, Eisenberg K. Effect of isocaloric substitution of chocolate cake for potato in type 1 diabetic patients. Diabetic Care 1990:888-92.

838) Peters AL, Davidson MB. Protein and fat effects on glucose responses and insulin requirements in subjects with insulin-dependent diabetes mellitus. Am J Clin Nutr 1993;58:555-60.

839) Petersen KR, Skouby SO, Vedel PV, Haaber AB. Hormonal contraception in women with IDDM. Diabetes Care 1995;18(6):800-806.

840) Peto R, Lopez AD, Boreham J, Thun M, Heath C Jr. Mortality from smoking in developed countries 1950-2000: indirect estimates from national vital statistics. Oxford: Oxford University Press, 1994.

841) Petrie HJ, Stover EA, Horswill CA. Nutritional concerns for the child and adolescent competitor. Nutrition 2004;20:620-31.

842) Peveler R, Boller I, Fairburn C, Dunger D. Eating disorders in adolescents with IDDM. Diabetes Care 10/1992;15:1356-60.

843) Peyrot MF, Pichert JW. Stress buffering and glycemic control. Diabetes Care 1992;7:842-846.

844) Pezzarossa A, Taddei F, Cimicchi MC, Rossini E, Contini S, Bonora A, Gnudi A, Uggeri E. Perioperative management of diabetic subjects. Subcutaneous versus intravenous insulin administration during glucose-potassioum infusion. Diabetes Care 1988;11/1:52-58.

845) Pfützner A, Kustner E, Forst T, Schulze-Schleppinghoff B, Trautmann ME, Haslbeck M, Schatz H, Beyer J. Intensive insulin therapy with insulin lispro in patients with type 1 diabetes reduces the frequency of hypoglycemic episodes. Exp Clin Endocrinol Diabetes 1996;104:25-30.

846) Pham-Short A, Donaghue KC, Ambler G, Chan AK, Hing S, Cusumano J, Craig ME. Early elevation of albumin excretion rate is associated with poor gluten-free diet adherence in young people with coeliac disease and diabetes. Diabet Med 2013;

847) Philotheou A, Araslanian S, Blatniczky L, Peterkova V, Souhami E, Danne T. Efficacy and Safety of Insulin Glulisine (GLU) vs Insulin Lispro (LIS) as Part of a Basal-Bolus Insulin (INS) Regimen in Children and Adolescents with Type 1 Diabetes (T1DM). Diabetes 2008;57(Suppl 1):A496 (abstract).

848) Pieber TR, Eugene-Jolchine I, Derobert E. Efficacy and safety of HOE 901 versus NPH insulin in patients with type 1 diabetes. The European Study Group of HOE 901 in type 1 diabetes. Diabetes Care 2000;23:157-62.

849) Pieber TR, Treichel HC, Hompesch B, Philotheou A, Mordhorst L, Gall MA, Robertson LI. Comparison of insulin detemir and insulin glargine in subjects with Type 1 diabetes using intensive insulin therapy. Diabet Med 2007;24:635–642.

850) Pinelli L, Mormile R, Alfonsi L, Gonfiantini E, Piccoli R, Chiarelli F. The role of nutrition in prevention of complications in insulin-dependent diabetes mellitus. Acta Paediatr 1999;88(Suppl):39-42.

851) Pinson M, Hoffman WH, Garnick JJ, Litaker MS. Periodontal disease and type 1 diabetes mellitus in children and adolescents. J Clin Periodontol 1995;22:118-23.

852) Plank J, Wutte A, Brunner G, Siebenhofer A, Semlitsch B, Sommer R, Hirschberger S, Pieber TR. A direct comparison of insulin aspart and insulin lispro in patients with type 1 diabetes. Diabetes Care 2002;25:2053-7.

853) Plank J, Bodenlenz M, Sinner F, Magnes C, Gorzer E, Regittnig W, Endahl LA, Draeger E, Zdravkovic M, Pieber TR. A double-blind, randomized, dose-response study investigating the pharmacodynamic and pharmacokinetic

properties of the long-acting insulin analog detemir. Diabetes Care 2005;28:1107-12.

854) Pocecco M, Ronfani L. Transient focal neurologic deficits associated with hypoglycaemia in children with insulin-dependent diabetes mellitus. Italian Collaborative Paediatric Diabetologic Group. Acta Paediatr 1998;87:542-44.

855) Pohl R, Hauser R, Li M, De Souza E, Feldstein R, Seibert R, Ozhan K, Kashyap N, Steiner S. Ultra-rapid absorption of recombinant human insulin induced by zinc chelation and surface charge masking. J Diabetes Sci Technol 2012;6:755-63.

856) Polak M, Beregszaszi M, Belarbi N, Benali K, Czernichow P, Tubiana-Rufi N. Subcutaneous or intramuscular injections of insulin in children; Are we injecting where we think we are? Diabetes Care 1996;19:1434-36.

857) Polonsky WH. Diabetes Burnout. McGraw-Hill Professional Publishing 1999.

858) Poortmans JR, Saerens P, Edelman R, Vertongen F, Dorchy H. Influence of the degree of metabolic control on physical fitness in type I diabetic adolescents. Int J Sports Med 1986;7:232-5.

859) Porter PA, Byrne G, Stick S Jones TW. Nocturnal hypoglycaemia and sleep disturbances in young teenagers with insulin dependent diabetes mellitus. Arch Dis Child 1996;75:120-3.

860) Pozzilli P, Visalli N. Signore A et al. Double blind trial of nicotinamid in recent-onset IDDM (the IMDIAB III study). Diabetologia 1995;38:848-52.

861) Price DE, Burden AC. Growth of children before onset of diabetes. Diabetes Care 1992; 15:1393-95.

862) Pryce R. Diabetic ketoacidosis caused by exposure of insulin pump to heat and sunlight. BMJ 2009;338:a2218.

863) Puczynski M, Puczynski S, Reich J, Kaspas JC, Emanuele MA. Mental efficiency and hypoglycemia. J Dev Behav Pediatr 1990;11:170-74.

864) Putz D, Kabadi UM. Insulin glargine in continuous enteric tube feeding. Diabetes Care 2002;25:1889-90.

865) Quillian WC, Cox DJ, Gonder-Frederick LA, Driesen NR, Clarke WL. Reliability of driving performance during moderate hypoglycemia in adults with IDDM. Diabetes Care 1994;17:1367-68.

866) Rabasa-Lhoret R, Garon J, Langelier H, Poisson D, Chiasson JL. Effects of meal carbohydrate content on insulin requirements in type 1 diabetic patients treated intensively with the basal-bolus (ultralente-regular) insulin regimen. Diabetes Care 1999;22:667-73.

867) Rabasa-Lhoret R, Bourque J, Ducros F, Chiasson JL. Guidelines for premeal insulin dose reduction for postprandial exercise of different intensities and durations in type 1 diabetic subjects treated intensively with a basal-bolus insulin regimen (ultralente-lispro). Diabetes Care 2001;24:625-30.

868) Raile K, Kapellen T, Schweiger A, Hunkert F, Nietzschmann U, Dost A, Kiess W. Physical activity and competitive sports in children and adolescents with type 1 diabetes. Diabetes Care 1999;22:1904-5.

869) Rami B, Zidek T, Schober E. Influence of a beta-glucan-enriched bedtime snack on nocturnal blood glucose levels in diabetic children. J Pediatr Gastroenterol Nutr 2001;32:34-36.

870) Rangawala S, Shah P, Hussain SZ, Goenka S, Pillai KK. Insulin stored in matka (earthen pitcher) with water for 60 days does not reduce in bio-activity. J Ped Endocrinol and Metab 1997;10 (suppl 2); 347 (abstract).

871) Rassam AG, Zeise TM, Burge MR, Schade DS. Optimal administration of lispro insulin in hyperglycemic type 1 diabetes. Diabetes Care 1999;22:133-6.

872) Rathod M, Saravolatz L, Pohlod D, Whitehouse F, Goldman J. Evaluation of the sterility and stability of insulin from multidose vials used for prolonged periods. Infect Control 1985;6:491-4.

873) Ratner RE, Hirsch IB, Neifing JL, Garg SK, Mecca TE, Wilson CA. Less hypoglycemia with insulin glargine in intensive insulin therapy for type 1 diabetes. U.S. Study Group of Insulin Glargine in Type 1 Diabetes. Diabetes Care 2000;23:639-43.

874) Ratner RE, Dickey R, Fineman M, Maggs DG, Shen L, Strobel SA, Weyer C, Kolterman OG. Amylin replacement with pramlintide as an adjunct to insulin therapy improves long-term glycaemic and weight control in Type 1 diabetes mellitus: a 1-year, randomized controlled trial. Diabet Med 2004;21:1204-12.

875) Rave K, Heise T, Herrnberger J, Bender R, Hirschberger S, Heinemann L. Intramuscular versus subcutaneous injection of soluble and lispro insulin: Comparison of effects in healthy subjects. Diab Med 1998;15:747-51.

876) Rave KM, Nosek L, de la Pena A, Seger M, Ernest CS, 2nd, Heinemann L, Batycky RP, Muchmore DB. Dose response of inhaled dry-powder insulin and dose equivalence to subcutaneous insulin lispro. Diabetes Care 2005;28:2400-5.

877) Raz I, Weiss R, Yegorchikov Y, Bitton G, Nagar R, Pesach B. Effect of a local heating device on insulin and glucose pharmacokinetic profiles in an open-label, randomized, two-period, one-way crossover study in patients with type 1 diabetes using continuous subcutaneous insulin infusion. Clin Ther 2009;31:980-7.

878) Read NW, Welch IM, Austen CJ. Barnish C et al. Swallowing food without chewing; a simple way to reduce postprandial glycemia. Br J Nutrition 1986;55:43-7.

879) Regber S, Kelly KB. Missed opportunities-adolescents with a chronic condition (insulin-dependent diabetes mellitus) describe their cigarette-smoking trajectories and consider health risks. Acta Paediatr 2007;96:1770-6.

880) Reichard P, Britz A, Rosenqvist U. Intensified conventional insulin treatment and neuropsychological impairment. Br Med J 1991;303:1439-42.

881) Reichard P, Nilsson B-Y, Rosenqvist U. The effect of long-term intensified insulin treatment on the development of microvascular complications of diabetes mellitus. N Engl J Med 1993;329:304-309.

882) Reichard P. Are there any glycemic thresholds for the serious microvascular diabetic complications? J Diab Compl 1995;9:25-30.

883) Reichard P, Pihl M, Rosenqvist U, Sule J. Complications in IDDM are caused by elevated blood glucose level: the Stockholm Diabetes Intervention Study (SDIS) at 10-year follow up. Diabetologia 1996;39:1483-8.

884) Reichel A, Rietzsch H, Kohler HJ, Pfutzner A, Gudat U, Schulze J. Cessation of insulin infusion at night-time during CSII-therapy: comparison of regular human insulin and insulin lispro. Exp Clin Endocrinol Diabetes 1998;106: 168-72.

885) Rewers M, Pihoker C, Donaghue K, Hanas R, Swift P, Klingensmith GJ. Assessment and monitoring of glycemic control in children and adolescents with diabetes. ISPAD Clinical Practice Consensus Guidelines 2009 Compendium. Pediatr Diabetes 2009: 10 (Suppl. 12): 71–81.

886) Richardson T, Kerr D. Skin-related complications of insulin therapy: epidemiology and emerging management strategies. Am J Clin Dermatol 2003; 4:661-7.

887) Richardson T, Weiss M, Thomas P, Kerr D. Day after the night before: influence of evening alcohol on risk of hypoglycaemia in patients with type 1 diabetes. Diabetes Care 2005;28:1801-2.

888) Riddell MC, Bar-Or O, Ayub BV, Calvert RE, Heigenhauser GJ. Glucose ingestion matched with total carbohydrate utilization attenuates hypoglycemia during exercise in adolescents with IDDM. Int J Sport Nutr 1999;9:24-34.

889) Riddell MC, Bar-Or O, Gerstein HC, Heigenhauser GJ. Perceived exertion with glucose ingestion in adolescent males with IDDM. Med Sci Sports Exerc 2000;32:167-73.

890) Riddell M, Iscoe K. Physical activity, sport, and pediatric diabetes. Pediatr Diabetes 2006;7:60-70.

891) Riddell M, Perkins B. Type 1 diabetes and vigorous exercise: Applications of exercise physiology to patient management. Can J Diab 2006;30:63-71.

892) Riddell MC, Milliken J. Preventing exercise-induced hypoglycemia in type 1 diabetes using real-time continuous glucose monitoring and a new carbohydrate intake algorithm: an observational field study. Diabetes Technol Ther 2011;13:819-25.

893) Rizzo TA, Dooley SL, Metzger BE, Cho NH, Ogata ES, Silverman BL. Prenatal and perinatal influences on long-term psychomotor development in offspring of diabetic mothers. Am J Obstet Gynecol 1995;173:1753-8.

894) Robertson KJ, Schoenle E, Gucev Z, Mordhorst L, Gall MA, Ludvigsson J. Insulin detemir compared with NPH insulin in children and adolescents with Type 1 diabetes. Diabet Med 2007;24:27-34.

895) Robertson K, Adolfsson P, Riddell M, Guinhouya B, Hanas R. Exercise in children and adolescents with diabetes. ISPAD Clinical Practice Consensus Guidelines 2014 Compendium. Pediatric Diabetes 2014.

896) Robinson N, Lloyd CE, Fuller J, Yateman NA. Psychosocial factors and the onset of type 1 diabetes. Diabetic Med 1989;6:53-8.

897) Rodin G, Craven J, Littlefield C, Murray M, Daneman D. Eating disorders and intentional undertreatment in adolescent females with diabetes. Psychosomatics 1991;32:171-6.

898) Rodin GM, Danman D. Eating disorders and IDDM. Diabetes Care 1992; 15:1402-12.

899) Rohlfing CL, Wiedmeyer HM, Little RR, England JD, Tennill A, Goldstein DE. Defining the relationship between plasma glucose and HbA1c: analysis of glucose profiles and HbA1c in the Diabetes Control and Complications Trial. Diabetes Care 2002;25:275-8.

900) Rönnemaa T, Viikari J. Reducing snacks when switching from conventional soluble to lispro insulin treatment: effects on glycaemic control and hypoglycaemia. Diabet Med 1998;15:601-7.

901) Roper NA, Bilous RW. Resolution of lipohypertrophy following change of short-acting insulin to insulin lispro (Humalog). Diabet Med 1998;15:1063-4.

902) Rosén T. Hypophysis failure from methadone and other opoids. Substans nr 4:7. Västra Götalandsregionen 2013.

903) Rosenbloom A, Beverly P, Giordano RN: Chronic overtreatment with insulin in children. Am J Dis Child 1977;131:881-885.

904) Rosenbloom AL. The cause of the epidemic of type 2 in children. Current Opinion in Endocrinology & Diabetes 2000;7:191-96.

905) Rosenbloom AL. Insulin Injection Lipoatrophy Recidivus. Pediatr Diabetes 2013;

906) Rosenn BM, Miodovnik M, Khoury JC, Siddiqi TA. Counterregulatory hormonal responses to hypoglycemia during pregnancy. Obstet Gynecol 1996; 87/4:568-74.

907) Rosenstock J, Park G, Zimmerman J. Basal insulin glargine (HOE 901) versus NPH insulin in patients with type 1 diabetes on multiple daily insulin regimens. Diabetes Care 2000;23:1137-42.

908) Rosskamp RH, Park G. Long-acting insulin analogs. Diabetes Care 1999; 22 Suppl 2:B109-13.

909) Rovet J, Alvarez M. Attentional functioning in children and adolescents with IDDM. Diabetes Care 1997;20:803-810.

910) Rovet JF, Ehrlich RM. The effect of hypoglycemic seizures on cognitive function in children with diabetes: a 7-year prospective study. J Pediatr 1999; 134:503-6.

911) Russell-Jones D, Simpson R, Hylleberg B, Draeger E, Bolinder J. Effects of QD insulin detemir or neutral protamine Hagedorn on blood glucose control in patients with type I diabetes mellitus using a basal-bolus regimen. Clin Ther 2004;26:724-36.

912) Rutledge KS, Chase HP, Klingensmith GJ, Walravens PA, Slover RH, Garg SK. Effectiveness of postprandial Humalog in toddlers with diabetes. Pediatrics 1997;100:968-72.

913) Ryan C, Yega A, Drash A. Cognitive deficits in adolescents who developed diabetes early in life. Pediatrics 1985;75:921-927.

914) Ryan CM, Atchison J, Puczynski SS et al. Mild hypoglycemia associated with deterioration of mental efficiency in children with insulin-dependent diabetes mellitus. J Pediatr 1990;117:32-38.

915) Ryan C. Lecture, IDF 2000, Mexico City.

916) Ryan EA, Paty BW, Senior PA, Bigam D, Alfadhli E, Kneteman NM, Lakey JR, Shapiro AM. Five-year follow-up after clinical islet transplantation. Diabetes 2005;54:2060-9.

917) Ryan CM. Diabetes and brain damage: more (or less) than meets the eye? Diabetologia 2006;49:2229-33.

918) Ryan CM. Why is cognitive dysfunction associated with the development of diabetes early in life? The diathesis hypothesis. Pediatr Diabetes 2006;7: 289-97.

919) Rydén O, Nevander L, Johnsson P, Westbom L, Sjöblad S. Diabetic Children and Their Parents: Personality Correlates of Metabolic Control. Acta Paediatr Scand 1990;79:1204-1.

920) Sackey AH, Jefferson IG. Interval between insulin injection and breakfast in diabetes. Arch Dis Child 1994;71:248-50.

921) Sacks DB, Bruns DE, Goldstein DE, Maclaren NK, McDonald JM, Parrott M. Guidelines and recommendations for laboratory analysis in the diagnosis and management of diabetes mellitus. Diabetes Care 2002;25:750-86.

922) Sacks FM, Bray GA, Carey VJ, Smith SR, Ryan DH, Anton SD, McManus K, Champagne CM, Bishop LM, Laranjo N, et al. Comparison of weight-loss diets with different compositions of fat, protein, and carbohydrates. N Engl J Med 2009;360:859-73.

923) Saleh TY, Cryer PE. Alanine and terbutaline in the prevention of nocturnal hypoglycemia in IDDM. Diabetes Care 1997;20:1231-36.

924) Salerno M, Argenziano A, Di Maio S, Gasparini N, Formicola S, De Filippo G, Tenore A. Pubertal growth, sexual maturation, and final height in children with IDDM. Diabetes Care 1997;20:721-24.

925) Salti I, Benard E, Detournay B, Bianchi-Biscay M, Le Brigand C, Voinet C, Jabbar A. A population-based study of diabetes and its characteristics during the fasting month of Ramadan in 13 countries: results of the epidemiology of diabetes and Ramadan 1422/2001 (EPIDIAR) study. Diabetes Care 2004;27:2306-11.

926) Samuelsson U, Johansson C, Ludvigsson J. Breast-feeding seems to play a marginal role in the prevention of IDDM. Diabetes Res. Clin. Pract 3/1993; 3:203-10.

927) Samuelsson U, Johansson C, Carstensen J, Ludvigsson J. Space-time clustering in insulin dependent diabetes mellitus (IDDM) in south-east Sweden. Int. J Epidemiol. 1994;23:138-142.

928) Samuelsson U, Ludvigsson J. When should determination of ketonemia be recommended? Diabetes Technol Ther 2002;4:645-50.

929) Samuelsson U. SWEDIABKIDS 2012 report.

930) Sandelin O, Rogberg N. Diving into the depth of prejudice. The Diving Journal 4/1989:28-29.

931) Sandoval DA, Guy DL, Richardson MA, Ertl AC, Davis SN. Effects of low and moderate antecedent exercise on counterregulatory responses to subsequent hypoglycemia in type 1 diabetes. Diabetes 2004;53:1798-806.

932) Sane T, Koivisto VA, Nikkanen P, Pelkonen R. Adjustment of insulin doses of diabetic patients during long distance flights. BMJ 1990;301:421-22.

933) Sane T, Helve E, Pelkonen R, Koivisto VA. The adjustment of diet and insulin dose during long-term endurance exercise in type 1 (insulin-dependent) diabetic men. Diabetologia 1988: 31: 35-40.

934) Sank A, Wei D, Reid J, Ertl D, Nimni M, Weaver F, Yellin A, Tuan TL. Human endothelial cells are defective in diabetic vascular disease. J Surg Res 1994;57:647-53.

935) Santiago J. Lessons from the Diabetes Control and Complications Trial. Diabetes 1993;42:1549-1554.

936) Sapone A, de Magistris L, Pietzak M, Clemente MG, Tripathi A, Cucca F, Lampis R, Kryszak D, Carteni M, Generoso M, et al. Zonulin upregulation is associated with increased gut permeability in subjects with type 1 diabetes and their relatives. Diabetes 2006;55:1443-9.

937) Saukkonen T, Vaisanen S, Akerblom HK, Savilahti E. Coeliac disease in children and adolescents with type 1 diabetes: a study of growth, glycaemic control, and experiences of families. Acta Paediatr 2002;91:297-302.

938) Savilahti E, Åkerblom HK, Tainio V-M, Koskimies S. Children with newly diagnosed insulin dependent diabetes mellitus have increased levels of cows' milk antibodies. Diabetes Res 1988;7:137-40.

939) Sawicki P, Didjurgeit U, Mühlhauser I, Bender R, Heinemann L, Berger M. Smoking is associated with progression of diabetic nephropathy. Diabetes Care 1994;17:126-131.

940) Sawka AM, Burgart V, Zimmerman D. Loss of awareness of hypoglycemia temporally associated with selective serotonin reuptake inhibitors. Diabetes Care 2001;24:1845-6.

941) Scaramuzza A, De Palma A, Mameli C, Spiri D, Santoro L, Zuccotti GV. Adolescents with type 1 diabetes and risky behaviour. Acta Paediatr 99:1237-41.

942) Schatz DA, Maclaren NK. Cows' milk and insulin-dependent diabetes. Innocent until proven guilty. JAMA 1996;276(8):647-8.

943) Schernthaner G, Wein W, Sandholzer K, Equiluz-Bruck S, Bates PC, Birkett MA. Postprandial insulin lispro. A new therapeutic option for type 1 diabetic patients. Diabetes Care 1998;21/4:570-3.

944) Scherstén B, Alm A, Berne C, Blohmé G, Eckerlund I, Edman L et al. A consensus document: vision-threatening retinal changes in diabetes. Lakartidningen 51-51/1991;88:4475-4478.

945) Schiavi RC, Stimmel BB, Mandeli J, Rayfield EJ. Diabetes mellitus and male sexual function: a controlled study. Diabetologia 1993;36:745-751.

946) Schiffrin A, Belmonte M: Multiple daily self-glucose monitoring: its essential role in long-term glucose control in insulin-dependent patients treated with pump and multiple subcutaneous injections. Diabetes Care 1982; 5: 479-84.

947) Schiffrin A, Suissa S. Predicting nocturnal hypoglycemia in patients with type 1 diabetes treated with continous insulin infusion. Am J Med 1987;82: 1127-32.

948) Schmauss S, König A, Landgraf R. Human insulin analogue [Lys(B28), Pro(B29)]: the ideal pump insulin? Diabetic Med 1998;15:247-9.

949) Schober E, Borkenstein M, Frisch H. Basic-bolus therapy of diabetic children and adolescents using Novo Pens. Wien Klin Wochenschr 1987;99: 312-3.

950) Schober E, Schoenle E, Van Dyk J, Wernicke-Panten K. Comparative trial between insulin glargine and NPH insulin in children and adolescents with type 1 diabetes mellitus. J Pediatr Endocrinol Metab 2002;15:369-76.

951) Schoenle EJ, Schoenle D, Molinari L, Largo RH. Impaired intellectual development in children with Type I diabetes: association with HbA(1c), age at diagnosis and sex. Diabetologia 2002;45:108-14.
952) Schreiber M, Steele A, Goguen J, Levin A, Halperin M. Can a severe degree of ketoacidosis develop overnight? J Am Soc Nephrol 1996;7:192-7.
953) Schroeder B, Hertweck SP, Sanfilippo JS, Foster MB. Correlation between glycemic control and menstruation in diabetic adolescents. J Reprod Med 2000;45:1-5.
954) von Schütz W, Fuchs S, Stephan S, Lange K, Heiming R, Hürter P. Incidence of severe hypoglycemia under conventional and intensive insulin therapy in diabetic children and adolescents. Diabetologia 1994;37 (Suppl 1):abstract 66.
955) Schuler G, Peltz K, Kerp L. Is the reuse of needles for insulin injection systems associated with a higher risk cutaneous complications? Diabetes Res Clin Pract 1992;16/3:209-12.
956) Schvarcz E, Palmér M, Åman J, Lindqvist B, Beckman K-W. Hypoglycemia increases the gastric emptying rate in patients with type-1 diabetes mellitus. Diabetic Med 1993;10:660-63.
957) Schvarcz E, Palmer M, Aman J, Horowitz M, Stridsberg M, Berne C. Physiological hyperglycemia slows gastric emptying in normal subjects and patients with insulin-dependent diabetes mellitus. Gastroenterology 1997; 113:60-6.
958) Seidl R, Birnbacher R, Hauser E, Bernert G, Freilinger M, Schober E. Brainstem auditory evoked potentials and visually evoked potentials in young patients with IDDM. Diabetes Care 1996;19:1220-4.
959) Sells CJ, Robinson NM, Brown Z, Knopp RH. Long-term developmental follow-up of infants of diabetic mothers. J Pediatr. 1994;125:1,S9-17.
960) Service FJ, O'Brien PC, Wise SD, Ness S, LeBlanc SM. Dermal interstitial glucose as an indicator of ambient glycemia. Diabetes Care 1997;20: 1426-9.
961) Seymour HR, Gilman D, Quin JD. Severe ketoacidosis complicated by 'ecstasy' ingestion and prolonged exercise. Diabet Med 1996;13:908-9.
962) Shah S, Malone J, Simpson N. A randomized trial of intensive insulin therapy in newly diagnosed insulin-dependent diabetes mellitus. N Engl J Med 1989; 320:550-54.
963) Shapiro AM, Lakey JR, Ryan EA, Korbutt GS, Toth E, Warnock GL, Kneteman NM, Rajotte RV. Islet transplantation in seven patients with type 1 diabetes mellitus using a glucocorticoid-free immunosuppressive regimen. N Engl J Med 2000;343:230-8.
964) Shapiro AM, Ricordi C, Hering BJ, Auchincloss H, Lindblad R, Robertson RP, Secchi A, Brendel MD, Berney T, Brennan DC, Cagliero E, Alejandro R, Ryan EA, DiMercurio B, Morel P, Polonsky KS, Reems JA, Bretzel RG, Bertuzzi F, Froud T, Kandaswamy R, Sutherland DE, Eisenbarth G, Segal M, Preiksaitis J, Korbutt GS, Barton FB, Viviano L, Seyfert-Margolis V, Bluestone J, Lakey JR. International trial of the Edmonton protocol for islet transplantation. N Engl J Med 2006;355:1318-30.
965) Shehadeh N, Kassem J, Tchaban I, Ravid S, Shahar E, Naveh T, Etzioni A. High incidence of hypoglycemic episodes with neurologic manifestations in children with insulin dependent diabetes mellitus. J Pediatr Endocrinol Metab 1998;11 Suppl 1:183-7.
966) Shield JPH, Baum JD. Advances in childhood onset diabetes. Arch Dis Child 1998;78:391-94.
967) Silink M. Sick day rules. In the book: Baba S, Kaneko T (Ed.). Diabetes 1994. Elsevier Science BV 1995.
968) Silink M (Ed.). APEG handbook on childhood and adolescent diabetes. Australian Pediatric Endocrine Group 1996.
969) Silva SR, Clark L, Goodman SN, Plotnick LP. Can caretakers of children with IDDM accurately measure small insulin doses and dose changes? Diabetes Care 1996;19:56-59.
970) Silverstein J, Klingensmith G, Copeland K, Plotnick L, Kaufman F, Laffel L, Deeb L, Grey M, Anderson B, Holzmeister LA, et al. Care of children and adolescents with type 1 diabetes: a statement of the American Diabetes Association. Diabetes Care 2005;28:186-212.
971) Sindelka G, Heinemann L, Berger M, Frenck W, Chantelau E. Effect of insulin concentration, subcutaneous fat thickness and skin temperature on subcutaneous insulin absorption in healthy subjects. Diabetologia 1994; 37:377-80.
972) Singh R, Barden A, Mori T, Beilin L. Advanced glycation end-products: a review. Diabetologia 2001;44:129-46.
973) Sinha RN, Patrick AW, Richardson L, Wallymahmed M, MacFarlane IA. A six-year follow-up study of smoking habits and microvascular complications in young adults with type 1 diabetes. Postgrad Med J 1997;73:293-4.
974) Sjöblad S. Hypoglycemia in children. Paediatricus 1988;18:90-101.
975) Sjöblad S (Ed.). Consensus guidelines for the treatment of childhood and adolescent diabetes. Swedish Pediatric Association 1996.
976) Sjolie AK, Stephenson J, Aldington S, Kohner E, Janka H, Stevens L, Fuller J. Retinopathy and vision loss in insulin-dependent diabetes in Europe. The EURODIAB IDDM Complications Study. Ophthalmology 1997;104:252-60.
977) Skogsberg L, Fors H, Hanas R, Chaplin JE, Lindman E, Skogsberg J. Improved treatment satisfaction but no difference in metabolic control when using continuous subcutaneous insulin infusion versus multiple daily injections in children at onset of type 1 diabetes mellitus. Pediatric Diabetes 2008;9 (in press).
978) Skyler JS, Krischer JP, Wolfsdorf J, Cowie C, Palmer JP, Greenbaum C, Cuthbertson D, Rafkin-Mervis LE, Chase HP, Leschek E. Effects of oral insulin in relatives of patients with type 1 diabetes: The Diabetes Prevention Trial-Type 1. Diabetes Care 2005;28:1068-76.
979) Skyler JS, Weinstock RS, Raskin P, Yale JF, Barrett E, Gerich JE, Gerstein HC. Use of inhaled insulin in a basal/bolus insulin regimen in type 1 diabetic subjects: a 6-month, randomized, comparative trial. Diabetes Care 2005;28:1630-5.
980) Sleeman F, Northam EA, Crouch W, Cameron FJ. Psychological adjustment of well siblings of children with Type 1 diabetes. Diabet Med 2010;27: 1084-7.
981) Slama G. Unpublished results 1990, personal communication.
982) Smith CP, Sargent MA, Wilson BPM, Price DA. Subcutaneous or intramuscular insulin injections. Arch Dis Childhood 1991;66:879-82.
983) Soedamah-Muthu SS, Fuller JH, Mulnier HE, Raleigh VS, Lawrenson RA, Colhoun HM. All-cause mortality rates in patients with type 1 diabetes mellitus compared with a non-diabetic population from the UK general practice research database, 1992-1999. Diabetologia 2006;49:660-6.
984) Solomon CG, Willett WC, Carey VJ, Rich-Edwards J, Hunter DJ, Colditz GA, Stampfer MJ, Speizer FE, Spiegelman D, Manson JE. A prospective study of pregravid determinants of gestational diabetes mellitus. JAMA 1997;278: 1078-83.
985) Soltész G, Ascádi G. Association between diabetes, severe hypoglycemia and electroencephalographic abnormalities. Arch Dis Child. 1989;64:992-96.
986) Somogyi M. Insulin as a cause of extreme hyperglycemia and instability. Weekly Bulletin of the St Louis Medical Society 1938;32:498-510.
987) Sonnenberg GE, Fredrickson L. DKA Prevention. In the book: Fredrickson L (Ed.). The Insulin Pump Therapy Book. Insights from the experts. MiniMed, Los Angeles 1995.
988) Sönksen PH, Tompkins CV, Srivastava MC, Nabarro JDN. A comparative study on the metabolism of human insulin and porcine proinsulin in man. Clin Sci Mol Med 1973;45:633-54.
989) Søvik O, Thordarson H. Dead-in-bed syndrome in young diabetic patients. Diabetes Care 1999;22 Suppl 2:B40-2.
990) Soon-Shiong P, Heintz RE, Meredith N, Yao QX, Zheng T, Murphy M, Moloney MK, Schmehl M, Harris M et al. Insulin independence in a type-1 diabetic patient after encapsulated islet transplantation. Lancet 1994;343: 950-51.
991) Steil GM, Rebrin K, Darwin C, Hariri F, Saad MF. Feasibility of automating insulin delivery for the treatment of type 1 diabetes. Diabetes 2006; 55(12):3344-50.
992) Steindel BS, Roe TR, Costin G, Carlson M, Kaufman FR. Continous subcutaneous insulin infusion (CSII) in children and adolescents with chronic poorly controlled type 1 diabetes mellitus. Diabetes Research and Clinical Practise 1995;27:199-204.
993) Steiner S, Hompesch M, Pohl R, Simms P, Flacke F, Mohr T, Pfutzner A, Heinemann L. A novel insulin formulation with a more rapid onset of action. Diabetologia 2008;51:1602-6.
994) Stenninger E, Åman J. Intranasal glucagon treatment relieves hypoglycemia with Type 1 (insulin-dependent) diabetes mellitus. Diabetologia 1993; 36:931-35.
995) Stettler C, Jenni S, Allemann S, Steiner R, Hoppeler H, Trepp R, Christ ER, Zwahlen M, Diem P. Exercise capacity in subjects with type 1 diabetes mellitus in eu- and hyperglycaemia. Diabetes Metab Res Rev 2005;
996) Stewart NL, Darlow BA. Insulin loss at the injection site in children with type 1 diabetes mellitus. Diabetic Medicine 1994;11:802-05.
997) Stickelmeyer MP, Graf CJ, Frank BH, Ballard RL, Storms SM. Stability of U-10 and U-50 dilutions of insulin lispro. Diabetes Technol Ther 2000;2:61-6.
998) Stiller R, Kothny T, Gudat UHK, Anderson JH, Seger M, Johnson RD, Richardson MS, Haslbeck M. Intravenous administration of insulin lispro versus regular insulin in patients with type 1 diabetes. Diabetes 1999; 48(suppl 1):abstract O497.
999) Strauss K. Insulin delivery devices and correct injection techniques. Becton-Dickinson 1997.
1000) Strauss K. Insulin injection techniques. Report from the 1st international Insulin Injection Technique Workshop, Strasbourg, France - June 1997. Pract Diab Int 1998;15:181-184.
1001) Strudwick SK, Carne C, Gardiner J, Foster JK, Davis EA, Jones TW. Cognitive functioning in children with early onset type 1 diabetes and severe hypoglycemia. J Pediatr 2005;147:680-5.
1002) Stuckey BG, Jadzinsky MN, Murphy LJ, Montorsi F, Kadioglu A, Fraige F, Manzano P, Deerochanawong C. Sildenafil citrate for treatment of erectile dysfunction in men with type 1 diabetes: results of a randomized controlled trial. Diabetes Care 2003 Feb;26(2):279-84.
1003) Suhonen L, Hiilesmaa V, Teramo K. Glycaemic control during early pregnancy and fetal malformations in women with type I diabetes mellitus. Diabetologia 2000;43:79-82.
1004) Sumnik Z, Kolouskova S, Malcova H, Vavrinec J, Venhacova J, Lebl J, Cinek O. High prevalence of coeliac disease in siblings of children with type 1 diabetes. Eur J Pediatr 2005;164:9-12.
1005) Sun WM, Houghton LA, Read NW, Grundy DG, Johnson AG. Effect of meal temperature on gastric emptying of liquids in man. Gut 1988; 29: 302-305.
1006) Sundberg F, Forsander G. Detection and treatment efficacy of hypoglycemic events in the everyday life of children younger than 7 yr. Pediatr Diabetes 2014;15:34-40.
1007) Sundkvist G. Autonomic neuropathy. In the book: Agardh CD, Berne C, Östman J (Ed.). Diabetes. Liber, Stockholm 2002;265-271.
1008) Sutherland D, Moudry-Munns K, Elick B. Pancreas Transplantation. In the book: Rifkin H, Porte D. Diabetes Mellitus, Theory and Practice. Elsevier 1990:869-79.
1009) Svenungsson B, Jertborn M, Wiström J. Prophylaxis and therapy of travelers' diarrhea. Nord Med 11/1992;107:272-73.
1010) Swedish National Board of Health and Welfare. Recommendations from an expert meeting: Treatment of insulin-dependent diabetes mellitus. Lakartidningen 42/1989;86:3585-3589.
1011) Swift PG, Hearnshaw JR, Botha JL, Wright G, Raymond NT, Jamieson KF. A decade of diabetes: keeping children out of hospital. BMJ 1993;307:96-8.
1012) Swift PGF, Waldron S, Glass S. A child with diabetes: distress, discrepancies and dietetic debate. Pract Diab Internat 1995;12:59-62.
1013) Swift PGF. Personal communication 2003.
1014) Tainio VM, Savilahti E, Arjomaa P, Salmenperä L, Perheentupa J, Siimes MA. Plasma antibodies to cows' milk are increased by early weaning and consumption of unmodified milk, but production of plasma IgA and IgM cows milk antibodies is stimulated even during exclusive breast feeding. Acta Paediatr Scand 1988;77:807-11.

1015) Tahara Y. Shima K. Response to Chantelau and Rech. Diabetes Care 1994;17:345.

1016) Tahara Y, Shima K. Kinetics of HbA1c, glycated albumin, and fructosamine and analysis of their weight functions aganst preceding plasma glucose levels. Diabetes Care 1995;18:440-47.

1017) Tallroth G, Karlson B, Nilsson A, Agardh CD. The influence of different insulin regimens on quality of life and metabolic control in insulin-dependent diabetics. Diabetes Res Clin Pract 1989;6:37-43.

1018) Tamás G, Tabák AG, Vargha P, Kerényi Z. Effect of menstrual cycle on insulin demand in IDDM women. Diabetologia 1996;39 (Suppl 1):A52 (abstract 188).

1019) Tan CY, Wilson DM, Buckingham B. Initiation of insulin glargine in children and adolescents with type 1 diabetes. Pediatr Diabetes 2004;5:80-6.

1020) Tanenberg RJ. Candidate Selection. In the book: Fredrickson L (Ed.). The Insulin Pump Therapy Book. Insights from the experts. MiniMed, Los Angeles 1995.

1021) Tansey MJ, Tsalikian E, Beck RW, Mauras N, Buckingham BA, Weinzimer SA, Janz KF, Kollman C, Xing D, Ruedy KJ, et al. The effects of aerobic exercise on glucose and counterregulatory hormone concentrations in children with type 1 diabetes. Diabetes Care 2006;29:20-5.

1022) Tattersall R. Brittle diabetes. Clin Endocr Metabol 1977;6:403-19.

1023) Tattersall RB, Gill GV. Unexplained death of type-1 diabetic patients. Diabetic Med. 1991;8:49-58.

1024) Tattersall R. Treatment of insulin-dependent diabetes – art or science. Lecture, Stockholm 1993.

1025) Temple MYM, Riddell MC, Bar-Or O. The reliability and repeatability of the blood glucose response to prolonged exercise in adolescent boys with IDDM. Diabetes Care 1995;18:326-332.

1026) Tenovuo J, Alanen P, Larjava H, Viikari J, Lehtonen OP. Oral health of patients with insulin-dependent diabetes mellitus. Scand J Dent Res 1986; 94:338-46.

1027) ter Braak EW, Woodworth JR, Bianchi R, Cerimele B, Erkelens DE, Thijssen JHH, Kurtz D. Injection site effects on the pharmacokinetics and glucodynamics of insulin lispro and regular insulin. Diabetes Care 1996;19: 1437-40.

1028) ter Braak EW, Appelman AM, van de Laak M, Stolk RP, van Haeften TW, Erkelens DW. Clinical characteristics of type 1 diabetic patients with and without severe hypoglycemia. Diabetes Care 2000;23:1467-71.

1029) Tesfaye S, Cullen DR, Wilson RM, Wooley PD. Diabetic ketoacidosis precipitated by genital herpes infection. Diab Res Clin Pract 1991;13:83-84.

1030) Tesfaye S, Malik R, Ward JD. Vascular factors in diabetic neuropathy. Diabetologia 1994;37:847-54.

1031) Thalange N, Bereket A, Larsen J, Hiort LC, Peterkova V. Treatment with insulin detemir or NPH insulin in children aged 2-5 yr with type 1 diabetes mellitus. Pediatr Diabetes 2011;12:632-41.

1032) Thernlund GM, Dahlquist G, Hansson K, Ivarsson SA, Ludvigsson J, Sjöblad S, Hägglöf B. Psychological stress and the onset of IDDM in children. Diabetes Care 1995;18:/10:1323-29.

1033) Thernlung G, Dahlquist G, Hägglöf B, Ivarsson SA, Lernmark B, Ludvigsson J, Sjöblad S. Psychological reactions at the onset of insulin-dependent diabetes in children and later adjustment and metabolic control. Act Pediatr 1996;85:947-53.

1034) Thorburn A, Brand J, Truswell S: The glycaemic index of foods: The Medical Journal of Australia, 1986;144:580-82.

1035) Thorburn AW, Brand JC, Truswell AS. Salt and the glycaemic response. Br Med J (Clin Res Ed) 1986;292:1697-9.

1036) Thordarson H, Sovik O. Dead in bed syndrome in young diabetic patients in Norway. Diabet Med. 1995 Sep;12(9):782-7.

1037) Thow JC, Johnson AB, Antsiferov M, Home PD. Effect of raising injection-site skin temperature on isophane (NPH) insulin crystal dissociation. Diabetes Care 1989;12:432-4.

1038) Thow J, Home P. Insulin injection technique. BMJ 1990;301:3-4.

1039) Thow JC, Johnson AB, Marsden S, Taylor R, Home PD. Morphology of palpably abnormal injection sites and effects on absorption of isophane (NPH) insulin. Diabetic medicine 1990;7:795-99.

1040) Thrailkill KM, Quattrin T, Baker L, Kuntze JE, Compton PG, Martha PM, Jr. Cotherapy with recombinant human insulin-like growth factor I and insulin improves glycemic control in type 1 diabetes. RhIGF-I in IDDM Study Group. Diabetes Care 1999;22:585-92.

1041) Torlone E, Pampanelli S, Lalli C, Del Sindaco P, Di Vincenzo A, Rambotti AM, Modarelli F, Epifano L, Kassi G, Perriello G, Brunetti P, Bolli G. Effects of the short-acting insulin analog [Lys(B28),Pro(B29)] on postprandial blood glucose control in IDDM. Diabetes Care 1996;19/9:945-52.

1042) Torsdottir I, Andersson H. Effect on the postprandial glycaemic level of the addition of water to a meal ingested by healthy subjects and type 2 (non-insulin-dependent) diabetic patients. Diabetologia 1989;32:231-5.

1043) Tsalikian E, Mauras N, Beck RW, Tamborlane WV, Janz KF, Chase HP, Wysocki T, Weinzimer SA, Buckingham BA, Kollman C, et al. Impact of exercise on overnight glycemic control in children with type 1 diabetes mellitus. J Pediatr 2005;147:528-34.

1044) Tubiana-Rufi N, Levy-Marchal C, Mugnier E, Czernichow P. Long term feasibility of multiple daily injections with insulin pens in children and adolescents with diabetes. Eur J Pediatr 1989;149:80-3.

1045) Tubiana-Rufi N, Prieur AM, Bourden R, Priollet P, Czernichow P. Early detection of limited joint mobility in diabetic children and adolescents. Diabete Metab 1991;17:504-11.

1046) Tubiana-Rufi N, de Lonlay P, Bloch J, Czernichow P. Remission of severe hypoglycemic incidents in young diabetic children treated with subcutaneous infusion. Arch Fr Pediatr 1996;3:969-76.

1047) Tubiana-Rufi N, Belarbi N, Du Pasquier-Fediaevsky L, Polak M, Kakou B, Leridon L, Hassan M, Czernichow P. Short needles (8 mm) reduce the risk of intramuscular injections in children with type 1 diabetes. Diabetes Care 1999;22:1621-25.

1048) Tubiana-Rufi N, Coutand R, Bloch J, Munz-Licha G, Delcroix C, Limal JM, Czernichow P. Efficacy and tolerance of insulin lispro in young diabetic children treated with CSII. Diabetologia 2000;43(suppl. 1):762 (abstract 762).

1049) Tuomilehto J, Tuomilehto-Wolf E, Virtala E, LaPorte RE: Coffee consumption as trigger for insulin-dependent diabetes mellitus in childhood. BMJ 1990;300:642-43.

1050) Tuominen JA, Karonen SL, Melamies L, Bolli G. Koivisto VA. Exercise-induced hypoglycaemia in IDDM patients treated with a short- acting insulin analogue. Diabetologia 1995;38:106-11.

1051) Tupola S, Rajantie J, Mäenpää J. Severe hypoglycemia in children and adolescents during multiple-dose insulin therapy. Diab Med 1998;15:695-99.

1052) Tupola S, Rajantie J. Documented symptomatic hypoglycaemia in children and adolescents using multiple daily insulin injection therapy. Diabet Med 1998;15:492-6.

1053) Turner BC, Jenkins E, Kerr D, Sherwin RS, Cavan DA. The effect of evening alcohol consumption on next-morning glucose control in type 1 diabetes. Diabetes Care 2001;24:1888-93.

1054) Twetman S, Johansson I, Birkhed D, Nederfors T. Caries incidence in young type 1 diabetes mellitus patients in relation to metabolic control and caries-associated risk factors. Caries Res 2002;36:31-5.

1055) Twyman S, Rowe D, Mansell P, Schapira D, Betts P, Leatherdale B. Longitudinal study of urinary albumin excretion in young diabetic patients– Wessex Diabetic Nephropathy Project. Diabet Med 2001;18:402-8.

1056) Tylleskär K, Tuvemo T, Gustafsson J. Diabetes control deteriorates in girls at cessation of growth: relationship with body mass index. Diabet Med 2001;18:811-5.

1057) Updike SJ, Shults MC, Gilligan BJ, Rhodes RK. A subcutaneous glucose sensor with improved longevity, dynamic range, and stability of calibration. Diabetes Care 2000;23:208-14.

1058) U.S. Pharmacopeia, 21st Rev. In the book: US Pharmacopeial Convention, Rockville, MD, 1985; p 1180.

1059) Vaag A, Handberg A, Lauritzen M, Henriksen JE, Damgaard Pedersen K, Beck-Nielsen H. Variation in absorption of NPH insulin due to intramuscular injection. Diabetes Care 1990;13:74-76.

1060) Vague P, Picq R, Bernal M et al. Effect of nicotinamide treatment on the residual insulin secretion in type-I (insulin-dependent) diabetic patients. Diabetologia 1989;32:316-21.

1061) Vague P, Selam JL, Skeie S, De Leeuw I, Elte JW, Haahr H, Kristensen A, Draeger E. Insulin detemir is associated with more predictable glycemic control and reduced risk of hypoglycemia than NPH insulin in patients with type 1 diabetes on a basal-bolus regimen with premeal insulin aspart. Diabetes Care 2003;26:590-6.

1062) Valenzuela GA, McCallum R. Etiology and diagnosis of gastroparesis:An introduction. Motility 1988;1:10-14.

1063) van Duinkerken E, Schoonheim MM, Sanz-Arigita EJ, RG IJ, Moll AC, Snoek FJ, Ryan CM, Klein M, Diamant M, Barkhof F. Resting-state brain networks in type 1 diabetic patients with and without microangiopathy and their relation to cognitive functions and disease variables. Diabetes 2012; 61:1814-21.

1064) Van Haeften TW. Clinical significance of insulin antibodies in insulin-treated diabetic patients. Diabetes Care 1989;12:641-8.

1065) Velho G, Froguel P. Genetic, metabolic and clinical characteristics of maturity onset diabetes of the young. Eur J Endocrinol 1998;138:233-9.

1066) Veneman T. Mitrakou A. Mokan M. Cryer P, Gerich J. Induction of hypoglycemia unawareness by asymptomatic nocturnal hypoglycemia. Diabetes 1993;42:1233-37.

1067) Verge CF, Simpson JM, Howard NJ, Mackerras D, Irwig L, Silink M. Environmental factors in IDDM. Diabetes Care 1994;17:1381-89.

1068) Verotti A, Chiarelli F, Blasetti A, Bruni E, Morgese G. Severe hypoglycemia in insulin-dependent diabetic children treated by multiple injection regimen. Acta Diabetol 1996;33/1:53-57.

1069) Vervoort G, Goldschmidt HMG, van Doorn LG. Nocturnal blood glucose profiles in patients with type 1 diabetes mellitus on multiple (> 1) daily insulin injection regimes. Diabet Med 1996;13:794-99.

1070) Vessby B, Gustafsson IB. Diet treatment. In the book: Diabetes. SPRI and Swedish Medical Society 1989:206-214.

1071) Viberti G. Mogensen CE. Groop LC. Pauls JF. Effect of captopril on progression to clinical proteinuria in patients with insulin-dependent diabetes mellitus and microalbuminuria. European Microalbuminuria Captopril Study Group. JAMA 1994;271:275-79.

1072) Virtanen SM, Räsänen L, Aro A, Ylönen K, Sippola H, Lounamaa R. Toumilehto J, Åkerblom HK. Feeding in infancy and the risk of type 1 diabetes mellitus in Finnish children. Diabetic Medicine 1992;9:815-19.

1073) Virtanen SM, Saukkonen T, Savilahti E, Ylönen K, Räsänen L, Aro A, Knip M, Toumilehto J, Åkerblom HK and the Childhood Diabetes in Finland Study Group. Diet, cows' milk protein antibodies and the risk of IDDM in Finnish children. Diabetologia 1994;37:381-87.

1074) Virtanen SM, Laara E, Hypponen E, Reijonen H, Rasanen L, Aro A, Knip M, Ilonen J, Akerblom HK. Cows' milk consumption, HLA-DQB1 genotype, and type 1 diabetes: a nested case-control study of siblings of children with diabetes. Childhood diabetes in Finland study group. Diabetes 2000;49:912-7.

1075) Virtanen SM, Virta-Autio P, Rasanen L, Akerblom HK. Changes in food habits in families with a newly diagnosed child with type 1 diabetes mellitus. J Pediatr Endocrinol Metab 2001;14 Suppl 1:627-36.

1076) Vlachokosta FV, Piper CM, Gleason R, Kinzel L, Kahn CR. Dietary carbohydrate, a Big Mac, and insulin requirements in type I diabetes. Diabetes Care 1988;11:330-6.

1077) Waernbaum I, Blohme G, Ostman J, Sundkvist G, Eriksson JW, Arnqvist HJ, Bolinder J, Nystrom L. Excess mortality in incident cases of diabetes mellitus aged 15 to 34 years at diagnosis: a population-based study (DISS) in Sweden. Diabetologia 2006;49:653-9.

1078) Wahren J, Felig P, Hagenfeldt L. Physical exercise and fuel homeostasis in diabetes mellitus. Diabetologia 1978;14:213-22.

1079) Waldron S. Childhood diabetes - current dietary management. Current Pediatrics 1993;3:138-41.
1080) Waldron S, Swift P, Oliver L, Foote D. The nutritional management of children's diabetes. In the book: Frost GF (Ed.). Dietetic Management of Diabetes. John Wiley, London 2003.
1081) Walker M, Marshall SM, Alberti KGMM. Clinical aspects of diabetic ketoacidosis. Diabetes/Metabolism Reviews 1989;5:651-63.
1082) Wallace TM, Meston NM, Gardner SG, Matthews DR. The hospital and home use of a 30-second hand-held blood ketone meter: guidelines for clinical practice. Diabet Med 2001;18:640-5.
1083) Wallberg-Henriksson H, Wahren J. Exercise. In the book: Agardh C-D, Berne C, Östman J. Diabetes. Almqvist & Wiksell, Stockholm 1992:97-107.
1084) Wallymahmed ME, Littler P, Clegg C, Haqqani MT, Macfarlane IA. Nodules of fibrocollagenous scar tissue induced by subcutaneous insulin injections: a cause of poor diabetic control. Postgrad Med J 2004;80:732-3.
1085) Walsh JM, Wheat ME, Freund K. Detection, evaluation, and treatment of eating disorders, the role of the primary care physician. J Gen Intern Med 2000;15:577-90.
1086) Walsh PA, Roberts R. Pumping insulin. Everything You Need for Success with a Smart Insulin Pump. 5th ed. Torrey Pines Press, San Diego, 2012.
1087) Walter M, Kaupper T, Adler K, Foersch J, Bonifacio E, Ziegler AG. No effect of the 1alpha,25-dihydroxyvitamin D3 on beta-cell residual function and insulin requirement in adults with new-onset type 1 diabetes. Diabetes Care 2010;33:1443-8.
1088) Walton C, Allan BJ, Hepburn DA. Tight glycemic control should be avoided post-partum because of increased risk of severe hypoglycemia. Diab Med 2000;17(suppl 1):A84 (abstract).
1089) Wanke T, Auinger M, Formanek D, Merkle M, Lahrmann H, Ogris E, Zwick H, Irsigler K. Defective endogenous opioid response to exercise in type I diabetic patients. Metabolism 1996;45:137-142.
1090) Warram J, Martin BC, Krolewski AS. Risk of IDDM in children of diabetic mothers decreases with increasing maternal age at pregnancy. Diabetes 1991;40:1679-1684.
1091) Warren RE, Zammitt NN, Deary IJ, Frier BM. The effects of acute hypoglycaemia on memory acquisition and recall and prospective memory in type 1 diabetes. Diabetologia 2007;50:178-85.
1092) Warshaw HS, Kulkarni K. Complete Guide to Carb Counting. ADA 2001, Virginia, USA.
1093) Wasserman D, Zinman B. Exercise in individuals with IDDM. Diabetes Care 1994;17:924-37.
1094) Watson J, Kerr D. The best defense against hypoglycemia is to recognize it: is caffeine useful? Diabetes Technol Ther 1999;1:193-200.
1095) Weinger K, Jacobson AM, Draelos MT, Finkelstein DM, Simonson DC. Blood glucose estimation and symptoms during hyperglycemia and hypoglycemia in patients with insulin-dependent diabetes mellitus. Am J Med, 1995 Jan, 98:1, 22-31.
1096) Weinger K, Kinsley BT, Levy CJ, Bajaj M, Simonson DC, Cox DJ, Ryan CM, Jacobson AM. The perception of safe driving ability during hypoglycemia in patients with type 1 diabetes mellitus. Am J Med 1999;107:246-53.
1097) Weinzimer SA, Ahern JH, Doyle EA, Vincent MR, Dziura J, Steffen AT, Tamborlane WV. Persistence of benefits of continuous subcutaneous insulin infusion in very young children with type 1 diabetes: a follow-up report. Pediatrics 2004;114:1601-5.
1098) Weinzimer SA, Steil GM, Swan KL, Dziura J, Kurtz N, Tamborlane WV. Fully automated closed-loop insulin delivery versus semiautomated hybrid control in pediatric patients with type 1 diabetes using an artificial pancreas. Diabetes Care 2008;31:934-9.
1099) Weinzimer SA, Ternand C, Howard C, Chang CT, Becker DJ, Laffel LM. A randomized trial comparing continuous subcutaneous insulin infusion of insulin aspart versus insulin lispro in children and adolescents with type 1 diabetes. Diabetes Care 2008;31:210-5.
1100) Weissberg-Benchell J, Glasgow A, Tynan D, Wirtz P, Turek J, Ward J. Adolescent diabetes management and mismanagement. Diabetes Care 1995; 18:77-82.
1101) Welch IM, Bruce C, Hill SE, Read NW. Duodenal and ileal lipids suppresses postprandial blood glucose and insulin responses in man: possible implications for the dietary management of diabetes mellitus. Clinical Science 1987;72:209-16.
1102) Wheeler ML, Fineberg SE, Gibson R, Fineberg N. Controlled portions of presweetened cereals present no glycemic penalty in persons with insulin-dependent diabetes mellitus. J Am Diet Assoc 1996;96:458-63.
1103) Whincup G, Milner RD. Prediction and management of nocturnal hypoglycaemia in diabetes. Arch Dis Child 1987;62:333-7.
1104) White NH, Cleary PA, Dahms W, Goldstein D, Malone J, Tamborlane WV. Beneficial effects of intensive therapy of diabetes during adolescence: outcomes after the conclusion of the Diabetes Control and Complications Trial (DCCT). J Pediatr 2001;139:804-12.
1105) White SA, Nicholson ML. Islet cell transplantation and type 1 diabetes mellitus. Diabet Med 2001;18 Suppl 1:6-9.
1106) Widom B, Simonson DC. Intermittent hypoglycemia impairs glucose counter-regulation. Diabetes 1992;41:1597-602.
1107) Wiesli P, Schmid C, Kerwer O, Nigg-Koch C, Klaghofer R, Seifert B, Spinas GA, Schwegler K. Acute psychological stress affects glucose concentrations in patients with type 1 diabetes following food intake but not in the fasting state. Diabetes Care 2005;28:1910-5.
1108) Wiethop BV, Cryer PE. Alanine and terbutaline in treatment of hypoglycemia in IDDM. Diabetes Care 1993;16:1131-6.

1109) Willi SM. Type 2 diabetes mellitus in adolescents. Current Opinion in Endocrinolgy & Diabetes 2000;7:71-76.
1110) Wilson DM, Beck RW, Tamborlane WV, Dontchev MJ, Kollman C, Chase P, Fox LA, Ruedy KJ, Tsalikian E, Weinzimer SA. The accuracy of the FreeStyle Navigator continuous glucose monitoring system in children with type 1 diabetes. Diabetes Care 2007;30:59-64.
1111) Wilson DM, Kollman. Relationship of A1C to glucose concentrations in children with type 1 diabetes: assessments by high-frequency glucose determinations by sensors. Diabetes Care 2008;31:381-5.
1112) Wise JE, Kolb KJ, Sauder SE. Effect of glycemic control on growth velocity in children with IDDM. Diabetes Care 1992;15:826-30.
1113) Wittesjö B, Stenström TA, Eitrem R, Rombo L. Every other traveller abroad risks diarrhea. Water and food are the most common sources of infection. Lakartidningen 1995;92:865-67.
1114) Wolever TMS. The Glycemic index. In the book: Bourne GH (Ed.). Aspects of some vitamins, minerals and enzymes in health and disease. World Rev Nutr Diet. Basel, Karger 1990;62:120-85.
1115) Wolever TM. American diabetes association evidence-based nutrition principles and recommendations are not based on evidence. Diabetes Care 2002;25:1263-4.
1116) Wolfsdorf J, Craig ME, Daneman D, Dunger D, Edge J, Lee WR, Rosenbloom A, Sperling MA, Hanas R. Diabetic ketoacidosis. Pediatr Diabetes 2007;8:28-43.
1117) Woodworth J. Howey D, Bowsher R, Lutz S, Sanat P, Brady P. [Lys(B28), Pro(B29) Human Insulin (K): Dose ranging vs. Humulin R (H). Diabetologia 1993;42(Suppl)1:54A.
1118) Woolderink JM, van Loon AJ, Storms F, de Heide L, Hoogenberg K. Use of insulin glargine during pregnancy in seven type 1 diabetic women. Diabetes Care 2005;28:2594-5.
1119) Würsch P, Pi-Sunyer FX. The role of viscous soluble fiber in the metabolic control of diabetes. A review with special emphasis on cereals rich in ß-glucan. Diabetes Care 1997;20:1774-80.
1120) Wyatt JW, Frias JL, Hoyme HE, Jovanovic L, Kaaja R, Brown F, Garg S, Lee-Parritz A, Seely EW, Kerr L, et al. Congenital anomaly rate in offspring of mothers with diabetes treated with insulin lispro during pregnancy. Diabet Med 2005;22:803-7.
1121) Wynne HA, Brown PM Sönksen PM. Acceptability and effectiveness of self-administered intramuscular insulin in juvenile-onset diabetes. Practical Diabetes 1985;2:32-33.
1122) Wysocki T, Meinhold PM, Taylor A, Hough BS, Barnard MU, Clarke WL, Bellando BJ, Bourgeois MJ. Psychometric properties and normative data for the parent version of the diabetes independence survey. Diabetes Educ 1996;22:587-91.
1123) Wysocki T, Harris MA, Mauras N, Fox L, Taylor A, Jackson SC, White NH. Absence of adverse effects of severe hypoglycemia on cognitive function in school-aged children with diabetes over 18 months. Diabetes Care 2003; 26:1100-5.
1124) Yki-Järvinen H, Helve E, Koivisto VA. Hyperglycemia decreases glucose uptake in type 1 diabetes. Diabetes 1987;36:892-96.
1125) Yki-Järvinen H. Glucose toxicity. Endocrine Reviews 1992;13:414-431.
1126) Yki-Järvinen H. Glucose toxicity - its pros and cons. Nord Med 1996;111: 80-3.
1127) Yosipovitch G, Hodak E, Vardi P, Shraga I, Karp M, Sprecher E, David M. The prevalence of cutaneous manifestations in IDDM patients and their association with diabetes risk factors and microvascular complications. Diabetes Care 1998;21:506-9.
1128) Young RJ, Hannan WJ, Frier BM, Steel JM, Duncan LJP. Diabetic lipohypertrophy delays insulin absorption. Diabetes Care 1984; 7:479-80.
1129) Zachrisson I, Brismar K, Hall K, Wallensteen M, Dahlquist G. Determinants of growth in diabetic pubertal subjects. Diabetes Care 1997;20: 1261-65.
1130) Zammitt NN, Warren RE, Deary IJ, Frier BM. Delayed recovery of cognitive function following hypoglycemia in adults with type 1 diabetes: effect of impaired awareness of hypoglycemia. Diabetes 2008;57:732-6.
1131) Zimmet P, Turner R, McCarty D, Rowley M, Mackay I. Crucial points at diagnosis. Type 2 diabetes or slow type 1 diabetes. Diabetes Care 1999;22 Suppl 2:B59-64.
1132) Zinman B, Tildesley H, Chiasson JL, Tsui E, Strack TR. Insulin Lispro in CSII: Results of a double-blind, crossover study. Diabetes 1997;46:440-43.
1133) Zinman B, Ross S, Campos RV, Strack T. Effectiveness of human ultralente versus NPH insulin in providing basal insulin replacement for an insulin lispro multiple daily injection regimen. A double-blind randomized prospective trial. The Canadian Lispro Study Group. Diabetes Care 1999; 22:603-8.
1134) Zipitis CS, Akobeng AK. Vitamin D supplementation in early childhood and risk of type 1 diabetes: a systematic review and meta-analysis. Arch Dis Child 2008;93:512-7.
1135) Zisser H, Jovanovic L. OmniPod Insulin Management System: patient perceptions, preference, and glycemic control. Diabetes Care 2006;29:2175.
1136) Zisser H. Quantifying the impact of a short-interval interruption of insulin-pump infusion sets on glycemic excursions. Diabetes Care 2008;31:238-9.
1137) Zisser HC, Bevier W, Dassau E, Jovanovic L. Siphon effects on continuous subcutaneous insulin infusion pump delivery performance. J Diabetes Sci Technol 2010;4:98-103.
1138) Zisser H, Wagner R, Pleus S, Haug C, Jendrike N, Parkin C, Schweitzer M, Freckmann G. Clinical performance of three bolus calculators in subjects with type 1 diabetes mellitus: a head-to-head-to-head comparison. Diabetes Technol Ther 2010;12:955-61.

Index

Entries in *italic* denote where the main information on the particular item can be found.